Pharmacology and Drug Management for Nurses

For Churchill Livingstone

Commissioning Editor: Ellen Green
Project Editor: Mairi McCubbin
Senior Project Controller: Neil A. Dickson
Project Controller: Nicola S. Haig
Design direction: Judith Wright
Sales Promotion Executive: Hilary Brown

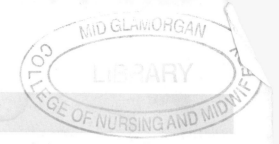

Pharmacology and Drug Management for Nurses

George Downie MSc MRPharmS
Trust Pharmacy Manager, Grampian Healthcare NHS Trust, Aberdeen

Jean Mackenzie BA RGN SCM DipN(Lond) RCT
Clinical Teacher, Foresterhill College, Aberdeen

Arthur Williams OBE FRPharmS
Chief Administrative Pharmaceutical Officer, Grampian, Orkney and Shetland Health
Boards, Aberdeen

CHURCHILL LIVINGSTONE
EDINBURGH LONDON MADRID MELBOURNE NEW YORK AND TOKYO 1995

CHURCHILL LIVINGSTONE
Medical Division of Longman Group Limited

Distributed in the United States of America by Churchill
Livingstone Inc., 650 Avenue of the Americas, New York,
N. Y. 10011, and by associated companies, branches and
representatives throughout the world.

First published 1995

ISBN 0 443 04477 5

British Library Cataloguing in Publication Data
A catalogue record for this book is available from the
British Library.

Library of Congress Cataloging in Publication Data
Downie, George, MSc.
    Pharmacology and drug management for
nurses/George Downie, Jean Mackenzie, Arthur
Williams.
        p.   cm.
    Includes index.
    ISBN 0-443-04477-5
    1. Pharmacology.   2. Nursing.   I. Mackenzie, Jean,
RGN.   II. Williams, Arthur, MPS.   III. Title.
    [DNLM: 1. Pharmacology—nurses' instruction.
2. Drug Therapy—nurses' instruction.   QV 4 0751p
1994]
RM301.D69   1994
615'.1'024613—dc20
DNLM/DLC
for Library of Congress   94-8716

The
publisher's
policy is to use
**paper manufactured
from sustainable forests**

Produced by Longman Singapore Publishers (Pte) Ltd.
Printed in Singapore.

Contents

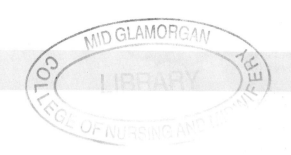

Preface

All nurses are involved in at least some aspect of the management of medicines from a very early stage in their career. Although their responsibilities in this regard increase and change with time, the safe and effective management of medicines remains a high priority for all practising nurses.

The importance of establishing a firm basis of learning during the pre-registration period is well recognised, as is the need to progress to wider aspects once registration has been reached. Thus the nurse progressively builds on the knowledge and skills she has acquired in preparation for the particular responsibilities and duties of her chosen branch of nursing.

As with all health professionals, the nurse has a responsibility to keep up to date and to make her contribution to professional issues of the day. We hope this book will be of value at all stages of the nurse's career, providing information and practical help as well as being a frame of reference for her own experience.

Nurses returning to the profession will, we hope, find a study of the book a useful adjunct to their refresher studies. The needs of the community nurse have also been addressed since by far the majority of medicines are prescribed for use in the community. While the book will not provide all the detailed knowledge the specialist nurse requires, it will form a sound basis and prepare the way for further study whether novice, practitioner or specialist nurse.

To maintain consistency throughout the text, an approach has been adopted in which nurses are referred to in the female gender and patients in the male gender.

Although it is recognised that the emphasis will vary, depending on the specialty in which the nurse works, the role of the nurse in drug therapy can, we believe, be summarised broadly under the following headings:

- to ensure that the correct dosage is given at the correct time and by the correct route
- to observe/report any side-effects and drug interactions, and to take action to alleviate unavoidable side-effects
- to observe and assess the patient so that medical and nursing decisions can be made
- to participate in education and guidance of patients (and in some cases their relatives) with regard to their drug therapy, in order to promote patient compliance and the achievement of therapeutic objectives
- to take action to help reduce, or remove, the need for drug therapy
- to contribute to the evaluation and development of new treatments, and/or the reassessment of existing treatments
- to follow recognised procedures for the control of medicines and pharmaceutical products at ward or department level and to contribute to the development of these procedures and controls in response to changing situations.

The nurse's role is much more than a mechanical achievement of objectives. It is a professional role requiring skill, judgement and commitment. In order to assist in the discharge of this role, the nurse should have access to a broadly-based book, which links together aspects of knowledge which are currently only available in separate publications.

Having outlined the current role of the nurse in drug therapy it is important to realise that many changes and developments are taking place within both health care and the health professions. These changes are having, and will continue to have, an increasing impact on the practising nurse whether in hospital or community. Some of the changes are as follows:

- changing patterns in the provision of health care
- increasing complexity of drug therapy in general
- increasing specialisation in the use of drugs, such as cytotoxic therapy and total parenteral nutrition
- the development of new drug delivery systems
- changes in drug presentation, improved packaging, and new drug distribution systems
- increasing concern regarding the side-effects of drug treatment
- a greater interest in alternative medicine
- an increasing emphasis on the need to use resources effectively
- the need to ensure that the person administering drugs is not harmed by them
- greater awareness of the need to ensure the safe and effective use of medicines by older people
- increasing use of computers in clinical practice, both in hospitals and the community
- an increasing emphasis on self-care
- the development of clinical pharmacy services
- professional aspirations of health care workers generally.

Developments within nursing which may affect or be affected by developments in the management of medicines include:

- primary nursing
- nursing models
- nurse prescribing
- nurses in general management posts
- ward managers and budget holders
- standard setting by nurses and/or with other disciplines
- changes in nurse education, e.g. preregistration and professional studies courses at diploma and degree level
- preparation of health care support workers with vocational qualifications.

The practising nurse is more aware than ever of the great benefits and the potential dangers of drug therapy. The level of importance attached to this aspect of health care can lead to a high level of anxiety amongst nurses. As each individual nurse is accountable for her clinical actions (or inactions), it is essential that she acquires well-founded confidence in what she does. Confidence is achieved through the mastering of practical skills supported by the necessary theoretical knowledge. No matter how careful and expert the prescribing doctor, or pharmacist, the consequences for the patient may be disastrous if the nurse is ill-equipped to discharge her vital role to the full. We hope that this book will serve both as a ready reference for nurses working in the practical situation and an educational tool for learning and teaching, with the patient being the ultimate beneficiary.

G. D.
J. M.
A. W.

Aberdeen 1994

Acknowledgements

We gratefully acknowledge the assistance we have been given in compiling this book. Our very sincere thanks go to contributing authors, Dr David M Levy, the late Miss May McGillivray and Mrs Ingrid G Starritt. We also wish to thank Grampian Health Board for permission to reproduce documents and Mr Gordon W Bell for preparing most of the diagrams. We also acknowledge the help of pharmaceutical companies in providing a number of illustrations.

Preparing a manuscript for publication requires many hours of work and re-work. This has been cheerfully and expertly undertaken by a team led by Miss Angela Ness. Angela's contribution deserves special mention and to her we say a particular 'thank you' for so dependably producing work of the highest standard.

Aberdeen 1994

G. D.
J. M.
A. W.

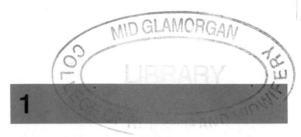

1

Medicines today

Mankind has always been subject to injury and disease. Our ancestors perhaps faced less self-inflicted illness than is seen today, but then, as now, medicines were needed to alleviate pain and suffering. Over the years our expectations of medicines have increased, just as they have in other technological aspects of our lives. Today, those who prescribe, administer and use medicines rightly demand safety, efficacy, economy and convenience from their medicines. Even after decades of very significant progress these demands cannot always be fully met. Great progress has been made on the safety of medicines, but events of recent years demonstrate that there is no room for complacency (Veitch & Talbot 1985). Efficacy has also improved, but we still have very few cures; indeed, effective treatment for a number of conditions still appears to be many years away. Nevertheless, we do have a range of products which help to control symptoms and improve the quality of life for many people. However, the very real advances of recent years have not been achieved without the expenditure of vast sums of money. The development of new drugs is a very high-risk business, and the costs of new treatments reflect this. An individual course of treatment can now cost several thousand pounds, and, even then, benefits to the patient are not always seen and certainly cannot be guaranteed. Just as the drugs have been improved so have the means of delivery, thus increasing convenience to the user and improving targeting.

On the establishment of the National Health

Service (NHS) in 1948, the range of safe and effective medicines available to the prescriber was very limited indeed, by today's standards. Most of the drugs that are now taken for granted were not even a gleam in the eye of the molecular chemist in 1948. Safe and effective cardiovascular drugs, anticancer agents, oral diuretics and psychoactive drugs simply did not exist. Even as recently as the early 1950s, heavy reliance was placed on simple, though not always harmless, inorganic and organic chemicals and products of very dubious composition derived from naturally occurring products such as roots, leaves and barks. Natural products remain a very important source of valuable medicines, but today we have sophisticated methods of extraction, purification and standardisation which, in the case of licensed medicines, guarantees the use and consistency in quality and performance. Methods of drug delivery were also very basic indeed, with oral solid dosage forms adequate but crude by today's standards. Simple oral liquid preparations were often poorly formulated, foul-tasting, poorly preserved and inconvenient to use. Although quality assurance procedures were in place, these were aimed at testing the final product rather than controlling the whole manufacturing process. The Medicines Act of 1968 marked a new beginning in the control of all aspects of the production, testing and marketing of medicines. Some idea of the progress made in the last 70 years can be gained from the summary shown in Table 1.1.

Table 1.1 Progress in drug development in the last 70 years

Decade	Drugs developed
1920s	Insulin
1940s	Penicillin and streptomycin
1950s	Chlorpromazine, prednisolone and thiazide diuretics
1960s	Benzodiazepines, ampicillin, vinblastine, melphalan, propranolol and cytarabine
1970s	Cephalexin, enflurane, doxorubicin, clotrimazole, naproxen, streptokinase and cimetidine
1980s	Clozapine, salmeterol, lisinopril, goserelin, erythropoietin and ranitidine
1990s	Monoclonal antibodies, colfosceril and lamotrigine; third-generation cephalosporins

There is no doubt that the efforts of the pharmaceutical industry will continue to be directed towards producing medicines that meet the needs of both patients and health professionals caring for them. Standards of production and quality assurance are very high indeed. Before a product can be given a product licence and be marketed, safety and efficacy must be established beyond all reasonable doubt.

Figure 1.1 gives an outline of the stages involved in bringing a new medicine into use in the United Kingdom. Only international companies with vast resources to draw on can hope to remain an effective force in this highly competitive business.

BENEFITS AND COSTS OF MODERN MEDICINES

Today, many patients are enjoying both a longer and better life as a result of drug treatment. Perhaps the most dramatic example of this is the control of infections which, 50 years ago, would have almost certainly been fatal. Drugs acting on the cardiovascular system, the newer insulins, oncolytic agents and psychotropic drugs have prolonged and improved life for many patients. Safer anaesthetic agents have played a major part in the surgical advances of recent years. At a time when the resources available for health care are under increasing pressure, health service managers are required to examine carefully all competing demands. The drug bill is no exception to this process. Unfortunately, techniques for economic evaluation of drug treatments have not been fully developed, and, as a result, the debate on cost–benefits of drug treatments tends to be limited to consideration of costs only. There is a need for an informed public debate on this aspect of health care. The pharmaceutical industry has an excellent record of innovation, and the new drugs produced must be sold in order to recover costs and make profits for further investment. Advertising and sales promotion may cause tensions and pressures within the NHS, but there are signs of improved understandings developing,

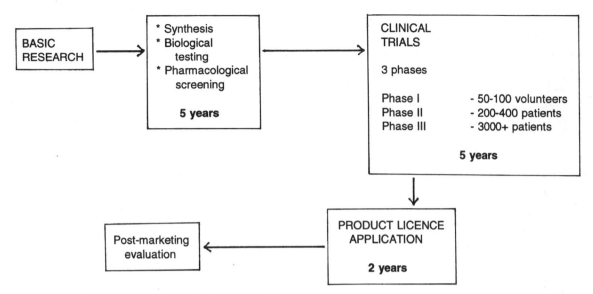

Figure 1.1 Stages in the development of a new medicine.

especially in the context of the development of formularies and prescribing policies.

PROBLEMS

Although many patients derive great benefit from their medicines, the search for the 'magic bullet' goes on. All medicines have the potential to cause harm to the patient, even when used in standard doses. Many patients, especially older patients, suffer from more than one condition resulting in multiple drug therapy or polypharmacy. The risk of drug interactions thus increases, but fortunately the risk of harm to the patient is quite low since the professionals involved in prescribing, dispensing and administration of medicines take steps to protect the patient from such eventualities. Chapter 26 describes in some detail the vital contribution made by the nurse in helping to ensure that the patient derives benefit from the prescribed treatment.

Abuse of chemicals is of growing concern throughout the world, a particular concern being the use of so-called recreational drugs. Much drug abuse is based on the use of illegal substances, but medicines can be abused with equally devastating outcomes for the abuser and his family. Dependency on chemicals (drugs) may arise as the result of bona fide medical treatment, but this is fortunately quite a rare occurrence. There is increasing concern about the extent to which patients may become dependent on benzodiazepines and other anxiolytic drugs. Legislation is of course in place to reduce the likelihood of drug abuse, but there can be no substitute for vigilance by all members of the health care team when involved in the prescribing, dispensing, storage and administration of drugs with an abuse potential, however slight this may be. Even in the best-regulated organisation there will always be a need to dispose of time-expired, surplus and obsolete drugs. Legal and environmental considerations require that such drugs are disposed of in a way that does not damage the environment. Incineration under controlled conditions, e.g. very high temperatures, is needed to meet the legal requirements.

PUBLIC PERCEPTIONS AND ATTITUDES

Health promotion resources are increasingly being targeted at prevention strategies, such as a healthy lifestyle, but the belief that health can be achieved or maintained by the use of medicines is still widely held. All health professionals must seek to ensure that these patients have realistic expectations of their drug therapy and where drug therapy is required.

Economic and other pressures have led to campaigns designed to encourage people to take more responsibility for their own health. One outcome of this is the increasing sales of proprietary medicines both of the traditional type and less orthodox remedies. There can be no doubt of the importance of self-medication in health care. Public health services would collapse if all the demands for medication had to be met from NHS resources. There are dangers in assuming that proprietary over-the-counter medicines are completely safe and can be treated as placebos. Many remedies contain aspirin, which has been implicated in harmful drug interactions.

One key element of the reformed NHS is the importance of providing patients with more information about all aspects of their treatment. Linked with this is the need to ensure that patients and their carers have all the necessary information to enable courses of drug treatment to be completed successfully. A co-ordinated approach between the professions is called for on the provision of relevant well-presented information. The recognition of the need for a wider range of information on treatment is a product of both consumer pressures and changing attitudes within the professions. However, care is needed to ensure that the information needs and views of ethnic minorities are recognised and responded to with sensitivity.

ALTERNATIVE AND COMPLEMENTARY THERAPIES

Interest in alternative complementary medicine is increasing. Patients seek relief from a range of problems such as pain, allergies, gastrointestinal and psychological conditions. In a study reported in the *British Medical Journal* (Moore et al 1985) it was found that patients interviewed were not 'cranks' and had not lost confidence in conventional medicine. A high percentage of patients often felt better after the treatment.

The range of alternative therapies is very wide, but only those involving the use of medicines are briefly discussed here. Homeopathy has been a source of help for many patients over the years, and homeopathic treatment is available via the NHS. Herbal remedies are used by many people in the belief that they are natural and completely safe. A number of studies have shown that this belief may be seriously flawed (MacGregor et al 1989). Side-effects arising from herbal treatments are well documented. Hepatotoxicity, pulmonary and veno-occlusive disease have been shown to be caused by herbal remedies. However, it should not be forgotten that many valuable and effective drugs are derived from natural sources. There appears to be no doubt that patients will continue to seek relief from alternative and complementary medicines. It is incumbent on all health professionals to ensure that at the very least these remedies do not harm patients.

THE FUTURE OF DRUG THERAPY

Based on our experience since the establishment of the NHS it can be confidently predicted that the search for new and more effective drug treatments will continue and that the search will be successful. At the same time, efforts will be made to ensure that drugs are more specific in their activities and can be delivered accurately to the required site.

Legislation controlling the development, marketing and introduction of new drugs will become even more stringent. Drug costs have always been a major cause for concern in the NHS. It appears certain that this concern will continue to test the mettle of those who provide and manage health services. As with all developments in health care, nurses in both community and hospital practice will continue to play a key role. The advent of nurse-prescribing (Department of Health 1989) will further reinforce that role, although the legislation to enable nurses to prescribe has not yet been passed.

REFERENCES

Department of Health 1989 Report of the advisory group on nurse prescribing. Crown Report

MacGregor F B, Abernethy V E, Dahabra S et al 1989 Hepatotoxicity of herbal remedies. British Medical Journal 299: 1156–1157

Moore J, Phipps K, Mareer D et al 1985 Why do people seek treatment by alternative medicine? British Medical Journal 290: 28–29

Veitch G B A, Talbot J C C 1985 The pharmacist and adverse drug reaction reporting. Pharmaceutical Journal 261: 107–109

General principles of pharmacology

2

Pharmacokinetics

Pharmacokinetics deals with the absorption, distribution, metabolism and excretion of drugs. In order to achieve the desired pharmacological response, a drug must first be available in a suitable form and then be given by an appropriate route. The drug will either have a local action or, as is often the case, must be absorbed and distributed via the circulation before reaching its site of action. For the effect to wear off, the drug must be metabolised and the metabolic products excreted from the body, although in certain instances the drug may be eliminated without being metabolised.

ABSORPTION OF ORAL DRUGS

The oral route is the most common, and a convenient, method of giving a drug. When a medicine is taken by mouth, both the amount absorbed and the rate of absorption are determined by many factors, in particular:

- the physical nature of the dosage form
- the presence of food in the stomach
- the composition of the gastrointestinal contents
- gastric or intestinal pH
- gastrointestinal motility
- mesenteric blood flow
- concurrent oral administration of other drugs.

Gastrointestinal absorption following administration of tablets and capsules takes place only after the dosage form has disintegrated and the released drug has been dissolved in the gastrointestinal fluids. With liquid dosage forms, disintegration, and, in many instances, dissolution, of drugs has already been accomplished; therefore, these drugs tend to be absorbed more rapidly. Gastrointestinal motility effects thorough mixing in the gastrointestinal tract and this increases the efficiency with which the drug is brought into contact with surfaces available for absorption. The level of mesenteric blood flow will affect the rate of removal of the drug from the site of absorption.

Drug absorption occurs mainly in the upper part of the small intestine. The absorption is facilitated by a combination of a large surface area created by the villi and their rich blood supply. Alterations in the rate of gastric emptying will result in corresponding alterations in the rate of absorption. In migraine, the rate of absorption of analgesics may be reduced because of reduced gastric motility, resulting in a delayed response to oral analgesics. This delay can be lessened by using metoclopramide, which increases the gastric emptying rate.

BIOAVAILABILITY

To produce therapeutic effects, the drug, after release from the dosage form, must reach an adequate concentration in the blood. 'Bioavailability' refers to the amount and rate of appearance of the drug in the blood after administration of the dosage form. The bioavailability of drugs administered intravenously is 100% because of direct introduction into the bloodstream. However, the bioavailibility of oral medications can vary greatly. Drugs which are poorly soluble in body fluids will have a low bioavailability. Furthermore, tablets containing the same active principle but produced by different manufacturers may differ in bioavailibility, depending on the degree of compression, or the nature of added substances (excipients), which, in turn, affect disintegration and dissolution. Some years ago one manufacturer was able to improve a formulation of digoxin tablets to such an extent that the new tablets were twice as effective as the old ones, although the drug content of the two was identical.

Another example where formulation can influence bioavailability is phenytoin tablets. The crystal size of the active ingredient and the excipients used can alter bioavailability. Control of manufacturing processes in the United Kingdom ensures that where the same product is produced by different companies, bioavailability is consistent. However, some patients prefer to continue to use a particular brand of a product rather than be given a different brand or product from another manufacturer. When faced with such preferences, the nurse should seek the advice of the clinical pharmacist.

EFFECTS OF FOOD

The bioavailability of a number of drugs (e.g. penicillins, erythromycin, rifampicin and thyroxine) is reduced by food. In such cases it is recommended that these preparations be taken half an hour before meals.

Drugs may also require to be taken before meals for specific reasons – for example, the local anaesthetic effect of oxethazaine, a constituent of the antacid Mucaine, will lessen oesophagitis as food passes through the oesophagus. Some drugs, including aspirin, levodopa, metformin, metronidazole, spironolactone or non-steroidal anti-inflammatory drugs, cause gastric symptoms if taken on an empty stomach. When taken with or immediately after a meal, these substances will mix with the food which gives a degree of protection from the gastric side-effects.

It is often assumed that food will, in general, delay drug absorption. However, this is an oversimplification since food may increase, decrease or have no consistent effect on the amount of drug absorbed. The absorption of preparations including aspirin, paracetamol, digoxin, bumetanide and frusemide, is delayed by food. This contrasts with an improvement in absorption of other drugs in the presence of food which may be due to an alteration in tablet disintegration and drug dissolution, or the variable effects of different types of meal on intestinal transit time.

The increase in bioavailability in the presence of food may be due to a number of factors:

- first-pass metabolism is reduced, e.g. metoprolol, propranolol
- drug poorly soluble in water but readily soluble in fat, e.g. griseofulvin
- delayed gastric emptying increases the time available for dissolution of poorly soluble tablets, e.g. nitrofurantoin, spironolactone.

It should be noted that if a patient is in a state of shock, stomach emptying may be delayed, sometimes for several hours, so that drugs given orally will not reach the small intestine and consequently will not be absorbed.

FIRST-PASS METABOLISM IN THE LIVER

Orally and rectally administered drugs which are absorbed from the gastrointestinal tract are carried by the hepatic portal vein to the liver. The liver acts as a 'poison filter', protecting the systemic circulation from potential toxins absorbed from the gastrointestinal tract. The liver has a large range of detoxicating mechanisms for natural toxins and these mechanisms may be active in detoxicating or metabolising drugs. As a result, for many drugs, of that which is absorbed from the gastrointestinal tract, only part may reach the systemic circulation intact. This is known as the 'first-pass effect' (Fig. 2.1), the second and subsequent passes being as the drug passes through the liver from the systemic circulation via the hepatic artery and therefore in much lower concentrations.

Those drugs which have a high hepatic extraction ratio exhibit marked first-pass effects, i.e. a large proportion of the drug is removed before it can enter the general circulation. For certain drugs, (e.g. glyceryl trinitrate if swallowed), the rate of hepatic metabolism is so rapid that the quantity of active compound reaching the systemic circulation after the first pass through the liver is only a small fraction of the dose. Some drugs which are extensively metabolised during the first pass through the liver may still be given orally if their metabolites are active, e.g. propranolol is metabolised to 4-hydroxypropranol which is pharmacologically active. By the intravenous route, propranolol produces a β-blocking effect in a single dose of about 5 mg, but an oral dose of about 100 mg would be required to produce a similar effect since 95% is lost by first-pass metabolism.

DISTRIBUTION OF DRUGS AND THEIR BINDING TO PLASMA PROTEINS

When a drug enters the bloodstream it is rapidly diluted and transported throughout the body. Movement from the blood to tissues is influenced by a number of factors which can greatly affect the resultant drug action. Plasma proteins, particularly albumin, can bind many drugs (Fig. 2.2). Only the *unbound* fraction of the drug is free to move from the bloodstream into tissues to exert a pharmacological effect. The bound drug is pharmacologically inactive because the drug–protein complex is unable to cross cell membranes (Fig. 2.2). It provides a reserve of drug since the complex can dissociate and quickly replenish the unbound drug as it is removed from the plasma. The degree of protein binding will thus affect the intensity and duration of a drug's action.

In addition, if a patient suffers from a disease in which plasma proteins are deficient (e.g. liver disease, malnutrition), more of the drug is free to enter the tissues. A normal dose of a drug could then be dangerous because so little is bound by available protein, thus increasing the availability of unbound drug (Table 2.1).

In practice, changes in the protein-bound drug, resulting in increased levels of unbound drug, are important only for highly bound drugs with a narrow therapeutic index, such as warfarin and phenytoin. In the case of a drug with a narrow therapeutic index, the toxic level is only slightly above the therapeutic level. An increase in unbound drug may therefore result in a toxic level being reached.

Different drugs may share the same protein-binding site. If two drugs are administered concurrently, the one with higher affinity will be preferentially bound and will displace the drug with lower affinity from the protein-binding

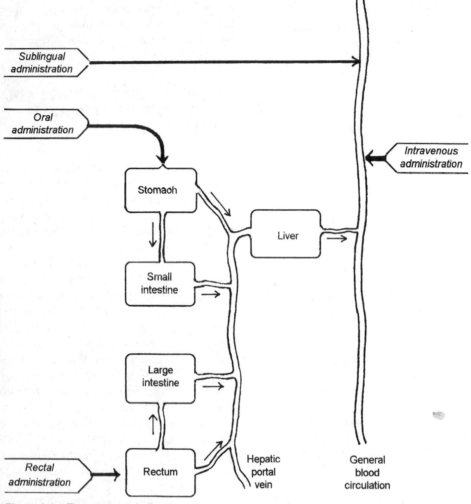

Figure 2.1 First-pass metabolism.

site (Fig. 2.2). For example, clofibrate will displace warfarin from protein-binding sites thus increasing the level of free warfarin and potentiating its pharmacological action. This may result in haemorrhage.

Other factors which affect the rate and extent of distribution are cardiac output and regional bloodflow. If the patient is nursed in a warm environment this will help to maintain a better blood circulation and improve drug distribution, an important factor in patients receiving antibiotics. Similarly, inflamed tissues have increased vascularity and permeability which leads to an increased rate of passage of drugs, especially antibiotics.

DRUG TRANSFER

Unbound drug is transported in circulating blood to body tissues. To diffuse into these tissues and exert its action, a drug must cross a lipid, i.e. fat, layer. If the drug is highly fat-soluble, it will pass across and be taken up rapidly by the tissues; the rapid distribution of such *lipophilic* drugs is especially pronounced in the CNS, which has the most efficient bloodflow

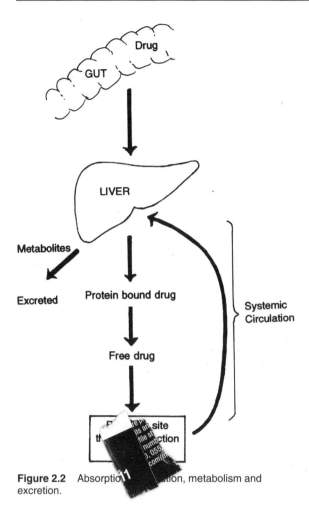

Figure 2.2 Absorption, distribution, metabolism and excretion.

Table 2.1 Percentage protein binding of some commonly used drugs

>95% Bound	>90–95% Bound	50–90% Bound	<50% Bound
Thyroxine	Glibenclamide	Aspirin	Chlorpropamide
Warfarin	Phenytoin	Chloroquine	Digoxin
Amitriptyline	Propranolol	Disopyramide	Insulin
Diazepam	Tolbutamide	Theophylline	Paracetamol
Frusemide	Valproate		

great proportion will be free to exert its pharmacological action. This may have a toxic effect.

TRANSFER BARRIERS

Most of the CNS is surrounded by a specialised membrane, that is, the blood–brain and blood–cerebrospinal fluid barriers. This membrane is highly selective for lipid-soluble drugs, e.g. the penicillins diffuse well into body tissues and fluids but penetration into the cerebrospinal fluid is poor, except when the meninges are inflamed. Chloramphenicol, because of its lipid solubility, is one of the few antibiotics which reaches the cerebrospinal fluid in appreciable concentrations. Dopamine in the treatment of Parkinson's disease cannot be given in this form since it does not cross the blood–brain barrier. It is administered orally as the precursor, levodopa, which is absorbed, crosses the blood–brain barrier, and is broken down to dopamine by the enzyme dopa decarboxylase.

During pregnancy the placenta provides a barrier between mother and fetus. Some drugs cross it relatively easily (e.g. ethanol, chlorpromazine, and morphine), while others (e.g. suxamethonium chloride) are not transferred. Since fetal liver and kidney are unable to metabolise or excrete drugs, and the fetus is likely to be more sensitive to them, drugs must be used with caution in pregnancy and, in general, few are used.

DRUG METABOLISM

As has been previously noted, drugs dissolve in gastric fluid, and in order to diffuse across membranes they must be lipid-soluble. The

in relation to tissue mass. Because of this, there is an almost immediate onset of general anaesthesia once an anaesthetic agent (e.g. thiopentone sodium) enters the systemic circulation. However, because of its great solubility in lipids, compared to its solubility in water, thiopentone sodium is also rapidly taken up by fat cells. This transfer is so marked that, some hours after administration of the drug, little remains in the bloodstream yet quite a large amount may still be present in the fat. The fat store thus helps to remove the drug from the bloodstream and shortens its action. This will also influence the effect of a second dose of the drug. If the fat stores are already saturated, the drug will not be removed from the bloodstream into the fat and a higher the solubility in lipids, compared to solubility in water (lipid/water coefficient), the more rapidly will the drug diffuse into the tissues. When drugs pass through the kidney, lipid-soluble drugs are re-absorbed at the distal tubule and return to the plasma. To get rid of these drugs the body must metabolise them into compounds which are less lipid-soluble and more water-soluble. These metabolites are not re-absorbed at the distal tubule and are excreted in the urine (Fig. 2.3).

The rate of metabolism will determine the duration of action of the drug. Metabolites formed are usually, but not always, less active than the parent compound. A few drugs are made active by metabolism, e.g. talampicillin is the pro-drug for ampicillin, and the cytotoxic agent cyclophosphamide is the pro-drug for several metabolites which produce the pharmacological effect. Many drugs, including imipramine, propranolol, and diazepam, are themselves active but also have active metabolites which contribute to the overall effect of the drug.

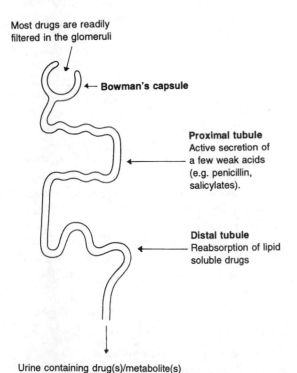

Most drugs are readily filtered in the glomeruli

← Bowman's capsule

Proximal tubule
Active secretion of a few weak acids (e.g. penicillin, salicylates).

Distal tubule
Reabsorption of lipid soluble drugs

Urine containing drug(s)/metabolite(s)

Figure 2.3   Filtration of drugs through the kidney.

Diamorphine is an active narcotic that is converted to morphine – which has approximately half the narcotic activity of its parent compound. Morphine is further metabolised to inactive products.

The main site of drug metabolism is the liver, but other tissues, e.g. lungs, kidneys, blood and intestine may also metabolise drugs. Isoprenaline is metabolised in the gut wall so that it must be given sublingually or by injection. In order to make them more water-soluble, some drugs undergo a variety of chemical reactions, e.g. oxidation, reduction or hydrolysis, of which oxidation is by far the most important. Other drugs are conjugated with naturally occurring substances such as glucuronic acid, sulphate or glycine. A number of drugs undergo chemical reaction and conjugation.

The metabolism of drugs in the liver is influenced by enzymes, whose activity can be increased, giving more rapid metabolism, or decreased, slowing metabolism, by a wide variety of drugs and chemicals. Barbiturates, phenytoin, and rifampicin increase the amount of enzyme that increases metabolism of corticosteroids. Thus, larger doses of corticosteroids require to be administered. This process, known as enzyme induction, is responsible for much of the tolerance which develops with chronic drug administration. Should a patient be on concurrent therapy of an enzyme inducer and warfarin, he will need a higher than normal dose of warfarin to give the desired degree of anticoagulation. Cessation of the inducer drug without a corresponding lowering of the warfarin dose could result in haemorrhage. If a patient is taking oral contraceptives, the oestrogen and progestogen may be rapidly degraded when there is enzyme induction and the level of steroids may be insufficient to give a contraceptive effect. Patients who are taking oral contraceptives and are prescribed enzyme-inducing drugs should be warned of the consequences and advised to use barrier methods of contraception.

Heavy cigarette smoking causes enzyme induction that results in faster metabolism of theophylline. Heavy smokers therefore require a higher dose of theophylline.

Conversely, drugs such as isoniazid and chloramphenicol inhibit the enzymes involved in the metabolism of phenytoin. Concurrent therapy would result in phenytoin toxicity if the dose of phenytoin is not lowered to take this factor into account. Patients in a state of malnutrition, or who have liver disease, suffer from a reduced rate of drug metabolism because their enzyme function is inadequate. The ability to metabolise drugs is reduced in the very young and, for some drugs, in the elderly. In both cases this is due to diminished hepatic microsomal enzyme activity.

The rate of metabolism for the same drug may vary between individuals because of genetic or racial factors. Isoniazid undergoes conjugation with acetyl coenzyme A to form acetylated isoniazid. This proceeds at different rates in different individuals, over half the population being slow acetylators and the remainder fast acetylators. The fast acetylators will require a higher dose than the slow acetylators in order to receive an equivalent therapeutic effect. Other drugs which are acetylated – such as procainamide, phenelzine and hydralazine – will be affected similarly.

DRUG EXCRETION

Most drugs are excreted by the kidney, either unchanged or after metabolism. Most drugs are lipid-soluble and will be re-absorbed at the distal tubule when they pass through the kidney. They must therefore be metabolised before elimination. Examples of drugs eliminated unchanged by active secretion at the proximal tubule include penicillin, digoxin and salicylates (see Fig. 2.3).

The rate of excretion varies greatly between drugs, some being excreted within an hour or two and others taking days or weeks. The elimination of penicillin can be delayed with probenecid, which inhibits the active secretion of penicillin at the proximal tubule thus prolonging its antibacterial action. It should be noted that if renal function is impaired, drugs which are primarily excreted unchanged or as active metabolites will be eliminated more slowly. This will have important consequences if the usual dosage is not reduced, since the plasma level of the drug will rise and may produce toxic effects,

e.g. high plasma levels of gentamicin are nephrotoxic and ototoxic.

In some cases the rate of excretion can be increased (e.g. by altering urinary pH). Aspirin excretion can be increased by the administration of sodium bicarbonate, which raises the urinary pH. Advantage is taken of this in the treatment of salicylate poisoning.

Although the kidney is the major pathway for excretion of drugs and their metabolites, other organs will excrete drugs too. Neomycin which is used for sterilisation of the large intestine when taken orally, is not absorbed and is eliminated in the faeces. General anaesthetics such as nitrous oxide and halothane are eliminated from the lungs. Some drugs and drug metabolites are excreted into the bile. Ampicillin and rifampicin are excreted in high concentrations in the bile, so they may be utilised in a biliary tract infection. Certain drugs undergo enterohepatic circulation (e.g. indomethacin and oestrogens); they are excreted in the bile, enter the gastrointestinal tract, and are subsequently absorbed from the intestine before returning to the circulation.

DOSE/EFFECT RELATIONSHIP

Safe and effective therapy can be achieved only with doses which produce optimal concentrations of a drug in the plasma and target tissues. Smaller doses will be ineffective, while larger doses will not increase the benefits and may have toxic effects. Between the minimal dose which gives the required therapeutic response and the dose at which toxic symptoms appear is a dose range called the therapeutic dose range. Some drugs have a narrow range whereas others have a wide therapeutic range.

After administration of a drug, its plasma level rises; the more rapidly the drug is absorbed, the faster its plasma level rises (Fig. 2.4).

As drug absorption decreases, and distribution, metabolism and excretion rates increase, the curve reaches its peak. It then descends, as elimination occurs more rapidly than absorption. As previously noted, the route of administration influences the time taken for the drug to reach maximal concentration. This is fastest with an

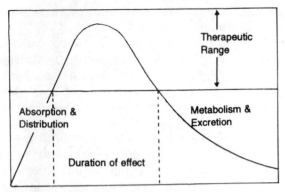

Figure 2.4 Effects of absorption, distribution, metabolism and excretion on the plasma concentration of an administered drug.

intravenous injection, and slower with intramuscular and subcutaneous injections, and oral doses.

As the dose of a drug is increased its therapeutic effect increases as more receptors are occupied. Eventually one reaches the dose that produces a maximal effect when all the receptors of the target organs are occupied by drug molecules. Increasing the dose further will therefore not increase the therapeutic effect.

HALF-LIFE OF DRUGS

The rate at which drugs are eliminated from plasma is commonly expressed in terms of the drug's half-life ($t^1/_2$). This is the time required for the concentration of the drug in the plasma to decrease to one-half of its initial value. The half-life of gentamicin is 2 hours. If the plasma concentration is measured and found to be 8 µg/ml, 2 hours later (one half-life), the level will be half, i.e. 4 µg/ml.

The plasma concentration of a drug at one half-life is 50% of its initial value, at two half-lives 25%, at three half-lives 12.5%, at four half-lives 6.25% and at five half-lives just over 3%. Returning to the original gentamicin concentration of 8 µg/ml, after one half-life (2 hours) the concentration will be 4 µg/ml, after two half-lives (4 hours) 2 µg/ml, after three half-lives (6 hours) 1 µg/ml, after four half-lives (8 hours) 0.5 µg/ml and after five half-lives (10 hours)

0.25 µg/ml. Thus, most of the drug (almost 97%) is eliminated in five half-lives, regardless of the dose or route of administration. This rule of thumb can be applied in calculating the time required to elapse when discontinuing one drug and starting another which may interact if given in conjunction with the first. It is also useful in estimating how long it will take a toxic plasma concentration (after overdosing) to clear the body.

Half-lives of different drugs vary widely, e.g. the $t^1/_2$ of theophylline is 3 hours, the $t^1/_2$ of aspirin is 6 hours, of metronidazole 9 hours, of digoxin about 36 hours, and that of phenobarbitone is about 5 days. A short half-life may result from extensive tissue uptake, rapid metabolism or rapid excretion, and a long half-life may be the consequence of extensive plasma protein-binding, slow metabolism, or poor excretion. The knowledge of half-lives of drugs is essential in determining the intervals between drug doses.

Certain conditions can be treated with a single dose of medication (e.g. analgesics for a headache). Many conditions, however, require continuous drug action (e.g. diabetes mellitus, infections, arthritis). This can be achieved through the administration of repeated doses at regular intervals. In such therapy the second, third and subsequent doses will add to whatever remains of the previous dose, causing gradual accumulation until stable concentrations are maintained (Fig. 2.5).

The level of drug in the plasma rises after absorption, reaches its peak, then falls to minimal effective concentration. Administration of the next dose raises the drug concentration to a

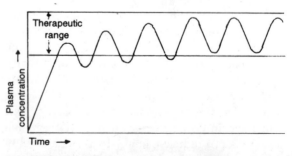

Figure 2.5 Concentration of drug after repeated dosage.

peak. The concentration falls as the drug is metabolised and excreted, then rises again after the next dose. If the interval between doses is too long, or the dose too small, the plasma concentration will have fallen below the therapeutic range before the next dose is given. As a result, the drug concentration is within the therapeutic range only for short intervals.

If a drug is administered too frequently or in too high a dose, the plasma concentration will rise above the therapeutic range and may give rise to toxic effects. In theory, the optimal dosage interval between drug administrations is equal to the half-life of the drug. Initially, the drug accumulates in the body. If 100 mg of drug is given with a half-life of 6 hours, when the second dose of 100 mg is given 6 hours later, 50 mg of the original dose will still be present in the body – giving a total of 150 mg. After a further 6 hours, 75 mg will remain when the third dose of 100 mg is administered, giving a total of 175 mg. At the next dose, 88 mg remains – giving a total of 188 mg. As can be seen, the rate of accumulation becomes less between doses, i.e. 50 mg after the second dose, 25 mg after the third dose, 13 mg after the fourth dose and, in practical terms, a steady-state maximal concentration is reached after approximately five doses. In the steady state the plasma level rises and falls between doses but remains within the therapeutic range – the quantity of drug supplied by each dose is equal to the amount eliminated between doses.

The time required to reach a steady concentration depends on the half-life of the drug. The shorter the half-life, the faster the steady state is reached, irrespective of the route of administration. Aspirin, with a half-life of 6 hours, will reach equilibrium in five half-lives, i.e. 30 hours.

A dosing interval equal to the half-life of a drug may be impractical for drugs with very short half-lives. Penicillin would have to be given every 30 minutes. This would be inconvenient (if not impossible) for the patient and would lead to poor compliance. Penicillin, however, has a wide therapeutic range, and high doses are relatively non-toxic, so that much higher doses can be given every 6–8 hours compared with the dose that would be given every 30 minutes. This ensures that the therapeutic level in the blood is maintained until the next dose. Short half-life drugs, such as lignocaine, which have a narrow therapeutic range, must be given by intravenous infusion since larger doses given infrequently would cause toxic effects.

Most drugs obey a simple relationship between steady-state concentration and dose. Usually the dose and steady-state concentration are directly proportional: if the dose is doubled, the steady-state concentration doubles. For some drugs, however (e.g. phenytoin, aspirin), the rate of clearance decreases with increasing serum concentrations. When dosages of these drugs are increased, steady-state concentrations increase more than expected. There are also drugs (e.g, disopyramide, sodium valproate), with the opposite effect, i.e. clearance increases with increasing concentration. In these cases, increased dosages will produce a smaller than expected increase in steady-state concentration.

LOADING DOSE

In certain conditions it is desirable to reach an effective level of drug in the blood without waiting for accumulation to take place (e.g. if a patient has an infection and requires antibiotic treatment). This can be achieved by giving the patient an initial dose which is twice the maintenance dose. The effective blood concentration is reached after the first dose (e.g. 500 mg) and maintained during subsequent dosing intervals by giving appropriate doses (e.g. 250 mg). With a drug which has a long half-life this regimen is impractical and may be dangerous. It is usually better to allow gradual accumulation following the usual dose and dosage intervals. The patient will then reach his individual steady-state concentration in due course.

PROLONGATION OF DRUG ACTION

Because most drugs are absorbed, then cleared from the body fairly quickly, therapeutic effects are maintained for a relatively short time. In order to prolong the therapeutic effect, the drug must be administered either frequently or by constant infusion. It may be desirable to reduce the frequency of dosage, for example, where compliance is poor, or to simplify regimens, where a number of drugs are being administered. Either or both may be achieved by regulating the release of the active drug from the dosage form in order to maintain therapeutic plasma concentrations (Fig. 2.6).

Absorption can be delayed and the drug's action correspondingly prolonged in a number of different ways. In local anaesthesia with lignocaine, the addition of adrenalin causes constriction of local blood vessels, thus delaying absorption of the anaesthetic into the bloodstream and prolonging its local effect. Delay can also be achieved by giving the drug as an insoluble suspension (e.g. insulin zinc suspension) which dissolves and is absorbed slowly (depot therapy).

In certain instances, extremely slow absorption may be desirable. In psychiatric practice, long-acting preparations can be used to avoid frequent drug administration to patients who find it difficult to remember, or who refuse to take their tablets. The introduction of oily injections of fluphenazine ensures that non-compliant chronic schizophrenic patients can be treated satisfactorily by single intramuscular injections at 4- or 6-weekly intervals. Similarly, long-lasting

contraception can be achieved with depot injections of progestogen. Single depot injections of 15 mg of vitamin D have proved successful in combating nutritional osteomalacia in elderly women in whom compliance with oral medication is often a problem.

Some longer-acting oral preparations

The sustained release of a drug can be achieved in a number of ways, as discussed below.

Coated granules

The active drug is contained in small granules packed in a gelatin capsule. Some granules have no coating and dissolve immediately. Other granules have coatings of varying thickness of materials such as waxes. The granules with thin coatings will dissolve and release the drug faster than those with thicker coatings. It is possible therefore for the active drug to be released over a longer period of time and a steady plasma level to be maintained by one dose instead of three or four individual doses of the conventional preparation.

Multilayer tablets

Sustained action can be achieved by manufacturing tablets which consist of a number of layers or several coats. The drug is dissolved immediately from one layer or the outer coat and more slowly from succeeding layers or coats.

Matrix preparations

The active ingredient is distributed throughout an inert wax or plastic matrix. The drug is slowly leached out of this network and its action may be sustained for up to 24 hours. A variation of this involves the active substance being embedded in a tablet surrounded by a porous coating. The pores are filled with water-soluble crystals, which dissolve on contact with aqueous liquids allowing the active ingredient to be released in a controlled manner by diffusion through the pores.

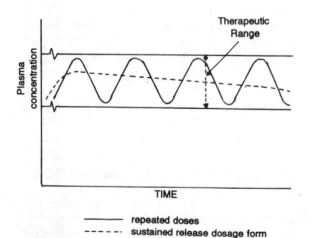

Figure 2.6   Prolongation of drug action.

Miniature osmotic pump

A novel method of achieving oral controlled release of a drug is the miniature osmotic pump. The traditional tablet structure is replaced by a tablet-sized structure made up of a semipermeable membrane which encloses the active drug and the osmotic driving agent (see Fig. 2.7). This system is used to provide a controlled release of salbutamol in the treatment of asthma and related conditions. As with other controlled release products it is important to explain to patients that the tablet must be taken whole with a glass of water and not chewed or crushed.

Controlled-release oral dosage forms may be more convenient than conventional preparations because they require less frequent administration, thus improving the patient's compliance. In addition, the gastric mucosa is exposed to a lower concentration of drug than would have been the case with immediate-release products. This may be important when the drug causes irritation or bleeding of the gastrointestinal tract. However, in practice, the results obtained from controlled-release dosage forms may be far from ideal and may vary between patients. The contents of sustained-release preparations may not be released completely and may tail off, giving therapeutic concentrations initially, but only subtherapeutic concentrations prior to the next dose.

Other methods of prolongation of drug action

Implants

Gentamicin impregnated copolymer beads for the treatment of chronic bone infections are left in situ in the bone cavity for 10–30 days, providing higher concentrations of the drug than would be attained by standard systemic therapy. Implants of other drugs, such as testosterone, have been used to achieve a very long-acting systemic effect (4–8 months).

Gentamicin and other antibiotics are included in bone cements used in orthopaedic surgery. This provides a very slow release designed to prevent local infection in a joint.

Ophthalmic prolonged release

Continuous application of drugs to the eye is necessary both to achieve an intense local action and to avoid systemic complications. If therapy is not regularly maintained, optimal therapy may not be achieved. A unit has been developed which can be placed comfortably in the conjunctival sac allowing slow diffusion of pilocarpine over several days. The system consists of a core reservoir of pilocarpine surrounded by a membrane which controls the drug's diffusion from the system into the tear fluid. The dose is lower than that required in eye drops, resulting in a marked reduction in side-effects. The device does not interfere with the use of other ophthalmic drugs.

Infusion systems

Currently being developed are miniaturised infusion systems which are suitable for implantation under the skin for the administration of insulin or heparin.

In the future it seems likely that more sophisticated drug-delivery systems will be developed with the aim of achieving maximum therapeutic benefit for the patient.

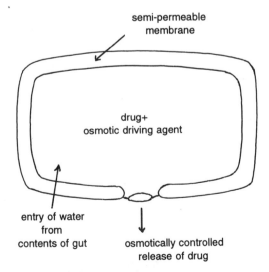

Figure 2.7 Miniature osmotic pump.

3

Pharmacodynamics

Pharmacodynamics is the process by which specific drug dosages produce biochemical or physiological changes in the body.

MECHANISMS OF DRUG ACTION

Drugs act by affecting either biochemical or physiological processes in the body or by controlling changes in these processes brought about by disease. In certain cases the medicine will bring about a normal physiological response where it is a replacement for a deficiency, for example:

- thyroxine is taken orally in hypothyroidism
- insulin is injected subcutaneously in diabetes mellitus
- hydroxocobalamin is injected intramuscularly in the treatment of pernicious anaemia
- ferrous salts are taken orally to treat anaemia due to iron deficiency
- electrolytes in aqueous solution may be administered orally in cases of severe diarrhoea.

The mechanisms of drug action will be considered under the following headings:

Receptor agonists
Receptor antagonists
Enzyme inhibitors
Drugs affecting transport processes
Chemotherapeutic agents
Miscellaneous

Receptor agonists

Receptors

The term 'receptor' can be used to mean any clearly defined target molecule with which a drug molecule has to combine in order to produce a specific effect. Receptors will interact only with those drugs that are exactly compatible structurally (Fig. 3.1). When the drug binds to the receptor a complex is formed which may produce two results. First, activation of the receptor may occur, producing a specific result (receptor agonist). The second type of effect is where a drug binds with a receptor preventing a naturally-occurring substance within the body combining with the receptor. In this way the normal response is blocked (receptor antagonist).

Receptor agonists can be used to alleviate a variety of conditions, examples of which are detailed below.

1. β_2-Adrenoceptor agonists. The main effect is a bronchodilator action directly on the β_2-adrenoceptors of smooth muscle, providing relief in asthma sufferers. Examples include terbutaline, salbutamol and rimiterol.

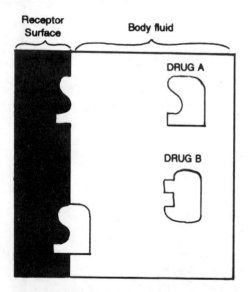

The receptors are compatible with drug A.
Drug B will not react with these receptors

Figure 3.1 Drug–receptor interaction.

2. Sumatriptan is a 5-HT$_1$ (hydroxytryptamine) agonist which is used in the treatment of migraine. Headaches that are a prominent feature of migraine are believed to result from excessive dilatation of extracerebral cranial arteries, arteriovenous shunts, or both. Sumatriptan is a novel selective agonist which blocks these mechanisms.

3. In Parkinson's disease, dopamine production in the brain is greatly reduced. Bromocriptine can be administered to alleviate this condition since it acts as a direct agonist, stimulating dopamine receptors. It has another action since it mimics the action of dopamine on the pituitary, which inhibits prolactin release and, as a result, lactation is suppressed.

Receptor antagonists, by preventing a naturally occurring substance combining with the receptor, produce therapeutic outcomes as illustrated by the following examples.

1. 5-HT$_3$ receptor antagonist. The major sites responsive to emetic stimuli are in the gut and in the brain, areas which are rich in 5-HT$_3$ receptors. Ondansetron is a potent 5-HT$_3$ receptor antagonist and, as such, blocks the emetic reflex responses.

2. β_1-Adrenoceptor antagonists. Atenolol blocks the β_1 actions of noradrenalin released from cardiac sympathetic stimulation and of circulating adrenalin. It is used to treat angina pectoris and hypertension. In angina pectoris, β-receptor antagonists reduce the force and contraction of the ventricle, resulting in a reduction in cardiac oxygen consumption, relieving anginal pain.

3. H$_1$ histamine receptor antagonists. There are two classes of histamine antagonists: H$_1$ receptor antagonists and H$_2$ receptor antagonists. The term 'antihistamine' conventionally refers to the H$_1$ receptor antagonists such as promethazine and terfenadine. They are used mainly to block the actions of histamine released during hypersensitivity reactions.

4. H$_2$ histamine receptor antagonists. Histamine has numerous actions, including a powerful stimulant effect on gastric secretion. Selective antagonists have been developed which have proved potent in blocking the stimulant action of

histamine on the acid-secreting parietal cells of the stomach. H_2 receptor antagonists such as cimetidine and ranitidine are capable of reducing gastric acid secretion by 70% or more.

Enzyme inhibitors

An enzyme is a protein which can promote or accelerate a biochemical reaction with a substrate. When the enzyme mistakenly identifies the drug as being the substrate, a drug–enzyme interaction occurs. This interaction could increase or decrease the rate of a biochemical reaction.

1. Carbidopa/benserazide. In Parkinson's disease, levodopa is given as the precursor to dopamine since it crosses the blood–brain barrier which dopamine is unable to do. It is then broken down to dopamine by dopa decarboxylase. However, dopa decarboxylase is present in the gut and liver – resulting in the breakdown of a proportion of the levodopa before it enters the brain. By combining the levodopa with either carbidopa or benserazide which inhibit the action of dopa decarboxylase, the breakdown of levodopa is reduced and a lower dose can be given.

2. Vigabatrin. δ-Aminobutyric acid (GABA) inhibits the spread of seizure activity by blocking synaptic transmission. GABA is metabolised by the enzyme GABA transaminase (GABA-T). The action of vigabatrin in the treatment of epilepsy is to inhibit GABA-T irreversibly, thus preventing the breakdown of GABA. The action persists until the new enzyme is synthesised.

3. Neostigmine. Neostigmine is used in the treatment of myasthenia gravis. Acetylcholine is broken down by the enzyme cholinesterase. Neostigmine inhibits the action of cholinesterase allowing an accumulation of acetylcholine at the muscle motor end-plate, thereby alleviating the block in neuromuscular transmission which occurs in this condition.

4. Omeprazole. Omeprazole reduces secretion of gastric acid by inhibiting an enzyme called H^+K^+-adenosine triphosphatase (the so-called gastric proton pump). This enzyme is responsible for the final stage in the production of acid in the parietal cells of the gastric mucosa. It pumps protons out from the cell into the gastric lumen in exchange for potassium ions. Once in the lumen the protons (hydrogen ions) meet up with chloride ions to form hydrochloric acid.

Drugs affecting transport processes

This mechanism of action can apply both to drugs introduced to the body and substances synthesized by the body.

1. Thiazide diuretics. The thiazide diuretics decrease the re-absorption of sodium in the renal distal tubule. This results in an increased excretion of sodium and water.

2. Probenecid. In gout there is an increase in the amount of uric acid in the body. Probenecid inhibits the transport of organic acids across epithelial membranes. The re-absorption of uric acid from the renal tubule is blocked by probenecid, resulting in an increased secretion and relief from the symptoms of gout.

3. Insulin. Insulin has a number of actions, one of which is to promote the transport of glucose into cells. This action results in a rapid fall in glucose levels in the blood in relieving hyperglycaemic diabetic coma.

Chemotherapeutic agents

In cancer chemotherapy, cytotoxic drugs act by interfering with cell growth and division. Ideally, a drug is required to have a selective action on all abnormal, rapidly dividing cells found in cancerous conditions with no toxic effect in normal cells. Such a drug is not yet available since currently used drugs attack normal growing cells as well as malignant cells. All cells which are synthesising deoxyribonucleic acid (DNA) go through a cycle which has several different phases. Different cytotoxic drugs act at different phases of the cell cycle:

- methotrexate inhibits the formation of folic acid which is important in the synthesis of DNA
- bleomycin damages DNA.

In infective disease an increasing number of drugs affect bacteria and other microorganisms:

- penicillins and cephalosporins inhibit synthesis of bacterial cell walls
- nystatin and amphotericin act by increasing the permeability of cell membranes of invading organisms
- chloramphenicol and erythromycin inhibit bacterial protein synthesis.

Miscellaneous

There is a significant number of drug actions which can be classed under this heading:

1. Antacids such as aluminium hydroxide and magnesium hydroxide have a direct neutralising effect on acid and reduce gastric acidity.

2. Ion-exchange resins such as calcium polystyrene sulphonate are used to remove excess potassium in mild hyperkalaemia. The sodium in the ion-exchange resin exchanges for potassium, which is removed from the body as the resin passes through and is excreted.

3. Desferrioxamine chelates ferrous iron in the treatment of iron poisoning.

4. Potassium citrate makes the urine alkaline and relieves discomfort in urinary-tract infections.

THE EFFECT OF PATHOLOGICAL STATE AND BIOLOGICAL VARIABILITY

The dose of drug administered may have to be altered when drug absorption, distribution, metabolism or elimination are abnormal because of age, genetic factors, functional state of the kidney, heart or liver, or the severity of the disease process affected by other drugs taken concurrently. Consequently, in some individuals the average or usual dose of a drug may result in plasma levels that are either too low and cannot produce the desired therapeutic effect, or are too high and produce toxic effects.

Liver disease

The liver is the main organ of metabolism for many drugs, and any disease process that results in damage of liver cells, slowing of hepatic blood flow, or decrease in plasma protein may raise plasma concentrations of many drugs. Toxicity of most drugs is related to their elevated concentration in plasma resulting from a decrease in the rate of metabolism. This occurs in hepatic disease. It may therefore be necessary to avoid certain drugs (e.g. lignocaine) or to reduce doses (e.g. of propranolol, aminophylline, chlormethiazole) and monitor plasma concentrations. Severe liver disease results in a low level of albumin in the blood. Drugs which have a high degree of protein binding, such as phenytoin and prednisone, will be bound to a smaller extent and consequently there will be more free drug available which may give rise to toxic effects. There will also be a reduction in the hepatic synthesis of blood clotting factors and this is indicated by a prolonged prothrombin time. Anticoagulants (e.g. warfarin) should therefore be avoided.

Chronic alcoholism

Chronic alcoholism induces microsomal oxidation enzymes which participate in the metabolism of certain drugs (e.g. theophylline). When these drugs are given in normal doses there will be a more rapid metabolism due to a higher level of enzymes. This will result in inadequate plasma concentrations. The opposite effect will occur in advanced cirrhosis of the liver, since the flow of blood through the liver will be impaired. Drugs such as propranolol, pentazocine and pethidine which are extensively metabolised by first-pass metabolism, will therefore reach the tissues in higher concentrations. Dosage should be altered accordingly. Monitoring of plasma concentrations of the drugs may be necessary to prevent overdosage and consequent toxic effects.

Renal disease

Renal disease has the potential to reduce the rate of elimination of drugs. The greater effect will be produced on drugs which are eliminated by the kidney entirely or partially in an unmetabolised form, or where the metabolites are pharmacologically active. As a result, the half-lives of such drugs may be considerably lengthened and plasma concentrations will rise – increasing the potential for toxicity. Dosage adjustment must take account of the extent of renal impairment and the relative toxicity of increased plasma concentrations. However, if only a small percentage of the drug is excreted by the kidney and the metabolites are not toxic, there will be little risk of accumulation in renal failure.

Based on these considerations no action would be required on drugs such as erythromycin and lignocaine which are eliminated principally after metabolism by the liver. A second group (e.g. benzylpenicillin, ampicillin), has a wide therapeutic range and only in severe renal impairment would dosages require lowering. Certain drugs (e.g. nitrofurantoin, allopurinol) should be avoided as toxicity is caused by their metabolites which accumulate to high concentrations in the plasma of patients with impaired renal function. Drugs with a narrow therapeutic range and which can cause problems of toxicity at plasma concentrations only slightly above those required for a therapeutic effect, must be monitored carefully and require lower dosages in all degrees of renal failure; these drugs include gentamicin, kanamycin, digoxin and procainamide. The total maintenance dose of a drug can be reduced either by reducing the size of the individual dose or increasing the interval between doses. For some drugs, if the size of the maintenance dose is reduced, it will be important to give a loading dose if an immediate effect is required, since it takes five half-lives to achieve steady-state plasma concentrations; otherwise, it may take many days to achieve therapeutic plasma concentrations. Nephrotoxic drugs (e.g. amphotericin) should be avoided where possible in patients with renal disease.

Altered doses

Since renal impairment results in a decreased capacity of the kidney to eliminate drugs, dosages must be adjusted to achieve drug therapeutic plasma levels.

The severity of renal impairment is expressed in terms of glomerular filtration rate (GFR), also known as creatinine clearance. Creatinine is an end-product of muscle metabolism and is eliminated from the body by the kidney. Creatinine clearance is obtained by measuring the plasma creatinine concentration in a 24-hour collection of urine. Where this is difficult to obtain, the serum creatinine clearance is used. Normal creatinine clearance is 100–120 ml/min for both men and women. Renal impairment is divided into three grades, as shown in Table 3.1. Renal function declines with age, and many elderly patients have a glomerular filtration rate of less than 50 ml/min.

If the glomerular filtration rate is only 50% of normal, the half-life of drug, eliminated in an unchanged form by the kidney, will be doubled. The dose can be adjusted either by being halved or by giving the normal dose at double the time intervals.

For drugs with a narrow therapeutic range, the predicted dosage schedule should be regarded only as a guide to initial treatment. The recommended intramuscular dose for gentamicin is 2–5 mg/kg daily in divided doses every 8 hours. In renal impairment the interval between successive doses should be increased to 12 hours when the creatinine clearance is 30–70 ml/min, to 24 hours when 10–30 ml/min and to 48 hours when 5–10 ml/min. Predicted dosage schedules should be regarded only as a guide to initial treatment and subsequent treatment must be adjusted according to the clinical response and the serum levels achieved.

DRUG TOLERANCE

'Drug tolerance' refers to a diminished response to a drug taken in the same dose and on a regular

Table 3.1 The three grades of renal impairment

Grade	Glomerular filtration rate (creatinine clearance)
Mild	20–50 ml/min
Moderate	10–20 ml/min
Severe	<10 ml/min

basis. In order to achieve a satisfactory therapeutic effect the dose must therefore be increased. Diamorphine and morphine, for example, induce tolerance to such an extent that doses must be continually increased to many times their initial level to control pain.

There are different reasons why drug tolerance occurs. Metabolic drug tolerance results from an increased rate of metabolism. This is due to induction of hepatic microsomal drug-metabolising enzymes. As the level of these enzymes increases, the drug is broken down more quickly, necessitating a higher dose of drug to achieve the same effect. Tolerance may also be due to a blocking action of a chemical which triggers drug receptors.

DRUG DEPENDENCE

The following chemicals are those most commonly subject to abuse:

- hypnotics and tranquillisers
- alcohol
- cannabis
- amphetamines and cocaine
- opiates.

Dependence on drugs involves a number of factors. Psychological dependence is a state in which a person becomes dependent on taking a drug to achieve a satisfactory everyday function or endpoint. If this person were to suffer physical withdrawal symptoms on discontinuation and, consequently, were to require the continued administration of the drug to prevent this, then physical dependence exists. The term 'drug addiction' encompasses both psychological and physical dependence.

Drug dependence most commonly occurs with the continued taking of opiates such as morphine and diamorphine (heroin). These initially may be abused by sniffing ('snorting') which may graduate to intravenous administration. A temporary state of euphoria is created. As tolerance develops the addict uses the intravenous route with increasing dosage in order to reverse withdrawal symptoms and to reproduce the euphoria and pleasurable body sensa-

tions resulting from high plasma drug concentrations.

Withdrawal symptoms begin about 8 hours after the last dose and peak at 36–72 hours. The initial symptoms include anxiety, depression, irritability, and drug craving. These progress to nausea, vomiting, abdominal cramps, muscle pain, diarrhoea, chill, goose-flesh, and insomnia which fade over about 5 to 10 days.

In Britain, increasing problems due to drug and alcohol abuse and addiction have given rise to increasing numbers of clinics in order to try to contain the problem. At these clinics addicts can receive advice, help and controlled amounts of drugs. One aim will be dosage reduction which may be accompanied by methadone maintenance therapy. The methadone, which is administered orally, is aimed at preventing withdrawal symptoms.

Needle-exchange centres have been set up in towns and cities in order to minimise the sharing of needles by addicts in administering intravenous drugs. This is one of a number of measures being taken to counteract the spread of the HIV virus.

DRUG ALLERGY

The incidence of drug allergy has increased with the rise in the number of people receiving multiple drug therapy. Although almost any drug can produce hypersensitivity, in practice it is the penicillins which are most commonly involved. In this type of reaction, previous exposure to the drug itself, or to a closely related drug, results in the formation of antibodies in the blood. When the drug is given on subsequent occasions, it reacts with the antibodies, and in turn releases chemicals, such as histamine, which can cause the allergic reaction.

IDIOSYNCRASY

Idiosyncrasy is an abnormal reaction which occurs owing to a genetic abnormality. It may alter the normal metabolic pathways of drugs and produce serious adverse reactions in certain individuals. Unlike drug allergy, this response does not require previous sensitisation. Two examples illustrate this condition:

1. Patients with a deficiency of a red blood cell enzyme, glucose 6-phosphate dehydrogenase, suffer haemolytic anaemia when administered drugs such as the sulphonamides or nitrofurantoin.

2. A deficiency in the enzyme cholinesterase greatly prolongs the action of the muscle relaxant suxamethonium.

4

Adverse drug reactions

It is well recognised that pharmaceutical preparations can be potentially harmful. This is one reason why most medicines are very strictly controlled and not available except on prescription. One notable incident occurred in the early 1960s and involved a hypnotic called thalidomide. This drug proved to be teratogenic, and many deformed babies were born to mothers who had taken this preparation in early pregnancy. This led to much more rigorous testing and evaluation of drugs prior to marketing and to a greatly increased awareness of adverse drug effects and methods of detecting them.

AGE-RELATED ADVERSE REACTIONS

Drugs in pregnancy

During the first 2 weeks of human gestation the fertilised ovum is already sensitive to drugs and, after this, drugs may produce congenital malformations in the first trimester in the fetus. The time of greatest risk is between the 3rd and 11th weeks of pregnancy when differentiation of organs occurs. The development of the embryo is very rapid, with continuous changes resulting from cell division, cell migration and cell differentiation. Each organ and each system undergoes a critical stage of differentiation at a precise period of prenatal development, e.g. the heart from day 20 to day 40, and limbs from day 24 to day 46. It is during this time that specific gross malformations can be produced by particular drugs.

Complete closure of the palate occurs in the fetus at 8 weeks, differentiation of the external genitalia between the 4th and 5th month, and further differentiation of the nervous system from the 4th month until after birth. Drugs administered around these times may interfere with the normal development of the genitalia and nervous system.

As a general principle, drugs should not be administered to a woman during pregnancy unless the potential benefit to the mother outweighs the risk to the fetus. However, serious illness can occur during pregnancy, and complications of pregnancy often need to be treated with drugs so that administration cannot always be avoided. The mother may suffer from a chronic condition which requires continuous medication. For example, patients with hypothyroidism require regular doses of thyroxine. Although the placenta is relatively impermeable to thyroxine, adequate replacement in hypothyroid patients is extremely important as it has been shown that children of women who had inadequate replacement therapy scored lower tests of mental and fine motor development when compared to the offspring of women with adequate replacement therapy.

The transfer of drugs across the placenta is accomplished in a similar manner to the distribution of drugs in body organs and tissues. Most drugs cross the placenta by simple diffusion from an area of high concentration to an area of low concentration. Biochemical and physiological changes occur in women during pregnancy and, therefore, drug distribution, metabolism and excretion may be altered. Metabolism of drugs in the maternal liver is reduced during pregnancy and an increase in plasma volume in conjunction with a reduction in albumin content may increase the amount of free drug in the plasma. Since the fetus is in equilibrium with the maternal circulation, drugs and metabolites which readily cross the placenta and enter the fetal circulation will also be in equilibrium and will then pass back into the mother's circulation when cleared by the fetus.

Care must be taken when drugs are administered shortly before term or during labour since these may not have been cleared from the fetus before birth. A drug can no longer pass from the fetal to the maternal circulation after the umbilical cord has been clamped, and this may cause adverse effects on the neonate after delivery due to problems of metabolism and excretion. If treatment is required, drugs preferred are those which have been used extensively. New or untried drugs should be avoided when an alternative with a known 'safe' history is available.

Since the thalidomide tragedy, drugs have been tested in animal studies for teratogenic effects and data collected when adverse effects occurred. Information on the possible or confirmed teratogenic effect of many drugs is now available from drug information centres and drug companies. Some drugs are used which are known to be teratogenic. For example, isotretinoin, used for systemic treatment of severe acne, causes serious central nervous system malformations in the fetus. It is *essential* to ensure that the patient is not pregnant at the time of starting treatment, and effective contraception must be carried out both during treatment and for at least 4 weeks after stopping treatment to allow drug clearance from the body to take place. Similarly, where acitretin is prescribed for treatment of severe psoriasis, effective contraception must be continued for two years after stopping treatment due to this drug's long half-life. Patients are advised not to donate blood during this period since the drug could be transferred to someone who is pregnant. Alkylating drugs and methotrexate also carry a high risk of teratogenicity.

Antibacterial drugs are frequently used in pregnancy for the treatment of maternal infection. The penicillins are probably the safest antibiotics for use in pregnancy. Tetracyclines are irreversibly incorporated into fetal teeth resulting in discolouration and a tendency to develop dental caries. Although the benefits of anti-epileptics to the mother may outweigh the risk to the fetus, there is an increased incidence of congenital malformation in infants born to mothers receiving anti-epileptic drugs. There is no evidence that general anaesthetics are harmful to the fetus provided that maternal hypotension and respiratory depression are avoided.

Although a great deal of work is now being done on the adverse effects of drugs administered during pregnancy, the effects of many drugs on the fetus have yet to be determined. Much of the work has been done on animals which may react differently to humans. In addition, studies conducted in humans are usually retrospective and it is difficult to attribute adverse effects on the fetus to a particular drug.

Drug treatment should be avoided whenever possible during pregnancy especially during the first trimester and prior to delivery. Care should also be taken in administering drugs to women of childbearing age as major harmful effects of drugs on the fetus will be produced very early in pregnancy, possibly before the woman realises she is pregnant.

Drug therapy in the young

All children, and particularly neonates, differ from adults in their response to drugs. The immaturity of organs involved in drug metabolism and excretion may alter not only the pharmacokinetics but also the toxicity of many drugs. Great variability exists in absorption, protein-binding, distribution, metabolism and excretion according to age and weight, and important differences have been observed in premature neonates, full-term babies and older children. These differences become more complex where congenital anomalies or disease states exist.

Absorption of drugs

Gastrointestinal tract The absorption of drugs from the gastrointestinal tract is influenced by the pH of the stomach contents and also by gastric emptying time. The pH of the stomach at birth is 6–8 but falls to a pH of 1–3 in the first 24 hours. (In premature neonates this fall does not occur because the acid-secreting mechanism has not fully developed.) The pH then returns to between 6 and 8 for 10–15 days since no more acid is secreted during this period. This relatively neutral pH of the stomach contents may result in higher blood levels of drugs such as penicillin

due to reduced chemical decomposition resulting in increased availability for absorption. The adult value of gastric pH (approximately 3) is gradually reached between 2 and 3 years of age.

The gastric emptying time may be as long as 6–8 hours in neonates, reaching adult values at 6–8 months. This prolonged emptying time may have an important influence on the absorption rate of orally-administered drugs.

Intramuscular injection The absorption rate of drugs following intramuscular injection is influenced by the changes in muscle blood flow which occur in the first days of life and by vasoconstriction resulting from temperature change or circulatory insufficiency.

Skin Percutaneous absorption is greatly increased in neonates and young infants who have thin, well-hydrated skin. This increased permeability has led to toxic effects associated with the use of hexachlorophane soaps and powders, and salicylic acid ointments. The dangers of absorption of corticosteroids from topical preparations are also widely recognised.

The binding of drugs by proteins

Neonates have reduced plasma protein binding of various drugs. This is because of a reduced plasma protein concentration and because neonatal albumin has a lower binding capacity for drugs than that of adults. These factors may vary in their effects and may lead to drug toxicity. On the other hand, the dose of digoxin required in infants is high compared to that for adults. An average daily maintenance dose for adults is 3–5 µg/kg body weight, whereas in infants it is 10–25 µg/kg. This higher dose is required because the digoxin has a lower binding affinity for digoxin receptors in the myocardium of neonates. In addition to reduced plasma protein binding, another factor affecting drug distribution is the total body water in neonates – which is 70%, compared to the adult value of 55%.

Hepatic metabolism of drugs

Drug metabolism by the liver can occur in a number of ways, for example, by acetylation or by conjugation. In the newborn the necessary enzyme systems are developed to varying extents. Conjugation involving glucuronidation is deficient in some newborn infants. A number of drugs, including chloramphenicol, are metabolised in this way. Where chloramphenicol is administered in 'normal' doses based on weight, serious toxicity can occur which may result in death ('grey syndrome'). This deficiency in metabolism disappears in the first or second week of life.

Excretion of drugs

At birth, all aspects of renal function are diminished but become comparable to that in adults between 6 months and a year. Full-term babies have a reduced glomerular filtration rate compared to adults. Compounds which are not extensively metabolised and depend on renal function for excretion are eliminated more slowly in neonates. The maintenance dose must be adjusted depending on the child's kidney function, increasing as the kidney function develops. On the other hand, drugs such as diuretics which depend on the glomerular filtration to produce a therapeutic effect will require a higher dose at birth when the creatinine clearance is approximately 20 ml/min, but at age 1 month, when the clearance rate is 60 ml/min, the dose would be reduced accordingly.

Drugs in breast milk

Breast milk is the only food the infant requires for the first 4–6 months of life. There are many benefits to be gained from breast-feeding. The composition of human milk is tailored to organ development and growth, and some protection against infection is obtained; compared with cow's milk, there is less likelihood of food allergy and it is more digestible. The advantages for the nursing mother, in addition to maternal bonding, are lower cost than substitute products and convenience. In 1975 only 24% of mothers were breast-feeding 6 weeks after the baby's birth but by 1990 this figure had risen to 63%.

When drugs are administered to nursing mothers there may be a number of adverse effects. The contact of the baby's sucking serves to keep prolactin levels high and may delay subsequent pregnancy. Prolactin secretion can be altered by drugs. It is decreased by levodopa and bromocriptine and increased by phenothiazines, methyldopa and theophylline. The production of milk can be affected by diuretics. Bendrofluazide has been shown to stop lactation. Spironolactone, however, can be used safely.

Although most drugs are excreted to some extent in breast milk, the significance of their effects depends on the amount excreted in the milk. The newborn metabolise and excrete drugs very inefficiently. Pre-term infants are at greater risk than others but the risk decreases as renal and hepatic functions mature. Since infants have poorly developed renal and hepatic functions, they may be particularly sensitive to the accumulation of drugs. Where possible, drugs should be avoided during breast-feeding and mothers should be warned of the possible dangers of self-medication.

Because of their potential toxicity, a number of drugs are absolutely contraindicated while the mother is breast-feeding. These include antithyroid drugs, radioactive isotopes, lithium, chloramphenicol, ergot alkaloids, iodides and most anticancer drugs. If some form of drug treatment is essential, then alternatives to these must be used or breast-feeding must be stopped. A number of other drugs are to be avoided or used with caution. For example, atropine may cause intoxication in sensitive infants, phenindione may cause haemorrhage, and calciferol, in high doses, may cause hypercalcaemia in the infant.

If drugs (e.g. penicillins) are secreted in milk in relatively low concentrations, the advantages of breast-feeding probably outweigh the marginal risks involved. Many drugs (e.g. cephalosporins) known to be excreted in breast milk do not appear to produce adverse effects in the infant.

Generally, the mother should breast-feed prior to taking medication. When a nursing mother takes a drug which is potentially hazardous to the infant, breast-feeding may be temporarily discontinued where a single dose or short course is involved. Attention should be paid to the half-life of the drug. In this situation breast milk should be expressed regularly to maintain lactation, and then discarded.

When drugs are prescribed for a nursing mother, a number of principles are adhered to by the doctor, and the nurse should be aware of these principles:

- never prescribe a drug unless it is essential
- use the safest drug where alternatives are available
- use the lowest effective dose for the shortest possible time.

If there is no alternative to drug therapy and the principles above are adhered to, adverse effects on the baby should not occur. The mother may need reassurance and general guidance so that she is alert for any recognisable effects on the baby.

Drugs in older people

With advancing years, illness becomes more prevalent and the need for drug treatment increases. It would be wrong to view older people as a homogenous group, although it must be recognised that physiological changes occur as we get older.

Distribution of drugs in the body

In most older people, total body mass, lean body mass and total body water decrease; total body fat increases. These changes in body composition can affect a drug's concentration in the body. A water-soluble drug such as gentamicin is distributed primarily in the aqueous parts of the body and lean body tissue. Because an older person has relatively less water and lean tissue, more of the water-soluble drug stays in the blood – leading to increased blood concentration levels; dosage reduction is therefore required.

The older patient has a higher proportion of body fat, and more of a fat-soluble drug is distributed to the fatty tissue. This produces misleadingly low blood levels and may cause dosage to be incorrectly increased. The fatty tissue slowly releases stored drug into the bloodstream and this explains why a fat-soluble sedative may produce a hangover effect.

A decrease in albumin results in a reduction in the plasma protein binding of some drugs (e.g. phenytoin, warfarin, tolbutamide). More non-bound drug is available to act at receptor sites and may result in toxicity. In these cases a dose reduction should be considered.

Metabolism of drugs in older people

Hepatic metabolism of some drugs would appear to be altered as a consequence of the ageing process which results in a reduction of liver blood flow and a reduction in liver mass. General rules cannot be formulated, but for some drugs it appears that decreased hepatic metabolism does result in longer half-life of the drug.

Renal excretion of drugs in older people

Whereas the effect on drug action of reduced hepatic metabolism is difficult to predict, the effect of reduced renal excretion is more readily determined. Glomerular filtration rate by the age of 80 may have fallen to 60–70 ml/min. Drugs or active metabolites of those which are mainly excreted in the urine will require to be administered in lower dose, particularly those with a narrow therapeutic index, e.g. digoxin, lithium, procainamide and the aminoglycosides (e.g. gentamicin). Tetracyclines are best avoided in older people because, in the presence of poor renal function, they accumulate, causing nausea and vomiting resulting in dehydration and further deterioration in renal function.

DOSE-RELATED ADVERSE REACTIONS

Not all individuals will react to the same dose of a drug in the same way. This may be due to pharmacokinetic or pharmacodynamic differences. A controlling dose of insulin in one person may cause hypoglycaemia in another. The anticholinergic effects of tricylic antidepressants (dry mouth, constipation, postural hypotension, urinary retention) may be more pronounced in some patients than others. Drugs with a wide therapeutic index will have a greater margin of safety than those with a narrow therapeutic index, where exceeding the therapeutic dose by a small margin may result in toxicity. Commonly used drugs with a narrow therapeutic index are as follows:

- aminoglycosides (e.g. gentamicin)
- digoxin
- lithium
- anti-arrhythmic drugs (e.g. lignocaine)
- theophylline and aminophylline
- anticoagulants.

Increasing the dosage of a drug previously tolerated at a lower dose may lead to adverse effects, particularly if the drug has a narrow therapeutic index. Adverse reactions may also occur as a result of reduced metabolism in liver disease (p. 24) or accumulation in renal diseases (p. 24).

DIETARY FACTORS

Substances in foods may interfere with the activity of certain drugs. For example, tyramine in some cheeses, beer and red wine can precipitate a hypertensive crisis when ingested while a patient is taking monoamine-oxidase inhibitors. On the other hand, by taking certain drugs with food, adverse effects can be reduced. For example, with NSAIDs there is a reduction in the incidence of gastrointestinal dicomfort, nausea, bleeding and ulceration than would otherwise be the case with an empty stomach.

DRUG-INDUCED SKIN DISORDERS

Drug-induced skin eruptions are likely to be the most frequent adverse reaction seen by a nurse since approximately 30% of reported drug reactions involve the skin.

Erythematous eruptions

This is a skin rash characterised by erythema (abnormal flushing of the skin) and is the most common type of drug-induced skin reaction. Erythematous rashes may be morbilliform (re-sembling measles) or maculopapular, i.e. consisting of macules (distinct flat areas, mostly discoloured) and papules (raised lesions). Early reactions start within 2 or 3 days of the administration of the drug and occur in previously sensitised patients, i.e. patients who have built up antibodies after receiving the drug on a previous occasion. In the late-type reaction the hypersensitivity develops during administration. The peak incidence is around the 9th day but rashes can occur as late as 3 weeks after starting treatment. A high incidence of erythematous rashes can be expected during or following treatment with penicillins, gold salts and non-steroidal anti-inflammatory drugs.

Pruritus

Pruritus may be the first sign of drug hypersensitivity and should act as an early warning for more severe skin reactions, such as those seen with gold therapy. Anal pruritus can be produced as a contact allergy following the local administration of ointments and suppositories.

Urticaria

Urticaria is referred to as 'hives' or 'nettle rash' and is an acute or chronic allergic reaction in which red weals develop. The weals itch intensely and may last for hours or days. Sometimes urticaria affects areas other than the skin, causing swelling of the tongue, lips and eyelids. This serious variety is called angioedema and requires urgent medical attention. Only acute urticaria is likely to be drug-induced, occurring straight away or shortly after the administration of a drug to a sensitised patient, and can be regarded as the cutaneous manifestation of anaphylaxis. Urticaria may arise following treatment with, for example, penicillins, vaccines, indomethacin, imipramine, aspirin, dextrans and X-ray contrast media.

Erythema multiforme

The lesions are erythematous maculopapules affecting the hands and feet more than the trunk.

They appear over a few days and fade within 1 or 2 weeks. Lesions which may be 1–2 cm after 48 hours can reach a size of up to 10 cm with the centre becoming cyanotic – a characteristic 'iris' or target-shaped lesion. Involvement of the mucosa is common. The drugs most likely to cause erythema multiforme are long-acting sulphonamides, penicillins, phenytoin, carbamazepine, NSAIDs and gold salts.

Exfoliative dermatitis

This condition usually starts a few weeks after the start of treatment with the drug concerned. It is characterised by a redness of the whole skin with widespread exfoliation (peeling) and may be caused by streptomycin, chloramphenicol, carbamazepine, gold salts or thiazide diuretics.

Lichenoid eruptions

In lichenoid drug eruptions the characteristic wide, flat, mauve pimples of lichen planus skin disease are present but can be associated with papular, scaling and eczematous lesions. The lesions are found mainly on the forearms, neck and between the thighs. Drugs which can cause this condition include phenothiazines, captopril, carbamazepine, gold salts, NSAIDs, penicillamine and thiazide diuretics.

Erythema nodosum

The lesions are painful subcutaneous nodules usually limited to extremities and may be preceded by transient erythema. Although not commonly drug-induced, erythema nodosum has been observed in women taking oral contraceptives. Other suspect drugs are sulphonamides, salicylates, penicillins and gold salts.

Photosensitivity

Increased sensitivity to light may be produced by

thiazide diuretics, sulphonamides, tetracyclines, phenothiazines and nalidixic acid.

DRUG-INDUCED BLOOD DYSCRASIAS

The exact incidence of drug-induced blood dyscrasias is difficult to assess but they are among the more common serious adverse effects of drug therapy. In most cases, withdrawal of the drug responsible for the reaction will improve the blood picture and return it to normal provided death does not occur due to complications.

Aplastic anaemia

This results from the suppression of all bone marrow function (hypoplasia). The defective production from differentiation of stem cells of red cells, white cells and platelets results in low plasma counts for all cells. It is the most serious type of blood dyscrasia with a high incidence of mortality. The clinical features vary with the severity of the aplastic anaemia. Anaemia (reduced red cells) gives symptoms of weakness, fatigue and shortness of breath on exertion. Neutropenia and agranulocytosis (reduced white cells) can produce sore throat, ulceration of the mouth and pharynx, fever, and infections of candida in the skin and mucous membranes. Thrombocytopenia (reduced platelets) can produce haemorrhage into the skin and bleeding from the gum and the alimentary tract.

Drug-induced aplastic anaemia can arise due to a direct, dose-related effect on cell division in the bone marrow by cytotoxic agents. Alternatively it can arise due to a sensitivity reaction which may not become apparent until several months after the drug has been stopped. The drug should never be re-administered as this might be fatal to a patient who is sensitised. Drugs commonly associated with aplastic anaemia are listed in Box 4.1.

Agranulocytosis

Neutropenia, a reduction in the number of circu-

Box 4.1 Drugs associated with aplastic anaemia, agranulocytosis and thrombocytopenia

Acetazolamide	Ethosuximide
Allopurinol	Frusemide
Antihistamines	Gold salts
Antineoplastic drugs	Mianserin
Captopril	Penicillamine
Carbamazepine	Phenothiazines
Carbimazole	Phenytoin
Chloramphenicol	Tolbutamide
Chloroquine	Tricyclic antidepressants
Chlorpropramide	

---

lating neutrophils, is often caused by drug-induced suppression of white cells. Agranulocytosis is complete absence of neutrophils in the blood. The body's ability to fight infection is compromised.

In acute neutropenia, fever, sore throat and painful mucosal ulcers are common symptoms. Patients receiving drugs with a high incidence of agranulocytosis (e.g. mianserin, penicillamine, gold and clozapine) should undergo regular blood screens and, where a problem arises, the drug should be withdrawn.

Thrombocytopenia

Thrombocytopenia is a reduction in the platelet count. This can be caused by destruction of platelets or decreased production in the bone marrow. The symptoms include widespread small haemorrhagic spots, nose bleeds (epistaxes) and bleeding from the gums. The mechanism of drug-induced thrombocytopenia is either selective marrow depression or an immune reaction, which results in antibodies active against platelets, which causes platelet agglutination. On withdrawal of the drug, the platelet count returns to normal. Since there are common mechanisms involved in drug-induced aplastic anaemia, agranulocytosis and thrombocytopenia, in the main, the same drugs can cause all three conditions (Box 4.1). However, heparin, paracetamol and rifampicin have caused only thrombocytopenia.

ADVERSE REACTIONS – CENTRAL NERVOUS SYSTEM

Nausea and vomiting

Chemotherapeutic agents may cause the release of 5-HT (see p. 140) in the small intestine initiating a vomiting reflex by activating 5-HT receptors. In addition, 5-HT may be released in the brain – which promotes emesis centrally. The emetogenic effect of cancer chemotherapy varies according to the dose and combination of drugs used. High-dose cisplatin therapy is highly emetogenic. Carboplatin is also emetogenic but less so than cisplatin. Other drugs cause gastrointestinal side-effects by a more direct irritant effect on the gut.

Headache

Vasodilators such as the nitrates can cause drug-induced headaches. Migraine headaches can be caused by drugs which increase 5-hydroxytryptamine levels, e.g. fluoxetine, fluvoxamine and tryptophan.

Dizziness

Dizziness is a symptom which can arise with most centrally acting drugs, including the antipsychotic drugs, antidepressants, benzodiazepines, anticonvulsants, NSAIDs and antihypertensives.

Tinnitus

This refers to any noise, such as ringing, in the ears. The reaction is dose-related and the dose must be reduced or the drug stopped. Tinnitus caused by the salicylates is an indication of a toxic reaction. Aminoglycosides are ototoxic.

Drowsiness

Many drugs have special labelling requirements because they cause drowsiness – 'This drug may cause drowsiness. If affected, do not drive or operate machinery'. Drowsiness is a common effect of many drugs that act on the central nervous system. All antipsychotic drugs can produce some sedation. Most tricyclic antidepressants produce sedation to varying degrees. This effect can be beneficial in depressed patients with sleeping difficulties where the antidepressant is given at night. Many of the long-established antihistamines cause drowsiness but newer ones have been developed where this is greatly reduced, e.g. terfenadine.

Parkinsonism

Parkinson's disease, due to a decrease in dopamine production, is characterised by tremor, rigidity and a poverty of spontaneous movements. Drug-induced parkinsonism resembles Parkinson's disease and occurs to varying degrees in patients treated with antipsychotic drugs. The phenothiazines (e.g. trifluoperazine, fluphenazine), the butyrophenones (e.g. haloperidol, droperidol) and the diphenylbutyl piperidines (e.g. pimozide, fluspirilene) are associated with a higher incidence of extrapyramidal effects. Drug-induced parkinsonism is reversible on dose reduction or drug withdrawal. Other drugs which have been implicated in parkinsonism include prochlorperazine, metoclopromide and tricyclic antidepressants.

ADVERSE REACTIONS – GASTROINTESTINAL SYSTEM
Gastrointestinal side-effects

Many drugs cause gastrointestinal upsets which may significantly interfere with the patient's treatment. Patients may discontinue the therapy, or absorption of the drug may be reduced. Gastrointestinal side-effects present in a number of ways. Drugs which are implicated in gastrointestinal disturbances are shown in Table 4.1.

Gastrointestinal side-effects can be minimised in a number of ways. Administration with food, or after a meal, may be helpful. Adjustment of dose, change of formulation or co-administration of an antacid should be considered. If this is necessary care must be taken to avoid drug interactions.

ALLERGIC EMERGENCY (ANAPHYLACTIC SHOCK)

This is a life-threatening reaction with abrupt onset caused by exposure of sensitised individuals to specific allergens. The mechanism in susceptible individuals involves the production of IgE antibody directed against the antigens. IgE binds to the surface of the mast cells and baso-

Table 4.1 Drugs causing gastrointestinal side-effects

Drug	Symptoms/notes
Antibiotics, e.g. tetracycline, amoxycillin	Nausea and vomiting; diarrhoea, indigestion
Corticosteroids, e.g. prednisolone	Dyspepsia, peptic ulceration, oesophageal ulceration
Oral contraceptives	Absorption of drug may be reduced where there is nausea and vomiting
Diflucan	Diarrhoea, flatulence, nausea
Ferrous sulphate (and other iron salts)	Anorexia, discomfort, constipation, diarrhoea, darkening of stools
Lisinopril	Abdominal pain, dry mouth, hepatitis
Methyldopa	Nausea, vomiting, distension, constipation and diarrhoea
Mefenamic acid	Diarrhoea
Morphine	Nausea, vomiting and constipation
Non-steroidal anti-inflammatory drugs (NSAIDs), e.g. naproxen, indomethacin	Nausea, vomiting, abdominal discomfort; gastrointestinal bleeding and peptic ulceration are rare but serious complications
Paroxetine	Dry mouth
Tricyclic antidepressants	Anticholinergic side-effects may cause constipation and paralytic ileus.

phils. Subsequent exposure to antigen triggers the release of various substances, predominant among which is histamine. This causes:

- vasodilation
- increased capillary permeability
- tissue oedema.

These changes give rise to:

- hypotension
- urticaria
- erythema of face and neck.

The reaction develops rapidly, reaching a maximum within 5–30 minutes. Individuals who experience an anaphylactic reaction may have a personal or family history of allergy.

In a severe reaction the signs and symptoms are:

- pallor or cyanosis with weakening pulse
- skin cold and clammy to touch
- swelling of the glottis
- bronchoconstriction
- feeling of faintness
- loss of consciousness.

Other less serious features include:

- nasal congestion
- rhinorrhoea
- hoarseness.

Death from anaphylactic shock is mostly due to respiratory tract obstruction resulting from laryngeal oedema and bronchoconstriction. The incidence of these serious reactions is low, but in their rarity lies danger.

Common causes include:

- drugs, particularly if given by injection
- blood products
- insect stings
- desensitising agents
- certain foods (nuts, fish, shellfish).

The following groups of drugs are most commonly implicated:

- vaccines
- antibiotics, particularly penicillins
- desensitising solutions

- heparin
- anti-inflammatory analgesics
- iron injections
- neuromuscular blocking drugs
- hydroxocobalamin
- cytotoxic drugs.

Anaphylaxis is more likely to occur as the result of an injection than from taking an oral preparation.

Prevention

The following actions may assist in prevention of an anaphylactic reaction:

- Ask the patient if he has suffered any previous reaction to drugs.
- Ask the patient if he is taking drugs currently, including both prescribed and non-prescribed drugs.
- Ask the patient if he has suffered from previous allergies such as asthma, hay fever, eczema.
- If in doubt, discuss with the doctor or other colleague before giving the drug.
- Consider giving a small, test dose and carefully observe the patient before giving the full dose.

Treatment

This takes the form of drug therapy and is directed towards antagonising the effects of chemical mediators, and preventing the further release of mediator substances.

First-line treatment includes laying the patient flat then restoring the blood pressure by administering 0.5–1 ml of adrenalin 1 in 1000 (0.5–1 mg) by the intramuscular route as quickly as possible. This is repeated every 10–15 minutes until improvement in the blood pressure occurs.

Adrenalin inhibits the release of mediator chemicals from mast cells, limiting the severity of anaphylaxis. It also stimulates the β_2 receptors in bronchial smooth muscle causing bronchodilation. Where there is a severe reaction, the adrenalin injection is followed by chlorpheniramine given by slow intravenous injection and continued for 24–48 hours to prevent a relapse. This is an antihistamine or H_1-receptor blocking drug. The effect of this is to block the H_1-receptor mediated actions of histamine, reducing vascular permeability and bronchospasm.

Corticosteroids such as hydrocortisone or prednisolone are of no value in the initial treat-

ment of anaphylaxis as onset of their therapeutic effect takes several hours. They can prove useful in preventing further deterioration in severely affected patients by inhibiting the release of inflammatory mediators and suppressing inflammatory reactions. Some patients with severe allergy to insect stings may be advised to carry

Table 4.2 Treatment of poisoning

Agent/method	Uses/indications
Acetylcysteine	This drug is given by intravenous infusion in the treatment of paracetamol poisoning. The dose is determined by reference to plasma paracetamol levels. Treatment with aceytylcysteine is designed to reduce the often fatal liver damage caused by paracetamol ingestion in high doses. Treatment must be commenced as soon as possible after ingestion. If a period of more than 24 hours has passed after ingestion the liver damage will be irreversible.
Charcoal (activated)	Used to bind poisons, thus reducing absorption. A single dose of up to 50 g reduces absorption, and repeated doses of activated charcoal enhance the elimination of certain drugs after absorption.
Desferrioxamine	This is a specific antidote for iron poisoning. The drug acts by chelating the iron. Administration is by mouth, intramuscular, or intravenous infusion, depending on the patient's condition.
Dicobalt edetate	This is a specific antidote used in the treatment of cyanide poisoning.
Dimercaprol	In poisoning by metals such as gold and mercury. Also in poisoning by arsenic and antimony.
Diuresis	Forced alkaline diuresis has been used for salicylate and barbiturate poisoning, but is not now recommended.
Fuller's earth (or bentonite)	To adsorb paraquat (a herbicide) by oral administration.
Haemoperfusion and haemodialysis	These techniques may be used in severely poisoned patients, particularly in the treatment of salicylate and barbiturate poisoning.
Ipecacuanha	Used to induce emesis. Available as a specially made up elixir for oral administration. Must be used with care, but is preferred to other emetics such as salt.
Methionine	Given orally in paracetamol poisoning.
Naloxone	Naloxone is a specific antidote for opioid overdosage. The intramuscular, intravenous or subcutaneous routes can be used, the dosage being determined in accordance with the patient's needs – e.g. 2 mg in 500 ml as an intravenous infusion, the rate of infusion depending on the patient's condition.
Penicillamine	Copper and lead poisoning by oral administration.
Pralidoxime	With atropine in the treatment of organophosphorus poisoning by intramuscular or slow intravenous injection.
Sodium calcium edetate	The treatment of lead poisoning by intravenous infusion.
Sodium nitrite and sodium thiosulphate	Used in combination in the treatment of cyanide poisoning.

Other drugs used in the treatment of poisoning include:
Atropine
Diazepam
Intravenous fluids and electrolytes
Anti-arrhythmic drugs
Benztropine
Procyclidine

an adrenalin inhaler or syringes prefilled with adrenalin solution.

TREATMENT OF POISONING

At the extreme end of the adverse drug reaction spectrum is poisoning. The treatment of acute poisoning, either intentional or accidental, presents a major challenge to clinical staff. Deaths from accidental poisoning have increased markedly in the last 30 years. Careless storage of medicines and household products is a common cause of accidental poisoning in children. Natural products, leaves, berries etc. may also be implicated. Intentional poisoning is a complex subject. Self-poisoning may be undertaken by a person determined to end his or her life. However, in some cases the ingestion of a poisonous substance, often a medicinal product, may be a 'cry for help' or form part of a manipulative personal situation. Many social factors contribute to the tragic situations that can arise, e.g. poverty, alcoholism, unemployment and broken homes.

The management of a patient who has been poisoned, whatever the cause or circumstances, must be directed towards the maintenance of respiration and circulation. Seldom are the symptoms of poisoning highly specific, but many clues are available to the observant doctor or nurse. Tablets may be found in the victim's possessions or at the scene of the tragedy. Family members and/or friends may be able to give useful information. The first priority of treatment is to maintain the patient's vital functions. If necessary, laboratory tests to determine the exact nature of the poison are undertaken at an appropriate time. National Poisons' Centres provide back-up, advice and guidance on clinical management in special situations. Key aspects in the treatment of poisoning are as follows:

- maintenance of respiration – physical methods
- maintenance of circulation – physical methods and drug treatment
- maintenance of body temperature – physical methods
- maintenance of fluid and electrolyte levels in accordance with biochemical tests
- removal of the poisons (gastric lavage/emesis/active elimination)
- inactivation of the poisons – use of activated charcoal to adsorb the poison
- correction of metabolic complications, e.g. metabolic acidosis.

Once the acute situation has been dealt with and the patient assessed it may be necessary to call in specialised psychiatric help.

Some poisons have specific antidotes, but these can be no substitute for general supportive measures outlined above. An outline of the agents available for the treatment of poisoning is given in Table 4.2. These agents will be used together with general supportive measures.

In considering the treatment of acute poisoning, it is important to recognise the place of prevention, especially in children. Some useful guidelines for parents are given in Box 4.2.

Box 4.2 Guidelines for preventing child poisoning

- Keep medicines locked away
- If your medicine is stored in a fridge fit a safety lock to the door
- Teach children not to play with medicines
- Never share medicines
- Warn children not to swallow anything unfamiliar
- Never pretend medicines are sweets
- Dispose of medicines at the pharmacy

If you think your child has swallowed a medicine or poison:
- Get the child to the nearest accident and emergency department as soon as possible
- Take the drug container with you so that the doctor knows what has been taken
- Do not try to make the child sick
- If the child is unconscious, lay on one side to ease breathing and stop choking

FURTHER READING

Breathnach S M 1993 Drug eruptions. Hospital Update 19(6): 344–351

Davenport D 1993 Structured support at a time of crisis. Treatment of paracetamol overdosage. Professional Nurse 8(9): 558–562

5

Drug interactions

When two or more drugs are administered at the same time they may exert their effect independently or they may interact. This may result in the action of one drug being more potent or being reduced due to an effect by the other drug. Many drug interactions are harmless, and a particular drug combination may only cause harm to a small proportion of individuals who receive it. The drugs most often involved in serious interactions are those with a narrow therapeutic range (e.g. aminoglycosides, phenytoin) and those where the dose must be closely monitored according to the response (e.g. anticoagulants, antidiabetic drugs). Patients at increased risk from drug interactions include those with impaired renal and liver function, and the elderly because of changes in physiology due to ageing and also because the elderly are prescribed proportionately more drugs than the young.

Drug interactions can be considered under three main headings:

- chemical interactions
- pharmacokinetic interactions
- pharmacodynamic interactions.

CHEMICAL INTERACTIONS

These may occur when incompatible drugs are mixed in syringes or added to infusion liquids prior to administration, or when the vehicle may be incompatible with the drug. Amphotericin must be diluted in glucose 5% injection with a pH greater than 4.2. Care must be taken when calcium salts and phosphate are added to an intravenous infusion since above certain concentrations a precipitate is formed.

PHARMACOKINETIC INTERACTIONS

These occur when one drug alters the absorption, distribution, protein-binding, metabolism or excretion of another, thus reducing the amount of drug available to produce its pharmacological effects.

Interactions affecting drug absorption

When iron and tetracycline are required they should be administered separately, as absorption is diminished when both are administered at the same time. The absorption of iron, tetracycline and several other drugs is affected by antacids.

An example of a beneficial absorption interaction is that between metoclopramide and analgesics in the treatment of an acute attack of migraine. Because nausea and vomiting may occur in acute attacks and may be associated with gastric stasis due to inhibition of gastric motility, metoclopramide not only relieves the nausea and vomiting, but, by increasing the speed of gastric emptying, improves the absorption of oral analgesics (mainly absorbed from the small intestine).

Interactions due to changes in protein-binding of drugs

The extent of effect of a drug depends on its level in the plasma since the higher the level the more will diffuse from the plasma to its site of action. A proportion of the drug after absorption will be free in the plasma and the remainder will be bound to plasma protein. Should a drug (e.g. warfarin) be displaced from plasma protein by another which has a stronger binding action (e.g. tolbutamide), there will be an increased concentration of unbound warfarin in the plasma which will result in a greater therapeutic effect. This is exacerbated since, in this particular reaction, warfarin metabolism is inhibited.

Interactions affecting drug metabolism

Many drugs are inactivated by metabolism in the liver. One drug may inhibit the metabolism of another due to competition by both drugs for a particular drug-metabolising enzyme. Inhibition leads to lengthening of the plasma half-life of the inhibited drug, elevated plasma concentrations and an enhanced pharmacological effect which may cause toxicity. The potentiation of warfarin by cotrimoxazole and dextropropoxyphene is due partly to this mechanism in addition to changes in plasma protein binding. Similarly, cimetidine affects phenytoin and diazepam metabolism.

Levodopa is metabolised to dopamine by the enzyme dopa decarboxylase. The inhibition of this enzyme by carbidopa or benserazide which is given concurrently, inhibits the breakdown of levodopa before it reaches its site of action and therefore allows a lower dose to be administered.

Certain drugs may cause enzyme induction, increasing the level of a particular enzyme. Drugs which are metabolised by this enzyme will therefore be broken down more quickly. Griseofulvin potentiates the enzymes which break down warfarin, and rifampicin potentiates those which break down oestrogens and progestogens. The latter interaction is important where the patient is taking oral contraceptives since these will be broken down more quickly and may not produce the desired effect.

Interactions affecting the renal excretion of drugs

Drugs are eliminated through the kidney both by glomerular filtration and by active tubular excretion. Competition can occur when drugs share the active transport mechanisms in the proximal tubule. Probenecid delays the excretion of all penicillins and some cephalosporins, which leads to their increased plasma levels. A combination of aspirin and methotrexate leads to a risk of toxicity from increased levels of methotrexate due to competition for tubular secretion.

PHARMACODYNAMIC INTERACTIONS

These interactions occur between drugs which have similar or antagonistic pharmacological effects or side-effects.

Interactions at receptor sites

These interactions occur when two drugs act on the same site either antagonistically or synergistically.

1. *Antagonism.* An example of this, which is therapeutically beneficial, is the reversal of the effects of opiates by naloxone.

2. *Synergism.* Aminoglycosides potentiate the action of competitive neuromuscular drugs such as tubocurarine, resulting in prolonged paralysis.

Interactions between drugs affecting the same system

Acetazolamide, carbenoxolone, corticosteroids and corticotrophin interact with thiazide diuretics, frusemide, bumetanide and ethacrynic acid, causing increased urinary potassium loss resulting in hypokalaemia. Antihypertensive drugs are potentiated by hypnotics, tranquillisers and levodopa which produce hypotension as a side-effect.

Interactions due to altered physiology

These interactions can occur in a number of ways, e.g. carbenoxolone and corticosteroids antagonise the effect of antihypertensive drugs due to fluid retention. Potassium-losing diuretics may give rise to digoxin toxicity due to increased potassium loss.

DRUG INTERACTIONS WITH ALCOHOL

Alcohol can interact with many drugs. It has a depressant effect on the nervous system and when administered concurrently with CNS depressants the effect is additive. Alcohol increases the risk of death from an overdose of these drugs. The vasodilator effect of alcohol increases the postural hypotension of antihypertensive drugs. It can cause postural hypotension with peripheral vasodilators (e.g. oxpentifylline) and anti-anginal drugs (e.g. nitrates, verapamil). This interaction can also occur with metronidazole and procarbazine. Some alcoholic drinks contain tyramine. If this is taken along with monoamine-oxidase inhibitors such as phenelzine or tranylcypromine there is a risk of a hypertensive crisis.

FURTHER READING

Aronson J 1993 Serious drug interactions. Practitioner 237: 789–791

Tully H P 1993 Iatrogenic disease in the elderly patient. Hospital Pharmacy Practice 3(3): 138–144

6

Autonomic nervous system

The autonomic or involuntary nervous system conveys all outputs from the central nervous system to the rest of the body, except for skeletal muscle. It controls the activities of the gastrointestinal tract, the respiratory and urogenital system, the heart and vascular system, the eyes and various secretory glands. The autonomic nervous system consists of two divisions, and most organs are supplied by nerves from both of these divisions. They are called the sympathetic and the parasympathetic systems. Each organ controlled by the autonomic nervous system can be stimulated or inhibited according to physiological needs, and the functions of the sympathetic and parasympathetic nervous systems can be regarded as having basically opposite effects.

ANATOMY

The sympathetic nervous system consists of a series of short nerve fibres from the thoracic and lumbar parts of the spinal cord passing to one of a chain of ganglia on either side of the vertebral column (Fig. 6.1). Here they form a synapse or junction, and other longer nerve fibres (the postganglionic fibres) pass out to the smooth muscle of the visceral organs.

The preganglionic parasympathetic nerve fibres originate in the midbrain, medulla and sacral parts of the spinal cord. They synapse in ganglia situated either in or close to the enervated organ. Consequently, the postganglionic parasympathetic nerve fibre is much shorter than the postganglionic sympathetic fibre (Fig. 6.1).

SYMPATHETIC NERVOUS SYSTEM

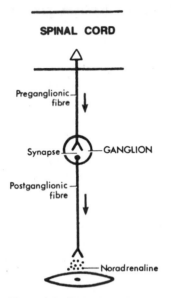

PARASYMPATHETIC NERVOUS SYSTEM

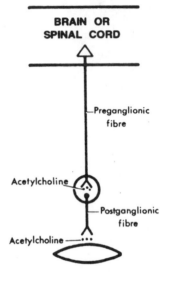

Figure 6.1 Neurotransmitter systems.

Transmitters

When an impulse passes from the central nervous system along a preganglionic fibre and reaches a ganglion, a messenger substance, acetylcholine, is liberated in order to carry the impulse across the ganglion to the postganglionic fibre. As soon as the impulse has passed, the released acetylcholine is immediately broken down by an enzyme, cholinesterase. The impulse continues along the postganglionic fibre and in the case of parasympathetic nerves, acetylcholine is released when the impulse reaches the point where the nerve joins the organ concerned. The acetylcholine acts on a receptor to produce the necessary response. The response is limited in duration and intensity by the rapid destruction of the acetylcholine, as occurred in the ganglion.

A similar process takes place in the sympathetic nervous system up to the junction of the nerve and tissue but, instead of acetylcholine being released, the neuro-transmitter is nor-adrenalin (Fig. 6.1). In addition, this is accompanied by a release of noradrenalin and adrenalin from the medulla of the adrenal gland. These substances enter the systemic circulation and produce widespread effects since they can act on a number of receptors, i.e. α, β_1 and β_2. The noradrenalin may be broken down by monoamine oxidase or may be taken back up into the nerve ending by a re-uptake mechanism. If this did not happen there would be continual stimulation of the receptors.

Receptors

Receptors are generally termed according to the

Table 6.1 Commonly used terms

	Sympathetic nervous system	Parasympathetic nervous system
Agonists	Sympathomimetics	Parasympathomimetics
Antagonists	Sympatholytics	Parasympatholytics

Table 6.2 Actions resulting from sympathetic and parasympathetic nerve stimulation

Organ	Sympathetic response	Sympathetic receptor type	Parasympathetic response
Heart	Rate and force of contraction increased	β_1	Rate and force of contraction decreased
Blood vessels			
skin	Vasoconstriction	α	Dilatation
skeletal muscle	Vasoconstriction	α	Dilatation
	Vasodilatation	β_2	
Lungs (bronchial muscles)	Relaxation	β_2	Contraction
Intestine			
motility and tone	Decreased	α and β_2	Increased
sphincters	Contraction	α	Relaxation
glands	No effect		Secretion
Urinary system			
bladder	Relaxed	β_2	Contracted
sphincter	Contracted	α	Relaxed
Eye			
pupil (radial muscle)	Dilatation	α	Constriction
ciliary muscle	Relaxation	β	Contraction
Salivary glands	Sparse, thick secretion	α	Profuse, watery secretion
Skin			
sweat glands	Secretion	α	No effect
Male sex organs	Ejaculation	α	Erection

transmitter which activates the receptor, i.e. cholinergic receptors are activated by acetylcholine and noradrenergic receptors by noradrenalin. A drug which acts on a receptor in a similar way to the transmitter is called an agonist; a drug which prevents the action of the transmitter at the receptor is an antagonist.

Some commonly used terms are given in Table 6.1.

Cholinergic agents are drugs that promote the function of the neurotransmitter acetylcholine. The cholinergics are also called parasympathomimetics because they produce effects that imitate parasympathetic nerve stimulation. Drugs which antagonise the effect of postganglionic parasympathetic nerve stimulation are called parasympatholytics.

Table 6.3 Sympathomimetics

Drug	Receptor-stimulated	Effect
Methoxamine	α	Causes vasoconstriction of peripheral blood vessels and is used to control blood pressure in anaesthesia
Dobutamine	β_1	Increases force of contraction of the heart in cardiac failure
Salbutamol Terbutaline	β_2	Bronchodilation in asthmatics

Table 6.4 Adrenergic blocking drugs

Drug	Receptor-blocked	Effect	Side-effects
Tolazoline	α	Causes vasodilation – used in peripheral vascular disease	Flushing, goose-flesh
Propranolol	β_1 and β_2	Slows the heart and reduces cardiac output; used in hypertension and angina	Bradycardia, bronchospasm (acts on β_2 receptors in lungs)
Metoprolol Atenolol	Mainly β_1	As for propranolol	More selective – less likelihood of bronchospasm

Table 6.5   Adrenergic neurone blocking drugs – these block the release of noradrenalin

Drug	Indication	Side-effects
Guanethadine Debrisoquine	Hypertension	Postural hypotension, failure of ejaculation, fluid retention, nasal congestion

Similarly, noradrenalin and drugs which mimic the effect of postganglionic sympathetic nerve stimulation are called sympathomimetics, and those which antagonise this effect are called sympatholytics.

SYMPATHETIC AND PARASYMPATHETIC NERVE STIMULATION

The activation of these two parts of the autonomic nervous system is of profound physiological importance. Often both systems act on the same organ (at different times) but produce opposite effects. In a healthy person the two parts of the system are in dynamic equilibrium in response to physiological needs. In order to understand how drugs affect the functioning of the autonomic nervous system it is necessary to know which organs respond to stimulation and which receptors are involved (Table 6.2).

Table 6.6   Parasympathomimetics – these mimic the effect of parasympathetic stimulation*

Drug	Action	Side-effects
Pilocarpine	Contracts ciliary muscle, improving drainage and relieving pressure in the eye in glaucoma	Constriction of pupil, blurring of vision
Carbachol	Relaxes bladder sphincter in urinary retention	Nausea, vomiting, blurred vision, sweating, flushing of skin, bradycardia and intestinal colic

*Parasympathomimetics are contraindicated in hyperthyroidism (cause glands to secrete), peptic ulcer, bronchial asthma, bradycardia, hypotension and parkinsonism.

Table 6.7   Anticholinesterase drugs – these drugs block the enzyme responsible for the breakdown of acetylcholine, i.e. cholinesterase

Drug	Action	Side-effects
Physostigmine	Contracts ciliary muscle improving drainage and relieving pressure in the eye in glaucoma	Blurring of vision
Neostigmine	Used to treat muscle weakness in myasthenia gravis	Salivation, sweating, gastric secretion, motility, diarrhoea

EFFECT OF DRUGS ON THE AUTONOMIC NERVOUS SYSTEM

Drugs are administered in order to mediate the autonomic nervous system. These drugs can act in a number of ways; they can:

- mimic the effect of sympathetic or parasympathetic stimulation
- interfere with the enzymatic destruction of transmitters and thus potentiate the natural response
- block the receptor to the transmitter and reduce or negate the effect of the neurotransmitter (noradrenalin or acetylcholine).

Adrenalin acts at a number of receptor sites and, following injection, various actions quickly become apparent:

Table 6.8   Parasympatholytics (anticholinergics) – these drugs block the receptor and have an effect opposite to that of parasympathomimetics

Drug	Action	Side-effects
Atropine	Antispasmodic; premedication to dry bronchial and salivary secretions	Hallucinations, ataxia; avoid in glaucoma
Hyoscine	Antispasmodic; premedication to dry bronchial and salivary secretions	Hallucinations, ataxia; avoid in glaucoma
Ipratropium	Relieves bronchoconstriction	Dry mouth; avoid high doses in glaucoma

- an increase in force and rate of the heart (β_1)
- an increase in systolic blood pressure due to increased output of blood by the heart (β_1)
- bronchodilation (β_2).

Because adrenalin is non-specific, its use is now restricted mainly to the treatment of anaphylaxis by intramuscular injection.

More selective drugs are now used in the treatment of various conditions in order to reduce side-effects. Examples of the types of drug affecting the autonomic nervous system are listed in Tables 6.3–6.8. Many of the side-effects of these drugs are due to their ability to alter the equilibrium of the autonomic nervous system.

Clinical pharmacology

SECTION CONTENTS

7

Drug treatment of gastrointestinal disorders

ANATOMY AND PHYSIOLOGY OF THE GASTROINTESTINAL TRACT

The gastrointestinal tract (GIT) consists of a long, tubular structure extending from the mouth to the anus via the oesophagus, stomach and intestines. Its purpose is to digest, absorb and eliminate substances following the ingestion of food. The process of digestion is assisted by three accessory organs, namely, the salivary glands, the pancreas and the liver.

Digestion

Food is digested both mechanically and chemically. Mechanical digestion results from voluntary and involuntary muscle action, i.e. nervous control; chemical digestion is produced by the action of enzymes and hormones. The digestive processes taking place in each section of the GIT are summarised in Table 7.1.

Absorption

The absorption of some nutrients begins in the stomach, and some absorption takes place in the large intestine. By far the most absorption, however, occurs in the small intestine (see Fig. 7.1). Table 7.2 summarises some aspects of the absorption of nutrient materials and drugs from the GIT.

Elimination

Undigested and unabsorbed foodstuffs, along with the bile pigment and bilirubin, are elimi-

Table 7.1	Stages of digestion	
Organ	**Mechanical**	**Chemical**
Mouth	Food taken in is masticated (chewed) by the teeth. The muscular action of the tongue and the presence of saliva converts the food into a moist bolus ready for swallowing.	Saliva is produced by the salivary glands under the control of the autonomic nervous system. It consists of water and the enzyme salivary amylase. Salivary amylase converts cooked starches into maltose.
Oesophagus	Bolus is propelled forward first by voluntary muscle action and then under autonomic nerve control.	No chemical action initiated in the oesophagus.
Stomach	The muscular layers produce a churning action and assist peristalsis. The semi-solid mixture produced is known as chyme.	Stimulated by the hormone gastrin, gastric juice is produced by the gastric mucosa. It is composed of: • water, which liquefies food • hydrochloric acid, which acidifies food, kills microorganisms and converts the enzyme pepsinogen secreted by the parietal cells into pepsin, an essential factor in the digestion of protein • intrinsic factor, necessary for absorption of vitamin B_{12} • mucus, which, as a lubricant, protects the stomach wall from the harmful effects of hydrochloric acid and protein-digesting pepsin.

Small intestine	Onward movement of contents by peristalsis and segmental movement.	The hormones secretin and cholecystokinin-pancreozymin (CCK-PZ) stimulate the secretion of pancreatic juice which consists of:
		• water
		• mineral salts
		• enzymes
		    pancreatic amylase, which converts starches not affected by salivary amylase to sugars
		    lipase, which converts fats to fatty acids and glycerol
		    trypsinogen and chymotrypsinogen, which convert polypeptides into amino acids.
		
		Stimulated by CCK-PZ, bile, secreted by the liver but stored in the gall bladder, passes into the duodenum after a meal has been taken. Bile consists of:
		• water
		• mineral salts
		• mucus
		• bile salts
		• bile pigment
		
		Bile is essential for the emulsification of fats and the absorption of vitamin K, and it colours and deodorises the faeces.
		
		Intestinal juice is secreted by glands in the small intestine and consists of:
		• water
		• mucus
		• the enzyme enterokinase

Large intestine	Intermittent waves of peristalsis known as mass movement often precipitated by the gastrocolic reflex following the entry of food into the stomach.	No secretion of enzymes – the last phase of digestion depends on the presence of bacteria in the colon. Bacteria: • ferment foodstuffs in faecal matter, producing gases which form flatus • break down other nutrients and give faeces their distinctive odour • decompose bilirubin, giving faeces their characteristic colour • synthesise vitamins

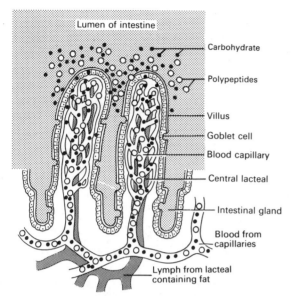

Figure 7.1 Absorption in the small intestine. (From Ross & Wilson 1990 Anatomy and physiology in health and illness, 7th edn. Churchill Livingstone.)

nated as waste from the body via the large intestine in the form of faeces. 'Defaecation' is the term used to describe the expulsion of faeces from the rectum and anal canal. Prior to the act of defaecation, several physiological processes take place; these are shown in Box 7.1.

The act of defaecation is voluntarily assisted by contraction of the diaphragm and the muscles of the abdominal wall. Relaxation of the external anal sphincter finally allows the faeces to be expelled.

COMMON DISORDERS OF THE GASTROINTESTINAL TRACT

The following are some common disorders:

- peptic ulcer disease
- Zollinger-Ellison syndrome
- gastro-oesophageal reflux disease
- inflammatory bowel disease
- constipation.

Peptic ulcer disease

Peptic ulcer disease remains a major cause of morbidity and mortality in spite of the great advances made in both the diagnosis and treatment of this condition. It is more common in men than in women. However, older women (over 74 years) are increasingly likely to suffer fatal consequences of peptic ulcer disease. Appropriate treatment will bring about control of this condition but, like other chronic conditions, a cure cannot be achieved. Unless patients are given maintenance therapy following healing of an ulcer, relapse is very common. The key diagnostic features of peptic ulcer disease are well localised epigastric pain and nocturnal pain. The

Table 7.2 Absorption in the gastrointestinal tract*

Organ	Site of absorption	Substances absorbed
Stomach	Walls of the stomach. Systemic absorption influenced by acid environment and gastric emptying time.	Water. Alcohol. Weak acids, e.g. aspirin, lipid-soluble non-ionised drugs.
Small intestine	The villi and microvilli into the capillaries and lacteals. Largest GI surface area for absorption. Alkaline environment may influence absorption of some substances.	Carbohydrates as monosaccharides. Proteins as amino acids. Fats as fatty acids and glycerol. Vitamins. Mineral salts. Some water (one-tenth only).
Large intestine	Predominantly the caecum and ascending colon.	Water (remaining nine-tenths). Mineral salts, especially sodium. Drugs not absorbed in small intestine may be absorbed to some extent.

*Absorption of drugs from the GIT is very complex and may be affected by a range of factors, including dosage form, pH, gut motility, presence/absence of food and pathology.

Box 7.1   Physiological processes prior to defaecation

Mass movement in pelvic colon
↓
Faecal matter enters rectum
↓
Rectal wall distended
↓
Pressure receptors in wall stimulated
↓
Nerve impulses transmitted to sacral cord
↓
Motor impulses transmitted back from cord via parasympathetic nerves
↓
Rectal muscles contract
↓
Pressure in rectum increases
↓
Reflex relaxation of internal anal sphincter
↓
Desire to defaecate

Table 7.3   Peptic ulceration – a comparison

Gastric ulcers	Duodenal ulcers
Rare in patients under 40	Prevalence highest in patients over 60 but occur in all age groups
Pain relief following food intake short-lived	Pain relieved by food intake Pain generally worse before meals
Anorexia and nausea more prominent than in duodenal ulcers	
Gastric acid secretion may be normal or even below normal	Gastric acid a major factor
Anti-secretory therapy produces healing but more slowly than with duodenal ulcers	Anti-secretory therapy often produces healing in 4 weeks Lesions smaller than in gastric ulcers
Healing can occur without active treatment	Ulcers recur when therapy stopped
Recurrence rate lower than with duodenal ulcers	
Helicobacter pylori infection present in 85% of cases	*Helicobacter pylori* infection present in 100% of cases
Very important to exclude gastric cancer in patients who present with symptoms of gastric ulcer	

pain is often relieved by food and antacids. In some patients the pain may be relieved by vomiting. There are significant differences between gastric and duodenal ulcers; these are summarised in Table 7.3.

Risk factors in peptic ulceration

The risk factors are summarised in Table 7.4.

In healthy people there is a balance between the damaging forces (e.g. acid, smoking, drugs, stress) and the protective and repair mechanisms. When these forces become out of balance, ulcers and erosions can occur.

Treatment of peptic ulcer disease

Various aspects of treatment are as follows:

- General measures — Control of smoking and drinking, and attention to diet (avoiding certain foods that the patient finds exacerbate symptoms).
- Simple antacids — Examples include: aluminium hydroxide mixture magnesium-containing compounds combined antacid preparations magnesium trisilicate mixture or powder

  Antacids can interact with other drugs (see p. 44) and may cause enteric-coated tablets to leak in the stomach. Antacids do often provide rapid relief of symptoms but have limited ulcer-healing properties.
- Combination antacid products — Antacids may be combined with anti-foaming agents (dimethicone) which are claimed to be of value in flatulence. Alginates (derived from certain seaweeds) form a gel-like 'raft' which is claimed to

Table 7.4 Risk factors in peptic ulceration

Acid	This is especially important in duodenal ulcer patients who often have twice as many parietal cells as normal subjects
Mucus	Reduced mucus production may be involved since the protective effect of mucus may be lost
Bacteria	*Helicobacter pylori* is known to be strongly associated with gastritis and peptic ulcer disease; antibacterial therapy designed to eradicate *H. pylori* reduces the risk of duodenal ulcer recurrence
Cigarette smoking	The smoking of cigarettes is a major risk factor; peptic ulcers in smokers heal more slowly and are more likely to recur than those in non-smokers
Drugs	Many NSAIDs (see p. 287) can cause serious gastric damage; the extent to which duodenal ulceration is caused by NSAIDs is still the subject of much debate and research
Stress	Stress has long been associated with peptic ulcer disease
Foods	Some foods have been associated with peptic ulcer disease – there is considerable variation between patients; avoidance of foods that cause problems is advocated
Hereditary factors	There is a proven hereditary component in duodenal ulcers

- **Atropine-like antisecretory agents**

be effective in reflux oesophagitis. Antimuscarinic agents have little antisecretory effects in doses that are practicable due to atropine-like side-effects. The more specific antisecretory drugs, the H_2 receptor antagonists, are the basis of the treatment of peptic ulceration.

- **Histamine H_2 receptor antagonists (see p. 22)**

The introduction of cimetidine and ranitidine has played a major part in improving the treatment of peptic ulcer disease. Cimetidine is given orally in a dose of 400 mg twice daily or as a single dose of 800 mg at night. A 4-week course is given in duodenal ulcer and a 6-week course in gastric ulcer. Once healing has been achieved, a maintenance dose must be given over a long period. Ranitidine is also given orally, 150 mg twice daily or 300 mg at night. The side-effect profile of ranitidine is lower than with cimetidine. The use of both these drugs has greatly reduced the need for surgical treatment of peptic ulcers. Parenteral forms of the drug are available for use in conditions where the oral route is inappropriate, for example, when there is bleeding, for the prevention of stress ulceration in seriously ill patients and prophylactically in patients thought to be at risk from acid aspiration syndrome. Although these two drugs have similar properties there are significant differences (Table 7.5).

- **Selective anti-muscarinic agents**

Pirenzepine is almost free from atropine-like side-effects and is effective in reducing gastric acid secretion. Dosage is 50 mg twice daily, which can be increased to 50 mg three times daily.

- **Chelates and complexes**

Tripotassium dicitratobismuthate (De-Nol) is thought to act by having an antibacterial action on *H. pylori*. Other actions attributed to this compound include the stimulation of the secretion of prostaglandin (a mucosal protective) and/or the stimulation of bicarbonate secretion. The usual dose is $2 \times$ 120 mg tablets twice daily. Sulcralfate (complex of aluminium hydroxide and sulphated sucrose) has only minimal antacid properties but is an effective treatment for both gastric and duodenal ulcer. The mode of action may be to protect mucosa from acid and pepsin attack.

- Prosta-glandin analogues (see also p. 287)

  Misoprostol is a synthetic compound similar to prostaglandin E_1. It acts by inhibiting acid secretion and it promotes the healing of both gastric and duodenal ulcer. It may be given to treat gastric ulceration caused by NSAIDs. Combination products (NSAID and misoprostol) are claimed to be safer than NSAIDs alone for 'at risk' patients.

- Carben-oxolone

  This drug improves the resistance of gastric mucosa to attack from acid. It is now used only rarely (for the treatment of gastric ulcers) since it has aldosterone-like activity which may cause problems in older patients due to oedema and hypokalaemia. Treatment of patients over 65 years of age with this drug is not recommended. The normal dosage range is 100 mg three times daily after meals.

- Proton-pump inhibitors

  Omeprazole (Losec) is a very effective treatment for both gastric and duodenal ulcer. The mode of action is based on the property of blocking the hydrogen–potassium adenosine triphosphate enzyme system (see Fig. 7.2) in the parietal cell. This is also a very effective treatment for Zollinger–Ellison syndrome (see p. 6) and reflux oesosphagitis. An oral dose of 20 mg daily for 4 weeks is often effective but can be increased in refractory cases to 40 mg daily. It should be noted that the degree of acid suppression achieved is directly related to the rate of ulcer healing. Omeprazole 20 mg daily can produce healing within 4 weeks. This rate of healing can be achieved with H_2 antagonists

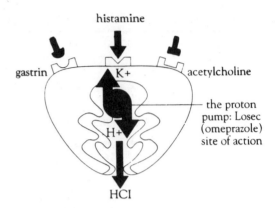

Figure 7.2   Proton pump.

given in higher doses, e.g. ranitidine 300 mg twice daily.

- Triple therapy

  This therapy is designed to eradicate *H. pylori* which will be achieved in 90% of cases. One approach to treatment is to give a 4-week course of an H_2 antagonist followed by a course of triple therapy to eradicate the bacteria and reduce the likelihood of relapse. Triple therapy is generally a 2-week course as follows: bismuth chelate 120 mg four times daily, metronidazole 400 mg three times daily, oxytetracycline 500 mg four times daily. If oxytetracycline is contraindicated (e.g. in renal impairment), amoxycillin 500 mg three times daily can be substituted. Careful monitoring of this therapy is essential. Resistance of *H. pylori* to metronidazole may occur and the therapy may cause serious gastrointestinal disturbances.

- Compli-cations of peptic ulceration

  Bleeding is a serious complication of peptic ulceration. As an uncontrolled ulcer develops, a blood vessel at the base of the ulcer is penetrated resulting in serious

Table 7.5   Similarities of, and differences between, cimetidine and ranitidine

	Cimetidine	Ranitidine
Mode of action	Selective histamine-H_2 receptor antagonists	As cimetidine
Indications	Peptic ulcer disease; Zollinger–Ellison syndrome	As cimetidine
Oral dose	400 mg twice daily	150 mg twice daily
Maintenance dose	400 mg at night	150 mg at night
Availability	Tablets, syrup; parenteral	As cimetidine – also granules
Contraindications and warnings	Dose reduced in patients with impaired renal function	As cimetidine
	Prolongs elimination of drugs metabolised by oxidation in the liver	Some changes (transient) have been reported in liver function
	May mask symptoms of gastric carcinoma	As cimetidine
	Some drug interactions, especially with oral anticoagulants and phenytoin (dosage reduction of these drugs may be needed)	Few drug interactions have been reported
	Rare reports of bradycardia and AV block	As cimetidine
	H_2 receptor antagonism may potentiate falls in blood cell counts caused by other factors, e.g. disease or other drug treatment	Leucopenia and thrombocytopenia have been rarely reported
	Gynaecomastia has been reported but is reversible on stopping treatment	Few reports with ranitidine

blood loss. Up to 20% of patients may suffer a bleeding episode and may experience haematemesis and/or melaena. The loss of blood may cause cardiovascular shock which must be treated urgently. Blood transfusion and resuscitative measures will be needed together with the combined skills of both physician and surgeon.

Role of the nurse in peptic ulcer disease

In view of the nature of the condition it is essential to ensure that patients comply with treatment regimes. Patient compliance can be improved by explaining to the patient the nature of his condition and the need to take the medication regularly over a period of time. The tendency some patients have to discontinue therapy once the symptoms ease must be recognised and appropriate action taken, otherwise a serious relapse may occur.

Many patients who present with peptic ulcer disease are elderly and may have co-existing diseases such as diabetes or cardiovascular problems. Nurses, as well as providing care, can encourage patients to adopt a more healthy lifestyle such as improved dietary intake, cessation of smoking and avoidance of stress. Patients with peptic ulcer disease may adjust doses of H_2 antagonists to control their symptoms. Some degree of freedom to adjust dosage may be an acceptable part of the patient's care. However, community nurses should be alert for any tendencies the patient may have to increase the dose prior to a planned episode of over-indulgence.

Zollinger–Ellison (ZE) syndrome

This condition is characterised by severe and often intractable ulceration caused by very high levels of acid secretion. The high levels of acid result from the continuous stimulation of the parietal cells by the hormone gastrin. Abnormal amounts of gastrin are produced by a gastrinoma (tumour) often situated in the pancreas. In two-thirds of cases the tumour is malignant.

Treatment of the ZE syndrome

Treatment of this condition is a matter for the specialist. H_2 receptor antagonists are used, as is omeprazole. Doses are higher than those used in the treatment of gastric or duodenal ulcer.

- Drug treatment of ZE syndrome
  Omeprazole 60 mg once daily initially, increasing up to 120 mg daily in divided doses, *or*
  Cimetidine 400 mg four times daily, *or*
  Ranitidine 150 mg three times daily, increasing to doses of up to 6 g daily.
- Surgical treatment
  Surgical treatment and/or cytotoxic therapy may be valuable if the growth of secondaries is not advanced.

Gastro-oesophageal reflux disease (GORD) (heartburn)

Patients presenting with GORD complain of a 'burning sensation' which is often accompanied by severe pains in the chest which may be difficult to distinguish from cardiac pain. Many patients admitted to hospital for suspected myocardial infarction are found to be suffering from GORD. In other patients the diagnosis creates no difficulty, especially where symptoms occur after a meal. Peptic ulcer disease may co-exist with GORD (as may cardiac disease) and it is also important to eliminate gastric neoplasm as a factor. Full diagnostic measures are used to establish the true nature of the patient's condition. Barium meal, endoscopic examinations and oesophageal pH monitoring are cornerstones of differential diagnosis together with a full history of the patient.

Treatment of GORD

The patient's dietary habits must be attended to. Weight loss, smoking cessation and reduction in alcohol intake are also vitally important. The head of the patient's bed should be raised by 20 cm.

Since the pain of GORD is caused by refluxing of gastric contents onto very sensitive oeso-phageal mucosa, it follows that antacids are the first-line agents. Combinations of antacids with alginates are very useful. If reflux does occur the stomach contents have been 'neutralised' to some extent and therefore are less likely to cause irritation. If simple antacid therapy does not provide relief, H_2 antagonists or omeprazole should be considered. Omeprazole is more effective than H_2 antagonists and is effective in a high proportion of patients, even where resistance to H_2 antagonists has occurred.

Metoclopramide may be useful since this drug improves gastric emptying and tightens the gastro-oesophageal junction. Cisapride increases lower oesophageal sphincter pressure and improves oesophageal motor activity. Cisapride has been shown to reduce the duration of reflux episodes. The dose is 10 mg three times daily and 10 mg at night. The mechanism of action of cisapride is thought to be based on enhancing the release of acetylcholine (see p. 48) from the myenteric plexus.

If medical treatment fails (this is rare), consideration has to be given to surgical intervention.

Inflammatory bowel disease (IBD)

The most common presenting symptom of IBD is chronic diarrhoea. However, it is important to recognise that diarrhoea may be due to one of a number of causes. Infection often presents as a sudden episode of diarrhoea but more sinister causes of diarrhoea are IBD or neoplastic disease. Differential diagnosis is vitally important so as to ensure that the treatment instigated does not mask the underlying condition. The two main conditions are Crohn's disease (CD) and ulcerative colitis (UC). These conditions have similar features and yet are distinctly separate diseases (Table 7.6.).

Diagnosis of Crohn's disease and ulcerative colitis

Differential diagnosis relies on clinical examination supported by histological examination. Differentiation can be very difficult as both condi-

Table 7.6   A comparison of the main features of Crohn's disease and ulcerative colitis

Crohn's disease (also known as ulcerative enteritis)	Ulcerative colitis
Can affect any part of the gastrointestinal tract from mouth to anus	Primarily involves large bowel
Most common sites are terminal ileum and ascending colon	
Rectum affected in approximately 50% of patients	Most patients have rectal involvement
Inflammatory process involves all layers of bowel	Inflammatory process mainly confined to mucosa
Presence of multiple granulomas	Multiple granulomas not seen
Clinical symptoms: bloody diarrhoea; anorexia; abdominal pain; fever; weight loss due to malabsorption	Clinical symptoms: similar to Crohn's disease but bloody diarrhoea less common; abdominal pain and fever more prominent; signs of malabsorption not seen
Neoplastic changes may be seen in cases of extensive disease	

tions can be mimicked by enteric infections and pseudomembranous colitis.

Drug treatment

Although the causes of IBD are not yet known, knowledge of the factors involved is increasing. Various theories have been put forward, including infection, diet and immunological causes. The fact that corticosteroids and immunosuppressants are beneficial in the treatment of IBD lends support to the theory that these diseases are due to an immunological disorder. An infection may be the 'trigger' for the immunological changes that occur in IBD. The pathogenesis of these conditions may be multifactorial with infection, genetic influences, diet and environmental agents combining in ways which are not fully understood. Prostaglandins (see p. 287) have been shown in animal studies to act with other agents such as histamine to alter lymphocyte function and increase vascular permeability. The treatments available do ameliorate the symptoms of IBD which can be very distressing and debilitating. Table 7.7 gives an outline of the main drugs used in the treatment of both main forms of IBD. In addition to drug treatment, attention must be given to diet, although direct links between diet and IBD are not clear. Foods that have a high residue content are best avoided.

Constipation

Constipation arises from decreased colonic activity. Bowel contents pass slowly through the colon, becoming dehydrated and hard with loss of faecal volume. Decreased colonic activity can arise in old age and with immobility, and is often associated with a low dietary fibre intake and dehydration.

In considering the causes of constipation, a detailed drug history should be taken. Drugs with anticholinergic activity (see p. 50) are especially liable to cause constipation. Constipation is often present in patients suffering from depression and confusional states. Certain metabolic disorders, such as hypercalcaemia and myxoedema, may also cause constipation. Constipation may occur when the call to stool is neglected. This has the effect of decreasing the sensitivity of rectal sensors. If the patient is too ill to respond to the call to stool or for some other reason is unable to respond, such as pressure of duties, the stimulus is gradually lost and the rectum becomes overloaded with faecal material.

All patients complaining of constipation should be carefully investigated so as to eliminate a more serious condition. Pain (arising from a malignant condition) on bowel evacuation may result in constipation. Whenever possible, constipation should be treated by attention to diet and exercise, and the encouragement of a healthy lifestyle. For example, the simple step of adding bran to food may be all that is required. If drug treatment is required a wide range of products is available.

Despite the 'homely' image of laxatives, it must not be forgotten that these are drugs with potentially serious adverse effects. Overuse of laxatives can cause hypokalaemia and an atonic

Table 7.7 Treatment of IBD		
Drug	**Dose**	**Notes**
ANTIDIARRHOEAL AGENTS ■ **Codeine phosphate** ■ **Loperamide**	15–30 mg three or four times daily 4 mg initially, then 2 mg after each loose stool with a maximum of 16 mg daily for 5 days	Reduce gastrointestinal motility; antidiarrhoeal agents should not be used in patients with acute ulcerative colitis
TETRACOSACTRIN ACETATE (ACTH)	1 mg intramuscularly daily or 1 mg every 12 hours in acute cases	Useful in patients who have not been receiving corticosteroids prior to admission and in patients who do not respond to normal doses of oral corticosteroids
CORTICOSTEROIDS ■ **PREDNISOLONE**	Variable dose depending on the condition; 10 mg three or four times daily is a typical dose given for 2–3 weeks. Above this level, side-effects may be troublesome	Small-bowel diarrhoea reduced by oral corticosteroids. Beneficial action thought to be due to anti-inflammatory and immunosuppressive action. Corticosteroids are especially useful in the acute phase of IBD
ANTIMICROBIAL AGENTS ■ **Metronidazole** ■ **Tetracycline** ■ **Cyclosporin**	Doses given in relation to body weight and carefully monitored by blood level determinations	Bacterial overgrowth in small bowel due to active Crohn's disease may cause diarrhoea which is amenable to treatment with antimicrobial agents in normal doses Potent immunosuppressive drug (see p. 264). Place in treatment of refractory Crohn's disease remains to be further investigated
IMMUNOSUPPRESSIVE THERAPY ■ **Azathiaprine**	3 mg/kg body weight per day reducing to smaller maintenance dose according to response	Not first-line therapy but reserved for patients who are intolerant of or who do not respond to corticosteroids. Used to reduce corticosteroid dosage levels in patients with ulcerative colitis. Has been reported to induce remission in patients with Crohn's disease. Adverse effects limit its use (see p. 264)
SALICYLATES ■ **Sulphasalazine**	1–2 g four times daily in acute attack. Maintenance dose of 500 mg four times daily. Corticosteroids may be needed in the acute phase	Used for the treatment of active Crohn's disease and is the first-line agent of choice for maintenance therapy in ulcerative colitis. Combination of a salicylate and a sulphonamide. Salicylate part of compound has desired therapeutic effect; sulphonamide part associated with side-effects. An enteric-coated tablet may be useful for patients who are intolerant of the uncoated tablet. Topical sulphasalazine also available in the form of suppositories or retention enema. Drug colours the urine yellow and patients should be warned about this
■ **Mesalazine** **(5-aminosalicylic acid)**	For acute ulcerative colitis 800 mg (two tablets) three times daily with corticosteroid therapy where necessary. Maintenance dose should be lowest that will maintain remission. 400 mg three times daily up to 800 mg three times daily may be required	Sulphasalazine is metabolised to sulphapyridine and 5-aminosalicylic acid, and it is thought that sulphapyridine component is the major cause of side-effects. Mesalazine is the active component of sulphasalazine. Presented for use as a tablet coated with special resin designed to release active ingredient in the terminal ileum and colon. Suppositories of 250 mg and 500 mg also available for use in patients with distal disease. The drug should not be given to patients with renal impairment; large doses have been shown to cause renal damage in experimental animals. Should not

Table 7.7 Cont'd		
Drug	**Dose**	**Notes**
		be given to patients with salicylate intolerance. Anti-inflammatory effect not achieved if intestinal transit time rapid due to diarrhoea
■ Olsalazine	For acute mild ulcerative colitis 1 g daily in divided doses up to maximum of 3 g daily over 1 week. 250 mg twice daily will often maintain patient in remission	Compound which is combination of two molecules of 5-aminosalicylic acid (5-ASA). Specifically designed to reach the colon where the compound breaks down to release 5-ASA. Almost no systemic absorption of 5-ASA; therefore available to act topically on colonic mucosa. Side-effects reported similar to other salicylates; gastrointestinal problems such as watery diarrhoea may occur

non-functioning colon. Inappropriate use of laxatives in situations where the diagnosis of the cause of the constipation is inadequate can be very dangerous. Local prescribing protocols may permit the prescription of laxatives by nurses. This is to be welcomed, but situations where nurses are allowed to prescribe laxatives must be well documented and agreed by all parties. Nurses have an important role to play in advising patients about their use of laxatives. Laxatives should be used only where other measures have failed. These would include attention to the amount of dietary fibre (whole wheat cereals, wholemeal bread and whole fruit), fluid intake and exercise. Attention to details such as the provision of warmth and privacy when attending to toileting needs and exploiting the gastrocolic reflex after breakfast can greatly assist the constipated patient. Where laxatives are indicated, patients should be encouraged to continue with these simple measures and to take only the recommended dose. Despite the best endeavours of nurses and pharmacists to limit the use of laxatives, a visit to a drug cupboard in a long-stay ward (or patient's medicine cabinet at home) will often show how ineffective these efforts have been. There are, of course, very important indications for the use of laxatives on a routine basis, especially in patients receiving opioids for palliative care. The main laxative drugs are listed in Table 7.8.

Treatment of haemorrhoids and other perianal conditions

Painful, itching and bleeding conditions of the perianal region are common. Usually the lesions are benign and may often be amenable to treatment by topical application of soothing, emollient, anti-inflammatory and anaesthetic agents, alone or in combination. The most common perianal condition is haemorrhoids. The condition may present in a variety of ways ranging from superficial bleeding to permanently prolapsed haemorrhoids. The causes of haemorrhoids are not fully understood but the condition is associated with congestion of the superior haemorrhoidal venous plexus. Surgical treatment or local injection with a sclerosing agent (oily phenol injection) may be required. Considerable relief can be obtained by the use of rectal ointments designed to relieve itching and pain. Application of the ointment is aided by using a rectal nozzle. In some cases a suppository with similar active ingredients to the ointments may be used. Some active ingredients of rectal ointments are listed in Table 7.9.

DRUG TREATMENT OF HEPATIC DISORDERS
Anatomy of the liver

The liver can be considered as the 'chemical factory' of the body. It is the largest organ in the

Table 7.8 Main laxative drugs

Drug	Dose	Notes
BULK-FORMING AGENTS **Ispaghula husk**	3.5 g twice daily with water	Important to ensure patient has good fluid intake to avoid intestinal obstruction. For ease of use can be made into a jelly
Methylcellulose	Available as 500 mg tablet. 3–6 tablets daily with 300 ml of water	Good fluid intake essential. Bulk-forming agents should be carefully swallowed with water and should not be taken immediately before going to bed
STIMULANTS **Bisacodyl**	5–10 mg orally at night. Also available as suppository	Like other stimulant laxatives, can cause local irritation and griping pain
Danthron	Available as co-danthramer (i.e. danthron 25 mg with poloxamer 200 mg in 5 ml). Normal dose 5–10 ml	Because of possible carcinogenic effects, reserved for use in older patients. Especially valuable where essential that bowel movements are not accompanied by straining. Also widely used in patients receiving opioids in palliative care
Docusate sodium	Orally up to 500 mg daily in divided doses	
Glycerol (glycerin)	Given in suppository form	Mild irritant
Senna	2–4 tablets, each containing 7.5 mg sennosides at night	Also used prior to radiological examination, endoscopy and surgery
Sodium picosulphate	Available as elixir containing 5 mg/5 ml. Dose: 5–15 ml at night	Similar indications to senna
FAECAL SOFTENERS **Arachis oil**	130 ml given as retention enema	Warmed before use. Used to soften impacted faeces. As with all enemas, should be used with caution in patients with intestinal obstruction
OSMOTIC LAXATIVES **Lactulose (a disaccharide)**	Available as an elixir containing 3.35 g in 5 ml. Initial dose 15 ml twice daily reducing when patient's condition warrants	Lactulose passes through the small intestine unchanged. It is broken down in the colon by bacteria to substances (acetic and lactic acids) which exert their osmotic effect in the gut lumen. May cause cramps and flatulence
MAGNESIUM SALTS **Magnesium sulphate**	5–10 g in water	Produces rapid bowel clearance (2–4 hours). Other magnesium salts also used, e.g. magnesium citrate and magnesium hydroxide
PHOSPHATES	Sodium acid phosphate 12.8 g and sodium phosphate 10.24 g in the form of an enema (128 ml)	Contraindicated in patients with ulcerative or inflammatory bowel conditions. Local irritation may occur, and sodium absorption can cause problems in patients who have a low sodium requirement
SODIUM CITRATE	Given in form of a microenema together with a surfactant	Small volume (5 ml) of these enemas makes for ease of use

Table 7.8 *Cont'd*

Drug	Dose	Notes
LUBRICANTS **Liquid paraffin**	The dose is variable, 10–30 ml being the usual range. Also available as an emulsion or in combination with magnesium hydroxide. Combinations of liquid paraffin emulsion and phenolphthalein are not advised as the phenolphthalein is recycled via the liver and as a result has a prolonged action	The long-term use of this may interfere with the absorption of fat-soluble vitamins (A, D and K). Lipid-aspiration pneumonia has been reported (inhalation of liquid paraffin following vomiting). Leakage of the oil from the anus often occurs. There is some evidence that the long-term use of liquid paraffin may cause cancer of the large bowel. Liquid paraffin is subject to an MCA warning in the BNF

body, weighing up to 2.3 kg (range 1–2.3 kg). The liver has four lobes situated in the upper part of the abdominal cavity in the right hypochondriac region (see Fig. 7.3). The most obvious lobes are the right and left lobes. Closely associated with the liver are the organs of the gastro-intestinal tract, large blood vessels and the gall bladder (see Fig. 7.4).

At the microscopic level hepatocytes make up the lobules, which are just visible to the naked eye.

Table 7.9 Active ingredients of rectal ointments and suppositories (often used in combination)

Ingredient	Normal strength in ointment	Action/notes
Allantoin	0.5%	Healing agent
Betamethasone*	0.05%	Anti-inflammatory
Bismuth compounds	various	Mild astringent
Cinchocaine	0.5%	Local anaesthetic
Hydrocortisone*	0.5%	Anti-inflammatory
Lignocaine	0.5%	Local anaesthetic; as with other anaesthetics, may be absorbed to produce toxic effects
Phenylephrine	0.1%	Vasoconstrictor
Prednisolone hexanoate*	0.19%	Anti-inflammatory
Zinc oxide	range 10–18%	Mild astringent

*All corticosteroid topical preparations should be used for limited periods to avoid absorption and possible side-effects (see p. 312).
A typical formulation for a rectal ointment is: betamethasone 0.05%, lignocaine 2.5%, and phenylephrine 0.1%; the base is usually of soft paraffin, which has a lubricant effect.

Physiology of the liver

The liver carries out a great range of chemical functions which are essential to health. These functions are summarised in Table 7.10.

Liver diseases disrupt the functions of the liver, which may have profound consequences for the patient.

Hepatic disease

The main diseases of the liver are potentially life-threatening but unfortunately some are not very amenable to drug treatment. Drug treatment in

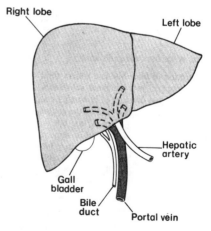

Figure 7.3 The liver. (From Chandler 1991 Tabbner's nursing care: theory and practice, 2nd edn. Churchill Livingstone.)

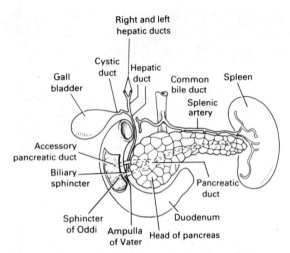

Figure 7.4 Associated organs. (From Chandler 1991 Tabbner's nursing care: theory and practice, 2nd edn. Churchill Livingstone.)

Table 7.10 Functions of the liver

Main function	Outline of functions
Amino acid metabolism	Breakdown of certain amino acids to form urea; formation of uric acid from nucleoprotein
Bile production	Bile salts, pigments and cholesterol produced in liver cells
Carbohydrate metabolism	Glucose is converted to glycogen (after a meal), and glycogen is broken down to glucose to meet energy requirements (see also Ch. 12)
Detoxification processes	Drugs and other noxious substances (e.g. toxins produced by microorganisms); also metabolises ethyl alcohol taken in alcoholic drinks (see p. 69)
Fat metabolism	Fat is converted into a form which can be used by the body as an energy source
Heat production	Since a great number of chemical processes are carried out in the liver, heat is produced, which is the main source of body heat
Inactivation	A wide range of hormones is inactivated, e.g. insulin, thyroid hormones, sex hormones and aldosterone
Storage functions	Vitamins, both fat- and water-soluble, iron and copper; glucose in the form of glycogen
Synthesis	Vitamin A, non-essential amino acids and blood-clotting factors

combination with general supportive measures, and alteration to diet, can help to ameliorate symptoms.

Hepatitis

Hepatitis may be caused by one of a number of viruses or by a toxic chemical, very often a drug. In both virus- and drug-induced hepatitis there is extensive cell damage throughout the liver, although there may be variation in the extent of the damage in different lobes of the liver.

Hepatitis due to the hepatitis A virus is generally not life-threatening, although the infection has a significant mortality level in patients over 60 years.

Hepatitis due to the B virus is a much more serious condition. In both forms of infection the symptoms are similar, although much more severe in the B form of the disease. Symptoms include chills, headache, general malaise, gastrointestinal disturbances and anorexia. Abdominal pain and dark urine will be followed by jaundice. Liver enlargement occurs, and the liver is often tender. The course of the A infection generally lasts 3–6 weeks. In view of the seriousness of hepatitis B, special attention must be given to protecting people at particular risk. Health workers should be protected by vaccination, and great care must be taken with all procedures involved in taking blood and other invasive techniques. Safe disposal of contaminated equipment is essential.

Treatment of hepatitis (acute)

Care must be taken to determine the cause of the condition. It is particularly important to exclude drugs as a cause. If a drug is implicated (see p. 34) the treatment should be stopped and further exposure to the drug avoided. Exposure to toxic chemicals in the workplace must also be considered as a possible cause. Key elements of the treatment of hepatitis are dietary measures and bed rest. It is important to maintain a high-calorie diet, although the patient's gastrointestinal problems may restrict the range of foods he is able to tolerate. Bed rest is very important so as to avoid exhaustion to which the patient may be especially prone. Fluid and electrolyte therapy should be given in the acute phase of the condition. Corticosteroids may be of value for their appetite-stimulating properties. However, the side-effects of corticosteroids are so hazardous that their use should be minimised. All drugs with a potential to cause liver damage must be avoided, as must alcohol, a well-recognised liver toxin. Corticosteroids are useful in the form of chronic hepatitis that is not due to viral infection. Interferon has also been used in chronic hepatitis B infection.

Hepatic failure

This is a very serious condition for which no specific treatment is available. Since the liver performs so many vital functions it follows that liver failure has very serious consequences. The usual cause of fulminant hepatic failure is an acute viral infection but it may be caused by drugs, pregnancy or Wilson's disease.

The symptoms of hepatic failure include cerebral disturbance. The cause of encephalopathy arises from the accumulation of toxic substances in the blood which arise because the damaged liver cannot metabolise the range of chemical substances a healthy liver can cope with. A wide range of neurological symptoms are seen, including restlessness, behavioural abnormalities, mania, drowsiness and coma. Jaundice develops and physical signs are abnormal. Mortality is age-related. Profound biochemical disturbances are common during the course of the illness, e.g. electrolyte disturbances, alkalosis and coagulation disorders.

Treatment plans include general supportive measures together with measures designed to sustain the patient in the hope that the hepatic tissue will regenerate. Nutritional needs should be met with glucose orally or parenterally. Nitrogen-producing bacteria in the colon should be suppressed with a suitable antibiotic, e.g. neomycin orally. Neomycin is a non-absorbable antibiotic but small amounts may be absorbed over time to produce potentially dangerous side-effects. Infection and electrolyte disturbances

must be treated, and, if renal failure occurs, haemodialysis and other measures may be required. The physical and biochemical parameters must be monitored and corrective measures taken. Disorders of blood coagulation may lead to bleeding from the gastrointestinal tract. Ranitidine by intravenous injection may be required to control this. Lactulose (orally) is used to acidify the colonic contents so as to reduce the level of nitrogen-producing bacteria.

Cirrhosis of the liver

Cirrhosis is caused by alcohol abuse, chronic hepatitis or biliary cirrhosis. Alcohol has a direct toxic effect on the liver. A daily substantial intake over a number of years will result in cirrhosis. Women are at greater risk than men from a prolonged and regular intake of alcohol. Other causes of cirrhosis include certain metabolic disorders, viral infections and drugs. Obstruction in the biliary network may also cause cirrhosis. Cirrhosis of the liver has a number of clinical features. The presentation of the condition varies, but often includes portal hypertension, blood disorders, ascites, circulatory changes and jaundice. Treatment of hepatic cirrhosis is based on attempting to halt the progression of the condition since there is no treatment that can reverse cirrhosis.

Substance abuse (alcohol and/or drugs) must be dealt with by complete abstinence. A high-calorie diet is advisable, together with bed rest. Fluid and sodium intake must be restricted. Diuretics should be used with care, in conjunction with monitoring of electrolytes and blood urea.

A common complication of hepatic cirrhosis is bleeding from oesophageal varices. These are caused by portal hypertension. Various techniques are used to deal with this condition. Pressure can be applied to the varices by special tubes with inflatable 'cuffs', or surgical treatment can be used. Any treatment designed to arrest bleeding by constriction of the splanchnic arterioles may be useful. Vasopressin is given by intravenous infusion in a dose of 20 units over a period of 15 minutes.

Blood transfusions may be required to correct losses from recurrent bleeds. The possibility of injecting the varices with a sclerosing agent may be worth considering.

Tumours of the liver

The treatment of malignant disease of the liver is discussed on p. 246.

BILIARY TRACT DISEASE

Gallstones are frequently asymptomatic, but gallstones can cause a variety of symptoms including biliary colic or cholecystitis. Most gallstones are made up of cholesterol, although some gallstones contain a high proportion of calcium in the form of salts of bilirubin. The reasons for the formation of gallstones are not fully understood.

Treatment is by surgical removal or, in the case of small stones, by the administration of cheno-deoxycholic acid or ursodeoxycholic acid. These drugs have no effect on large radiopaque stones. Ultrasound has been used as a non-invasive method of breaking up gallstones.

FURTHER READING

Betts A 1993 Peptic ulceration. Practice Nursing September/October: 20–21
Brian H, Ferguson A 1993 Inflammatory bowel disease. Practice Nursing June/July: 11–12
Murrell A 1993 Unlocking the virus. Providing support and treatment for people with hepatitis. Professional Nurse 8(12): 780–783

Ronayne C 1993 The use of aqueous cream to relieve pruritus in patients with liver disease. British Journal of Nursing 2(10): 527–531
Shafik A 1993 Constipation. Pathogenesis and management. Drugs 45(4): 528–540

8

Drug treatment of cardiovascular disorders

ANATOMY AND PHYSIOLOGY OF THE CARDIOVASCULAR SYSTEM

The heart

The heart lies between the lungs, behind the lower sternum, in front of the oesophagus and above the diaphragm, on which it rests. It is roughly conical in shape with a base and an apex. It consists of four chambers: the right and left atria above, and the right and left ventricles below. The atria and ventricles are separated by, on the right side, the tricuspid valve and, on the left side, the mitral valve. The walls of the heart have three layers – outermost, a fibrous envelope called the pericardium, in the middle, a thick muscle known as the myocardium, and the innnermost layer, a smooth lining called the endocardium (Fig. 8.1).

Venous blood returns from various parts of the body to the heart. It enters the right atrium via the superior and inferior venae cavae and passes through the tricuspid valve to the right ventricle. The right ventricle pumps the blood to the lungs, via the pulmonary artery. In the lungs the blood is oxygenated and carbon dioxide is removed. The blood then returns via the four pulmonary veins into the left atrium from where it passes through the mitral valve into the left ventricle. The left ventricle pumps the oxygenated blood through the aortic valve into the aorta and out into the body.

The heart derives its own blood supply from the two main coronary arteries which originate from the aorta just above the aortic valve.

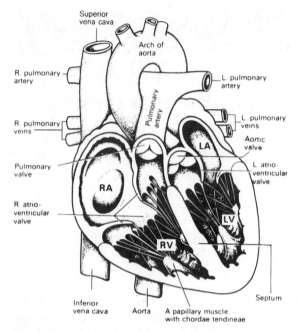

Figure 8.1 The heart. (From Ross & Wilson 1990 Anatomy and physiology in health and illness, 7th edn. Churchill Livingstone.)

The activity of the heart is rhythmical, consisting of contraction ('systole') and relaxation ('diastole'). The impulse to contract is generated by a clump of specialised tissue situated at the junction of the superior vena cava and the right atrium, known as the sinoatrial (SA) node. The wave of excitation spreads throughout the muscle layer of both atria causing them to contract, forcing blood into the ventricles. The impulse is picked up by another collection of specialised cells called the atrioventricular (AV) node situated in the septal walls of the right atrium. It is relayed by the fibres of Purkinje down the bundle of His and along the right and left branches causing the ventricles to contract and drive blood into the pulmonary artery and the aorta. The heart then relaxes, refills with venous blood, and awaits the next stimulus for contraction. Although the heart initiates its own impulse to contract, the fine adjustments to its activity needed to meet the body's constantly changing needs derive from the autonomic nervous system. Sympathetic nerves increase the heart rate and parasympathetic nerves slow the heart rate.

The SA node is normally the pacemaker for the heart because of its rapid firing rate of 60–100 electrical discharges per minute. Although the specialised cells at the AV node and at the bundle of His are also capable of spontaneously producing an electrical discharge and taking over control of the rhythm, they are normally required to do so only if the SA node fails or becomes unduly slow. The cells of the AV node emit discharges at 50 per minute and those of the ventricles at 40 or less per minute.

Every time the heart beats, approximately 70 ml of blood is pumped out of each ventricle. The heart rate is normally 70 beats per minute. These two figures multiplied together are termed the cardiac output.

The blood vessels

The blood is transported round the body via the blood vessels which comprise arteries and arterioles, veins and venules, and capillaries. As a rule, arteries convey oxygenated blood and veins convey deoxygenated blood which has a high percentage of carbon dioxide. Arteries convey blood away from the heart; veins transport blood back to the heart. Capillaries are tiny blood vessels in the periphery of the arteriovenous system. It is through the capillary walls that oxygen and nutrients pass to the tissues and cells, and waste products return from the cells into the circulation.

Like the heart, the walls of the blood vessels consist of three layers – the fibrous outer tunica adventitia, the middle muscular layer, the tunica media, and the smooth lining of the tunica intima. The outer coat of an artery allows it to stand open, whereas a vein collapses when it is cut. The proportion of muscle tissue depends on the size of the vessel, with much more in arteries than in veins. Some veins have valves which allow the blood to flow back to the heart but prevent flow in the opposite direction. The walls of the capillaries are only one cell thick; this readily facilitates gaseous and nutrient exchange.

Blood pressure

Blood pressure may be defined as the force exerted on the walls of the blood vessels. Arterial blood pressure is the pressure exerted when the heart pumps blood into the already full aorta. The factors determining the blood pressure are:

- cardiac output
- blood volume
- peripheral resistance
- viscosity of the blood
- venous return.

Blood pressure is maintained by sensory receptors found in several of the arteries close to the heart. These baroreceptors convey information to the vasomotor centre in the medulla of the brain in response to changes in the blood pressure. The vasomotor centre in turn transmits impulses via the sympathetic nervous system to the smooth muscle in the walls of the arterioles which are stimulated to contract. The chemical transmitter between neurone and muscle is noradrenalin. The arterioles are kept in a state of partial vasoconstriction by the vasomotor centre. If the vasomotor activity increases, the blood vessels will constrict and the blood pressure will rise; and vice versa.

COMMON DISORDERS OF THE HEART

The disorders of the heart most frequently encountered by nurses are:

- cardiac failure
  left ventricular failure
  biventricular failure
  right ventricular failure
- ischaemic heart disease
  angina pectoris
  myocardial infarction
- disorders of conduction
  atrial fibrillation
  ventricular fibrillation
  heart block
- infective endocarditis

Cardiac failure (heart failure)

The volume of blood passing through the heart per minute is known as the cardiac output. This output varies considerably depending on the needs of the body, being low at rest and rising with exercise. The healthy heart has a great functional reserve and can cope with the demands for increased output which occur from time to time. In cardiac failure the cardiac output is reduced. At first this may be apparent only on exercise, but as the condition progresses it may be insufficient for the needs of the body even at rest. As a result, the tissues and organs receive an inadequate blood supply and therefore insufficient oxygen and nutrients.

Drug therapy can control the symptoms of cardiac failure, but the natural course of the condition is often one of progressive deterioration. Cardiac failure is common, affecting 1–2% of the population, and is becoming more prevalent as elderly people form a larger part of the population.

Types and causes of heart failure

Heart failure is not a diagnosis in itself, rather a 'state' that patients can move in and out of. For example, in otherwise healthy people a profound anaemia, hyperthyroidism or an overwhelming infection may precipitate heart failure. As these conditions are treated, so the failure will improve. For many patients, however, heart failure exists to a greater or lesser extent as the result of a specific condition and this will dictate which part of the heart's pumping mechanism is failing and therefore which features present. Table 8.1 summarises the types of heart failure, what causes them to develop, and the resulting clinical features.

Ischaemic heart disease

Ischaemia arises when the normally smooth endothelial surface of one or more of the coronary arteries becomes roughened. Narrowing occurs as a result of fatty deposits (atheroma) which partly occlude the artery. The resulting

Table 8.1   Types of heart failure

Causes	Clinical features

Left heart failure
Hypertension
Aortic valve disease
Coronary artery disease
	Those associated with increased venous pressure:
	  dyspnoea (in acute pulmonary oedema, the patient will also be acutely anxious, sweating, pale and very ill-looking)
	
	  cough (this may or may not be accompanied by sputum; sputum is generally copious, frothy and tinged with blood)
	
	  cyanosis
	
	Those associated with low cardiac output and poor peripheral perfusion:
	  tiredness
	
	  weakness

Right heart failure
Chronic lung disease (e.g. chronic bronchitis)
Pulmonary valve disease
Congenital defects
	These are predominately the result of increased venous pressure:
	  raised jugular venous pressure
	
	  hepatomegaly, jaundice
	
	  anorexia, nausea, vomiting
	
	  constipation
	
	  peripheral oedema

Biventricular failure (congestive cardiac failure)
(Fig. 8.2)
Left heart failure
	Those associated with left heart failure:
	  dyspnoea
	
	  cough
	
	  cyanosis
	
	Those associated with increased venous pressure:
	  raised jugular venous pressure
	
	  hepatomegaly, jaundice
	
	  constipation
	
	  peripheral oedema
	
	Those associated with insufficient cardiac output:
	  mental confusion, Cheyne–Stokes respirations
	
	  oliguria, proteinuria
	
	  fatigue

reduction in blood flow leads to a reduction of oxygenated blood supply to the myocardium.

Angina pectoris

Angina pectoris is the clinical sign of transient myocardial ischaemia. It occurs when the metabolic demands of the heart for oxygen exceed the ability of diseased coronary arteries to supply adequate blood flow to the myocardium (physical exercise, anaemia). Angina is one of the principal symptoms of coronary heart disease. It is characterised by tightness of the chest which may or may not radiate to the jaw, down one or both arms or through into the back. The pain tends to occur during exertion and is of an alarming nature.

Chronic stable angina is by far the commonest form, and is characterised by brief (10 minute) episodes of pain closely related to precipitants which increase cardiac output, such as exertion, emotion and, less commonly, heavy meals. The treatments used have little or no effect on the

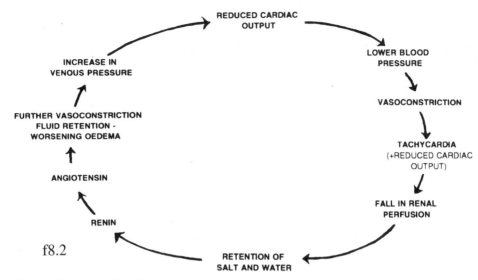

f8.2

Figure 8.2 Cycle of heart failure.

obstructed coronary artery itself but prevent angina by reducing or limiting the work of the heart. As its name suggests, this form of angina often follows a stable pattern for many years but may be complicated by myocardial infarction, unstable angina or sudden death.

Unstable angina presents as a worsening pattern of pre-existing angina, or with episodes of pain which are prolonged (30 minutes or longer) or which occur spontaneously. It is caused by a non-occlusive thrombus forming on an atherosclerotic plaque which has developed a fissure or had a haemorrhage into its substance. Unstable angina is a threatening condition because it confers a high risk of myocardial infarction or sudden death within weeks or months.

Myocardial infarction (MI)

In Western countries heart attacks are responsible for 30–50% of all deaths. The incidence increases with age and is greater in men. Factors which may contribute to the development of myocardial infarction include:

- family history of coronary heart disease
- stress
- cigarette smoking
- hypertension

- raised serum cholesterol
- obesity
- oral contraceptives
- diet rich in saturated fats and cholesterol.

Myocardial infarction occurs when there is a prolonged reduction in the oxygen supply to a region of myocardium (heart muscle). Tissue death follows and the area is said to be infarcted. This occurs primarily in patients with coronary artery disease where there is significant narrowing of one or more of the three major coronary arteries. As a result of turbulent blood flow at the site of the atheroma, platelets aggregate to form thrombi and blockage of the coronary artery occurs.

Typically, the symptoms of myocardial infarction are severe chest pain which is sudden in onset and prolonged. The pain is characteristically tight or 'band like' and may radiate to the jaw, shoulders, neck, back or arms. If is often associated with breathlessness, anxiety, weakness, sweating, nausea and vomiting.

The diagnosis is made primarily on the individual's history supported by evidence from an electrocardiogram and biochemical tests. As infarcted myocardium breaks down, enzymes are liberated into the blood stream and these can be measured. The three enzymes most frequently assayed are creatine kinase, lactate dehydrogenase and aspartate aminotransferase. Each enzyme has a particular time course for release from damaged myocardial cells during MI.

General treatment for myocardial infarction Treatment of acute MI comprises:

- relief of pain
- treatment of arrhythmias
- limiting of heart muscle damage
- treatment of cardiogenic shock
- correction of heart failure.

The most common causes of sudden death following an MI are ventricular fibrillation, heart block (blockage of electrical conduction in the heart) or asystole (total absence of heart beat).

Disorders of conduction

Under certain circumstances the cycle of contraction and relaxation of the heart may be disturbed. These disturbances are known as cardiac arrhythmias. There are several types of arrhythmia for which anti-arrhythmic drugs are used. An anti-arrhythmic drug is a drug which is used to control or correct abnormal rhythms of cardiac action. These drugs may be used for several different types of cardiac arrhythmia and it is essential that the specific type of arrhythmia is diagnosed by ECG prior to commencement of treatment.

Supraventricular arrhythmias

These are:

- atrial flutter
- atrial fibrillation
- ectopic beats
- supraventricular tachycardias.

As their name implies, these involve arrhythmias arising from above the ventricles and are normally tachyarrhythmias (i.e. faster than normal). The most common of these are atrial flutter and atrial fibrillation, which are often a result of ischaemic heart disease.

Atrial flutter This is very rapid, but regular, contractions of the atria of the heart which the ventricles may follow accurately, producing a very fast, regular pulse.

Atrial fibrillation This type of arrhythmia, which may develop following atrial flutter, involves very rapid (400–600 per minute) disordered contractions of the atria. This results in irregular stimulation of the AV node and, coupled again with AV block, a fast irregular pulse. Either of these conditions may lead (sometimes rapidly) to exhaustion of the myocardium, other arrhythmias and cardiac failure.

In both atrial flutter and atrial fibrillation, AV block develops because of, and its degree is determined by, the refractoriness of the bundle of His and the AV node. After each stimulation there is a period during which the fibres cannot be re-stimulated, and this is known as the 'refractory period'.

In atrial fibrillation and flutter, messages from the atria will reach the AV node during this refractory period and hence be missed. The length of the refractory period will determine how many atrial beats are blocked for each that is passed and hence the ventricles may only contract for every second, third, fourth or more atrial beats.

Ectopic beats Ectopic beats, also called premature beats or extrasystoles, arise from a focus other than the pacemaker. They rarely require drug treatment but it should be remembered that they may precipitate other types of arrhythmia. In certain cases they do become troublesome and may be treated with β-adrenoceptor blocking drugs.

Supraventricular tachycardias These tachycardias may arise for a number of reasons, e.g. following myocardial infarction, in patients with thyrotoxicosis or in patients suffering from Wolff–Parkinson–White syndrome. (This is a condition whereby impulses are conducted not only through the AV node but also through an anomalous pathway connecting the atria to the ventricles.) Paroxysmal supraventricular tachycardia (coming on in sudden bursts) does not usually require drug treatment and normal rhythm can often be achieved by e.g. respiratory manoeuvres, prompt squatting or pressure over one carotid sinus.

Ventricular arrhythmias

Ventricular tachycardia is potentially more dangerous than supraventricular tachycardias. These arrhythmias are common following acute myocardial infarction or can be precipitated by supraventricular tachycardias. A ventricular ectopic beat may initiate ventricular tachycardia followed by ventricular fibrillation with loss of cardiac output and death.

Bradycardia

Bradycardia is a slowing of the heart, is supraventricular in origin, and may occur, for example, following myocardial infarction or can be a side-effect of β-adrenoceptor blocking drugs.

Infective endocarditis

Sub-acute bacterial endocarditis is an uncommon condition but one which has a high mortality rate. It arises in patients with a history of rheumatic heart disease or congenital heart disease who develop an infection in the bloodstream following dental extraction. Bacteria settle on the previously damaged heart valves and, together with fibrin and platelets, cause a build-up of vegetation. The valve(s) in time become further damaged and there is risk of vegetation embolus leading to a stroke.

COMMON DISORDERS OF THE BLOOD VESSELS

The most common disorders are:

- atheroma and arteriosclerosis
- thrombophlebitis
- varicose veins
- hypertension
- hypotension

Atheroma

This starts at an early age and consists of abnormal plaques of fatty compounds which develop in the muscular layer of an artery. As they grow they project into the lumen of the artery, thus reducing blood flow.

Arteriosclerosis

This is a progressive degenerative condition which is much more common than atheroma. It is also a disorder of the arterial walls but is characterised by thickening, loss of elasticity and calcification resulting in a decreased blood supply.

Thrombophlebitis

This is a venous condition in which there is damage to the endothelium as the result of inflammation of the vein accompanied by formation of a clot. Thrombophlebitis of a superficial vein can be caused by prolonged intravenous catheterisation. Deep-vein thrombosis is more likely to affect a vein in the calf following immobilisation and is a more serious condition because of the greater risk of embolism.

Varicose veins

These are veins which have become so dilated and tortuous that the valves are rendered incompetent, leading to a backward flow of blood. There is a familial tendency to develop varicose veins, although in some people obesity, increased pressure, or standing for long periods may be predisposing factors.

Hypertension

Physicians have difficulty agreeing what constitutes hypertension. An elevation of the resting blood pressure above the 'normal' for the patient's age, weight and height is a broadly acceptable definition. This would be the result of taking several readings under resting conditions. Some 95% of all cases are described as essential hypertension for which there is no known cause. The remainder of cases are associated with renal disorder, adrenal disorder, coarctation of the aorta or toxaemia of pregnancy. In many instances there are no symptoms. Some cases are picked up on routine examination or when the patient presents with one of the complications of hypertension such as stroke, ischaemic heart disease or renal failure. Malignant hypertension is a rare condition which affects fairly young males. It has a rapid onset and causes severe headache, dizziness, left ventricular failure and papilloedema. The diastolic blood pressure may be as high as 140 mmHg.

Hypotension

Although some people have a naturally low blood pressure and come to no harm, when the blood pressure is unusually low there is an inadequate blood supply to the brain which causes the person to faint. Where this is caused by shock or haemorrhage the patient may lose consciousness and die. In older people, postural hypotension can result from rising from bed or chair too quickly and may provide the reason for some falls. Delay in baroreceptor response may account for this.

DRUGS USED IN THE TREATMENT OF DISEASES OF THE CARDIOVASCULAR SYSTEM

Positive inotropic drugs

Cardiac glycosides

These drugs are used almost exclusively in two conditions:

- cardiac failure
- cardiac arrhythmias.

Digoxin In chronic congestive cardiac failure, digoxin is given to improve myocardial contractility, hence increasing cardiac output for any given filling pressure. The use of digoxin in atrial flutter and fibrillation depends on two actions:

- digoxin may sensitise the sinoatrial (SA) node to vagal (inhibitory) impulses and in larger doses may directly depress its excitability, resulting in slowing of the heart
- digoxin delays conduction through the AV node and the bundle of His, allowing fewer of the excitatory transmissions from the atria to pass and hence slowing ventricular rate and restoring rhythm.

Mode of action of digoxin The actions of digoxin are complex and revolve around its ability to inhibit sodium transport out of cells through inhibition of the enzyme Na^+, K^+-ATPase, which allows increased intracellular myocardial calcium concentrations. This in turn improves contractility.

Pharmacokinetics Digoxin may be given orally as either tablets or as a liquid preparation. However, these preparations are not necessarily directly equivalent since digoxin tablets are only about 65% bioavailable. The liquid preparation has a bioavailability of about 85%. Digoxin may also be given intramuscularly or intravenously. Intramuscular digoxin should always be avoided since the drug is dissolved in propylene glycol which produces tissue damage at the injection site. Digoxin is poorly water-soluble and is therefore precipitated out of solution at the injection site, resulting in poor and varied bioavailability. Where parenteral administration is necessary the intravenous route is the preferred route, but this should be relatively rare. Intravenous digoxin should always be given very slowly to minimise the risks of exposing the myocardium to localised high concentrations which may induce arrhythmias. It is often simpler to add the digoxin to an intravenous infusion of 0.9% sodium chloride and administer this by intravenous infusion pump over 1 hour. Since digoxin is 80% renally eliminated, the dose must be adjusted according to renal function in order to minimise the risks of toxicity. In the elderly, who have a lower renal clearance than young healthy adults, a lower maintenance dose is therefore required. The elimination half-life of digoxin in a patient with normal renal function is 36 hours – which means that up to 7 days may be required after any dosage alteration to ensure that a steady state is reached.

Dose Where patients have mild failure, a loading dose is not required and a satisfactory plasma concentration can be achieved over a period of about a week using a dose of 125–250 µg orally twice a day which may then be reduced having special regard to renal function. Because of its long half-life, maintenance doses need be given only once daily. The maintenance dose in atrial fibrillation can usually be governed by ventricular response – which should not normally be allowed to fall below 60 beats per minute. If urgent digitalisation is required (i.e. very severe atrial fibrillation with very fast ventricular rate and danger or presence of other arrhythmias) digoxin may be given intravenously in a digitalising dose of 0.75–1 mg, preferably as an infusion over 2 or more hours (too rapid a rate is associated with nausea and risk of arrhythmias). Digoxin plasma concentrations are commonly measured and provide an indicator of toxicity and patient compliance. They relate only partially to the therapeutic effect because so many other factors can contribute to myocardial excitability, e.g. electrolyte concentrations, catecholamines and hypoxia but generally:

1–2 µg/l   therapeutic
>2 µg/l   possibly toxic

Although digoxin is still used to a large extent for congestive heart failure, its main indication is atrial fibrillation and certain other supraventricular arrhythmias. The use of digoxin in congestive heart failure is often questioned as its effects tend to be transient and it is very toxic. Moreover, less toxic drugs, e.g. diuretics, can give good results, and the effect of digoxin on the heart in sinus rhythm is poor. Digoxin is excreted mainly by the kidneys and therefore in patients with poor renal function, and in the elderly, a lower maintenance dose must be given.

Complications of digoxin therapy Digoxin treatment is particularly hazardous because the toxicity of digoxin is difficult to recognise and it has the potential to cause fatal arrhythmias. The drug's toxicity is more pronounced in the presence of metabolic and electrolyte disturbances (especially hypokalaemia, but also hypomagnesaemia hypercalcaemia, alkalosis, hypothyroidism and hypoxia). The patient's renal function should be taken into account when deciding the digoxin dose in order to minimise the risk of toxicity. Excessive digoxin dose should be considered in any patient who is unwell or who has suddenly deteriorated. Important signs of toxicity are abdominal pain, nausea/anorexia, tiredness/weakness, diarrhoea, confusion and any change in vision, mobility or mood. Toxicity can often be managed by discontinuing therapy and correcting hypokalaemia if appropriate. Serious occurrences require urgent specialist management. Digibind, digoxin-specific antibody fragments in injectable form, is available for reversal of life-threatening overdosage. The serious toxicity coupled with the obvious risks of accumulation in some patients with compromised renal function has meant that digitoxin is occasionally preferred. Other than the $t^{1}/_{2}$, plasma concentrations (140 h and 20–35 µg/l) and dose, the pharmacology of digoxin applies equally to digitoxin – with one exception. Digitoxin is metabolised by the liver rather than excreted by the kidney. This means that despite its longer $t^{1}/_{2}$ (6 days versus 1.5) there is less risk of unexpected accumulation, especially in the elderly.

Interactions Hypokalaemia predisposes to toxicity, so that diuretics used with digoxin should be either potassium-sparing or given with potassium supplements. Drugs such as amiodarone, verapamil and nifedipine may cause an increase in plasma digoxin concentrations and increase the risk of toxicity.

Physiology of the kidney

Each kidney is made up of approximately one million nephrons, each nephron comprising a glomerulus, and a proximal and distal tubule which are connected by the loop of Henle. The glomerulus consists of a group of capillaries and as the blood passes through these it is filtered. A large amount of water and dissolved salts is filtered from the blood and passes on to the tubules. In the tubules a selective re-absorption takes place. Glucose is normally completely re-absorbed. Water and electrolytes including sodium, potassium, chloride, and bicarbonate are selectively re-absorbed and pass back into the circulation. Urea, excess water, salts and other unwanted substances are excreted as urine. The exact amount of each substance excreted in the urine is controlled in order to maintain the composition of the body fluids at normal levels. The urine is further concentrated and, depending on the electrolyte balance, more sodium is absorbed in exchange for potassium. In the distal tubule, antidiuretic hormone (vasopressin) excreted by the posterior pituitary gland is an important controlling factor. Increased ingestion of water results in an increased urine flow. When water is absorbed in the GI tract, it causes the plasma to become more dilute and this, in turn, decreases the release of antidiuretic hormone (ADH) by the posterior lobe of the pituitary gland. Less ADH reaches the kidney and this causes the tubules to re-absorb less water so that more is excreted as urine.

Disease states resulting in oedema

In health the kidney maintains the composition of the blood within narrow limits. Disease can upset this delicate balance. Where the blood supply to the glomerulus is reduced because of impaired blood circulation, filtration slows.

However, tubular re-absorption continues at the normal rate and excess water and salts accumulate in the body tissues resulting in oedema. This can arise in cardiac failure. Oedema can also arise in renal disease (nephrotic syndrome) and cirrhosis of the liver.

Diuretics are used in the treatment of these conditions and also in the treatment of hypertension. They cause a net loss of sodium and water from the body by decreasing the re-absorption of sodium and chloride. Since a large proportion of the salt and water which passes into the tubule is re-absorbed, a small decrease in re-absorption can result in a marked increase in excretion.

Diuretics

There are a number of different diuretics which produce the same end result but through a different mode of action (Fig. 8.3). We consider the following diuretics:

- thiazide and related diuretics
- loop diuretics
- potassium-sparing diuretics
- osmotic diuretics
- carbonic anhydrase inhibitors.

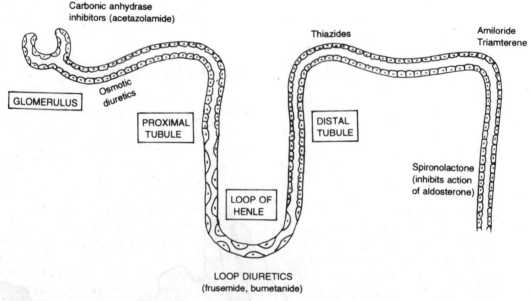

Figure 8.3 Sites of action of diuretics.

Thiazide and related diuretics

Mode of action Thiazide diuretics act by inhibiting the re-absorption of sodium and chloride in the distal tubule of the nephron, resulting in increased sodium, chloride and water secretion. There is also an increased secretion of potassium. The mode of action in relieving hypertension is unclear.

Pharmacokinetics These diuretics are well absorbed orally and are excreted unchanged by the kidney. Compared with loop diuretics (see later) the potency is lower with a slow onset and longer duration of action. Since the duration of action is about 12 hours, a thiazide diuretic should be given in the morning.

Indications Thiazide diuretics are used to treat hypertension and oedema resulting from cardiac failure, liver disease and nephrotic syndrome (see Table 8.2).

Adverse effects The most important adverse effects are hypokalaemia, hyponatraemia and dehydration. Hypomagnesaemia may also occur. Impotence is reversible on withdrawal of treatment. Competition with uric acid for secretion into the proximal tubule may cause hyperuricaemia and this may result in gout. Impaired glucose tolerance can occur.

Table 8.2   Some commonly used thiazide diuretics

Drug	Dose
Bendrofluazide	Oedema: initially 5–10 mg in the morning, daily or on alternate days Maintenance: 2.5–10 mg 1–3 times weekly Hypertension: 2.5 mg in the morning
Cyclopenthiazide	Oedema: initially 0.5–1 mg in the morning Maintenance: 500 µg on alternate days Hypertension: 250–500 mcg in the morning
Chlorothiazide	Oedema: initially 0.5–1 g once or twice daily Maintenance: 0.5–1 g daily on alternate days Hypertension: 0.5–1 g daily in single or divided doses
Metolazone	Oedema: 5–10 mg in the morning to a maximum of 80 mg in resistant cases Hypertension: initially 5 mg in the morning Maintenance: 5 mg on alternate days

Hypokalaemia Hypokalaemia is a common side-effect of thiazide diuretics, particularly at higher doses. Combination products are available containing diuretic plus potassium, but the quantity of potassium is insufficient to correct hypokalaemia. Where potassium supplements are necessary these should be given routinely in tablet or liquid form. Alternatively, the addition of a potassium-sparing diuretic can alleviate the need for supplementation.

Interactions Lithium excretion is reduced by thiazide diuretics, and dosages should be halved initially and adjusted with careful plasma concentration monitoring. Hypokalaemia potentiates the effects of digoxin and toxicity may result.

Loop diuretics

Mode of action This group of diuretics gets its name because sodium and chloride re-absorption in the ascending limb of the loop of Henle is inhibited. In addition, potassium secretion in the distal tubule is increased (greater with frusemide than with bumetanide).

Pharmacokinetics Bumetanide and ethacrynic acid are both almost completely absorbed after oral administration, while frusemide is 60–70% absorbed. Bumetanide is partially metabolised in the liver, and about 80% of a dose is excreted in the urine – 50% as unchanged drug. Ethacrynic acid is metabolised in the liver to the active cysteine conjugate. Approximately two-thirds of the dose is excreted in the urine. Frusemide is excreted primarily unchanged in the urine. Onset of action occurs in 30 minutes after an oral dose and within a few minutes of intravenous administration. The duration of action lasts between 3 and 6 hours after an oral dose.

Indications The loop diuretics (see Table 8.3) are the most potent diuretics available. They are used in:

- pulmonary oedema (may arise due to left ventricular failure)
- congestive heart failure no longer responding to thiazide diuretics
- oedema associated with nephrotic syndrome, especially if there is some degree of renal failure; very large doses may be used

Table 8.3 Examples of loop diuretics

Drug	Dose
Frusemide	Oral: oedema, 20–80 mg daily Oliguria: 250 mg to maximum of 2 g Intravenous: 20–50 mg by slow injection
Bumetanide	1–5 mg once daily orally or intravenously
Ethacrynic Acid	Oral: 50 –150 mg daily Slow intravenous injection or infusion, 50–100 mg

- hepatic disease
- acute and chronic renal failure.

Adverse effects The most important adverse effects are hypokalaemia, hyponatraemia and dehydration. Hypokalaemia may be treated with potassium supplements or potassium-sparing diuretics. Other side-effects include hypotension, nausea, gastrointestinal disturbances, hyperuricaemia. Tinnitus and deafness may occur with large parenteral doses and rapid administration, particularly with frusemide. Ethacrynic acid is used only rarely because of differing and more serious adverse reactions, including gastrointestinal intolerance and bleeding, and tissue irritation on exposure to the drug.

Interactions Hypokalaemia potentiates the effects of cardiac glycosides. Lithium excretion is diminished by frusemide and the dose should be halved. Frusemide also potentiates the nephrotoxic and ototoxic effect of the aminoglycosides.

Potassium-sparing diuretics

Mode of action Amiloride and triamterene cause increased sodium and chloride excretion in the distal tubule resulting in an increase in water excretion. The secretion of potassium in the distal tubule is inhibited (unlike thiazide and loop diuretics). The potassium-sparing diuretics have weaker diuretic and antihypertensive effects than other diuretics, but they have the advantage of conserving potassium. For this reason they are often prescribed with thiazide or loop diuretics.

Pharmacokinetics Following oral administration, approximately 50% of triamterene and 20% of amiloride are absorbed. Triamterene is extensively metabolised by the liver, but amiloride is excreted unchanged in the liver and faeces.

Indications Amiloride and triamterene are used on their own or more usually in combination with thiazide or loop diuretics in the treatment of oedema.

Dose Amiloride is given 5–20 mg orally, daily; triamterene is given 150–250 mg daily, reducing to alternate days after 1 week.

Adverse effects The more common adverse effects are hyperkalaemia, dehydration and hyponatraemia. Other adverse effects include gastrointestinal disturbances, dry mouth, rashes, confusion and hypotension.

Aldosterone antagonist – potassium-sparing diuretic

Sprinolactone is also a potassium-sparing diuretic.

Mode of action Spironolactone is metabolised to canrenone which is an antagonist of the action of aldosterone on the distal tubule of the nephron. Aldosterone promotes the retention of sodium and the excretion of potassium by the kidneys. Canrenone reverses this effect causing increased excretion of sodium and water, and retention of potassium.

Pharmacokinetics Spironolactone is well absorbed (approximately 70%). It is metabolised to its active form, canrenone, in the liver. The onset of action occurs in 2–4 hours. It has a long duration of action (up to 96 hours) and its maximum effect takes several days to occur.

Indications This diuretic is used to treat fluid retention due to cardiac failure, the nephrotic syndrome and hepatic disease. In the first two conditions it is usually used in combination with a thiazide or loop diuretic. In oedema caused by excessive aldosterone activity, e.g. cirrhosis of the liver, primary aldosteronism, it counteracts these effects by competing with aldosterone for receptor sites.

Dose Oral, 100–200 mg daily, increasing to 400 mg where required.

Adverse effects Hyperkalaemia is the major risk, and potassium supplements must not be given with spironolactone as the body potassium could rise to a dangerous level. Gastrointestinal disturbances and gynaecomastia may occur.

Osmotic diuretics

Osmotic diuretics are pharmacologically inert substances that are not metabolised in the body. An example is mannitol. If given as a 20% injection, mannitol passes through the glomerulus and is not re-absorbed in the renal tubules. The resulting osmotic effect prevents re-absorption of water from the tubules back into the blood and therefore increases the output of urine. Mannitol injection is used mainly in emergency situations:

- acute renal failure
- where toxic substances are present in the tubules to facilitate their excretion by forced diuresis
- cerebral oedema.

Carbonic anhydrase inhibitors

Carbonic anhydrase inhibitors act as enzymatic blocking agents that reverse the hydration of carbon dioxide, producing a bicarbonate diuresis that promotes the excretion of sodium, potassium and water. They have a limited diuretic effect and are not used to treat oedema. Instead, carbonic anhydrase inhibitors such as acetazolamide are used primarily to decrease intraocular pressure in glaucoma.

General precautions to be observed in the use of diuretics

Caution must be exercised when administering diuretics to patients with impaired liver or kidney function and also in patients suffering from diabetes. The patient should always be observed for signs of fluid and electrolyte imbalance.

Diuretics can cause acute toxic reactions in patients to whom digitalis glycosides or non-depolarising muscle relaxants have already been administered, by depleting serum potassium. They also enhance the effects of antihypertensive drugs, e.g. methyldopa, hydralazine, and this enables the dose of these drugs to be reduced when treating hypertension.

Many diuretics, in particular the thiazides and loop diuretics, lead to potassium depletion. In these cases, especially if treatment has to be carried on for more than 1 week, potassium supplements must be given.

Potassium supplements

The potassium loss produced by many diuretics may lead to a severe degree of hypokalaemia with its associated muscle weakness, mental disturbances, cardiac effects and increased risks of digitalis toxicity. Potassium supplements should therefore be given with the thiazide and loop diuretics when these drugs are administered on a regular basis.

Potassium chloride in solution is poorly tolerated because of its nauseous effects and it is not often used. Slow release preparations, e.g. Slow K, are well tolerated and are widely used. Apart from the use of diuretics, deficiency of potassium may occur for various reasons – for example, ulcerative colitis, diarrhoea, vomiting, but the most common cause is diuretic therapy.

Drugs for arrhythmias

The different types of arrhythmias are described on pages 76–77. Anti-arrhythmic drugs are used to treat abnormal electrical activity of the heart (see Tables 8.4–8.7). These drugs limit cardiac electrical activity to normal conduction pathways and decrease abnormally fast heart rates. They may be classified in a number of ways:

- those that act on supraventricular arrhythmias, e.g. verapamil
- those that act on both supraventricular arrhythmias and ventricular arrhythmias (e.g. quinidine)
- those that act on ventricular arrhythmias (e.g. lignocaine)
- by the Vaughan Williams classification, which classifies drugs into four distinct classes according to their effects on the electrical

Table 8.4 Treatment of supraventricular arrhythmias

Drug/drug group	Treatment
Cardiac glycosides	Treatment of choice in slowing ventricular response in atrial flutter or atrial fibrillation (see p. 76)
Verapamil	Is usually effective for supraventricular tachycardias. An initial intravenous dose may be followed by oral treatment. It should not be injected into patients recently treated with beta-blockers because of the risk of hypotension and asystole
Adenosine	This drug causes rapid reversion of sinus rhythm of paroxysmal supraventricular tachycardias. It is given by rapid intravenous injection into a large peripheral vein. Dose: 3 mg over 2 seconds with cardiac monitoring. If required, this is followed by 6 mg after 1–2 minutes then by 12 mg after a further 1–2 minutes. Adverse effects include transient facial flush, dyspnoea, light-headedness, choking sensation and nausea.

Table 8.5 Treatment of supraventricular and ventricular arrhythmias

Drug	Indications
Amiodarone	Used to treat tachycardia associated with the Wolff–Parkinson–White syndrome as it has an inhibiting effect on both the anomalous and normal conduction pathways. It should be initiated only under hospital or specialist supervision when used for treatment of other arrhythmias where previous treatments have failed, e.g. paroxysmal supraventricular, nodal and ventricular tachycardias, atrial fibrillation and flutter, and ventricular fibrillation.
Beta-blockers	Act as anti-arrhythmic drugs for the control of inappropriate sinus tachycardia or supraventricular arrhythmias provoked by conditions of high catecholamine excretion, e.g. emotion, exercise or anaesthesia. They are also used to control tachycardias following myocardial infarction and digitalis induced cardiac arrhythmias. Propranolol is the standard drug for oral therapy as it possesses membrane-stabilising properties in addition to its adrenergic inhibition properties. (see p. 90 for additional information on beta-blockers)
Disopyramide	Is very effective against ventricular extrasystoles and is also used for ventricular arrhythmias, especially where myocardial infarction is suspected or has been proven. It suppresses the frequency of ectopic ventricular beats as well as the frequency and duration of self-limiting bursts of ventricular tachycardia.
Flecainide	It is of value for serious symptomatic ventricular arrhythmias and paroxysmal atrial fibrillation. It delays intracardiac conduction (should be initiated in hospital). Like quinidine, it may precipitate serious arrhythmias in certain patients.
Procainamide	Used to control ventricular arrhythmias.

behaviour of myocardial cells during activity (termed the 'action potential').

To understand the actions of these drugs it is necessary first to examine the cardiac action potential itself (Fig. 8.4).

The cardiac action potential

Phase 4 Phase 4 is the resting phase in cells normally capable of spontaneous depolarisation (cells in SA node, AV node and His–Purkinje system). There is a voltage difference across the surface membrane of all myocardial cells which is called the resting transmembrane voltage or potential. During the resting phase there is a slow drift from the maximum negative potential (around –90 mV) to a potential of about –70 mV. This is due to a small influx of sodium ions into the cell and a small efflux of potassium ions. This depolarisation is spontaneous and continues until it reaches the threshold at which action potential is initiated automatically (phase 0). Atrial and ventricular cells do not normally exhibit spontaneous depolarisation, but remain at rest (diastole) until stimulated by a propagatory impulse.

Phase 0 When the threshold potential is reached and the cell is stimulated, there is a very rapid influx of sodium ions into the cell causing a rapid rise in transmembrane potential (depolarisation) until it reaches a given value (above +20 mV in Purkinje fibres). This inward current of sodium is very intense and very brief.

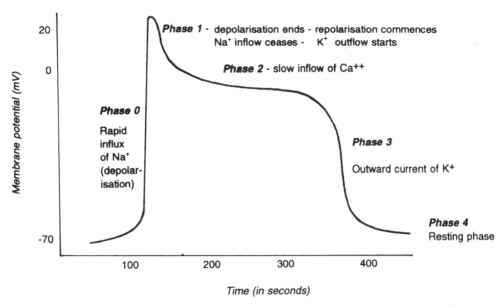

Figure 8.4 Phases of an action potential in the Purkinje fibre cell and the cationic changes which take place.

Phase 1 The potential starts to fall rapidly as repolarisation takes place until it plateaus.

Phase 2 This phase is known as the plateau phase. There is a slow current of calcium ions into the cell which is balanced by a small outward current of potassium ions. These calcium ions are important to the strength of cardiac contraction, which is discussed under calcium antagonists (pp 98–99).

Phase 3 Repolarisation continues marked by an outward flux of potassium ions. As the transmembrane potential falls to its maximum negative value the outward flux is terminated and phase 4 commences with sodium ions entering the cell and potassium ions leaving the cell.

Refractory period

During phases 1 to 3 (repolarisation), depolarisation cannot normally occur. This period is called the refractory period, although when about 50% of repolarisation has occurred a larger than normal stimulus can cause depolarisation.

Vaughan Williams classification of anti-arrhythmic actions

The classification categorises drugs by their action on cardiac conduction. A drug may show more than one of the classes of anti-arrhythmic action. Its main function is to define drugs with similar modes of action and to identify possible anti-arrhythmic compounds by their effects on cardiac conduction. The clinical value of this classification is limited and it excludes some anti-arrhythmic agents such as the cardiac glycosides. The four classes are as follows.

Class 1 drugs are those with local anaesthetic properties which act as membrane-stabilising agents. Depolarisation of the cardiac cell membrane is depressed by restricting entry of the fast sodium current. This reduces the rate of rise of phase 0 of the action potential and depresses the rate of phase 4 depolarisation. These effects tend to:

- reduce the automatic initiation of the action potential
- reduce the speed of conductivity
- increase the effective refractory period.

Table 8.6   Details of drugs used to treat supraventricular and ventricular arrhythmias

Drug	Pharmacokinetics	Dose	Adverse effects	Notes
Amiodarone	Slowly absorbed at widely varying rates. Onset of action occurs within 1 to 3 weeks. It has a long half-life (30–45 days) and effects can be seen months after the drug is withdrawn.	Oral: 200 mg three times daily for 1 week, reduced to 200 mg twice daily for 1 week then maintenance usually 200 mg daily. Intravenous infusion: 5 mg/kg over 20–120 minutes with ECG monitoring.	Causes corneal microdeposits on long-term therapy not requiring withdrawal which is reversible on discontinuation, (may cause dazzle to night drivers), photosensitisation (sun screen advisable), may cause hypothyroidism or hyperthyroidism, reversible peripheral neuropathy and myopathy, diffuse pulmonary alveolitis and fibrosis, hepatitis.	Contraindicated in sinus bradycardia, SA heart block, thyroid dysfunction, pregnancy and breast-feeding. Liver and thyroid function tests are required in long-term therapy. Contains 37% iodine which affects thyroid hormone metabolism.
Disopyramide	90% absorbed from gastrointestinal tract, metabolised in liver, 50% excreted unchanged in urine. Onset of action 30 minutes to 3 hours after oral administration.	Oral: 300–800 mg daily in divided doses. Slow intravenous infusion – 2 mg/kg over at least 5 minutes to a maximum of 150 mg with ECG monitoring followed immediately either by 200 mg by mouth then 200 mg every 8 hours for 24 hours or 400 µg/kg/hour by intravenous infusion.	The negative inotropic effect may cause hypotension and aggravate cardiac failure and it is important to avoid rapid infusion during the loading dose. Anticholinergic side-effects include dry mouth, blurred vision and urinary retention. May exacerbate glaucoma.	Contraindicated in heart block and SA dysfunction (unless pacemaker fitted). Caution in glaucoma, prostatic enlargement, hepatic and renal impairment, pregnancy, the elderly.
Flecainide	Well absorbed, reaching peak concentration in 2–3 hours.	Oral: 50–100 mg twice daily to maximum of 300 mg. Slow intravenous injection – 2 mg/kg over 10–30 minutes – maximum of 150 mg.	Dizziness and visual disturbances, jaundice, ataxia, peripheral neuropathy, pulmonary fibrosis.	Contraindicated in heart failure, long-standing atrial fibrillation, history of MI. Caution in patients with pacemakers, the elderly, hepatic and renal impairment.
Procainamide	90% absorbed from gastrointestinal tract. 50% is excreted unchanged, the other 50% metabolised including the active metabolite N-acetylprocainamide (NAPA), the quantity depending on whether the patient is a fast or slow acetylator. Doses should be reduced in hepatic disease and renal failure.	Oral: up to 50 mg/kg daily in divided doses. By slow intravenous injection – up to 50 mg/minute, 100 mg with ECG monitoring repeated at 5 minute intervals until arrhythmia controlled – max 1g.	Cardiac adverse effects include heart failure, hypotension and ventricular arrhythmias; nausea, diarrhoea, rashes and fever may occur; lupus erythematosus-like syndrome and agranulocytosis have been noted.	Contraindicated in heart failure and hypotension. Caution in the elderly, hepatic and renal impairment, asthma and myasthenia gravis.

Table 8.6 *Cont'd*				
Drug	**Pharmacokinetics**	**Dose**	**Adverse effects**	**Notes**
Quinidine	Almost completely absorbed. Onset of action is 30 minutes to 3 hours.	Oral: 200 mg test dose to detect hyper-sensitivity reactions. 200–400 mg 3–4 times daily.	Adverse effects are very common and have limited its usefulness. See under procainamide. In addition thrombocytopenia and haemolytic anaemia. Also cinchonism with tinnitus, visual disturbances, headache, flushing, confusion, dizziness, vomiting and abdominal pain.	Contraindicated in heart block. Quinidine inhibits renal tubular secretion of digoxin and the digoxin dose should be lowered accordingly. Enzyme inducers including rifampicin, phenytoin and phenobarbitone increase the metabolism of quinidine, therefore increased dose is required. Should not be used in combination with procainamide, amiodarone or disopyramide because of prolonged effect.

Clinical differences between the various drugs in class 1 necessitated their subdivision:

Class 1a   quinidine, procainamide, disopyramide
Class 1b   lignocaine, mexiletine, tocainide, phenytoin
Class 1c   flecainide, propafenone

Class 1a drugs moderately prolong the effective refractory period. Class 1b drugs shorten the action potential duration and prolong the effective refractory period to a greater extent than do Class 1a drugs. Class 1c drugs have little effect on the action potential duration, but increase the His–ventricular conduction time.

Class 2 contains drugs with antisympathetic activity. Adrenalin can cause ventricular extrasystoles and even fibrillation by its effect on the pacemaker potential and the slow inward current, carried by calcium ions, in myocardial cells. Ventricular dysrhythmias following myocardial infarction are partly due to increased sympathetic activity.

The beta-blockers act as competitive antagonists and block receptor sites in the conduction system of the heart. This slows the triggering of the SA node and the conductivity of the AV node and other cells. The beta-blockers also exert a significant negative inotropic effect. By decreasing myocardial oxygen demand, myocardial ischaemia may be reduced. As ischaemia abates, myocardial cells lose their automaticity and this effect suppresses atrial and ventricular ectopy. Examples are propranolol, metoprolol and acebutolol.

Class 3 drugs greatly prolong the duration of the action potential and the effective refractory period in both atrial and ventricular tissue. Bretylium and amiodarone are class 3 drugs.

Class 4. Calcium ions play an essential part in the process of contraction of vascular and myocardial smooth muscle. In the heart this occurs during phase 2 (plateau) of the action potential. The entry of calcium ions into the cells causes fibre shortening and increased myocardial wall tension. The degree of this contraction (or positive inotropic state) is regulated by the amount of calcium ions that reach the contractile proteins. Calcium antagonists block the entry of calcium ions through the slow calcium channels. This blockade greatly increases the effective refractory period of the AV node and slows the conduction rate between atria and ventricles. Verapamil is in Class 4.

Treatment of arrhythmias

Quinidine exerts general depressant actions on all the functions of the heart which tend to cause slowing and better filling of the heart between beats. It may be effective in suppressing supra-

Table 8.7   Drugs used in the treatment of ventricular arrhythmias

Drug	Indication	Pharmacokinetics	Dose	Adverse effects	Notes
Bretylium	Given by injection as an anti-arrhythmic in resuscitation.	Available only as an injection because gastrointestinal absorption is erratic. Active within minutes of intravenous injection in treatment of ventricular tachycardia and ectopy; onset of action takes 20 minutes to 6 hours. Half-life is 5–10 hours. Excreted unchanged by the kidneys over several days.	Intramuscular injection: 5 mg/kg repeated after 6–8 hours if necessary. By slow intravenous injection 5–10 mg/kg over 8–10 minutes with ECG and blood pressure monitoring. May be repeated.	Severe hypotension, nausea and vomiting.	Contraindicated in phaeochromo-cytoma. Adrenalin or other sympathomimetic amines should not be given.
Lignocaine	First choice in emergency. Effective in suppressing ventricular tachycardia and reducing the risk of ventricular fibrillation following myocardial infarction.	Not available in oral form because most of absorbed drug undergoes first-pass metabolism in the liver. Exerts anti-arrhythmic effect in 1–2 minutes after intravenous administration.	By intravenous injection 100 mg as a bolus over several minutes followed by infusion of 2–4 mg/minute. Lower doses in congestive heart failure, hepatic failure.	Central nervous system disturbances, including confusion, convulsions, drowsiness, paraesthesia.	
Mexiletine	Has a similar action to lignocaine and may be given as slow intravenous injection if lignocaine is ineffective.	Well absorbed from gastrointestinal tract. Onset of action is 30 minutes to 2 hours.	Oral: 400–600 mg followed after 2 hours by 200–250 mg 3 or 4 times daily. Intravenous injection: 100–250 mg at 25 mg/minute with ECG monitoring followed by infusion.	Adverse cardiovascular and central nervous system effects may limit the dose tolerated. Nausea and vomiting may prevent an effective dose being given by mouth. Side-effects include bradycardia, hypotension, confusion, convulsions.	Action antagonised by hypokalaemia; rifampicin accelerates metabolism.
Phenytoin	Was formerly used in ventricular arrhythmias, particularly those caused by cardiac glycosides but this use is now obsolete.				

Table 8.7	Cont'd				
Drug	**Indication**	**Pharmacokinetics**	**Dose**	**Adverse effects**	**Notes**
Propafenone	Prophylaxis and treatment of ventricular arrhythmias.	Rapidly absorbed after oral administration. Extensive hepatic metabolism. Half-life approximately 4–5 hours. Steady concentration attained after 3–4 days. Slow intravenous injection – works within minutes.	Oral: 150–300 mg three times daily after food under hospital supervision with ECG monitoring and blood pressure control.	Antimuscarinic side-effects include constipation, blurred vision, dry mouth. May also experience nausea, vomiting, diarrhoea, dizziness, headache, fatigue, postural hypotension, SA and AV block.	Contraindicated in uncontrolled congestive heart failure, severe bradycardia, electrolyte, imbalance, marked hypotension, myasthenia gravis. Caution in obstructive airways disease due to beta-blockers, hepatic and renal impairment, pacemaker patients, pregnancy.
Tocainide	Limited to treatment of ventricular tachyarrhythmias associated with left ventricular function where other therapy ineffective.	Well absorbed from gastrointestinal tract; metabolised in liver to active metabolites; onset of action is less than 30 minutes.	Oral: 1.2–2.4 g daily in 3 divided doses.	High incidence of side-effects severely limits use. CNS effects, gastrointestinal effects, fever and rash, pulmonary fibrosis, blood disorders.	Contraindicated in severe AV block unless a pacemaker is in operation. Regular blood counts are essential.

ventricular and ventricular arrhythmias, but may precipitate rhythm disorders. It is not used much now due to the development of effective drugs with less side-effects.

Beta-adrenoceptor blocking drugs

Adrenalin and noradrenalin, which are produced by the adrenal glands and at sympathetic nerve endings, exercise their physiological actions via alpha and beta-adrenoceptors. Beta-adrenoceptors are widely distributed in the body, being present in the heart, bronchi, blood vessels, eyes, pancreas, liver and gastrointestinal tract. The beta receptors can be divided into two groups:

- beta$_1$ receptors, which predominate in the heart
- beta$_2$ receptors, which are found mainly in the airways and blood vessels.

Beta-adrenergic blocking agents interfere with catecholamine binding at beta-adrenoceptors. Several beta-blockers (acebutolol, atenolol, esmolol, betaxolol, bisoprolol and metoprolol) are said to be cardioselective. These agents have the ability to antagonise the action of catecholamines at beta$_1$ receptors at smaller doses than required to block beta$_2$ receptors. They are not, however, cardiospecific. They have a smaller effect on airways' resistance but are not free of this side-effect. Others block both beta$_1$ and beta$_2$ receptors (i.e. cardiac + bronchial + peripheral blood vessel receptors) and are called non-selective beta-blockers. Blocking beta$_2$ receptors causes bronchospasm, which may be of little consequence in normal subjects but in asthmatic patients may make bronchospasm worse and increase dyspnoea. Beta-blockers should only be used in patients with asthma or a history of obstructive airways disease where no alternative treatment is available.

Some beta-blockers (acebutolol, prindolol, oxprenolol, penbutolol and carteolol) demonstrate various degrees of intrinsic sympathomimetic activity (ISA) which represents the capacity of beta-blockers to stimulate as well as block adrenergic receptors. These drugs cause a slight agonist response at the beta-receptor while blocking the effect of endogenous catecholamine. Patients given a drug with ISA experience a smaller reduction in resting heart rate than those receiving a beta-blocker without ISA. They tend to cause less bradycardia and less coldness of the extremities than the other beta-blockers, which is a problem particularly in patients with peripheral vascular disease.

Some beta-blockers are water-soluble and some are lipid-soluble. Lipophilic beta-blockers are able to cross the blood–brain barrier and exert effects on the central nervous system. Nightmares and hallucinations are more of a problem with the lipophilic agents. The most water-soluble are atenolol, nadolol and sotalol. They are less likely to enter the brain and may therefore cause less sleep disturbances and nightmares. Water-soluble beta-blockers are excreted by the kidneys and dose reduction may be required in renal impairment.

All beta-blockers slow the heart; the output of blood is reduced and the work done by the heart is thus decreased. They should not therefore be given to patients with heart failure or heart block.

Labetalol is a mixed alpha, and non-selective beta adrenergic antagonist which reduces peripheral resistance but has little effect on heart rate or cardiac output. Positive hypotension occurs. Labetalol may be useful in hypertension of pregnancy and in patients with renal failure.

Hypertension

Beta-blockers are effective antihypertensives. The mechanism of hypotensive action of the beta-blockers is not fully understood. Reduction of cardiac output, resetting of baroreceptors, suppression of renin (which is directly responsible for the production of angiotensin, a circulating vasoconstrictor hormone), release of vasodilator prostaglandins, prejunctional beta receptor blockade and a direct action on the central nervous system have all been proposed. It may be due to a combination of several of these theories. Blood pressure can usually be controlled with few side-effects in 30–50% of patients when used as a monotherapy. Combined thiazide/beta-blockers are available but should be used only when blood pressure is not adequately controlled by a thiazide or a beta-blocker alone.

Angina

Beta-blockers prevent angina mainly by reducing the cardiac output and limiting the work of the heart during exercise. When a beta-blocker is to be stopped it should be reduced gradually as sudden withdrawal may cause an exacerbation of angina.

Myocardial infarction

When given intravenously within 12 hours of symptom onset, beta-blockers have been shown to reduce both infarct size and the incidence of complex ventricular arrhythmias. Early mortality, the incidence of reinfarction and cardiac arrest have all been reduced. Beta$_1$ selective blockers including acebutolol, betaxolol, bisoprolol and esmolol may be advantageous as well as beta blockers with alpha$_1$ antagonistic properties such as celiprolol and labetalol, compared with other beta-blockers. Where there is pre-existing heart failure, hypotension, bradyarrhythmias or obstructive airways disease this group of drugs is unsuitable.

Other uses of beta-blockers

Beta-blockers (see Table 8.8) are used in pre-operative preparation for thyroidectomy 4 days before surgery. Propranolol reverses clinical symptoms of thyrotoxicosis. The thyroid is rendered less vascular, making surgery easier. Beta-blockers are also used:

- to relieve anxiety – patients with palpitations, tremor and tachycardia respond better

Table 8.8 Features of some beta-blockers

Drug	Feature of selectivity	Dose – oral
Propranolol	$\beta_1+\beta_2$	80–320 mg daily in divided doses
Acebutolol	$\beta_1>\beta_2$	400–1200 mg daily in divided doses
Atenolol	$\beta_1>\beta_2$	50–100 mg daily
Betaxolol	$\beta_1>\beta_2$	20–40 mg daily
Bisoprolol	$\beta_1>\beta_2$	10–20 mg daily
Esmolol	$\beta_1>\beta_2$	Intravenous only
Labetalol	$\alpha_1+\beta_1+\beta_2$	100–800 mg daily in divided doses
Metoprolol	$\beta_1>\beta_2$	50–300 mg daily in divided doses
Nadolol	$\beta_1+\beta_2$	40–240 mg daily
Oxprenolol	$\beta_1+\beta_2$	40–160 mg daily in divided doses
Sotalol	$\beta_1+\beta_2$	80–320 mg daily
Timolol	$\beta_1+\beta_2$	10–60 mg daily

- in prophylaxis of migraine (p. 139)
- topically in glaucoma (p. 296)

Pharmacokinetics

Beta-blockers are usually well absorbed from the gastrointestinal tract (atenolol is an exception – about 50%). Acebutolol, labetolol, metoprolol, propranolol and timolol undergo extensive first-pass metabolism in the liver. The duration of action ranges from 4 hours for oral timolol to 24 hours for oral atenolol.

Hypertension

Blood pressure changes with emotion, posture, exercise etc. In such circumstances, the changes are brought about by reflex adjustments the aim of which is to keep the pressure at the most appropriate level for the body's needs. In patients with hypertension these controls are not able to maintain the blood pressure at the normal level. This may be due to a number of factors:

- rigidity of blood vessels due to atheroma which inevitably occurs with age
- hormonal changes which alter peripheral resistance or blood volume
- other factors which may set the baroreceptors at the wrong level.

If there is an identified cause for hypertension, this must be treated, e.g. phaeochromocytoma, but this is rare. In the relatively few cases where a cause can be found the hypertension is designated as secondary hypertension. In the majority of patients where no specific cause for the raised blood pressure can be found, this is termed primary or essential hypertension.

Hypertension requires to be treated since serious cardiovascular complications may result – such as stroke, heart failure, renal failure or myocardial infarction. Where the cause cannot be removed, high blood pressure is treated with antihypertensive agents. The methods by which these are effective are based on the fact that blood pressure depends on:

- the peripheral vascular resistance
- the output of blood from the heart
- the volume of blood within the circulation.

By decreasing one or more of these it is possible to lower the blood pressure.

Aetiological factors in hypertension

A family history of hypertension is common in patients who present with raised blood pressure. There is also a positive correlation between obesity and blood pressure. It is accepted that a reduction in body weight will reduce blood pressure in hypertensive patients. A high salt and high alcohol intake may elevate blood pressure and these should be corrected.

Antihypertensive therapy

Antihypertensive therapy is recommended by the British Hypertension Society for patients whose diastolic blood pressure averages 100 mm of mercury or higher when measured on three different occasions or 100 to 109 mm of mercury when measured repeatedly over 4 to 6 months. The aim of antihypertensive treatment is to reduce the blood pressure to within normal limits, thereby reducing the number of subsequent cardiovascular events.

Diuretic therapy

Thiazide diuretics are regarded as first- or second-choice drugs for hypertension. The hypotensive effect of thiazides is not solely related to their promotion of salt and water loss, they also dilate arterioles – leading to reduced resistance. Only low doses are needed for maximal hypotensive effect, and increasing the dose merely increases the incidence of adverse effects. Drugs such as bendrofluazide 2.5–5 mg or hydrochlorothiazide 25–50 mg are often used because they are inexpensive and allow once-daily dosing. Routine use of low doses minimises adverse effects such as hypokalaemia, hyperuricaemia, glucose intolerance, insulin resistance and elevation of serum cholesterol and calcium. Thiazides are contraindicated in gout, diabetes and hypercalcaemia. Important interactions occur with lithium (lithium toxicity), digoxin (risk of arrhythmia) and non-steroidal anti-inflammatory drugs (hypotensive action reduced).

Loop diuretics have less antihypertensive action than thiazides in uncomplicated patients and are not routinely used for hypertension. They have a valuable role in patients with resistant hypertension, renal impairment, co-existent heart failure and in patients taking the potent vasodilator minoxidil (for further information on diuretics see pages 80–83).

Beta-adrenoceptor blocking drugs

These are used on their own, or where not effective, in combination with a thiazide diuretic (see p. 81).

Calcium-channel blockers

These have efficacy similar to that of beta-blockers and thiazide diuretics and are normally used if these prove unsuccessful. Within the calcium-channel blocking group of drugs, which includes diltiazem, verapamil, nifedipine, nicardipine and amlodipine, there are important differences (see pp 98–99).

Angiotensin-converting enzyme inhibitors (ACE inhibitors)

These drugs are commenced at low doses since they may cause a profound fall in blood pressure after the first dose, particularly in patients with renal impairment or receiving diuretic therapy. Diuretic therapy should be ceased 3 days before commencing ACE inhibitor treatment (for further details see pp 95–97).

Other drugs

Vasodilators (diazoxide, hydralazine, minoxidil) (see Table 8.9), alpha-adrenoceptor blocking drugs (prazosin, terazosin, doxazosin), and centrally acting drugs (methyldopa) are generally reserved for patients whose blood pressure is not controlled by, or who have contraindications to, the drugs already mentioned.

Systolic hypertension

Systolic blood pressure averaging over 160 mm of mercury is associated with increased risk of stroke and coronary events particularly in those over 60 years. Low-dose thiazide is an effective treatment with the addition of a beta-blocker where necessary.

Hypertension in pregnancy

This can be safely treated with methyldopa. Beta-blockers may cause intrauterine growth retardation early in pregnancy but are safe from the third trimester onwards.

Malignant hypertension (accelerated hypertension)

Malignant hypertension (diastolic blood pressure in excess of 140 mm of mercury) requires urgent hospital treatment. Although it is desirable to reduce diastolic blood pressure below 120 mm of mercury within 24 hours this can normally be achieved by oral therapy. If it is lowered too rapidly, cerebral blood flow may fall and brain damage and death can occur from cerebral anoxia, cerebral oedema and cerebral infarction. Normal treatment should be with a beta-blocker (atenolol or labetalol) or a calcium-channel blocker (nifedipine). Only rarely is parenteral treatment necessary, e.g. in patients

Table 8.9 Information on vasodilators

Drug	Pharmacokinetics	Dosages	Adverse effects	Notes
Diazoxide	Available only as injection. Metabolised in liver to inactive metabolites. One-third excreted unchanged in kidneys. It acts in a few minutes, its action lasting from 3 to 12 hours.	Rapid intravenous injection: 1–3 mg/kg to maximum 150 mg. May be repeated.	Headache, nausea, tachycardia, hyperglycaemia, sodium and water retention.	Caution in pregnancy, heart disease and impaired renal function.
Hydralazine	Readily absorbed from the gastrointestinal tract. Oral preparations act in 20–30 minutes and much faster by injection.	Oral: 25–50 mg twice daily. Slow intravenous injection: 5–10 mg.	Tachycardia, nausea, vomiting, diarrhoea, fluid retention.	Contraindicated in systemic lupus erythematosus since at higher doses over longer term it can cause a systemic lupus erythematosus-like syndrome. Caution in coronary disease, pregnancy and breast-feeding.
Minoxidil	Well absorbed from gastrointestinal tract. Onset of action is approximately 30 minutes. Its therapeutic action may last several days.	Initially 5 mg daily, increasing by 5–10 mg every 3 days as required. Maximum: 50 mg.	Vasodilatation is accompanied by increased cardiac output, tachycardia and sodium and water retention occur. For this reason a beta-blocker and a diuretic (usually frusemide in high dosage) are required. Other side-effects include weight gain and hypertrichosis.	Contraindicated in phaeochromocytoma, porphyria. Caution in angina, pregnancy, after myocardial infarction.

with acute dissection of aortic aneurysm, hypertensive encephalopathy. Sodium nitroprusside by infusion is the drug of choice.

Mode of action of sodium nitroprusside

Sodium nitroprusside has a direct relaxant effect on the smooth muscle of veins and arteries. The resultant peripheral vasodilation produces a hypotensive effect.

Pharmacokinetics of sodium nitroprusside

The half-life of sodium nitroprusside is only a few minutes. Its effects can therefore be accurately controlled when administered by infusion.

Dose

In patients not already receiving antihypertensives, sodium nitroprusside is given at a dose of 0.3–1 µg/kg/minute by infusion in 5% glucose and increased as required to a maximum of 8 µg/kg/minute. Patients on current antihypertensive therapy require a lower dose. The infusion should be protected from light.

Adverse effects

The following effects may occur but will reduce on slowing the infusion rate: headache, dizziness, nausea, retching, abdominal pain, perspiration and palpitations.

Vasodilator antihypertensive drugs

Diazoxide, hydralazine and minoxidil are potent drugs, especially when used in combination with a beta-blocker or a thiazide. However, they are generally reserved for patients whose blood pressure is not controlled by, or who have contraindications to, the drugs previously described – thiazides, beta-blockers, calcium-channel blockers and ACE inhibitors.

Mode of action

Diazoxide, hydralazine and minoxidil cause peripheral arteriolar dilatation by a direct relaxing effect on vascular smooth muscle. The peripheral dilation causes a fall in blood pressure. This in turn may cause a resultant reflex tachycardia negating the fall in blood pressure. This reflex tachycardia can be prevented by administering along with hydralazine or minoxidil a beta-blocker which potentiates their action. For this reason combination therapy is common when these vasodilators are used.

Centrally acting antihypertensive drugs

Methyldopa

Methyldopa is converted in the body to methylnoradrenalin. In the central nervous system this compound stimulates the alpha-adrenergic receptors which results in decreased activity of the sympathetic system. Vascular peripheral tone and arteriolar vasoconstriction are decreased which lowers standing and supine blood pressures. There is little effect on cardiac output and there is less orthostatic hypotension compared with peripherally acting agents.

Indications

Methyldopa is effective in the treatment of hypertension and is easy to use because the fall in blood pressure is not precipitous. It is no longer widely used because of a number of adverse effects. However, it is safe in asthmatics, in heart failure and in pregnancy.

Pharmacokinetics

Methyldopa is well absorbed from the gastro-intestinal tract. The onset of action is immediate when given intravenously and takes 3 to 6 hours after oral administration.

Dose

By mouth, 250 mg two or three times daily increased gradually at intervals of 2 or more days to a maximum of 3 g. By intravenous infusion, 250–500 mg repeated after 6 hours if required.

Adverse effects

Central nervous system adverse effects include depression, and drowsiness. It may also cause dry mouth, diarrhoea, fluid retention, failure of ejaculation, liver damage, and rarely haemolytic anaemia. In patients with severe renal impairment, dosage should be reduced. Methyldopa is contraindicated where there is active liver disease, history of depression and phaeochromocytoma. Where fluid retention is a problem this can be controlled by a diuretic.

Clonidine

Mode of action

The central action of clonidine is different from that of methyldopa. Clonidine stimulates alpha-adrenergic receptors in the medulla resulting in decreased sympathetic tone and resistance in the peripheral arterioles, lowering the standing and supine blood pressures and decreasing heart rate and output. It also produces peripheral vasodilation.

Indications

Clonidine produces a moderate fall in blood pressure with little postural hypotension. Adverse effects have led to a decline in its use.

Pharmacokinetics

Clonidine is well absorbed and acts within 30 to 60 minutes. The duration of action is approximately 8 hours, but it may be longer in some patients.

Dose

By mouth, 50–100 µg 3 times daily increased as required every second or third day. Maximum daily dose: 1.2 mg.

Adverse effects

Drowsiness and dry mouth are common. May also cause depression, sedation, fluid retention, bradycardia, headache, dizziness and constipation. When treatment is discontinued, dosage should be gradually tailed off since sudden withdrawal results in severe hypertension.

Adrenergic neurone blocking drugs

Guanethidine, bethanidine and debrisoquine are adrenergic neurone blocking drugs. They prevent the release of noradrenalin from postganglionic adrenergic neurones. Guanethidine also depletes the nerve endings or noradrenalin. These drugs do not control supine blood pressure and may cause postural hypotension. They are therefore rarely used now, only in combination with other therapy in resistant hypertension.

Alpha-adrenoceptor blocking drugs

The drugs to be considered in this section are doxazosin, indoramin, phenoxybenzamine, phentolamine, prazosin and terazosin.

Angiotensin-converting enzyme inhibitors (ACE inhibitors)

Mode of action

ACE inhibitors act by inhibiting the enzyme dipeptidyl carboxypeptidase that converts angiotensin I to angiotensin II, a powerful vasoconstrictor. This causes arteriolar and venous dilatation, resulting in reductions of peripheral resistance and arterial blood pressure. The inhibition decreases aldosterone release by the adrenal cortex, preventing sodium and water retention. The overall result, in a patient with hypertension, is a decreased blood pressure.

Table 8.10 Alpha-adrenoceptor blocking drugs: mode of action and indications

Drug	Mode of action	Indications
Prazosin	Selectively blocks alpha$_1$ receptors, interfering with sympathetic stimulation and directly relaxing arteriolar smooth muscle. This interference reduces peripheral vascular resistance and produces vasodilation without causing tachycardia or reducing cardiac output	Hypertension, congestive heart failure, Raynaud's syndrome, benign prostatic hyperplasia.
Terazosin	As for prazosin	Mild to moderate hypertension, benign prostatic hyperplasia
Indoramin	As for prazosin	Hypertension usually in conjunction with a thiazide or beta-blocker, benign prostatic hyperplasia
Doxazosin	As for prazosin	Hypertension usually in conjunction with a thiazide or beta-blocker.
Phentolamine	Acts directly on both alpha$_1$ and alpha$_2$ adrenoceptors, blocking the pharmacological action of noradrenalin-producing vasodilation by reducing peripheral resistance. Its action is not selective on alpha$_1$ receptors and reflex tachycardia occurs	Hypertensive crisis due to phaeochromocytoma or tyramine–MAOI interaction, clonidine withdrawal, acute left ventricular failure
Phenoxybenzamine	As for phentolamine	Used with beta-blockers for short-term management of severe hypertensive episodes associated with phaeochromocytoma. It is also used in the management of severe shock unresponsive to conventional therapy

Table 8.11   Alpha-adrenoceptor blocking drugs

Drug	Dose	Adverse effects	Notes
Prazosin	Hypertension, oral: 500 µg 2–3 times daily, increased to 1 mg 2–3 times daily after 3–7 days, further increased to a maximum 20 mg daily.	Dizziness and loss of consciousness may occur following the first dose because of profound hypotension. The initial dose should be taken in bed. Other common effects include drowsiness, weakness, headache, urinary frequency.	Reduce initial dose in renal impairment.
Terazosin	Oral, 1 mg at bedtime, dose doubled after 7 days if necessary, usual maintenance dose 2–10 mg daily.	Dizziness, lack of energy, peripheral oedema, urinary frequency. Initial dose taken at bedtime as for prazosin	
Indoramin	Hypertension, oral: usually in conjunction with a thiazide diuretic or a beta-blocker – initially 25 mg twice daily increased by 25–50 mg daily at intervals of 2 weeks; maximum daily dose 200 mg in 2–3 divided doses.	Drowsiness, dizziness, depression, dry mouth, weight gain, extra-pyramidal effects, failure of ejaculation.	Avoid alcohol (enhances absorption). Caution in Parkinson's disease, epilepsy, history of depression, hepatic or renal impairment.
Doxazosin	Oral, 1 mg daily increased after 1–2 weeks to 2 mg daily. Maximum 16 mg daily.	Postural hypotension, dizziness, headache, fatigue, oedema.	
Phentolamine	Intravenous injection 5–10 mg, repeated if necessary.	Hypotension, tachycardia, dizziness, nausea, diarrhoea, nasal congestion.	Monitor blood pressure and heart rate.
Phenoxybenzamine	Oral – phaeochromocytoma – 10 mg daily increased by 10 mg daily – usual dose 1–2 mg/kg daily in 2 divided doses.	Postural hypotension, dizziness, compensatory tachycardia, lassitude, nasal congestion, inhibition of ejaculation.	Caution in renal impairment, pregnancy, elderly, heart failure, ischaemic heart disease.

Indications

ACE inhibitors are used to control hypertension particularly when thiazides and beta-blockers are contraindicated or ineffective. Since, in some patients, all cause a very rapid fall in blood pressure, diuretic therapy should be stopped for several days before commencing ACE inhibitors in order to avoid an additive effect. This is termed first-dose hypotension and treatment should be commenced at low dose, being taken at bedtime.

ACE inhibitors are also used in the treatment of heart failure, either as an adjunct to diuretics or in cases where there is no response to diuretics. They may also be used, where appropriate, with digoxin. Dilatation of the arterioles reduces the load on the heart and improves its function. Potassium-sparing diuretics or potassium supplements should not be given concomitantly with ACE inhibitors as dangerous hyperkalaemia may result.

Pharmacokinetics

Captopril is well absorbed from the gastrointestinal tract, although the presence of food reduces absorption to 50%. Enalapril is approximately 60% absorbed, similar to cilazapril, while fosinopril is lower at 36%. The half-life of captopril is 3 hours, its duration of action ranging from 6 to 12 hours, necessitating a twice-daily dosage. Other ACE inhibitors, such as cilazapril, enalapril, fosinopril, cisinopril, perindopril, quinapril and ramipril, have half-lives which are approximately twice as long as that of captopril and they require only once-daily dosing.

Table 8.12 Dosages of several ACE inhibitors

Drug	Dose
Captopril	6.25–25 mg twice daily
Cilazapril	1–5 mg daily
Enalapril	2.5–20 mg daily
Lisinopril	2.5–20 mg daily
Quinapril	5–40 mg daily

Dosages (see Table 8.12)

Treatment is started at low dosage to minimise hypotension. The special-risk group of patients should have treatment commenced in hospital.

Adverse effects

The most important side-effect is a persistent dry cough, often troublesome at night, affecting 10–20% of patients. This may be associated with voice change and throat discomfort. Rashes are common and may be accompanied by fever and eosinophilia. Taste disturbance, which is usually transient, occurs in about 5% of patients. Other side-effects include proteinuria and neutropenia (which may progress to agranulocytosis).

Cautions

Severe renal failure is an important safety concern. It is essential to measure serum creatinine before and during ACE inhibitor treatment.

Contraindications

ACE inhibitors should be avoided in pregnancy, advanced renovascular disease and aortic stenosis, and must be used cautiously in patients with renal impairment or peripheral vascular disease.

Nitrates

Indications

The nitrates are used in the prophylaxis and treatment of angina pectoris and also to treat left ventricular failure. Beta-blockers and calcium-channel blockers are widely used to treat angina; however, short-acting nitrates retain an important role both for prophylactic use before exertion and for chest pain occurring during exercise. Angina pectoris occurs when the oxygen requirements of the myocardium greatly exceed the oxygen available to it.

Mode of action

Nitrates have several mechanisms of action:

- dilatation of vessels in the venous system decreases venous return and thus the preload to heart; the reduced preload prevents the left ventricle from overfilling and reduces the symptoms of cardiac failure
- dilatation of arterioles lowers peripheral resistance and left ventricular pressure, reducing myocardial work and oxygen demand
- dilatation of coronary arteries increases blood supply (and therefore oxygen supply) to the myocardium.

Pharmacokinetics

Glyceryl trinitrate undergoes extensive first-pass metabolism and has very little activity when taken orally. It is therefore administered sublingually as tablets or a metered aerosol. The onset of action occurs within a minute and lasts for 20–30 minutes. Transdermal delivery is used to prolong the effect either in the form of patches or as an ointment. The ointment has an onset of action of about 1 hour and lasts for 4–8 hours, while the transdermal patch delivery system may be effective for up to 1 day. Higher doses of organic nitrates are used to overcome the effect of first-pass metabolism, and high doses of oral glyceryl trinitrate in a sustained release form can be effective (sustac, nitrocontin continus).

Isosorbide dinitrate and mononitrate are effective when taken orally as they are less readily metabolised than glyceryl trinitrate in the liver. Isosorbide dinitrate is active, but has a short half-life (0.5 to 1 hour). It is metabolised to mononitrates, which are also active, but with longer half-lives (2 to 4.5 hours). Isosorbide dinitrate is also active sublingually. No matter which long-acting nitrate preparation is used the dose has to be titrated to attain the desired response or until the dose is limited by side-effects such as headache. The dose varies greatly between patients (see Table 8.13).

Nitrate tolerance

Nitrate tolerance refers to the loss of anti-anginal efficacy despite constant plasma levels of nitrate. Development of tolerance can be avoided by allowing the plasma nitrate concentration to fall at some period during the 24 hours. A nitrate-free gap of at least 6 hours in each 24-hour period can be achieved by removing glyceryl trinitrate patches for a period of 6 hours. A dosage schedule in which an oral nitrate is taken three times daily, but with the last dose at the time of the evening meal, allows an appropriate interval to counter the development of tolerance. Sustained release nitrate preparations provide a nitrate-free interval if given once daily.

Glyceryl trinitrate or isosorbide mononitrate may be tried by intravenous injection when the sublingual form is ineffective in patients with chest pain due to myocardial infarction or severe ischaemia. Intravenous injections are also useful in the treatment of acute left ventricular failure.

Calcium-channel blockers

The activation of smooth muscle is linked with an increase in the intracellular level of calcium, which is brought about by an influx of calcium into the cells via calcium channels. In the heart this muscle stimulation increases both heart rate and myocardial oxygen demand. If the oxygen demand becomes excessive, coronary irregularities, coronary artery spasms and angina may result.

Calcium-channel antagonists restrict the movement of calcium ions, and, by reducing the cardiac muscle excitability, lower the heart rate and cardiac load as well as reducing the myocardial oxygen demands. They also bring about a dilatation of the coronary and peripheral blood vessels and so have a spectrum of activity that in some ways resembles that of the beta-adrenergic blocking agents. All of the calcium-channel blocking agents have the same basic action, but have little chemical or structural similarity. Some are more effective in cardiac arrhythmias, some in angina and hypertension, and some in cerebral ischaemia (Table 8.14).

Nicardipine has similar effects to nifedipine. Amlodipine and felodipine also resemble nifedipine and nicardipine in their effects, but

Table 8.13   Nitrate information

Drug	Dose	Adverse effects	Notes
Glyceryl trinitrate	Sublingually, 0.3–1 mg repeated as required. Oral: 2.6–6.4 mg as modified-release tablets 2–3 times daily. Severe angina – 10 mg 3 times daily. Intravenous infusion 10–200 µg per minute. Spray: 1–2 doses under tongue.	Throbbing headache, flushing, dizziness, postural hypotension, tachycardia.	Glyceryl trinitrate tablets should be supplied in glass containers containing no cotton wool wadding. They should be discarded 8 weeks after first opening the container. Contraindicated where marked anaemia, closed-angle glaucoma, cerebral haemorrhage. Caution in hypotensive conditions.
Isosorbide dinitrate	Sublingually, 5–10 mg. Oral: daily in divided doses. Angina: 30–120 mg. Left ventricular failure: 40–160 mg. Intravenous infusion 2–10 mg/hour.	As for glyceryl trinitrate.	Contraindications and cautions as for glyceryl trinitrate.
Isosorbide mononitrate	Initially 20 mg 2–3 times daily (half this in those who have not received nitrates previously). Up to 120 mg daily in divided doses where required.	As for isosorbide dinitrate.	As for isosorbide dinitrate.

Table 8.14   Calcium-channel blockers

Drug	Indications and action	Pharmacokinetics	Dose	Adverse effects	Notes
Verapamil	Supraventricular arrhythmias, angina, hypertension. It reduces cardiac output, slows heart and may impair AV conduction.	Well absorbed but subject to 85% first-pass metabolism. Onset of action 30–60 minutes. Anti-arrhythmic effect begins within minutes of intravenous administration. Half life 5–7 hours.	Oral: 40–120 mg three times daily. Up to 480 mg daily in divided doses in hypertension. Slow intravenous injection 5–10 mg.	May impair atrioventricular conduction. It may precipitate heart failure, exacerbate conduction disorders and cause hypotension at high doses. Constipation is the most common side effect. Less commonly nausea, vomiting, flushing, headache.	Should not be used with beta-blockers since cardiac failure and hypotension may result from their combined use. Verapamil decreases the renal clearance of digoxin.
Nifedipine	Prophylaxis and treatment of angina, hypertension. Relaxes vascular smooth muscle, and dilates coronary and peripheral arterioles. Does not depress AV or sinus nodes so is of no value in arrhythmias.	Well absorbed, subject to 30% first-pass metabolism. Onset of action after oral dose is 10 minutes. Half-life 3–4 hours.	Oral: 10–20 mg three times a day with or after food. May bite capsule and release liquid for immediate effect in angina. Modified release 10–40 mg twice daily.	Commonest adverse effects are related to vasodilatation and include headache, flushing and dizziness. Also ankle swelling.	
Diltiazem	Effective in treatment of angina, longer-acting formulations used for hypertension.	Well absorbed, from gastrointestinal tract, subject to 60% first-pass metabolism. Anti-anginal effects start 30 minutes after an oral dose. Half-life 3–4 hours.	Angina 60–120 mg three times daily.	Bradycardia, hypotension, SA and AV block, headache, hot flushes, ankle oedema.	Dose reduced in hepatic or renal impairment.

have a longer duration of action and can be given once daily. Nicardipine, nifedipine and amlodipine are all used for the treatment of angina and hypertension. They are useful in conjunction with beta-blockers to treat severe symptoms or as an alternative treatment to beta-blockers where difficulties have arisen with the latter. Felodipine and isradipine are used only for hypertension. Isradipine has a higher affinity for calcium channels in arterial smooth muscle than for those in the myocardium. It therefore has the ability to cause dilatation of the coronary, peripheral and cerebral arterioles without any notable depression of cardiac activity.

Nimodipine has preferential and direct vasodilatory action on the cerebral circulation and little effect on the vascular circulation. It is partic-ularly useful for the treatment of subarachnoid haemorrhage as the subsequent cerebral artery spasm that occurs may lead to cerebral ischaemia and damage.

Peripheral vasodilators

The blood supply to the limb may be diminished by disease or spasm of the peripheral arteries. This leads to an inadequate oxygen supply to the muscle and thus pain in the muscle on walking (intermittent claudication). The cause of this is occlusion of the vessels either by spasm or sclerotic plaques. Vasodilators may increase blood flow at rest but have not been shown to be of benefit during exercise.

Since most vasodilators dilate the blood vessels to the skin rather than the muscle, they are more useful in the treatment of Raynaud's syndrome where spasm is a major factor in poor circulation. It is important that non-drug measures are carried out, e.g. stopping smoking, reducing weight and fat intake, increasing exercise to improve muscle efficiency and prevent build up of metabolites, avoidance of exposure to the cold.

Many of these drugs have unpleasant side-effects such as gastrointestinal disturbances, headache, dizziness. They may adversely affect patients suffering from angina, recent myocardial infarction (by diverting blood from ischaemic areas), those taking antihypertensives (by potentiating their effects) and diabetics (may potentiate insulin and oral hypoglycaemics). Examples of drugs in this class include cinnarizine, nicotinic acid derivatives, oxypentifylline, thymoxamine and naftidrofuryl oxalate (also a cerebral vasodilator).

Cerebral vasodilators

These drugs have been claimed to improve mental function. However, the drugs have not been shown to be of much benefit in dementia. Examples of this group of drugs are co-dergocrine mesylate and naftidrofuryl oxalate.

Co-dergocrine mesylate. This is claimed to improve the utilisation of oxygen and glucose in the brain. There may be some improvement in mental alertness, confusion and depression. The improvement is only slight and there is no evidence of long-term benefit.

Naftidrofuryl oxalate. This produces an increase of ATP levels and a decrease in lactic acid levels in ischaemic conditions, evidence for enhancement of cellular oxidative capacity. It is a powerful spasmolytic agent.

SYMPATHOMIMETICS

In this section inotropic and vasoconstrictor sympathomimetics will be discussed.

Inotropic sympathomimetics

The properties of the sympathomimetics vary according to whether they act on alpha or on beta adrenergic receptors. Adrenalin acts on both alpha and beta receptors:

alpha effect – vasoconstriction
$beta_1$ effect – increase in heart rate and contractility
$beta_2$ effect – peripheral vasodilatation.

Although a powerful sympathomimetic agent, adrenalin is used less frequently as more selective drugs are available. It is of value in anaphylaxis and bronchospasm and is the first drug given in cardiac arrest. In the latter indication it has a direct myocardial stimulatory effect, improving the quality of ventricular contraction and improving cardiac output. Adrenalin 1 in 10 000 (1 mg per 10 ml) is recommended in a dose of 10 ml by central intravenous injection.

Dopamine is a naturally occurring substance which is changed to noradrenalin in the body. However, dopamine has pharmacological actions of its own:

- $beta_1$ effect: potent inotropic action, i.e. it increases the force of contraction more than the rate of the heart
- stimulates alpha receptors in the peripheral vascular system causing vasoconstriction at higher doses
- stimulates dopamine receptors in the mesenteric, coronary, intracerebral and renal vascular systems; this causes dilatation, and, in the renal system, blood flow and urinary output are increased, which is useful in shock where there is a decline in renal function – this effect occurring at low dosage
- causes release of noradrenalin from sympathetic nerves.

Dopamine is used in cardiogenic shock in infarction or cardiac surgery. It is administered by intravenous infusion ($2.5–10\ \mu g/kg/minute$), the dose being adjusted according to response. Its use requires considerable care as higher doses cause sinus tachycardia, ectopic beats and other arrhythmias, vasoconstriction and a risk of angina, hypertension and renal impairment. Once the condition is under control the drug should be withdrawn slowly.

Dobutamine has a more selective action than dopamine, acting mainly on the beta-adrenoceptors, and it does not cause release of noradrenalin. It produces an increase in the force of contraction of the heart and at high doses causes peripheral vasodilatation. For the latter reason it is not appropriate in the treatment of shock where there is marked hypotension. However, it is preferable to dopamine if blood pressure is normal.

Xamoterol also acts on beta$_1$ receptors but is a partial agonist and is used in mild chronic heart failure for patients who are not breathless at rest, but who are limited by symptoms on exertion. It should be initiated in hospital and is contraindicated in moderate or severe heart failure as some patients have shown deterioration on xamoterol.

Dopamine stimulates:

- beta$_2$ receptors in cardiac muscle, producing a positive inotropic effect
- peripheral dopamine receptors, increasing mesenteric and renal perfusion.

Dopexamine is not an alpha adrenergic agonist and does not cause vasoconstriction. It is indicated for short-term intravenous administration to patients who require peripheral vasodilator (after-load reduction), renal vasodilator and mild positive inotropic therapy in the treatment of heart failure associated with cardiac surgery.

Isoprenaline is less selective and increases both heart rate and contractility. It is now used only as emergency treatment of heart block or severe bradycardia.

Vasoconstrictor sympathomimetics

Vasoconstrictor sympathomimetics raise blood pressure by acting on alpha-adrenergic receptors to constrict peripheral vessels. They are used in emergencies to raise blood pressure. They are also used in general and spinal anaesthesia to control blood pressure since spinal and epidural anaesthesia may result in sympathetic block with resultant hypotension (see Tables 8.15 and 8.16).

Blood coagulation

Platelets, disc-shaped cells 2–3 μm in diameter, are formed in the bone marrow under the control of a regulator called thrombopoietin. Aggregation of platelets occurs in response to blood-vessel injury and the platelets plug the disrupted vessel wall. Platelet aggregates are reinforced by precipitation of the insoluble protein called fibrin from soluble precursors in the plasma. Erythrocytes then become enmeshed within this fibrin framework. The formation of fibrin depends on the activation of the clotting cascade along an extrinsic and an intrinsic pathway (Fig. 8.5).

Exposure of collagen in damaged blood vessels initiates the action of factor XII and this leads to activation of the intrinsic pathway. The extrinsic part of the cascade is stimulated by

Table 8.15 Receptor activity, action and use of vasoconstrictor sympathomimetics

Drug	Receptor activity	Action	Use
Ephedrine	Alpha	Constricts peripheral vessels	Hypotension in anaesthesia with associated bradycardia
	Beta	Accelerates the heart	
Metaraminol	Alpha greater than beta	Mainly constriction of peripheral vessels	Acute hypotension
Methoxamine	Alpha	Increased peripheral resistance due to vasoconstriction; no direct action on heart	Hypotension in anaesthesia; when the hypotension occurs in association with tachycardia methoxamine is the drug of choice
Noradrenalin	Alpha greater than beta$_1$	Vasoconstriction	Acute hypotension, cardiac arrest
Phenylephrine	Alpha, beta (weak)	Vasoconstriction	Acute hypotension

Table 8.16   Dose, adverse effects and notes of vasoconstrictor sympathomimetics

Drug	Dose	Adverse effects	Notes
Ephedrine	Reversal of hypotension from spinal or epidural anaesthesia by slow intravenous injection 3–6 mg repeated every 3–4 minutes to maximum 30 mg. Prevention of hypotension from spinal anaesthesia. Intramuscular injection 15–30 mg.	Tachycardia, anxiety, restlessness, insomnia, tremor, arrhythmias, dry mouth, cold extremities.	Caution in hyperthyroidism, diabetes mellitus, ischaemic heart disease, hypertension, elderly, may cause acute retention in prostatic hypertrophy.
Metaraminol	By intravenous infusion 15–100 mg adjusted according to response.	Tachycardia, arrhythmias, reduced renal blood flow.	Extravasation at injection site may cause necrosis. Contraindicated in myocardial infarction and pregnancy.
Methoxamine	Intramuscular injection 5–20 mg Slow intravenous injection 5–10 mg.	Headache, hypertension, bradycardia.	Caution in hyperthyroidism, pregnancy.
Noradrenalin	Intravenous infusion 8 µg/ml of noradrenalin acid tartrate at 2–3 ml per minute adjusted according to response. Rapid intravenous or Intra-cardiac injection 0.5–0.75 ml of a solution of noradrenalin acid tartrate 200 µg/ml.	Headache, palpitations, bradycardia.	See metaraminol.
Phenylephrine	Subcutaneous or intramuscular injection 5 mg. Slow intravenous injection 100–500 µg. Intravenous infusion 5–20 mg in 500 ml adjusted according to response.	Hypertension with headache, palpitations, vomiting, tingling and coolness of skin, tachycardia or reflex bradycardia.	Contraindicated in hypertension, hyperthyroidism, myocardial infarction and pregnancy. Extravasation at injection site may cause necrosis.

tissue thromboplastin released from damaged tissue which activates factor VII. Once triggered the coagulation process accelerates. Platelet aggregation leads to release of various mediators including phospholipid factor III, which is a major accelerating influence upon blood coagulation. Thrombin generation also acts as a further stimulus to platelet aggregation. Thrombin (IIa) stimulates the conversion of fibrinogen to fibrin in the presence of calcium ions. The initial fibrin clot is soluble and is converted to an insoluble polymer when factor XIII is activated by thrombin and calcium. The initial conversion of fibrinogen to fibrin is rapid, the conversion to the polymer is slow and complete cross-linking takes several hours.

Eventually the process terminates because of the action of physiological inhibitors of coagulation factors (e.g. antithrombin) as well as through the inactivation of factors V and VII by high concentrations of thrombin. Phagocytosis facilitates the removal of precipitated fibrin complexes. Fibrin thrombus undergoes

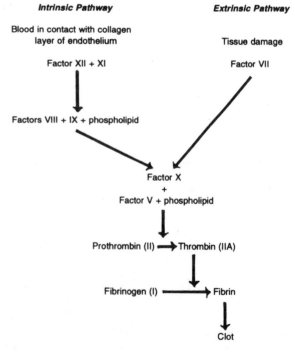

Figure 8.5   Blood coagulation system.

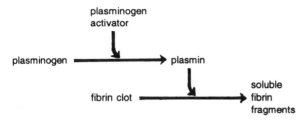

Figure 8.6   Action of plasmin in fibrinolysis.

enzymatic digestion to soluble polypeptides by the process of fibrinolysis. The proteolytic enzyme involved is called plasmin.

Plasminogen is incorporated in the clot and is converted to plasmin when the activators diffuse into the clot (Fig. 8.6). In addition to converting fibrin clot to soluble fragments, plasmin acts on fibrinogen, prothrombin, and factors V and VIII, rendering them ineffective in the coagulation system, thus preventing excessive coagulation.

ANTICOAGULANTS

In this section parenteral and oral anticoagulants will be considered.

Parenteral anticoagulants

Mode of action

Heparin promotes the action of antithrombin III which, in turn, inhibits factor X at low (prophylactic) doses, and factors IX and XI in anticoagulant doses. The outcome is the inhibition of prothrombin to thrombin and this prevents the conversion of fibrinogen to fibrin. This results in the prolongation of clotting time.

Indications

Heparin is used as an anticoagulant in the treatment of deep-vein thrombosis and pulmonary embolism or in the prevention of deep-vein thrombosis (DVT).

Pharmacokinetics

Heparin is not well absorbed from the gastro-intestinal tract so it must be administered parenterally. The intravenous route is preferred for high-dose treatment of acute thrombotic episodes, while the subcutaneous route is preferred for low-dose prophylactic therapy. The intramuscular route should be avoided because of the danger of local bleeding. With intravenous administration, the onset of action of heparin is almost immediate, and peak concentration levels occur within minutes. The patient's clotting time will return to normal within 2–6 hours after administration of an intravenous bolus. With subcutaneous administration, onset is delayed for about 2 hours. The serum half-life of heparin is dose-related, the duration of action being extended with higher doses.

The enzyme heparinase metabolises heparin in the liver. Half-life, approximately 1–1.5 hours, is dose-related. Low-molecular-weight heparin has a longer half-life, which facilitates once-daily dosing. The anticoagulant effect is measured by the activated partial thromboplastin time (APTT) test and the partial thromboplastin time. Dosage is adjusted daily with laboratory monitoring and adjusted according to the APTT.

Dose

By intravenous injection, loading dose of 5000 units followed by continuous infusion of 1000–2000 units/hour adjusted daily by laboratory monitoring or 5000–10 000 units by intravenous injection every 4 hours.

By subcutaneous injection, prophylaxis of deep-vein thrombosis, 5000 units 2 hours before surgery then every 8–12 hours until the patient is ambulant.

Treatment of deep-vein thrombosis, initially 10 000–20 000 units every 12 hours adjusted daily by laboratory monitoring.

Adverse effects

Haemorrhage, thrombocytopenia, hypersensitivity reactions, osteoporosis after prolonged use, alopecia.

Contraindications in haemophilia and other haemorrhagic disorders, thrombocytopenia, peptic ulcer, cerebral aneurysm, severe hypertension, severe liver disease.

Low-molecular-weight heparin

Low-molecular-weight heparins are used for prophylaxis of deep-vein thrombosis by subcutaneous injection, particularly in high-risk orthopaedic surgery. A number of brands are available, the timing of the first dose varying from 12 hours before surgery to 1–2 hours before surgery. Low-molecular-weight heparin has a longer half-life than heparin, necessitating only once-daily dosing. The regimen is therefore continued daily for 7–10 days or until the patient is ambulant.

Heparin flushes

These are used to maintain the potency of cannulae intended to be in place for longer than 48 hours. They are available as solutions of 10 units per ml and 100 units per ml.

Protamine sulphate

Bleeding due to overdosage may occur with heparin. As with all anticoagulants, this often first appears as haematuria but may develop from any site. Protamine sulphate is a strong base that neutralises acidic heparin by binding with it to form a stable compound with no anticoagulant effect. One milligram of protamine sulphate will neutralise approximately 100 units of heparin. The dose to be given should be carefully calculated bearing in mind the short half-life of heparin. The maximum dose is 50 mg. Protamine sulphate is given slowly by intravenous injection. Rapid injection can cause complications such as dyspnoea, flushing, bradycardia and hypotension. If used in excess, protamine has an anticoagulant effect. It is derived from fish sperm and hypersensitivity reactions may occur in patients with allergies to fish.

ORAL ANTICOAGULANTS

There are three substances in the coumarin group, warfarin, nicoumalone and phenindione. The drug of choice is warfarin, the others being seldom used.

Warfarin

Mode of action

Warfarin is effective by mouth. It antagonises the synthesis of vitamin K-dependent clotting factors in the liver, including prothrombin and Factors VII, IX and X. The resulting therapeutic anticoagulant effect does not occur until the already circulating clotting factors are depleted. This takes from several hours for Factor VII to 2–3 days for prothrombin. It therefore takes several days before the anticoagulant effect develops and heparin is used until warfarin is effective. Liver disease, in which synthesis of clotting factors is defective, potentiates warfarin.

Indications

Warfarin is indicated for:

- prophylaxis and treatment of venous thrombosis and pulmonary embolism
- prophylaxis of embolisation in rheumatic heart disease and atrial fibrillation
- prophylaxis after insertion of a prosthetic heart valve.

Pharmacokinetics

Warfarin is absorbed rapidly and almost completely after oral administration; it is highly protein-bound, although binding and half-life may vary considerably between patients. Dosage must therefore be individualised. The anticoagulant effect must be carefully monitored when other drugs which alter protein binding or metabolism are introduced or withdrawn.

Dose

Whenever possible, the base-line prothrombin

should be determined before the initial dose is given. An initial dose of 10 mg is given once daily for 2 days with daily measurements of International Normalised Ratio (INR) for prothrombin time and adjustments as required. The maintenance dose is usually 3–9 mg taken at the same time each day.

Adverse reactions

The main adverse reaction of all oral anticoagulants is haemorrhage. The level of INR at which bleeding occurs varies from patient to patient. However, an INR of 8 or over is considered dangerously high and usually necessitates the administration of plasma and possibly blood if haemorrhage has already occurred. Phytomenadione (vitamin K) 5 mg by slow intravenous injection will counteract the effects of warfarin but it is not ideal since it takes up to 6 hours to act and will render the patient resistant to anticoagulants for several weeks. Where the INR is raised but to a lesser extent (4.5–7 without haemorrhage) it may be sufficient to withdraw warfarin for 1 or 2 days then review. Anticoagulant treatment books are supplied by the pharmacist and must be carried by the patient.

Warfarin is contraindicated in pregnancy since it is teratogenic. It is also contraindicated in peptic ulcer, severe hypertension and bacterial endocarditis.

Interactions

Drug interactions occur commonly with warfarin for a number of reasons, for example:

- protein-binding displacement – warfarin is highly bound and is displaced by salicylates and sulphonamides, which enhances its action
- inhibition of metabolism increases its effect – metronidazole, cimetidine
- induction of metabolism by drugs which induce microsomal enzymes (including phenytoin, rifampicin, carbamazepine) reduces the effect of warfarin.

Antiplatelet drugs

Arterial thrombosis, such as occurs in coronary thrombosis and strokes, is partly due to an aggregation of platelets which ultimately form plugs in blood vessels. By decreasing platelet aggregation, dipyridamole and aspirin may inhibit thrombus formation on the arterial side of circulation (anticoagulants have little effect on arterial thrombus and antiplatelet drugs have little effect in venous thromboembolism). Dipyridamole is used orally as an adjunct to warfarin for prophylaxis of thromboembolism associated with prosthetic heart valves. The dose is 300–600 mg daily in 3–4 divided doses before food. The most common adverse effects are headache and diarrhoea. Peripheral vasodilatation may result in facial flushing and hypotension.

Aspirin is used in the prophylaxis of cerebrovascular disease or myocardial infarction; 300 mg is given daily. Low-dose aspirin (75 mg daily) is given following bypass surgery. Adverse reactions include gastrointestinal bleeding and bronchospasm. It is contraindicated in children under 12 and in breast-feeding because of the risk of Reye's syndrome.

Fibrinolytic drugs

Fibrinolytic drugs act as thrombolytics by activating plasminogen to form plasmin which degrades fibrin and breaks up thrombi. Three agents, streptokinase, alteplase (recombinant human tissue type plasminogen activator) and anistreplase (anisoylated plasminogen streptokinase activator complex) are well established and licensed for the treatment of myocardial infarction. Streptokinase is, in addition, indicated for deep-vein thrombosis, pulmonary embolism, acute arterial thromboembolism and thrombosed arteriovenous shunts.

Streptokinase remains the thrombolytic gold standard as an agent which is efficacious and relatively inexpensive. The principal advantage of tissue plasminogen activator is its lack of antigenicity compared with streptokinase, resulting in lower allergic reactions in primary use and its greater efficacy when a patient needs a subsequent dose. The principal advantage of anistreplase may be its ease of administration, which makes it particularly appropriate for use in the community. Urokinase has the advantage of being non-immunogenic.

The potential for benefit in myocardial infarction lessens as the delay from onset of major symptoms increases, the value of treatment within the first 12 hours being well established. In the case of streptokinase, aspirin has an additive effect in the reduction in mortality. Immediate heparin is necessary to obtain full efficacy from alteplase. An alternative to streptokinase or anistreplase should be used in patients who have received therapy in the previous 12 months or where an allergic action has occurred.

Streptokinase is an enzyme made by haemolytic streptococci. Most patients have antibodies to streptokinase, and a large loading dose is 250 000 units by intravenous infusion over 30 minutes in 0.9% sodium chloride. The maintenance dose is 100 000 units every hour for 24–74 hours.

The most common adverse effects are nausea, vomiting and bleeding.

Antifibrinolytic drugs and haemostatics

Tranexamic acid has the opposite effect of streptokinase by inhibition of plasminogen activation and fibrinolysis. It is useful in stemming haemorrhage in dental extraction or prostatectomy and in streptokinase overdose.

Aprotinon inhibits the action of plasmin. It is indicated for blood conservation in open-heart surgery. A loading dose is given after induction of anaesthesia and maintained by intravenous infusion until the end of the operation.

Lipid-lowering drugs

The hyperlipidaemias are frequently associated with atherosclerotic vascular disease. In these there are very high plasma concentrations of cholesterol or triglycerides or both. There are indications that lowering of low-density lipoprotein (LDL) cholesterol and raising high-density lipoprotein (HDL) cholesterol reduces the progress of coronary atherosclerosis. This can be achieved by weight loss and diet (decreased intake of animal fat and replacement with vegetables) and cessation of smoking.

Lipid-lowering drugs should be reserved for patients with coronary disease or a high risk of developing this. There are a number of groups:

- anion exchange resins: cholestyramine and colestipol bind to bile acids, preventing re-absorption and thus promote hepatic conversion of cholesterol to bile acids
- clofibrate group: e.g. bezafibrate, gemfibrozil – decrease serum triglycerides
- nicotinic acid group: inhibit synthesis, resulting in lower cholesterol and triglycerides, e.g. nicofuranose
- simvastatin and pravastatin are effective in lowering LDL cholesterol.

FURTHER READING

Becker R C, Gore J M 1991 Cardiovascular therapies in the 1990s – an overview. Drugs 41(3): 345–357

Grace R, Hunt B J 1993 Thromboprophylaxis. British Journal of Hospital Medicine 49(10): 720–726

Hinstridge V, Speight T M 1991 An overview of therapeutic interventions in myocardial infarctions. Drugs 42(suppl. 2): 8–20

Kulka P J, Tryba M 1993 Inotropic support of the critically ill patient. A review of the agents. Drugs 45(5): 654–667

McMurray J 1993 ACE inhibitors: optimal therapy for heart failure. Prescriber 4(10): 19–25

Rees Jones D 1993 It's never too late to treat hypertension. Care of the Elderly 5(6): 225–226

Sanai L, Armstrong I R, Grant I S 1993 Supraventricular tachydysrhythmias in the critically ill. British Journal of Intensive Care 3(10): 358–364

Sproat T T, Lopez L M 1991 Around the beta blockers, one more time. Annals of Pharmacotherapy 25: 962–971

Surawicz B 1990 What determines the choice of treatment in patients with supraventricular tachycardia. Cardiology Clinics 8(3): 523–533

Tait E W, Shepherd J 1989 Hyperlipidaemia: its pathogenesis, clinical significance and treatment. Pharmaceutical Journal 242: 134–137

Wikstrand J 1992 Reducing the risk for coronary heart disease and stroke in hypertensives – comments on mechanisms for coronary protection and quality of life. Journal of Clinical Pharmacy and Therapeutics 17: 9–29

9

Drug treatment of respiratory disorders

ANATOMY AND PHYSIOLOGY

The organs of the respiratory system comprise the nose, pharynx, larynx, trachea, bronchi, bronchioles, alveoli and lungs (Fig. 9.1).

The main functions of respiration are to take in oxygen and to give off carbon dioxide. In health the respiratory epithelium is protected by a mucous blanket of secretions, and ciliary activity ensures that the airways remain clear to allow the transport of gases between the alveoli and the atmosphere. The commonest disorders of the respiratory system are the result of:

- upper respiratory infection
- inhaled irritants
- allergens
- intrinsic causes

Changes to mucus production and cilia lead to cough, while narrowing of the airways produces dyspnoea and, in some cases, wheezing. Depending on the body's capacity to compensate for diminished oxygen intake the patient may or may not become cyanosed. Drug treatment is primarily directed towards getting the airways functioning normally. A variety of pulmonary function tests assist the doctor both in making a diagnosis and in selecting the appropriate drug therapy. Before discussing the drug groups used, a brief outline of the common disorders is given.

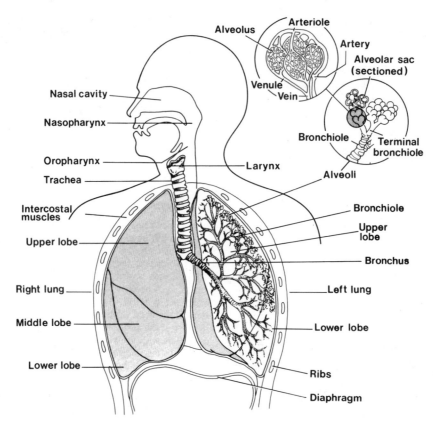

Figure 9.1 The lungs and an alveolus. (From Chandler 1991 Tabbner's nursing care: theory and practice, 2nd edn. Churchill Livingstone.)

COMMON DISORDERS OF THE RESPIRATORY SYSTEM

Acute bronchitis

Acute bronchitis is an inflammation of the trachea and the bronchi. It is usually bacterial in origin and frequently occurs as the result of respiratory viral infections. Cough is the main symptom. When initially only the largest airways are inflamed there is little or no obstruction to respiration; however, as the disorder progresses and smaller bronchi become involved so the cough worsens. Some degree of respiratory distress may also be noted which can progress from tightness in the chest to various degrees of dyspnoea and wheezing.

Chronic bronchitis

Chronic bronchitis results from repeated trauma to the lower respiratory tract. Irritants can be partly responsible, the most important of which is tobacco smoke. Environmental hazards are an important factor, although the results of these may take years to show full effects. Industrial factors include dust, smoke and fumes; social factors include dampness, cold, very dry air or poor nutritional state.

Chronic bronchitis usually occurs in middle age and beyond. The victim is subjected to attacks of acute bronchitis which become more frequent, recovery from each attack taking longer and often being incomplete. Eventually, repeated trauma produces irreversible damage to the bronchial and alveolar tissues and signs of obstructive airways disease emerge. The patient becomes permanently disabled with coughing, wheezing and shortness of breath, unable to lead a normal life.

Asthma

The characteristic symptom of asthma is wheezing resulting from narrowing of the bronchi and bronchioles. Asthma can be divided into two broad types:

- early onset, which occurs in childhood or adolescence, is allergy-related and occurs in patients who develop allergic disorders such as eczema or hay fever; there is a strong familial tendency
- late onset, which affects older people, has no allergic cause and is often referred to as intrinsic asthma.

Various factors can aggravate both types, and these include dust, tobacco smoke, environmental pollution, rapid changes in humidity or temperature, respiratory tract infection and stress.

While allergic asthma often resolves after a few years, intrinsic asthma rarely does. Severe acute asthma is a medical emergency clinically recognised by severe wheeze, inability to speak sentences without pausing for breath and a pulse rate over 110 per minute in the adult.

Allergic conditions

Allergic conditions vary from mild forms of hay fever, skin rashes and eczema to more severe forms such as asthma and anaphylactic shock. Allergens which provoke this response in certain individuals include pollen, animal hair, dust, components of various foods, such as fish and eggs, and some food dyes, notably tartrazine, drugs, feathers etc.

Initial exposure to allergen inhaled or ingested into the body stimulates the production and release of IgE from lymph nodes in atopic individuals. The IgE becomes fixed to mast cells (sensitised mast cells) which, on a second exposure to the allergen, causes release of inflammatory mediators, histamines and serotonin.

Histamine is a major factor in allergic and anaphylactic reactions; it causes:

- contraction of smooth muscle in the bronchial tract
- a short lasting fall in blood pressure due to dilatation of the arterioles
- increased permeability of the capillaries, leading to formation of weals and blisters (all actions on H_1 receptors)
- increased secretion of exocrine glands, e.g. acid in stomach (H_2 receptors).

THE MAIN GROUPS OF DRUGS

The main groups of drugs used in the treatment of respiratory disorders are:

- bronchodilators
- corticosteroids
- cromoglycate and related therapy
- antihistamines
- respiratory stimulants
- respiratory surfactants
- oxygen
- mucolytics
- inhalations
- cough preparations
- systemic nasal decongestants.

BRONCHODILATORS (Table 9.1)

Beta$_2$-adrenoceptor stimulants (beta$_2$ sympathomimetics)

These drugs cause bronchodilatation by acting on beta$_2$-adrenoceptors in bronchial tissue. When used in the recommended dosage their effect on cardiac beta$_1$-adrenoceptors is much reduced. This means that they are less likely to produce undesired cardiac side-effects. These selective beta$_2$-adrenoceptor stimulants are safe and effective and will therefore normally be the first-choice bronchodilator in the:

- rapid relief of an asthmatic attack
- maintenance treatment of chronic asthma, chronic bronchitis, emphysema.

There are some differences but little to choose between the various selective beta$_2$-adrenoceptor drugs.

Table 9.1 Bronchodilators

Clinical feature	Disordered physiology	Drug therapy	Action/benefits	Side-effects	Cautions
Dyspnoea	Constriction of smooth muscle of bronchi and bronchioles	Adrenoceptor stimulant	Relaxation of smooth muscle – β_2 effect	Tachycardia, headache, nervous tension, hypokalaemia (high doses) peripheral vasodilation	Hypertension, arrhythmias, myocardial insufficiency, hyperthyroidism
		Antimuscarinics	Relaxation of smooth muscle by blocking action of acetylcholine	Dry mouth, constipation	Glaucoma at higher doses, prostatic hypertrophy, pregnancy
		Theophylline	Smooth muscle relaxation	Tachycardia, nausea, palpitations, headache, insomnia, arrhythmias, gastrointestinal disturbances	Liver disease, cardiac disease, elderly

Drugs used in this group

Salbutamol
Terbutaline
Rimiterol
Fenoterol
Salmeterol

Formulation

Salbutamol and terbutaline, the most commonly used drugs in this group, are available in the widest range of formulations:

- aerosol inhalation
- dry powder inhalation
- respirator solution (for use in a nebuliser)
- tablets
- modified release tablets
- syrup
- injection
- intravenous infusion.

Duration of action and usage

The beta$_2$-adrenoceptor stimulants differ in their duration of action. The shortest acting beta$_2$-stimulant is **rimiterol**, followed by **salbutamol**, **terbutaline and fenoterol** with a duration of action of 3–5 hours.

Salmeterol has a slow onset but is long-acting (12 hours), which makes it suitable for twice-daily administration. It is not suitable for use in an acute asthma attack and should be used in conjunction with corticosteroid therapy. It is considered as an additional bronchodilator and not as a replacement for existing therapy.

Administration

Adrenoceptor bronchodilators are best given by **pressurised aerosol inhaler** as a rapid action ensues and side-effects are minimal.

The action is quick since, on inhalation, the medicament immediately reaches the site of action.

Absorption is rapid because of the large surface area of the alveoli, single layer of epithelial cells, and the rich blood supply.

Salbutamol and terbutaline may also be administered as respirator solution via a nebuliser.

Oral therapy has a much slower action since the drug must be absorbed into the blood circulation, pass through the liver and be transported through the body, including the lungs, where the required effect will take place.

Dosage

Inhalers are used on an as-required basis or as regular treatment in a dose of one to two puffs four times a day in the adult – maximum 12 puffs in 24 hours. The inhaled dose is small (**salbutamol**: 100 µg; **terbutaline**: 250 µg) and although only 12% reaches the airways, this is enough to be effective. The dose prescribed by nebuliser is substantially higher. One salbutamol nebule (single dose container) contains 2.5 mg in 2.5 ml, which is equivalent to 25 puffs of a salbutamol inhaler.

Although inhalation of beta$_2$-adrenoceptor stimultants is the preferred route (fewer side-effects), for those who experience difficulty with this method oral preparations are available. **Oral doses** have to be much higher because a considerable proportion of the drug is broken down in the liver and also because of the dilution factor. A 4 mg single dose of **salbutamol** will therefore be 40 times greater than a single aerosol inhalation. Consequently, side-effects are more likely to be experienced with oral therapy.

Modified release preparations, e.g. Ventolin CR tablets, Volmax tablets, Bricanyl SA tablets, may be of value in patients with nocturnal asthma as an alternative to modified release theophylline (see p. 114).

Side-effects

Side-effects are rarely experienced with beta$_2$-adrenoceptor stimulants inhaled from a pressurised aerosol inhaler but may occur with the much higher doses needed in oral therapy and treatment with a nebuliser. Possible side-effects include fine tremor (usually hands), nervous tension, headache, peripheral vasodilatation, tachycardia, hypokalaemia after high doses, and hypersensitivity reactions.

Important points

Warn patients treated by inhalation via a nebuliser that it is dangerous to exceed the stated dose. If the desired effect is not reached with the usual dose the patient should seek medical attention.

Instruct patients in the correct mechanical use of their inhaler (see pp 443–444).

Other adrenoceptor stimulants

These non-selective or partially selective beta-adrenoceptor stimulants, such as ephedrine, isoprenaline and orciprenaline, are now regarded as less safe and are therefore not used any more.

Antimuscarinic bronchodilators

Ipratropium bromide, an atropine analogue, relieves bronchoconstriction associated with chronic bronchitis. Traditionally regarded as more effective, it may provide some bronchodilation in patients who fail to respond to treatment with a selective beta$_2$-adrenoceptor stimulant. It may also be used in combination with a beta$_2$-adrenoceptor stimulant with a reduced dose of the beta$_2$-adrenoceptor.

Oxitropium bromide has a similar effect and is also used in chronic bronchitis.

Formulation

Ipratropium bromide is available as a pressurised metered dose inhaler (aerosol inhaler), and as a nebuliser solution.

Duration of action

The onset of action is slow and reaches its maximal effect after 30–60 minutes and lasts for 3–5 hours.

Dosage

Inhaler: two puffs four times daily (0.02 mg per puff); nebuliser solution: 2 ml four times a day (0.025 mg/ml).

Side-effects

Side-effects are rare, but occasionally the following atropine-like symptoms may occur: dry mouth, urinary retention, constipation.

With the recommended dose there is no effect on sputum viscosity.

Important points

Higher doses should not be used if the patient has glaucoma.

In patients on nebulised ipratropium bromide, ensure that no nebulised solution escapes from masks and reaches the patients' eyes.

Instruct patients in the correct mechanical use of their inhaler (see pp 443–444)

Xanthine bronchodilators

These drugs cause bronchodilation by relaxation of plain muscle of the bronchial tree. They also have a slight diuretic effect. They are used in the treatment of severe acute asthma attacks and chronic asthma, in particular control of nocturnal asthma and early morning wheezing.

Drugs used in this group

Theophylline
Aminophylline (a combination of theophylline and ethylenediamine)

Formulation

Aminophylline and **theophylline** are available as intravenous injection, modified release tablets and capsules, rapid release tablets, syrup.

Preparations from different manufacturers will have different release mechanisms resulting in the rate of release or quantity released varying to some extent. Consequently these controlled release preparations are not interchangeable without retitration of dosage.

Aminophylline suppositories are now not used any more because of their unpredictable response and their ability to cause proctitis.

Dosage

Theophylline has a low toxic:therapeutic ratio. The therapeutic plasma concentration lies between 10 and 20 mg/litre. **Theophylline** is metabolised in the liver and has a considerable variation in its half-life; therefore the dosage has to be adjusted individually. Ideally, plasma levels should be checked if one or more of the following factors are present (see metabolism of drugs p. 14).

Factors which increase the half-life:
- hepatic impairment
- heart failure
- concurrent use of
  cimetidine
  ciprofloxacin
  oral contraceptives
  erythromycin

Factors which decrease the half-life:
- smoking
- heavy drinking
- concurrent use of
  rifampicin
  barbiturates
  carbamazepine
  phenytoin

Elimination is delayed in the elderly and in neonates, but is more rapid in children than in adults.

In severe attacks of asthma, **aminophylline** may be given by **slow intravenous injection** (over 20 minutes) in doses of 250–500 mg. Reduced doses and measurement of plasma concentration are necessary if **oral theophylline** is already being taken. The average **oral dose** (slow release) is 200–400 mg twice daily.

Side-effects

Side-effects are dose-related and become more common above 20 mg/litre plasma concentration. The side-effects include arrhythmias, hypotension, convulsions, gastrointestinal disturbances, headache, insomnia, nausea and palpitations.

Important points

Take oral preparations with or immediately after food to avoid gastric disturbances.
Watch out for side-effects.

Peak flow meters

Peak flow meters are used in helping to diagnose airflow obstruction, as in chronic obstructive airways disease (COAD) and asthma, and in measuring the effectiveness of treatment prescribed for the individual patient.

Peak flow or the **peak expiratory flow rate (PEFR)** is the maximum flow of air achievable while breathing out as hard as possible. It is an indication of how wide the airways are at the time the measurement is taken. The speed of air passing through the meter is measured in litres per minute (l/min) and will vary according to sex, age and height (Table 9.2). Peak flow readings are usually higher in men than in women. Peak flow varies throughout the day and the morning reading is often lower than that of the evening. It is the difference between these two readings that is important. When asthma is out of control great swings occur with the morning readings being much lower and the evening readings much higher than normal.

Types of peak flow meter

The **Mini-Wright peak flow meter** (Fig. 9.2) is now available on prescription. Patients are instructed to take readings at the same time every morning and evening, and to keep a careful record of them to show to their doctor at the outpatient clinic.

Patients admitted to hospital with an acute asthma attack are more likely to use a **Wright's peak flow meter** (Fig. 9.3). The nurse records the results on a graph.

The use of peak flow meters

The use of peak flow meters is the same whichever type is used. The marker is first set to zero. Those able to stand to use the meter are advised to do so. Patients in hospital are likely to be sitting in bed or in a chair. The meter is held in front of the patient, preferably by the patient. The patient breathes in as fully as possible and then with the lips firmly around the mouthpiece, breathes out as hard and as fast as possible. The sequence is repeated twice more, keeping a note each time of the readings. The highest reading of all three measurements is regarded as the peak flow at that time. Peak flow readings are taken immediately before inhaler or nebuliser treatment and approximately 15 minutes after.

Nursing points

The patient should be instructed in the use of the

Table 9.2 Table of predicted peak flow (litres/min)*

Height	Age									
	25	30	35	40	45	50	55	60	65	70
Males										
5'3" (160 cm)	572	560	548	536	524	512	500	488	476	464
5'6" (167 cm)	597	584	572	559	547	534	522	509	496	484
5'9" (175 cm)	625	612	599	586	573	560	547	533	520	507
6'0" (183 cm)	654	640	626	613	599	585	572	558	544	530
6'3" (191 cm)	679	665	650	636	622	608	593	579	565	551
Females										
4'9" (144 cm)	377	366	356	345	335	324	314	303	293	282
5'0" (152 cm)	403	392	382	371	361	350	340	329	319	308
5'3" (160 cm)	433	422	412	401	391	380	370	359	349	338
5'6" (167 cm)	459	448	438	427	417	406	396	385	375	364
5'9" (175 cm)	489	478	468	457	447	436	426	415	405	394

Standard deviation: 60 1/min. Negligible ethnic variation.
* A severe asthmatic attack is recognised when the peak expiratory flow is less than 40% of the predicted peak flow. (Figures produced by the National Asthma Campaign.)

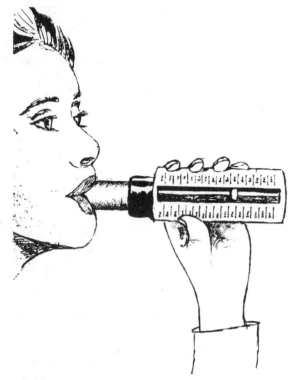

Figure 9.2 Mini-Wright peak flow meter.

peak flow meter and should be supervised until competent. Wherever possible the patient should be encouraged to use the flow meter independently.

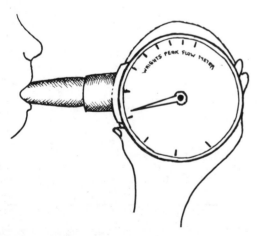

Figure 9.3 Wright's peak flow meter.

CORTICOSTEROIDS (Table 9.3)

Corticosteroids act in different ways: they have anti-inflammatory effects, thereby decreasing bronchial oedema and hypersecretion of mucus; they modify allergic reactions; they enhance the actions of beta$_2$-adrenoceptor stimulants.

Drugs used in this group

Inhaled drugs
  beclomethasone dipropionate
  budesonide

Oral drugs
  prednisolone

Usage

Corticosteroids are used in:

- the emergency treatment of a severe acute asthma attack (see p. 120)
- the treatment of mild to moderate acute asthma attacks (see p. 120)
- the prophylactic treatment of chronic asthma (see p. 120).

Inhaled therapy should be used in preference to oral therapy to avoid systemic side-effects. Corticosteroid inhalations must be used regularly to obtain maximum benefit, alleviation of symptoms usually occurring 3–7 days after initiation.

Dosage and formulations

The standard dose of **beclomethasone dipropionate** by aerosol inhaler is 200 µg (two puffs) twice daily or 100 µg (one puff) 3–4 times daily.

High-dose inhalers (2–5 times more potent) are available for patients with reduced response to a standard dose.

The maximum dose by aerosol inhaler is 500 µg 4 times daily.

Beclomethasone and **budesonide** are both available as dry powder formulations and may be tried by patients unable to use the aerosol inhaler (see administration of inhaled drugs).

A short course of oral corticosteroid, as sometimes needed in an acute asthma attack (see

Table 9.3 Corticosteroids

Clinical feature	Disordered physiology	Drug therapy	Action/benefits	Side-effects	Cautions
Dyspnoea ± wheezing	Inflammation of bronchial mucosa and hypersecretion of mucus	Corticosteroids – inhaled and oral	Anti-inflammatory – reduce oedema and hypersecretion of mucus	Candida of mouth and throat, and hoarseness (inhalation). Moon face, obesity, purple skin striae, hypertension, osteoporosis, diabetes mellitus, susceptibility to infections, acne, weight gain, gastrointestinal disturbances, mood changes	High-dose oral treatment should be reduced gradually

p. 120), starts with a high dose of e.g. **prednisolone** 40 mg for a few days gradually reduced once the attack has been controlled. Oral corticosteroids should be taken in the morning to reduce interference with circadian cortisol secretion.

Side-effects

Systemic side-effects associated with long-term oral and high-dose inhaled therapy are: moon face, obesity, purple skin striae, hypertension, osteoporosis, diabetes mellitus, susceptibility to infections and adrenal suppression.

With standard-dose inhaled therapy, systemic side-effects do not usually occur. The most common dose-related side-effects experienced with the use of corticosteroid aerosol inhalers are candidiasis of the mouth and throat, and hoarseness.

The use of a spacing device increases airways deposition and reduces oropharyngeal deposition, resulting in a marked reduction in the incidence of candidiasis and of systemic absorption (see administration of inhaled drugs).

Important points

Patients on regular oral or higher inhaled doses should carry a steroid card.

If the patient is having concurrent bronchodilator and corticosteroid therapy, the bronchodilator should be used first.

Ensure that patients are knowledgeable and competent in using their inhaler devices (see administration of inhaled drugs).

It is essential that the patient understands that beclomethasone gives no relief in an acute asthma attack and should be taken regularly.

Advise the patient to clear out as much mucus as possible before inhalation.

Advise the patient to rinse the mouth or to drink liquid after inhalation of a corticosteroid.

CROMOGLYCATE AND RELATED THERAPY (Table 9.4)

These drugs, also known as mast-cell stabilisers, block the release of mediators such as histamine and serotonin from sensitised mast cells in the lung. By stabilising the mast-cell membranes they can reduce the incidence of asthma attacks, particularly in children and young adults, and they allow dose reduction of bronchodilators and oral corticosteroids. They do not cause bronchodilation and are therefore of no value in the treatment of acute attacks of asthma.

Drugs used in this group

Sodium cromoglycate
Nedocromil sodium
Ketotifen

Formulations and dosage

Sodium cromoglycate is available as: (i) an *aerosol inhalation*: two puffs (= 10 mg) 4 times daily, increased to 6–8 times daily if necessary; maintenance: one puff (5 mg) 4 times daily. For the prevention of an exercise-induced attack a

Table 9.4 Cromoglycate and related therapy

Clinical feature	Disordered physiology	Drug therapy	Action/benefits	Side-effects	Cautions
None as such; used prophylactically to reduce incidence of asthma attack	Mast cells in lung have become sensitised	Sodium cromoglycate	Blocks release of histamine and serotonin from sensitised mast cells in lung	Dry powder may cause coughing, transient bronchospasm and throat irritation	No value in treatment of asthma attack

single dose is inhaled half an hour beforehand. (ii) *Autohaler* (see administration of inhaled drugs): dry powder inhalation in the form of a 20 mg gelatine capsule (spincaps) for use with a special turbohaler (spinhaler). The capsule is placed in the spinhaler, which punctures the capsule. When the patient places the turbohaler in his mouth and inhales, the capsule spins and vibrates, causing the micronised powder to be inhaled. Of the 1 to 2 mg cromoglycate inhaled into the lung, only about 12% is absorbed systemically. (iii) *2 ml ampoules* (10 mg/1 ml) for administration by nebuliser (see administration of inhaled drugs).

Nedocromil sodium is available as aerosol inhalation.

Ketotifen is available only in oral preparations (syrup and tablets).

Side-effects

Side-effects are rare; however, dry powder inhalation may cause bronchospasm. The use of a beta$_2$-adrenoceptor stimulant such as salbutamol or terbutaline a few minutes before the sodium cromoglycate inhalation can prevent that.

Ketotifen is an antihistamine said to resemble sodium cromoglycate. However, side-effects such as dry mouth and drowsiness make it less useful.

Important points

Advise the patient in the correct use of the inhaler (see administration of inhaled drugs).
Advise the patient that spincaps are for inhalation only and should not be swallowed.

Advise the patient that the drug is not suitable for the relief of an acute asthma attack.
Advise the patient that the drug should be administered regularly.

ANTIHISTAMINES

Antihistamines compete with histamine and block its action at histamine receptor sites. They do not reverse histamine effects once established. Some antihistamines have anti-emetic properties.

Usage

Antihistamines are used in the treatment of allergic skin rashes, nasal allergy, particularly the seasonal type (hay fever), pruritus, insect bites and stings, drug allergies and anaphylactic shock (see pp 37–40) and for the prevention of urticaria and motion sickness.

Drugs used in this group

1. Non-sedative
   Astemizole
   Loratadine
   Terfenadine

2. Sedative
   Azatadine maleate
   Brompheniramine maleate
   Chlorpheniramine maleate
   Clemastine
   Promethazine hydrochloride

Formulation and dosage

Most antihistamines are available only in the oral

form. Following oral administration, symptomatic relief of allergic reactions and side-effects may begin within 15 to 30 minutes, lasting for 3 to 6 hours.

Chlorpheniramine and **promethazine** are also available as injections to treat severe conditions. **Chlorpheniramine** can be administered by subcutaneous or intramuscular injection (10–20 mg) or by slow intravenous injection (10–20 mg) over 1 minute diluted in the syringe with 5 to 10 ml of blood (see anaphylactic shock pp 37–40).

Side-effects

Influence on the central nervous system (CNS), namely, drowsiness and dulling of mental alertness.

In newer antihistamines (group 1), sedative and psychomotor impairment effects are much reduced.

Headache.

Antimuscarinic effects such as urinary retention, dry mouth, blurred vision and gastrointestinal disturbances.

Interactions

Antihistamines may enhance sedative effects of central nervous system depressants such as alcohol, barbiturates, analgesics, sedatives and tranquillisers.

The newer antihistamines (group 1) do not seem to potentiate the effect of alcohol.

Caution

Antihistamines should be used with caution in epilepsy, prostatic hypertrophy, glaucoma and hepatic disease.

Important points

Advise patients to take antihistamines with or after food to avoid gastric disturbances.
Keep antihistamines out of reach of children to prevent poisoning.

Hyposensitisation

Except for wasp and bee sting allergy, the value of specific hyposensitisation is uncertain. Since the majority of patients are also sensitive to a wide range of other allergens (except wasp and bee sting allergy), hyposensitisation with an extract of a single allergen is, in most cases, no more than partially successful.

Hyposensitisation may precipitate severe allergic reactions; the risk is particularly high in children.

Treatment of reversible airways obstruction

Emergency treatment of severe acute asthma (status asthmaticus) Severe acute asthma can be fatal and must be promptly and rigorously treated. Symptoms include exhaustion, restlessness, pulse rate over 100/min in the adult and persistent dyspnoea with conventional bronchodilator therapy having little effect.

Nebulised solution of salbutamol or terbutaline (see p. 447) administered preferably with oxygen is quick-acting and should be commenced at once.

The patient should then be given a corticosteroid – either hydrocortisone 200 mg intravenously or 40 mg of prednisolone orally; children have half of these doses.

If the response is poor, consideration should be given to additional treatment: ipratropium by nebuliser (see p. 447); aminophylline by slow intravenous injection where the patient has not been receiving theophylline orally (see p. 114); beta$_2$- adrenoceptor stimulant intravenously.

Patients who do not respond to the above treatment might need intermittent positive pressure ventilation.

Acute, mild to moderate attack of asthma Acute intermittent asthma attacks are treated with a beta$_2$-adrenoceptor stimulant (see p. 113) by inhalation. Ipratropium (see p. 113) by inhalation is an alternative but is better reserved for the regular treatment of asthma. Beta$_2$-adrenoceptor stimulants may also be used prophylactically (e.g. before exercise) to prevent an attack.

If the effect of the treatment with a beta$_2$-adrenoceptor stimulant is not sufficient, a short course of oral corticosteroids (see p. 197) might be required. The course normally starts with a high dose of e.g. prednisolone 40 mg for a few days; this should be reduced gradually once the attack has been controlled.

Chronic asthma Maintenance therapy of chronic asthma should begin with a beta$_2$-adrenoceptor stimulant (see p. 112) by aerosol; ipratropium (see p. 113) can be added or used as an alternative. If this combined treatment is not sufficient, an oral theophylline (see p. 114) can be added.

Patients who do not respond sufficiently may require long-term treatment with either an inhaled or an oral corticosteroid or a combination of both. In order to keep the oral dose as low as possible, a high dose of inhaled corticosteroid should be continued.

RESPIRATORY STIMULANTS (ANALEPTICS)

The use of these drugs has declined, and they now only have a place in certain specific conditions (e.g. in ventilatory failure due to chronic obstructive airways disease) and then only under expert supervision in hospital.

Administration and dosage

Doxapram is given by continuous intravenous infusion in a dosage of 2 mg/minute with frequent monitoring.

Contraindications

Respiratory stimulants should not be used in severe acute asthma or in respiratory depression caused by drug overdose or diseases of the nervous system.

Nikethamide and **ethamivan** are no longer recommended as respiratory stimulants since the therapeutic dose is near the dose causing toxic effects, especially convulsions.

RESPIRATORY SURFACTANTS

Improved neonatal health care and the advent of mechanical ventilation techniques have markedly reduced infant mortality from respiratory distress syndrome. Replacement therapy with **colfosceril palmitate** can further reduce the morbidity and mortality associated with this condition. Used either prophylactically in infants at risk of developing respiratory distress syndrome or as rescue therapy in infants with the established condition, **colfosceril palmitate** improves the clinical outcome in infants weighing 700 g or more at birth.

Neonatal respiratory distress syndrome

This is a condition caused by pulmonary immaturity affecting approximately 10% of infants born at less than 37 weeks' gestation. It is characterised by tachypnoea, expiratory grunting and cyanosis.

The primary pathogenic feature is a deficiency of endogenous lung surfactant. Surfactant is necessary to lower surface tension forces at the air–alveolar interface in order to prevent the alveoli collapsing during expiration. In the absence of surfactant the infant tires, and progressive pulmonary failure develops.

Administration

Respiratory surfactant is given by endotracheal tube, 67.5 mg/kg, which may be repeated after 12 hours. Continuous monitoring of heart rate and arterial oxygenation is required to avoid hyperoxaemia due to a rapid improvement in arterial oxygen concentration.

Side-effects

The incidence of pulmonary haemorrhage may be increased. Obstruction of the endotracheal tube may occur due to mucous secretions.

OXYGEN

Oxygen, which comprises approximately 21% of

air, is essential to all forms of animal life. Medical uses of oxygen include maintaining tissue oxygenation during anaesthesia; treatment of diseases, including chronic lung disease, myocardial infarction, and pulmonary embolism; treatment of cardiopulmonary arrest; and the treatment of newborn babies with respiratory distress.

Administration of oxygen

Oxygen should normally be prescribed by a doctor, stating: the word 'oxygen'; the type of appliance to be used (e.g. mask, nasal cannulae), and, in the case of a mask, the appropriate percentage of oxygen, the flow rate of oxygen (e.g. litres per minute) and the frequency of administration.

Oxygen may be delivered to the patient using either a low-flow system or a high-flow system. These terms refer to the rates of oxygen delivered by the equipment. Low-flow systems which include nasal cannulae and standard masks deliver oxygen at flow rates that supplement the oxygen concentration in room air. The range can vary from as low as 21% to as high as 90%. High-flow systems include masks and nebulisers incorporating the Venturi principle, provide the person's total inspiratory needs, and can deliver a precise and accurate flow rate.

Oxygen may be administered on a nurse's own initiative only in a life-threatening situation as it has potentially harmful effects in some patients.

Devices for the administration of oxygen

Face masks These are the commonest method for administering oxygen. A variety of masks is available which are lightweight, efficient, and, for most patients, comfortable, and which allow for observation of lip colour. Care must be taken to ensure that the mask fits snugly and that its position is maintained for effective delivery. Redness and sores can result from pressure and chafing from the mask over the bridge of the nose and from the elastic strap over the temporal region and above the ears. When discomfort persists after adjusting the tension of the elastic,

this may be relieved by inserting a neat layer of cotton wool between the appliance and the skin. In the course of time, the mask can become moist and sticky, and patients appreciate having it removed for a few moments to allow the face and the mask to be wiped clean and dry. Unless it is given at a concentration greater than 40%, oxygen taken through a mask does not require to be humidified as the air with which it mixes on inspiration contains sufficient water vapour.

Nasal cannulae These have an advantage over face masks in that they do not interfere to the same extent with feeding and communication. In addition, those patients who experience feelings of claustrophobia with a mask may find nasal cannulae acceptable. Before inserting nasal cannulae the patient is asked to blow his nose, or else the nostrils are cleaned with moist cotton-tipped applicators.

Oxygen tents and hoods These are used in paediatric wards as very young children do not tolerate oxygen masks. A nurse can do much to help a child overcome feelings of isolation by staying close by and making physical contact with him through the appropriate openings in the apparatus.

Safety

Oxygen administration is a potentially dangerous procedure and every precaution must be taken to ensure that standards of safety are maintained.

Although in many hospitals today oxygen is piped to the bedside or operating theatre, portable cylinders still have to be used, for example, on patient trolleys and in emergencies outside the ward. All nurses must therefore be able to identify a cylinder of oxygen correctly, i.e. black with a white shoulder and marked with the word **OXYGEN**. Since the oxygen in cylinders is in compressed form, valves or flow meters should only be removed by those trained to do so and in accordance with local policy. This noisy procedure should take place outside patient areas. At all times cylinders should be supported in a stand so that they cannot be knocked over, and they should be stored away from direct heat to prevent explosion. Nurses require to anticipate when a replacement cylinder will be needed, taking into account that there will be a rapid decrease in pressure as the gauge reaches the empty mark. Sufficient time also needs to be allowed for a new supply to be delivered to the ward.

Emergency equipment should be checked daily!

Precautions

Since oxygen supports combustion and can convert a spark into a flame, precautions must be taken in the immediate area of its use.

The patient involved, the surrounding patients and any visitors should have these precautions explained to them.

Printed warnings should be in evidence.

Items likely to be a danger should be removed – for example, matches and cigarette lighters, electric shavers and battery-operated or friction toys.

Care should be exercised when bedmaking and combing hair to reduce risk of sparks created by static electricity.

Observations

Periodic observations must be made by the nurse as long as the patient is receiving oxygen.

A check should be made of the patient's condition, generally, and his respirations, specifically. It is important to recognise whether the oxygen is benefiting the patient.

Acute hypoxaemia produces alterations to rate and depth of respiration; bounding pulse; high blood pressure; cyanosis; restlessness; and confusion.

Other observations include the flow of oxgyen; the volume of oxygen remaining in the cylinder; and the general environment to ensure that safety is being maintained.

In a study of 206 in-patients receiving oxygen, it was found that one in five had an incorrectly set flow rate. When working with the patient receiving oxygen, care should be taken to prevent obstruction of the oxygen tubing by, for example, a cot side, backrest or the patient himself.

Nursing points

To counteract the drying effect of oxygen, the patient should be assisted and encouraged to increase his fluid intake. For the same reason, the frequency of oral and nasal hygiene should be increased. Since flammable materials such as oils are unsafe to use in the presence of oxygen, water-soluble lubricants such as glycerin should be used for soothing the lips or nasal mucosa. Soft paraffin is ill-advised.

The education of patients

Patients with chronic obstructive airways disease may require to have oxygen therapy continued on their discharge from hospital. Time must be spent with the patient and, if possible, a member of his family, giving clear instructions on the safe and effective use of oxygen. The community nursing service should be informed so that a domiciliary visit may be arranged. A register is maintained of community pharmacists who stock oxygen cylinders and administration sets. These are supplied on prescription to patients who require to use oxygen or to have it on standby. Consideration is being given to supplying the more cost-effective oxygen concentrators for domiciliary use to those patients who would otherwise require many cylinders. Clearly, education of the patient and family in the safe use of oxgyen in the home is an important aspect of the work of community nurse, doctor and pharmacist.

MUCOLYTICS

Mucolytics such as **acetylcysteine** are used to ease expectoration by reducing sputum viscosity in chronic asthma and bronchitis. Their therapéutic value, however, is doubtful. Steam inhalation is beneficial in some cases.

INHALATIONS

Decongestants such as **steam** and **menthol** may be helpful when breathed in from a Nelson-type inhaler.

Nursing points

Take every possible precaution to prevent the patient from scalding himself while receiving an inhalation.

Make a careful assessment of the patient's capabilities.

The following groups of patients must be closely supervised:

psychiatric and mentally handicapped patients

the elderly and children

weak and febrile patients

patients suffering from cerebral hypoxia.

COUGH PREPARATIONS

Cough suppressants

The cough reflex is important in maintaining an open airway. A productive cough expels secretions and foreign material and should not be suppressed.

Cough suppressants act directly on the medullary mechanism in the brain, suppressing the cough reflex.

Usage and drugs used in this group

The effectiveness of the cough suppressants is dubious. Therefore they are only occasionally useful in the treatment of:

- a dry, hacking, non-productive cough which disturbs sleep **(codeine, dextromethorphan and pholcodine)**
- an extremely distressing cough associated with lung cancer; in this case the most powerful narcotics are used, e.g. **methadone (physeptone) linctus, morphine mixture or linctus.**

Side-effects and contraindications

All cough suppressants tend to cause constipation.

Large doses cause respiratory depression and are contraindicated in patients suffering from asthma.

Important point

Cough suppressants are not recommeded for children under the age of 1 year, and only occasionally in older children.

Expectorants

Theoretically, the expectorants liquefy mucus and facilitate its removal from the lungs through coughing. There is no scientific basis for this; however, the use of mixtures such as **ammonia** and **ipecacuanha** may serve a useful placebo function.

Demulcents

Demulcent cough preparations contain soothing, moistening substances such as **syrup** or **glycerol**. Some patients find this useful in relieving a dry irritating cough. A demulcent such as **simple linctus** is harmless and inexpensive.

NASAL DECONGESTANTS

Local nasal decongestants cause vasoconstriction and reduce congestion and oedema of the nasal mucosa.

Systemic decongestants also cause bronchodilation.

Preparations used in this group

Local preparations such as nasal drops and sprays contain e.g. **ephedrine, xylometazoline**.

Systemic preparations contain mixtures of paracetamol, antihistamines, and nasal decongestants such as **pseudoephedrine**. These preparations are of doubtful therapeutic value.

Side-effects

Local decongestants are subject to tolerance and rebound vasodilation and cause damage to the nasal mucosa and cilia. They are not generally effective for more than a few days and therefore have limited usefulness.

The sympathomimetic (e.g. pseudoephedrine) component in systemic preparations may cause tachycardia and a rise in blood pressure.

The antihistamine component may cause drowsiness and affect the ability to drive or operate machinery.

Caution

Systemic nasal decongestants should be avoided in patients with hypertension, hyperthyroidism, coronary heart disease, diabetes (interfere with blood sugar control) and in patients taking monoamine-oxidase inhibitors (MAOIs).

FURTHER READING

Morice A 1993 Bronchodilator: types, clinical uses and efficacy. Prescriber 4(11): 35–57

10

Drugs acting on the central nervous system

ANATOMY AND PHYSIOLOGY OF THE CENTRAL NERVOUS SYSTEM

The central nervous system comprises the brain, spinal cord and peripheral nerves. There is a vast number of nerves, otherwise termed neurones, each consisting of a nerve cell and its processes, axons and dendrites. The neurones conduct nerve impulses which are akin to tiny electrical charges. Axons, which are usually longer than dendrites, carry nerve impulses away from the cell. Large axons are surrounded by a myelin sheath. Dendrites are nerve fibres which carry impulses towards nerve cells. They form synapses with dendrites of other neurones or terminate in specialised sensory receptors such as those in the skin (Fig. 10.1).

Synapse and chemical transmitters

A synapse is where nerve impulses are transmitted from one neurone, called the presynaptic neurone, to another neurone, called the postsynaptic neurone. The axon of one neurone breaks up into tiny branches. Those terminate in presynaptic knobs which are in close proximity to the dendrites and the cell body of the next neurone. The space between them is the synaptic cleft. Chemical transmitters carry nerve impulses across the synaptic cleft (Fig. 10.2). Noradrenalin, gamma aminobutyric acid (GABA), acetylcholine, dopamine and 5-hydroxytryptamine act as chemical transmitters. The endings of autonomic nerves supplying smooth muscle and glands

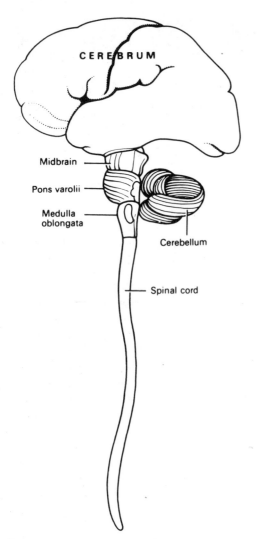

Figure 10.1 The brain. (From Ross & Wilson 1990 Anatomy and physiology in health and illness, 7th edn. Churchill Livingstone.)

release a transmitter substance which stimulates or depresses the activity of the structure.

The brain

The parts comprising the brain are the:

- cerebrum
- midbrain
- pons varolii   } brain stem
- medulla oblongata
- cerebellum

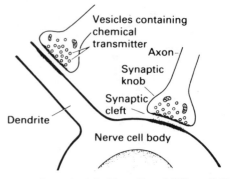

Figure 10.2 Synaptic cleft. (From Ross & Wilson 1990 Anatomy and physiology in health and illness, 7th edn. Churchill Livingstone.)

The peripheral part of the cerebrum is composed of nerve cells or grey matter forming the cerebral cortex, and the deeper layers consist of nerve fibres or white matter. The types of activity associated with the cerebral cortex are:

- mental activities – memory, reasoning, learning
- sensory perception – pain, temperature, touch, sight, hearing, taste, smell
- control of voluntary muscle contraction

The midbrain consists of nerve cells and fibres connecting the cerebrum with lower parts of the brain and with the spinal cord. The medulla oblongata extends from the pons varolii and is continuous with the spinal cord. The vital centres, comprising groups of cells associated with the autonomic reflex activity, lie within the medulla oblongata; they are listed in Table 10.1.

The cerebellum coordinates voluntary muscle movement, posture and balance. The sensory input is derived from the muscles, joints, eyes and ears. Damage to the cerebellum results in uncoordinated muscular movement such as staggering gait.

COMMON DISORDERS

Some common disorders are:

- insomnia
- anxiety

Table 10.1 The vital centres of the brain

Centre	Effect of stimulation
Cardiac centre	Sympathetic stimulation increases the rate and force of the heartbeat; parasympathetic stimulation has the opposite effect
Respiratory centre	Controls rate and depth of respiration
Vasomotor centre	Controls diameter of blood vessels; the vasomotor centre may be stimulated by baroreceptors, body temperature, emotion
Reflex centre	Irritating substances in the stomach or respiratory tract cause nerve impulses to pass to the medulla oblongata which initiate reflex actions such as vomiting, coughing or sneezing

- depression
- migraine
- nausea and vertigo
- epilepsy
- Parkinson's disease

INSOMNIA

Normal sleep is of two kinds:

- Slow wave sleep (SWS)
    heart rate, blood pressure, respiration are
        steady or in decline
    muscles are relaxed
    growth hormone secretion is maximal

- Rapid eye movement (REM)
    heart rate, blood pressure, respiration
        fluctuate
    cerebral blood flow increases above that
        during wakefulness
    skeletal muscles are profoundly relaxed
        though body movements are more
        pronounced (dreaming sleep)

A 'normal night' consists of a sleep latency period which varies from person to person (the 'dropping off' stage) followed by SWS sleep for about 1 hour, REM sleep for about 20 minutes, SWS for approximately 90 minutes, REM sleep for about 20 minutes and the rest of the night alternates between SWS and REM sleep until

wakefulness. Both kinds of sleep appear necessary for normal health.

Insomnia affects most of us at some time in our lives. For the majority it is transient but for some people insomnia becomes a chronic problem. Many people who sleep badly complain of tiredness during the day and mood disturbance. Insomnia may be characterised by:

- difficulty in falling asleep
- difficulty in staying asleep
- short unrefreshing sleep.

However, individual requirements differ, some people finding that only 4–6 hours is adequate, whereas others require 8 or 9 hours to feel refreshed the following day. In general, the elderly require less sleep than the young.

Hypnotics are often prescribed without adequate clinical evaluation to recognise underlying emotional or physical causes that may respond to specific psychotherapy or pharmacotherapy.

Where insomnia is caused by the following symptoms, treatment of these primary symptoms may relieve the problem: pain; dyspnoea; cough; frequency of micturition; excitatory drugs, e.g. caffeine; pruritus.

Insomnia is a common feature of psychiatric illness, particularly in anxiety states and depressive illness. Difficulty in getting to sleep is found in both depression and anxiety, and early morning awakening is common in depression. Choosing a medication to treat the illness with a secondary hypnotic activity can assist in alleviating the insomnia. For example, in depressed patients with early wakening a sedative antidepressant, e.g. amitriptyline, may be sufficient.

Certain drugs may produce insomnia, particularly the methylxanthines (theophylline and caffeine), the amphetamines and selegiline. Sleep disturbance is likely to be experienced in the early stages of treatment, and medication may need to be reviewed if problems persist.

Three main types of insomnia have been identified according to their duration:

- Transient insomnia. This may occur in those who normally sleep well, due to factors such as jet lag, shift work or acute stress and lasts only for a few days. Only one or two doses of a hypnotic should be given.

- Short-term insomnia. This is usually related to an emotional problem such as bereavement, problems at work or with marital relations. A hypnotic should not be given for more than 3 weeks, omitting doses when not required.
- Long-term (chronic) insomnia. This can have many causes. Prescription of hypnotics in long-term insomnia is rarely beneficial.

Non-drug treatment

A regular bedtime routine helps to induce sleep. Warm, milky drinks (not tea or coffee) can help. Relaxation exercises or relaxing with a book may be beneficial. An equable environmental temperature will be conducive to sleep.

Drug treatment

Hypnotics and anxiolytics

Hypnotic drugs are thought to inhibit excitatory pathways in the brain. Benzodiazepines facilitate transmission of gamma-aminobutyric acid (GABA), an inhibitory neurotransmitter.

Benzodiazepines Benzodiazepines reduce the latent period and prolong the duration of sleep. Approximately 25% of total normal sleep time is REM sleep. This can be reduced by as much as 75% by the administration of benzodiazepines. When the benzodiazepine is stopped, there is a rebound increase in REM sleep as if the body required to recover what has been lost. Nightmares occur with severe rebound and it is at this point that many people resort to restarting the medication. The rebound increase in REM sleep does revert to normal over a period of weeks after ceasing medication, but it is a major factor in the development of dependence on this group of drugs.

Benzodiazepines that are promoted for use as hypnotics may be divided into those with a short or longer duration of action. Shorter-acting benzodiazepines (temazepam and lormetazepam – half-lives of 5–6 hours) are indicated for

patients for whom residual effects are undesirable and they are generally preferred when insomnia is not accompanied by daytime anxiety. They are also the most suitable benzodiazepine hypnotics for elderly people, although caution is still required. It should be noted that half-lives of benzodiazepines may be greatly extended in the elderly where hepatic and renal function are known to deteriorate with age. The dosage should therefore be reduced accordingly. Benzodiazepines, such as nitrazepam, which have long half-lives should be avoided, particularly in the elderly; the same is true where the metabolites of benzodiazepines have long half-lives. Benzodiazepines have hangover effects such as drowsiness and lightheadedness the following day, confusion and ataxia particularly in the elderly.

Interactions Alcohol and benzodiazepines taken concomitantly may result in greater impairment of psychomotor function than either agent alone. The usual effect of the combination of alcohol and benzodiazepines is an increase in the sedative effects of the benzodiazepine.

Dependence Dependence on benzodiazepines does occur and is now regarded as a serious problem, particularly with longer term treatment and in patients with some types of personality disorder. Patients taking these drugs, even in therapeutic doses, may develop a physical withdrawal syndrome. The main symptom of this is anxiety, which usually subsides in 2–4 weeks, but sometimes lasts longer, although many patients would have been prone to anxiety prior to treatment. In addition, depression, nausea, depersonalisation, and perceptual changes such as intolerance of loud noises, bright lights or touch may occur. Insomnia may also be expected but the symptoms are variable. Occasionally, epileptic seizures, confusion and visual hallucinations may occur.

Stopping treatment with short-acting benzodiazepines leads to withdrawal symptoms within about 2–3 days, whereas with longer-acting drugs there may be a delay of 7 days. Patients being weaned from benzodiazepines need close supervision and support, and the drugs should be withdrawn slowly over weeks or even months.

Benzodiazepine withdrawal The benzodiazepine is substituted with an equivalent dose of diazepam, e.g. diazepam 10 mg is equivalent to temazepam 20 mg or nitrazepam 10 mg. Diazepam is used because of its long half-life. The withdrawal symptoms from diazepam appear to be less severe with little associated craving. There may be a problem with daytime sedation.

Once substitution has been achieved a gradual reduction of the diazepam dosage should follow. Diazepam is available in 2 mg, 5 mg and 10 mg tablets, all of which can be halved, and in an elixir of 2 mg in 5 ml. Stepwise reductions in dosage should be made weekly, fortnightly or even monthly, depending on the patient's response. These reductions can be in steps of 1 mg, 2 mg or 2.5 mg fortnightly. If withdrawal symptoms occur the dose is maintained until symptoms improve. As the dose is reduced small reductions are made as it is better to reduce too slowly than too quickly.

Once the patient is at a dosage of 0.5 mg daily, the dose interval can be increased to every 2 or 3 days. Many long-term benzodiazepine users can successfully withdraw without experiencing significant withdrawal symptoms. A number of patients may find it extremely difficult to withdraw completely.

Chloral derivatives Drugs such as chloral hydrate and chloral betaine have been used as hypnotics for a long time, particularly for elderly patients. Gastric irritation has been reported, the incidence being higher with chloral hydrate than with triclofos sodium.

Chloral hydrate can displace anticoagulants such as warfarin from plasma protein binding sites, and may produce excessive prolongation of prothrombin time and a risk of haemorrhage in anticoagulated patients. Chloral derivatives should therefore be avoided in those patients. Use of chloral derivatives can also lead to dependence.

Chlormethiazole Chlormethiazole has both hypnotic and anticonvulsant properties. There is a danger of respiratory depression in overdose, especially in combination with alcohol. It has a short half-life and may cause less confusion than benzodiazepines in the elderly. It may also be useful if benzodiazepines are ineffective or not tolerated.

Antihistamines Antihistamines are commonly prescribed as hypnotics and sedatives in paediatric practice. Caution should be exercised as these drugs can produce a paradoxical hyperexcitability in children. In general, hypnotics should not be used for children except for occasional use in night terrors and sleepwalking. Promethazine is occasionally used short-term in children.

Zopiclone The hypnotic effect of zopiclone is similar to the benzodiazepines. It was originally claimed to have less potential for dependence. However, a bulletin from the Committee on the Safety of Medicines states that the drug has the same potential as the benzodiazepines for causing adverse psychiatric reactions, including dependence.

Table 10.2 indicates the half-lives and dosages of commonly used hypnotics.

Summary

The ideal hypnotic does not exist, and hypnotics should be reserved for people whose insomnia is debilitating. They should be prescribed for short courses and only when all underlying causes of insomnia have been investigated and treated.

Table 10.2 Half-lives and dosages of commonly used hypnotics*

Drug	Elimination half-life (hours)	Hypnotic dose
Benzodiazepines		
Diazepam	20–100 (36–200)	5–10 mg
Loprazolam	6–12	1 mg
Lormetazepam	10–12	1 mg
Nitrazepam	15–38	5–10 mg
Temazepam	8–15	10–30 mg
Non-benzodiazepines		
Zopiclone	5–6	7.5–15 mg
Chloral hydrate	(8)	0.5–1 g
Chlormethiazole	4	192–384 mg
Antihistamines		
Promethazine	12	50 mg

* The figure in brackets is the half-life of pharmacologically active metabolite. Doses are adult doses. Dosage should be reduced in the elderly.

ANXIETY

Anxiety is a normal reaction we all experience when faced with major events in our lives, such as moving house, attending interviews, etc. It only becomes a medical problem when it is excessive or inappropriate. It can then be described as anxiety neurosis.

Anxiety neurosis is twice as common in women as in men; it is most prevalent in young women. The patient may describe a sensation of fear or dread, varying from mild to an overwhelming feeling of terror, the latter leading to panic attacks.

Physical symptoms include tremor, tensing of muscles, perspiration (particularly of the hands and forehead), hypertension, palpitations, gastrointestinal disturbances (such as frequency of defaecation), back pain, chest pain, dizziness and dyspnoea. These symptoms are very marked in panic attacks.

Treatment

Treatment of anxiety neurosis includes psychotherapy (relaxation, behavioural and reassurance techniques), as well as drug therapy. The decision whether to use psychotherapy, drug therapy or a combination of both is determined by the practitioner.

Drug treatment relies mainly on the use of anxiolytics such as benzodiazepines and buspirone, but beta-blockers, antidepressants with a sedative action (such as clomipramine) and antipsychotics (such as zuclopenthixol) have also been used, with varying degrees of success.

Benzodiazepines Benzodiazepines have both anxiolytic and hypnotic effects. Their relative safety in overdose and proven anxiolytic actions have led to widespread use.

The decision to start giving benzodiazepines for anxiety should normally be limited to patients whose anxiety is causing unacceptable distress. Treatment should usually be for a limited period only because of the increasing risk of dependence developing. The shorter-acting drugs such as oxazepam or lorazepam have sometimes been preferred for acute anxiety, although withdrawal symptoms may be more of a problem with these drugs.

In view of the similarities between different benzodiazepines, a limited list of drugs available for NHS prescription has been introduced. It includes diazepam, chlordiazepoxide, lorazepam, oxazepam, and some drugs marketed as hypnotics (nitrazepam, loprazolam, lormetazepam and temazepam).

Buspirone has a structure entirely different from that of other anxiolytics. The recommended dose range is 15–30 mg a day in divided doses. Buspirone is not very effective in patients who have not responded to benzodiazepines, and its anxiolytic effect is relatively slow to develop, which may be a disadvantage in some circumstances.

Side-effects are not usually severe, although gastrointestinal upset, dizziness and headache have occurred. No withdrawal symptoms have been reported on stopping treatment after 6 weeks to 6 months, and there is no evidence of tolerance. Buspirone does not appear to have an additive effect with alcohol. Diazepam remains the drug of choice for anxiety neurosis.

Antipsychotic drugs Antipsychotic drugs, also known as neuroleptics, are used in the symptomatic treatment of psychoses, including schizophrenia and the manic phase of manic depressive illness. Drugs in this group act primarily to produce emotional calmness and relaxation without significant sedation, hypnosis, motor impairment or euphoria. Antipsychotics can also be used to quieten mentally retarded children and agitated elderly patients. Shortly after administration of antipsychotics, a quieting and calming effect occurs. After several days, formerly fearful schizophrenic patients are no longer bothered by delusions and hallucinations; withdrawn patients become more responsive to communication. After several weeks' therapy, the patient becomes more coherent, and hallucinations and delusions frequently disappear.

The mechanism of action is complex, and many details remain to be established. Antipsychotic drugs inhibit the action of dopamine on certain post-synaptic dopamine receptors.

This causes parkinsonism adverse effects. Various peripheral effects are also attributable to their antimuscarinic properties and peripheral alpha-adrenergic blockade.

Antipsychotics can be classified on the basis of chemical structure. The phenothiazines can be divided into three main groups on the basis of difference in adverse effects (see Table 10.3).

The non-phenothiazine antipsychotics tend to have adverse effects similar to those of the phenothiazines of group 3. They can be divided into several classes of drug (Box 10.1).

Box 10.1   The non-phenothiazine antipsychotic drugs

Butyrophenones	Benperidol, droperidol, haloperidol and trifluperidol
Diphenylbutylpiperidines	Fluspirilene and zuclopenthixol
Phenylpiperazine	Oxypertine
Dibenzodiazepines	Loxapine and clozapine

Clozapine differs in that it is sedative with fewer extrapyramidal effects.

An oral preparation will produce effects in 2 to 4 hours, and an intramuscular injection in 15 to 30 minutes. Although the onset of action and tranquillising effects usually occur in a few hours, the antipsychotic effects (normalising of thoughts, moods and actions) may take several weeks to appear.

Choice of therapy

Chlorpromazine is widely used. It has significant sedating effects and is useful for controlling violent patients without causing stupor. Some antipsychotic drugs have mild antidepressant activity while others exacerbate depression.

- Antidepressant action
    chlorpromazine
    flupenthixol
    thioridazine

- Exacerbate depression
    fluphenazine
    pimozide
    pipothiazine

Chlorpromazine is also used to treat nausea, vomiting and intractable hiccups. Photosensitisation is more common with chlorpromazine than other antipsychotics. Thioridazine is useful for treating the elderly as there is a reduced incidence of extrapyramidal symptoms. Sulpiride in lower doses has an alerting effect on apathetic, withdrawn schizophrenics. Clozapine is used to treat patients unresponsive or intolerant to other antipsychotic drugs. Agranulocytosis is particularly troublesome and regular blood counts must be performed. Withdrawal of antipsychotics after long-term therapy should always be gradual.

Table 10.3   Adverse effects of phenothiazines

Group	Adverse effects Sedative	Antimuscarinic	Extrapyramidal
Group 1 Chlorpromazine Methotrimeprazine Promazine	Pronounced	Moderate	Moderate
Group 2 Pericyazine Pipothiazine Thioridazine	Moderate	Pronounced	Low
Group 3 Fluphenazine Perphenazine Prochlorperazine Trifluoperazine	Low	Low	Pronounced

Adverse effects

Antipsychotic drugs commonly produce adverse reactions to various degrees.

Extrapyramidal effects

These are common and depend partly on dosage and partly on the susceptibility of patients.

- Dystonia. This is characterised by spasms of the tongue, face, neck and back. Torticollis (a twisted position of the neck), grimacing, tongue protrusion and drooling can occur. This usually disappears with dosage reduction, or benztropine or biperiden may be administered. In acute dystonic reaction procyclidine is administered intravenously.
- Akathisia. This is a continuous restlessness or inability to sit or stand still. It is more common in elderly females.
- Tardive dyskinesia. This arises from long-term use and is characterised by chewing, lip smacking and rhythmic darting of the tongue. Elderly females receiving excessive doses are most at risk and in some cases the condition is permanent, even when antipsychotic drugs are withdrawn.
- Parkinsonism. This results from a direct blockade of dopamine receptors by antipsychotic agents producing muscle tremors, shuffling gait, drooling, bradykinesia and akinesia. These symptoms can be alleviated by lowering the dose. Antimuscarinics must be used with caution as care is needed with regard to glaucoma, urinary retention and drowsiness. They should not be used routinely as there is an increased risk of developing tardive dyskinesia.

Alpha blockade

Vasodilation leads to postural hypotension, reflex tachycardia and loss of body temperature control which can lead to hypothermia or, in hot weather, hyperthermia.

Antimuscarinic effects

These include dry mouth, urinary retention, constipation and blurring of vision.

Antipsychotic depot injections

Depot injections (see Table 10.4) have been a major breakthrough in psychiatric care and have enabled numerous patients to be treated at home and in day-care centres. Apart from aiding compliance, intramuscular routes sustain a more predictable therapeutic level. Patients should be given a small test-dose as undesirable side-effects are prolonged. In general not more than 2–3 ml should be administered at any one site. When transferring from oral to depot therapy, oral dosage should be gradually phased out. Extrapyramidal symptoms occur frequently.

Antimanic drugs Lithium salts have a narrow therapeutic/toxic ratio. It is essential to monitor serum levels, starting weekly until the required level is established, then monthly for 3 months, thereafter 3-monthly. The therapeutic range is 0.5–0.8 mmol per litre, taken 12 hours after the last dose. The drug should be started at a low dose 250–400 mg daily. In an acute attack of mania, treatment in tandem with an antipsychotic drug is usually required because it may take a few days for lithium to exert its antimanic effects, after which treatment with the antipsychotic is tailed off.

The side-effects of lithium include gastrointestinal upset (particularly early in treatment), fine tremor, weight gain and hypothyroidism. Toxicity can occur at levels above 1.2 mmol/litre, causing an increase in the above symptoms with a coarse tremor and ataxia. This may lead to coma and death.

Table 10.4 Equivalent doses of depot antipsychotics

Antipsychotic	Dose (mg)	Interval
Flupenthixol decanoate	40	2 weeks
Fluphenazine decanoate	25	2 weeks
Fluphenazine enanthate	25	2 weeks
Haloperidol decanoate	100	4 weeks
Pipothiazine palmitate	50	4 weeks
Zuclopenthixol decanoate	200	2 weeks

Interactions Lithium toxicity is made worse by sodium depletion so that the concurrent use of diuretics (particularly thiazides) should be avoided. NSAIDs also cause an increase in lithium levels. Every patient taking lithium should have a lithium card. The information on the card needs to be discussed with the patient and the lithium brand name recorded (Fig. 10.3). Carbamazepine may be used for the prophylaxis of manic depressive illness on patients unresponsive to lithium.

DEPRESSION

We tend to feel unhappy when things are going badly and it is normal to suffer from depression at these times. However, a person will be considered to be suffering from depressive illness only when they have experienced several symptoms of depression each day for a period of over 2 weeks. The symptoms of depression are as follows:

- Variability in mood. There is a general feeling of miserableness. The feeling of sadness may

A

THINKING ABOUT STARTING A FAMILY?

Because Lithium can affect the unborn baby do NOT become pregnant without first talking to your doctor. If you are pregnant tell your doctor now.

Published by the Royal Pharmaceutical Society of Great Britain, 1 Lambeth High Street, London, SE1 7JN.
Printed July 1991

KEEP YOUR TABLETS IN A SAFE PLACE WELL OUT OF THE REACH OF CHILDREN.

PLEASE RECORD YOUR BLOOD LEVEL OF LITHIUM

DATE TAKEN	BLOOD LEVEL	DAILY DOSE

LITHIUM TREATMENT CARD

CARRY THIS CARD WITH YOU AT ALL TIMES. SHOW IT TO ANY DOCTOR OR NURSE WHO TREATS YOU AND ANY PHARMACIST YOU BUY MEDICINES FROM.

NAME ....

PREPARATION
OF LITHIUM ....

Should a different proprietary product be prescribed, the card must be suitably endorsed.

B

HOW SHOULD I TAKE THE TABLETS?

Swallow each tablet whole or broken in half, with water. Do NOT chew or crush it. Try to take the dose at the same time each day.

WHAT SHOULD I DO IF I MISS A DOSE?

Do NOT double your next dose. If you find you have missed a few doses, start taking your usual dose on the day you remember and tell your doctor.

WHY MUST I HAVE A BLOOD TEST?

This is to check the amount of lithium in your blood. It is very important to have the correct amount because too much can be dangerous. Take the blood test ABOUT 12 HOURS AFTER the last dose of lithium.

CAN I DRINK ALCOHOL?

It is safe to drink SMALL quantities.

CAN I TAKE OTHER MEDICINES WITH LITHIUM?

Some medicines can change the amount of lithium in the blood. These include diuretic (water) tablets and capsules, some pain killers and some indigestion mixtures and laxatives. So check with your doctor or pharmacist before taking other medicines.

Please note: it is safe to take paracetamol but not ibuprofen.

WHAT ELSE ALTERS THE LITHIUM LEVEL?

The level can be altered by the amount of fluids you drink, changes in the amount of salt in your food, sweating more than usual (in hot weather, fever or infection), severe vomiting, severe diarrhoea and a low salt diet. Check with your doctor if any of these things happen.

SIGNS OF A HIGH LITHIUM LEVEL

Vomiting, severe diarrhoea, unusual drowsiness, muscle weakness and feeling very giddy may mean that your level of lithium is too high. Stop taking the tablets and talk to your doctor IMMEDIATELY.

DOES LITHIUM HAVE SIDE EFFECTS?

Some slight effects (such as sickness, shaking) may occur at first but they usually wear off if blood tests are normal. Discuss this with your doctor. Some patients may gain weight but this can be prevented with a sensible diet.

HOW LONG WILL I HAVE TO TAKE LITHIUM?

Lithium is a way of preventing illness so you may have to take it for many years. Never stop taking the tablets without asking your doctor.

Figure 10.3 Lithium treatment card. A. Front. B. Reverse.

not be alleviated by circumstances normally causing happiness, e.g. hearing good news. Often there are mood changes throughout the day (diurnal variation of mood) with transient brighter periods – stimulation of work or congenial company.

- Lack of interest and enjoyment (anhedonia). There is no longer interest in hobbies, and no pleasure from day-to-day living.
- Sleep disturbance/insomnia. Difficulty falling asleep and early morning wakening are experienced. Patients usually waken unrefreshed even where a long sleep has occurred.
- Slowness (psychomotor retardation). There may be a general slowing of activity, movement and speech.
- Decreased energy and tiredness. Everything becomes an effort. Routine tasks are not carried out and personal appearance is neglected which may result in an unkempt appearance. Loss of libido is common.
- Impaired appetite. It is common to experience a loss of appetite, resulting in weight loss. Constipation may become a problem. However, in certain cases excessive eating and weight gain may occur.
- Anxiety. The patient may have many symptoms of anxiety. He may be agitated and irritable, with a feeling of restlessness. These may be accompanied by a sense of worthlessness. The patient can see little reason for living (the rates of suicide are increased among depressed patients). Outlook is entirely pessimistic and this may be accompanied by guilt feelings from the past. Minor indiscretions or problems get blown out of all proportion. There is seen to be no future, only bleakness.

Types of depression

The term 'reactive depression' is used to describe situations where the depression is a reaction to circumstances beyond the individual's control. Endogenous depression is where the depression has no obvious cause, but appears to come from within. Reactive depression presents as an illness of mild to moderate severity in which many of the symptoms mentioned above are present. Endogenous depression is regarded as a more severe form of the illness. In addition to the symptoms described above being very marked and of great intensity, the sufferer may also have hallucinations and delusions.

Causes of depression

The biochemial disorders causing depression are not yet fully understood. There are indications that reduced levels of monoamines (noradrenalin and 5-hydroxytryptamine) in the brain occur in patients with depression.

- Reserpine depletes brain monoamines and can cause depression.
- Drugs which increase monoamine levels relieve the symptoms of depression, e.g. monoamine-oxidase inhibitors inhibit the metabolism of noradrenalin, 5-hydroxytryptamine and dopamine.
- It has been found that brain 5-hydroxytryptamine levels are lower in depressed suicide patients than in controls dying from other causes.

In addition to reserpine, other drug treatments that have been reported to cause depression include methyldopa, nifedipine and clonidine.

The length of the illness is variable, but it frequently lasts up to 9 months. Some people will get better without treatment and some will respond, or respond only partially, to tricyclic antidepressants, the standard in terms of antidepressant efficacy.

Tricyclic and related antidepressant drugs

It is believed that tricyclic antidepressants produce their therapeutic effect by preventing the reuptake of noradrenalin and 5-hydroxytryptamine. Some of the antidepressants inhibit noradrenalin uptake more than 5-hydroxytryptamine uptake (e.g. desipramine, nortriptyline), some the reverse (e.g. imipramine, amitriptyline, clomipramine) while others are non-selective for the two amines. Mianserin does not inhibit monoamine uptake at all.

Tricyclic antidepressants have in the past been the drug treatment of choice for depressive illness. A clinical response to these drugs takes place slowly over a period of 2–4 weeks. This in conjunction with the side-effect profile accounts for a high rate of non-compliance in the short term. The pharmacist has an important counselling role here in order to encourage the patient to take the medicine. A reasonable trial for a clinical response should be at least 4–6 weeks at an adequate dose. This may be too long to wait where severe depression or threat of suicide is hazardous and referral to hospital for electroconvulsive therapy may be required.

There are many side-effects associated with the tricyclic antidepressants. The most common are anticholinergic side-effects, e.g. dry mouth, blurred vision, and constipation. More serious and occurring less frequently are failure to pass urine, closed-angle glaucoma, jaundice, depression of the white blood cell count and convulsions. Cardiac effects include postural hypotension, arrhythmias and tachycardia.

To avoid a high incidence of unpleasant side-effects, the starting dose should be low, at about 25–50 mg of amitriptyline at night. Over a period of 2–3 weeks the dosage is increased to an adequate therapeutic level of 125–150 mg, or higher if required. Treatment should be continued for at least a month at the optimal level before any attempt is made at dose reduction. Treatment should not be withdrawn prematurely otherwise symptoms are likely to recur. An average course of antidepressants would be for 6 months to 1 year and should be given for at least 3 months after recovery.

Care must be taken in withdrawing antidepressants following treatment. Reduction in dosage should be carried out gradually over a period of about 4 weeks otherwise withdrawal symptoms will be experienced. These include gastrointestinal symptoms of nausea, vomiting and anorexia accompanied by headache, dizziness and insomnia. Panic anxiety and motor restlessness may also occur.

Many tricyclic antidepressants have a long half-life (e.g. amitriptyline 32–40 hours) which allows them to be taken as a single daily dose. Many also have sedative properties so that they can be prescribed at night to help treat insomnia in the short term. This also helps to alleviate the anticholinergic side-effects. The return of a more normal sleep pattern results as depression is alleviated. Taking more than one tricyclic antidepressant at the same time is not recommended. There is no evidence that side-effects are minimised. Examples of tricyclic and related antidepressants are listed in Table 10.5.

Monoamine-oxidase inhibitors (MAOIs)

Monoamine oxidase has a variety of isoenzymes which have been classified as type A (present in the gut and liver) and type B (present in the brain). The different isoenzymes have different selectivities for amine substrates:

- Monoamine oxidase A – metabolises 5-hydroxytryptamine (5-HT) and noradrenalin
- Monoamine oxidase B – metabolises phenylethylamine and benzylamine
- Dopamine and tyramine are metabolised by both the type A and type B enzymes

Since monoamine oxidase is one of the two main enzymes involved in the metabolism of 5-hydroxytryptamine, noradrenalin and dopamine, the MAOIs cause an increase of these substances in the brain. It is this effect that is thought to be the primary action of MAOIs in relieving depression. The MAOIs are not used as commonly as the tricyclic antidepressants, mainly because of problems associated with treatment. The most commonly prescribed are phenelzine and tranylcypromine. As with the tricyclics the dose needs to be built up gradually to a therapeutic level. There will be a time lag of 4–6 weeks to achieve full antidepressant effect. The MAOIs can cause anticholinergic side-effects, especially tranylcypromine. They are very alerting causing sleep disturbance. To avoid this, the last dose should be taken at lunchtime. Postural hypotension and weight gain can occur. As with all antidepressants, drug treatment

Table 10.5 Tricyclic and related antidepressants

Drug	Sedative/less sedative	Notes
Amitriptyline	Sedative	Probably the most widely used tricyclic antidepressant. Can be taken once daily, best at night. It is metabolised to nortriptyline. Half-life 32–40 hours. Suitable for anxious and agitated patients.
Amoxapine	Less sedative	Side-effects include tardive dyskinesia. Overdosage has been associated with seizures.
Clomipramine	Sedative	Particularly effective in patients with obsessional disorders and in some phobic states. Half-life 17–28 hours.
Dothiepin	Sedative	Similar to amitriptyline with no significant advantages. Cardiovascular side-effects are common. Dothiepin is very dangerous in overdose.
Doxepin	Sedative	It is less likely than other tricyclics to cause arrhythmias, and it has less marked anticholinergic side-effects – which may be an advantage in older patients or in the presence of cardiovascular disease. Half-life 8–25 hours.
Imipramine	Less sedative	Widely used. Half-life 6–20 hours. Metabolised to desipramine which has a longer half-life. Used in withdrawn apathetic patients.
Lofepramine	Less sedative	Has fewer and milder anticholinergic side-effects compared with amitriptyline. Hyponatraemia has been reported.
Nortriptyline	Less sedative	Similar to amitriptyline, but less sedative. Rarely used.
Protriptyline	Stimulant	Similar to imipramine, but cardiovascular side-effects are more common.
Trimipramine	Sedative	Cardiovascular and anticholinergic side-effects are more common than with other tricyclics.
Maprotiline	Sedative	Lower incidence of anticholinergic side-effects, but rashes are more common and convulsions can occur in patients with or without a history of epilepsy.
Mianserin	Sedative	Has a lower incidence of cardiovascular and anticholinergic side-effects than older antidepressants but has caused blood dyscrasias more frequently. Also causes jaundice. A full blood count should be carried out 4-weekly during the first 3 months of treatment, thereafter at longer intervals.
Trazodone	Sedative	Reported to reduce anxiety as well as depression. Similar to lofepramine but has sedative properties. Toxic confusional states have been reported. Taking with food slows down absorption resulting in reduced side-effects.

needs to be continued at least 3 months after the full antidepressant effect has become apparent. When no longer required, the drug should be withdrawn over a period of 4 weeks. Because of drug and food interactions, MAOIs are usually reserved for patients who have failed to respond to other forms of drug therapy.

Adverse effects

Hypertensive crisis is a rare but severe side-effect. It is due to MAOIs preventing metabolism of tyramine in tyramine-rich food or drink. A hypertensive crisis may also arise with sympathomimetic drugs.

Tyramine Irreversible MAOIs block the ability of monoamine oxidase to inactivate tyramine in the gastrointestinal tract and liver for a long period of time. The tyramine is present in foods such as cheese, salted fish, broad bean pods, Bovril, Oxo, Marmite, shrimp paste, paté and drinks including red wine, beer, ale, and non-alcoholic beers and lagers. Excess tyramine enters the bloodstream and releases noradrenalin from its storage sites located in the sympathetic nerve endings. This can cause vasoconstriction and an increase in blood pressure which can result in a potentially fatal reaction characterised by severe hypertension associated with severe headache, sweating, flushing, nausea, vomiting and palpitation. Patients on MAOIs are restrained to a low tyramine diet. They are given a treatment card (Fig. 10.4).

Sympathomimetics Sympathomimetics such as

TREATMENT CARD

Carry this card with you at all times. Show it to any doctor who may treat you other than the doctor who prescribed this medicine, and to your dentist if you require dental treatment.

INSTRUCTIONS TO PATIENTS

Please read carefully

While taking this medicine and for 14 days after your treatment finishes you must observe the following simple instructions:-

1　Do not eat CHEESE, PICKLED HERRING OR BROAD BEAN PODS.

2　Do not eat or drink BOVRIL, OXO, MARMITE or ANY SIMILAR MEAT OR YEAST EXTRACT.

3　Eat only FRESH foods and avoid food that you suspect could be stale or 'going off'. This is especially important with meat, fish, poultry or offal. Avoid game.

4　Do not take any other MEDICINES (including tablets, capsules, nose drops, inhalations or suppositories) whether purchased by you or previously prescribed by your doctor, without first consulting your doctor or your pharmacist.

　　NB *Treatment for coughs and colds, pain relievers, tonics and laxatives are medicines.*

5　Avoid alcoholic drinks and de-alcoholised (low alcohol) drinks.

Keep a careful note of any food or drink that disagrees with you, avoid it and tell your doctor.

Report any unusual or severe symptoms to your doctor and follow any other advice given by him.

| M A O I | Prepared by The Pharmaceutical Society and the British Medical Association on behalf of the Health Departments of the United Kingdom |

Printed in the UK for HMSO 8217411/150M/9.89/45292
Revised Sep. 1989

Figure 10.4　MAOI treatment card.

pseudoephedrine and phenylpropanolamine, which release noradrenalin at nerve endings, may be potentiated by MAOIs. A severe hypertensive crisis may result. An early warning symptom may be a throbbing headache. Sympathomimetics are present in many cough mixtures and decongestant nasal drops, and patients must be warned not to use these medicines. The danger of the reaction persists for up to 14 days after treatment with MAOIs has been discontinued.

Dopamine receptor agonists Levodopa may cause similar hypertensive reactions in patients taking non-selective MAOIs and should be avoided.

Tricyclic antidepressants Since tricyclic anti-depressants inhibit noradrenalin re-uptake by nerve endings, the combination of tricyclics with MAOIs is hazardous. MAOIs should not be started until at least a week after tricyclics and related antidepressants have been stopped and 2 weeks after cessation of 5-HT re-uptake inhibitors (5 weeks for fluoxetine). Similarly, other antidepressants should not be given to patients for 14 days after treatment with MAOIs has been discontinued.

Selective monoamine-oxidase inhibitors

Since the transmitters considered to play a role in depression are serotonin, noradrenalin and dopamine, the antidepressant effects are thought to depend largely or exclusively on inhibition of MAO-A (Fig. 10.5).

Drugs which reversibly affect mainly MAO-A are known as reversible inhibitors of MAO-A (RIMAs) (Fig. 10.6) as distinguished from the previously discussed irreversible MAOI (Fig. 10.7). A RIMA, which preferentially inhibits MAO-A, interferes less with the metabolism of tyramine. Reversible inhibition of MAO-A does not provoke an increase in blood pressure for two reasons. First, by preferentially inhibiting MAO-A, it leaves MAO-B free to metabolise ingested tyramine. Second, when an excess of tyramine is ingested, the RIMA inhibitor will dissociate with MAO-A, allowing the enzyme to metabolise the excess. An example of this type of drug is moclobemide.

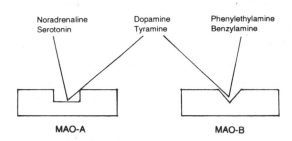

Figure 10.5　Metabolism of transmitters by monoamine-oxidase A and B.

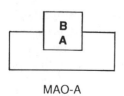

MAO-A   MAO-B

Figure 10.6 Selective MAOI.

Table 10.6	5-Hydroxytryptamine re-uptake inhibitors

Drug	Average daily dose/range
Fluoxetine	20 mg
Fluvoxamine	100–200 mg
Paroxetine	20–40 mg
Sertraline	50–100 mg

Moclobemide

Moclobemide is comparable in its effect to the tricyclic antidepressants and the MAOIs. It is equally effective against endogenous and non-endogenous depression. The usual dosage range is 300–450 mg daily in two or three divided doses. There is 95% absorption but extensive first-pass metabolism results in an oral bioavailability of 45–60%. The half-life is 1–2 hours.

Moclobemide is well tolerated, largely devoid of anticholinergic effects, postural hypotension or weight gain. The main side-effects include dizziness, headache, dry mouth, tremor, insomnia and nausea.

5-Hydroxytryptamine re-uptake inhibitors

The 5-HT re-uptake inhibitors, a relatively new class of antidepressant, include fluvoxamine, fluoxetine, paroxetine and sertraline (Table 10.6). They appear to be as effective as the tricyclic antidepressants with a similar time lag of 4–6 weeks before achieving the full antidepressant effect. They have a narrower spectrum of adverse effects with the potential, therefore, of better compliance and a lower incidence of relapse. The drugs are less sedating than the tricyclics, have low cardiotoxicity and have few antimuscarinic side-effects. So far they have not been shown to

cause any problems in overdosage. The main problems are nausea, vomiting and diarrhoea.

MIGRAINE

Migraine affects at least 10% of the population of the United Kingdom. Attacks generally start in the teens or 20s. After puberty, migraine affects more women than men. During the reproductive period about 20% of women suffer, particularly those in their early 40s. Headache is only one symptom of migraine which has been defined as 'episodic headaches lasting between 2 and 72 hours with each attack accompanied by visual and/or gastrointestinal disturbance'. Migraine's most common accompanying symptoms are photophobia, nausea and vomiting.

Migraine is classified into two main types:

- Migraine without aura (common migraine)
- Migraine with aura (classical migraine)

Only 10% of attacks are preceded by an aura. Patients who experience an aura can start their migraine treatment during this phase. Visual aura takes the form of blind spots. Other symptoms are sensory disturbances such as 'pins and needles' in one arm moving up to the face.

Triggers

Several factors need to be present to trigger a migraine attack. The triggers are not the same for everyone. The triggers are:

Hormonal factors (women)
pregnancy
oral contraception
hormone replacement therapy
menstruation

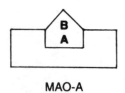

MAO-A   MAO-B

Figure 10.7 Non-selective MAOI.

Environmental factors
   bright or flickering lights
   overexertion
   travel
Emotional factors
Head and neck pain
Insufficient food – missed meals
Specific foods
   cheese
   chocolate
   caffeine
   citrus fruits.

Treatment

Early treatment during attacks with effective drugs is of the utmost importance as the efficacy of oral medication during migraine is impaired by gastric stasis. Patients should carry medication at all times. A drop in blood sugar precedes a migraine attack and food is an important part of treatment. If patients feel too nauseous the attack is being treated too late. For many, sleep is the best natural remedy and applications of hot and cold compresses can help ease the pain.

Drug treatment

This includes analgesics, anti-emetics, ergotamine and sumatriptan. Simple analgesics such as paracetamol and aspirin may be insufficient. There are specific 'over the counter' migraine preparations such as Migraleve (contains buclizine, paracetamol and codeine). Where these are unsuccessful, an anti-emetic with an effect on gastric motility is used with analgesics. Metoclopramide by mouth, or if vomiting is likely, by intramuscular injection relieves the nausea.

Ergotamine is available in oral, sublingual, suppository and inhaler form for use either separately or in addition to the above. It is thought to relieve migraine headache by constricting cranial arteries. Nausea is a common side-effect but can be relieved by adding an anti-emetic. Other adverse reactions include tingling and numbness, abdominal pains, cold peripheries and general malaise. Doses of 6–8 mg per attack and 10–12 mg per week should not be exceeded. Ergotamine treatment should not be repeated at intervals of less than 4 days. More regular use of ergot can result in limb pains, venous thrombosis, gangrene and ergotism. It is contraindicated for patients with circulatory disorders, heart disease, hypertension, impaired renal or hepatic functions and in pregnant women.

Sumatriptan is available as a subcutaneous autoinjector device for self administration and also in tablet form. It is a $5-HT_1$ agonist which appears to be of considerable value in the treatment of an acute attack. Side-effects include sensations of tingling, heat, heaviness, pressure or tightness in any part of the body, flushing, dizziness and drowsiness. It is contraindicated in patients with ischaemic heart disease, previous myocardial infarction or uncontrolled hypertension and should not be given to patients receiving concurrent treatment with MAOIs, selective re-uptake inhibitors and lithium.

Prophylaxis

Some patients require prophylactic medication taken daily to prevent migraine, usually given if the patient has more than two migraine attacks per month. Drugs used are listed in Table 10.7.

Clonidine and methysergide have been used but the former is probably little better than a placebo and the latter has dangerous side-effects, e.g. fibrosis of the heart valves and pleura.

Table 10.7   Drugs used to prevent migraine

Drug	Class	Dose
Pizotifen	Antihistamine and serotinin antagonist	0.5–3 mg daily
Propranolol	Beta-blocker	10–40 mg three times daily
Amitriptyline	Tricyclic antidepressant	10–50 mg at night
Cyproheptadine	Antihistamine with serotonin antagonist and calcium channel blocking properties	4 mg at night

NAUSEA AND VERTIGO

Nausea and vomiting

Anti-emetics relieve nausea and vomiting from a variety of causes. The group of nuclei known collectively as the vomiting centre is located in the medulla oblongata in the brain stem and can receive stimuli from various sources. The nausea response can be initiated when the upper GI tract sends nerve impulses to the vomiting centre along the vagus and sympathetic nerves. This can be stimulated, e.g. by irritation of mucosal receptors in the GI tract, radiation therapy injury of the GI mucosa or malignant disease of the GI tract.

Another collection of nuclei called the chemo-receptor trigger zone (CTZ) is located in the area postrema. Activation of the CTZ can stimulate the vomiting centre which, in turn, causes nausea or initiates emesis. Motion sickness results from stimulation of the vestibular apparatus of the ear which activates the vomiting centre via the CTZ. People who know they may experience motion sickness under certain circumstances can use an anti-emetic prophylactically to avoid this.

Labyrinthitis resulting from inflammation of the vestibular apparatus of the ear causes nausea, vomiting, dizziness and hearing loss. Ménière's disease which involves dilatation of the endolymphatic channels in the cochlea also produces nausea as well as dizziness, tinnitus and hearing loss.

Cancer chemotherapy can directly or indirectly (through the CTZ) stimulate the vomiting centre causing severe nausea and vomiting. Narcotics can cause nausea and vomiting either by stimulating the CTZ or sensitising the vestibular apparatus of the ear.

Nausea and vomiting are frequent and often distressing side-effects connected with anaesthesia and surgery. Various factors may be involved including inhalation agents, premedication, post-operative pain, opioid analgesia and movement.

The main neurotransmitters in the area postrema, those thought to have a role in emesis, are:

- acetylcholine
- histamine
- dopamine
- 5-hydroxytryptamine

The actions of certain anti-emetics indicate that acetylcholine and histamine are more important in motion sickness than in other types of emesis. Many anti-emetics are antidopaminergic, and this may lead to the occurrence of extrapyramidal reactions.

Drug treatments

Hyoscine

Hyoscine acts on the vomiting centre in the medulla where it has an antimuscarinic action. Its efficacy in motion sickness is due to an effect on the vestibular apparatus.

Phenothiazines

The phenothiazines are dopamine antagonists and act centrally by blocking the CTZ. They are rapidly absorbed after oral administration. Rectal or parenteral administration is required if vomiting has already started. Prochlorperazine, perphenazine, trifluoperazine and thiethylperazine are less sedating than chlorpromazine. Long-term use is limited by side-effects, including extrapyramidal reactions and antimuscarinic effects. Patients should be advised about drowsiness and warned not to drive or operate machinery. Side-effects include hypotension, cholestatic jaundice, skin rash and leucopenia. The sedative effects are potentiated by alcohol and other sedative drugs.

Metoclopramide

Metoclopramide blocks peripheral and central dopamine receptors when in high doses, and it also acts on peripheral and central 5-HT$_3$ receptors, which is of value in the prevention of nausea and vomiting associated with cytotoxic drug therapy. Metoclopramide also reduces oesophageal reflux and enhances gastric emptying, which is useful in treating gastric hypomotility found in migraine. Side-effects are usually mild, transient and reversible on discontinuation of therapy. CNS side-effects include dizziness, drowsiness, anxiety and depression. Extrapyramidal symptoms may also occur including akathisia, parkinsonism and acute dystonia.

Domperidone

Domperidone acts on the CTZ and has anti-emetic properties, and its effects on gastro-intestinal motility are similar to those of metoclopramide. It causes little extrapyramidal side-effects and is less sedating than metoclopramide; it is therefore useful in treating patients with Parkinson's disease where nausea and vomiting associated with levodopa or bromo-criptine are troublesome.

Antihistamines

These act on the vestibular apparatus, the vomiting centre and the CTZ. They potentiate CNS depressants such as alcohol, phenothiazines and benzodiazepines.

Selective 5-HT$_3$ antagonists

The 5-HT$_3$ antagonists, including ondansetron, granisetron and tropisetron act peripherally on vagus nerve endings and centrally in the CTZ. They have no action on other receptor types. The lack of therapeutic activity on dopamine receptors indicates that, unlike metoclopramide, anti-emetic activity can be achieved without dose-limiting extrapyramidal side-effects. These drugs are mainly used to treat nausea and vomiting in patients on highly emetogenic chemotherapy such as cisplatin, although ondansetron is also licensed for use in post-operative vomiting. A single intravenous dose is recommended immediately before chemo-therapy. If vomiting is not adequately controlled the drug should be continued orally or intra-venously for up to 5 days (granisetron is avail-able only in injectable form). Adverse effects include constipation and headache. These drugs are expensive.

Drug treatment of nausea and vomiting in particular situations

Motion sickness

Hyoscine is the most effective drug for the prevention of motion sickness. It is available both in tablet form and as a transdermal patch providing a slow continuous absorption into the bloodstream. A 300 µg tablet is taken 30 minutes before the start of the journey or a 500 µg patch is applied to a hairless area of skin behind the ear 5–6 hours before a journey and replaced after 72 hours if necessary. Side-effects such as drowsiness, blurred vision, dry mouth and urinary retention do not occur to any great extent at the doses used.

An alternative to hyoscine in motion sickness is the antihistamines such as cinnarizine, cycli-zine, dimenhydrinate and promethazine; the sedative effect and the times of administration of these four drugs are shown in Table 10.8.

Drowsiness may affect performance of skilled tasks such as driving or operating machinery. Effects of alcohol are enhanced.

Drug-induced nausea and vomiting

Lowering the dose or withdrawal of the drug should be considered. If the drug has to be continued, choice of treatment depends on drug-induced emesis. Local gastric irritation may be reduced by increasing dosage frequency and lowering the dose, and also by taking the drug with food. Domperidone is used for nausea and vomiting induced by drugs such as levodopa and bromocriptine in the treatment of Parkin-son's disease. Central effects such as opiate-induced vomiting may be treated with a pheno-thiazine such as prochlorperazine. Cyclizine is

Table 10.8 Administration and sedative effect of some antihistamines

	Taken before journey	Sedative effect
Cinnarizine	2 hours	Mild
Cyclizine	0.5 hour	Mild
Dimenhydrinate	0.5 hour	Moderate
Promethazine	0.5 hour	Moderate

often effective, and a combination of cyclizine and morphine is available as cyclimorph.

Postoperative vomiting

Postoperative nausea and vomiting may cause electrolyte imbalance and dehydration. Patients may have difficulty with food and fluid intake, and oral drug therapy can be disrupted. Metoclopramide or a phenothiazine can be used. More recently, ondansetron has been used to treat nausea and vomiting where not controlled by less expensive drugs.

Pregnancy

Drug therapy of vomiting in pregnancy should be reserved for severe cases and, where possible, treatment should be avoided during the first trimester. Vomiting is usually most troublesome during this period, reaching a peak at about 10 weeks. Promethazine has been widely used and appears to be free from teratogenic effects.

Cytotoxic drug therapy

Nausea and vomiting occur frequently during the treatment of cancer with cytotoxic drugs or irradiation. Not all cytotoxic agents cause vomiting but those that frequently do include cisplatin, doxorubicin, cyclophosphamide and nitrosoureas. Prochlorperazine may be effective in mild to moderate cases. Metoclopramide in higher doses is also effective, but dosage is limited by side-effects. Nabilone, an oral synthetic cannabinoid with anxiolytic properties, has been used but is limited by side-effects (drowsiness, hallucinations, psychosis, blurred vision and depression). Vomiting due to highly emetogenic drugs can often be alleviated by parenteral corticosteroids (dexamethasone and methylprednisolone). Adding a sedative such as lorazepam may help, and combination with high-dose metoclopramide is often effective.

When vomiting persists, 5-HT$_3$ antagonists are effective.

Vestibular disorders

Acute labyrinthine disorders are distressing for the patient. The symptoms of nausea, vomiting and vertigo usually respond to prochlorperazine. Antihistamines and phenothiazines may be helpful in treating chronic vertigo. Age-related loss of postural stability should not be treated with agents (notably phenothiazines) whose side-effects include postural hypotension, mental confusion and parkinsonism. Betahistine and cinnarizine are useful in treating Ménière's disease. In an acute attack, cyclizine or prochlorperazine may be given rectally or by intramuscular injection.

EPILEPSY

The term 'neurone' describes the nerve cells and their processes which are situated in the brain. These neurones behave like a small electrical source and, when nerve impulses are generated, the impulses pass along the axon to the neuromuscular junction and from there they energise the muscle fibres. During an epileptic seizure the nerve impulses generated are greatly in excess of normal and are uncoordinated. An epileptic seizure is defined as an intermittent disturbance of behaviour, emotion, motor function or sensation resulting from an abnormal electrical discharge originating within the cortex of the brain. Epilepsy describes a condition where an individual suffers repeated seizures.

Anticonvulsants act to prevent the spread of neuronal excitation by exerting a stabilising effect on excitable cell membranes or by enhancing the activity of neurotransmitters such as gamma-aminobutyric acid (GABA) which inhibit the spread of seizure activity by blocking synaptic transmission.

Classification

Many different terms have been used to describe the various types of epilepsy. A classification has been produced by the International League Against Epilepsy. In this classification, seizures are divided into two types: generalised and partial (or focal). An abbreviated version is as follows.

Generalised seizures

- Absence seizures (petit mal)
  This type of seizure occurs most commonly in childhood, often resolving during puberty. Absence seizures consist of brief episodes of unconsciousness with little or no motor accompaniment.
- Myoclonic seizures. These consist of single or multiple sudden or uncontrollable jerks.
- Tonic/clonic seizures (grand mal). The most commonly encountered seizure type, this disorder is characterised by a sudden loss of consciousness followed by muscle rigidity (the tonic phase), which, in turn, is followed by a period of jerking of the limbs (clonic phase). The patient then enters a deep coma, with consciousness usually being fully regained within 1 hour. There may be a period of confusion prior to full recovery. Urinary and faecal incontinence may occur during the tonic phase.

Partial (focal) seizures

- Simple partial seizures. These seizures result from a focal epileptic discharge in a localised area of the brain. A simple partial seizure may be motor (e.g. abnormal movement of limb), sensory (e.g. abnormal sensation) or both. It is not accompanied by unconsciousness and is usually of short duration. The nature of the symptoms depends largely on the anatomical site of seizure discharge. A partial seizure is often preceded by abnormal symptoms (an aura) such as an unpleasant taste or smell.
- Complex partial seizure. This seizure type may have a simple partial onset followed by impaired consciousness as it spreads throughout the brain to become secondarily generalised. This may result in bizarre or inappropriate behaviour (e.g. lip smacking, tearing of clothing).

Treatment

Drug treatment aims at achieving control of seizures without impairing mental or motor function. Anticonvulsants have a fairly narrow therapeutic index and dosages must be carefully tailored in order to maximise efficacy while minimising adverse effects. A major cause of treatment failure is poor compliance. It is essential that the patient understands the importance of regular medication. For improved compliance once-a-day dosage would be preferable but this may not be possible due to too short a half-life. Most anti-epileptic drugs can be given twice daily at the most.

Medication should be initiated with a single drug and very often at reduced dosage gradually increasing until the clinically effective level is reached. This is in order to minimise toxic effects. If this drug fails to provide adequate control of seizures another drug will be substituted. A second drug should be added to the regimen only if seizures continue despite high plasma concentrations or toxic effects. In order to attain the correct dose, plasma drug concentrations should be monitored where appropriate, e.g. phenytoin.

Drugs of choice in the treatment of particular types of epilepsy are listed in Table 10.9.

Table 10.9   Drugs of choice in treatment of epilepsy

Type of epilepsy	First choice	Other major drugs
Absence seizures (petit mal)	Ethosuximide	Sodium valproate
Myoclonic seizures	Sodium valproate	Clonazepam Ethosuximide
Tonic/clonic seizures (grand mal)	Carbamazepine	Phenytoin Sodium valproate Phenobarbitone Primidone Lamotrigine Vigabatrin
Simple partial seizures	Carbamazepine	Phenytoin Sodium valproate Vigabatrin Lamotrigine Phenobarbitone
Complex partial seizures	Carbamazepine	Phenytoin Phenobarbitone

Carbamazepine Carbamazepine should be introduced at a low dose (200 mg/day) increasing weekly by 100 mg/day until control is established or toxicity occurs. Visual symptoms are common at high doses – diplopia and blurred vision occurring at daily doses above 1200 mg. This may be minimised by giving in divided doses or by use of a controlled release formulation. Other adverse effects may include sedation, dizziness, headache, skin rashes, bone marrow suppression and hyponatraemia.

The drug is a powerful inducer of liver enzymes and its own clearance rate increases with the result that the half-life may reduce significantly over the first few weeks of treatment. Carbamazepine induces metabolism of several other drugs given concurrently, e.g. other anti-epileptics, oral contraceptives. Metabolism of carbamazepine is inhibited by certain drugs, including ciprofloxacin, verapamil and diltiazem, which may result in increased carbamazepine levels and toxicity.

Phenytoin Phenytoin, although a highly effective anti-epileptic is generally less suitable for many patients compared with carbamazepine due to a high incidence of side-effects and a difficulty in dosage optimisation because of its complex pharmacokinetics. Side-effects which may limit its use in children and women are gingival hyperplasia, hirsutism, acne and coarsening of facial features. Phenytoin is also associated with deficiencies of calcium, vitamin D and folic acid; hence, replacement therapy may be required. Dose-related adverse effects include nystagmus, diplopia and ataxia. These problems may be minimised if phenytoin plasma levels are maintained within the drug's therapeutic range (10–20 mg/litre). The pharmacokinetics of phenytoin are important, as the relationship between dose and plasma level is very variable, with the result that seizure control is related to plasma level, but not to dosage. The capacity of the liver to metabolise the drug may become saturated at or around the therapeutic range. Small increases in dosage will then produce large increases in plasma level as the additional drug cannot be metabolised. Therapeutic monitoring is therefore of great importance in the use of phenytoin.

Sodium valproate Sodium valproate is effective against all types of seizure and is the drug of choice in myoclonic seizures. It should be used with caution in children and those with liver disease. Side-effects include gastric irritation, nausea, ataxia and tremor.

Lamotrigine and vigabatrin Lamotrigine is a newer anti-epileptic for the adjunctive treatment of partial seizures and secondary generalised tonic-clonic seizures which are not satisfactorily controlled by other anti-epileptics. Side-effects include rashes, diplopia, blurred vision, dizziness, drowsiness and headache. Vigabatrin can be used in chronic epilepsy not satisfactorily controlled by other anti-epileptics. Side-effects are similar to those of lamotrigine.

Phenobarbitone and primidone Phenobarbitone is an effective drug for tonic and partial seizures but is rarely first choice. The major side-effect is sedation in adults and may cause behavioural disturbances in children. Primidone is largely converted to phenobarbitone in the body and this is probably responsible for its anti-epileptic action.

Dosages and therapeutic plasma concentration ranges of several anti-epileptics are shown in Table 10.10.

Drug withdrawal

Reduction in withdrawal should be carried out in stages. The changeover from one anti-epileptic drug regimen to another should be done with care, building up the second drug to a therapeutic range while gradually decreasing the first.

Driving

Epilepsy sufferers may drive a motor vehicle (not heavy goods or public service) provided they have had a seizure-free period of 2 years or, if subject to attacks only while asleep, have established a 3-year period of asleep attacks without awake attacks. Patients affected by drowsiness should not drive or operate machinery.

Table 10.10   Dosages and therapeutic plasma concentration range of anti-epileptic drugs

Drug	Initial dose	Usual adult dose	Therapeutic plasma concentration range
Carbamazepine	100–200 mg once or twice daily	0.8–1.2 g daily in divided doses	4–12 mg/litre
Ethosuximide	500 mg daily	1–1.5 g daily	40–100 mg/litre
Phenytoin	150–300 mg daily as one or two divided doses	300–400 mg daily	10–20 mg/litre
Sodium valproate	600 mg daily in divided doses	1–2 g daily	50–100 mg/litre
Phenobarbitone		60–180 mg at night	15–40 mg/litre
Primidone	125 mg daily at bedtime	500–1000 mg daily	Monitored by measuring phenobarbitone

Status epilepticus

This is a condition where there are recurrent fits without recovery of consciousness between attacks. It is a medical emergency and requires urgent treatment aimed at stopping seizures as quickly as possible. A nurse must stay with the patient. An airway should be established and the patient should be in a physical environment where he cannot hurt himself. Diazepam emulsion 10–20 mg should be administered intravenously over 3–6 minutes. This is repeated in 30 minutes if necessary, which may be followed by intravenous infusion to a maximum of 3 mg/kg over 24 hours. Caution should be exercised because of the risk of respiratory depression. Small doses of diazepam can be administered by rectal solution.

To prevent recurrence of seizures after the initial diazepam injection, phenytoin may be given by slow intravenous injection in a dose of 15 mg/kg with ECG monitoring in case of cardiac arrhythmias. If status epilepticus continues or returns chlormethiazole may be given by slow intravenous injection, monitoring respiration carefully, particularly if following on

diazepam. Paraldehyde may be given when other agents have failed to control seizures. Some 5–10 ml should be given by intramuscular injection. The dose may be repeated after 1 hour. Paraldehyde may cause muscle necrosis. Doses of 10 ml should be split into 2×5 ml doses in separate muscles.

Phenobarbitone can be given in a dose of 50–200 mg by slow intravenous injection, i.e. over about 5 minutes. This may be repeated after 6 hours if necessary. Prolonged sedation or respiratory depression may be a problem.

PARKINSON'S DISEASE

The disease gets its name from a description by Sir James Parkinson in 1817 in *An Essay on the Shaking Palsy*. The key symptoms of idiopathic Parkinson's disease are:

- tremor, present when the patient is at rest and when severe 'pill rolling' may be seen
- rigidity; on standing the patient may exhibit stooped posture, arms slightly bent, weight on ball of foot, knees flexed
- bradykinesia
  general slowness in daily activities
  difficulty initiating movement particularly walking
  difficulty in rising from a chair
- walking problems
  the patient's weight is on the ball of the foot and there appears to be a loss of heel strike
  reduction in length of stride
  the patient leans forward before commencing to walk and flexes knees to prevent falling forward
- balance problems
  frequent falls can occur
  difficulty in turning

Other features of Parkinson's disease include excessive salivation, dysphagia – frequently in older people, anxiety, depression and a fixed staring appearance.

Dopamine, working in balance with another chemical messenger, acetylcholine, is responsible for the mechanisms which control programmes of movements (Fig. 10.8). Imbalances in the neurotransmitters lead to movement disorders. In Parkinson's disease, degeneration of certain cells in the substantia nigra leads to a deficiency in the production of dopamine so that the normal balance between the neurotransmitters, dopamine and acetylcholine, is altered (Fig. 10.9).

The symptoms of Parkinson's disease do not appear until some 80% of the capacity to produce dopamine has been lost. The level of dopamine will continue to fall over subsequent years. However, each person with Parkinson's disease is very different, and the rate and character of the progression may vary greatly from one person to another. The disease usually presents in middle or old age.

Drug treatment

The main aim of drug therapy is to restore the balance between dopamine and acetylcholine. This can be achieved by:

- replacing dopamine
- use of dopamine agonists to stimulate surviving dopamine receptors
- prolonging action of dopamine by inhibiting metabolism
- use of antimuscarinic drugs.

Replacing dopamine

Administration of dopamine is ineffective since it cannot cross the blood–brain barrier into the brain cells where it is required to produce an effect. It is necessary to give its precursor, levodopa, which crosses the blood–brain barrier and is subsequently broken down to dopamine by the enzyme dopa decarboxylase. However, levodopa requires to be given in high concentrations since over 90% is decarboxylated in the liver and

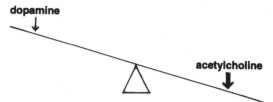

Figure 10.9 Dopamine deficiency with resultant cholinergic over-activity leading to symptoms of the disease.

gut prior to its reaching the brain. This results in peripheral side-effects such as nausea, vomiting, anorexia and postural hypotension.

Levodopa is rarely given alone. It is usually given in combination with an inhibitor of extra-cerebral dopa-decarboxylase, such as carbidopa (Sinemet) or benserazide (Madopar). This prevents the peripheral degradation of levodopa to dopamine and so increases effective brain levels. This allows the dose of levodopa to be reduced markedly, resulting in a reduction in side-effects.

Levodopa is the drug of choice in the treatment of Parkinson's disease and is tolerated by most patients who experience considerable improvement for several years, especially where stiffness and slowness of movement are concerned. It is initiated at low doses (50–100 mg twice daily with benserazide) since some feelings of nausea are common. These are usually mild and pass as the body adjusts to the drug. Taking levodopa with or after meals helps to minimise these effects.

Domperidone may be useful in controlling nausea where this is severe. The dosage regimen is gradually increased, the final dose being a compromise between increased mobility and incidence of side-effects. There is a small percentage of people who cannot tolerate levodopa because of severe sickness or other side-effects such as confusion, hallucinations and mood swings.

Levodopa usually provides very effective control of Parkinson's disease for a number of years, after which a deterioration in response often occurs. This is probably related to increasing degeneration of nigrostriatal neurones.

Interactions can occur with drugs which affect central monoamines, and MAOIs should be withdrawn at least 14 days before instituting

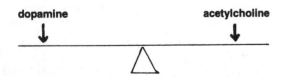

Figure 10.8 Dopamine and acetylcholine in balance.

levodopa treatment. Antipsychotic drugs, such as the phenothiazines, should not be administered concurrently as they would exacerbate the disease. Caution should be exercised in patients with open-angle glaucoma.

Dopamine agonists

Dopa agonists (bromocriptine, lysuride, pergolide) act by direct stimulation of surviving dopamine receptors. They are usually used in conjunction with levodopa to smooth out control of symptoms in patients whose response to treatment is beginning to fluctuate. Treatment is begun at low dosage, taken with food and gradually increased to a maintenance dose. The use of dopa agonists allows a reduction in the levodopa dosage and the effects of the combination should be carefully balanced. Drop-out rates can be high due to adverse effects. Gastrointestinal upset, postural hypotension, dizziness and headache are common. With bromocriptine, patients are best advised to refrain from excessive alcohol consumption as alcohol may reduce tolerance of the drug and lead to increased side-effects.

Apomorphine produces a direct effect on dopamine receptor sites in the brain. It can be tried in addition to current therapy in patients who experience sudden fluctuations in their symptoms despite all efforts to adjust their medication. It is given by subcutaneous injection and acts very quickly and reliably, bringing relief to those with extreme variations in mobility or severe involuntary movements, its effect lasting about 2 hours. It is not generally available and helps only those patients who are still responding to levodopa. Its effectiveness is limited by nausea, which can be minimised by domperidone.

Prolongation of dopamine action

Selegiline is a drug which prolongs the action of dopamine at the receptor by inhibiting its enzymatic degradation. It is a monoamine oxidase B inhibitor and its use therefore does not involve dietary restriction. The usual dose is 5 mg in the morning, increasing to 10 mg if necessary. It can

cause hypotension, nausea, vomiting, confusion and agitation, and the side-effects of levodopa may be increased. Its use may allow the concurrent levodopa dose to be reduced by 20 to 50%.

Antimuscarinic drugs

Antimuscarinic drugs (e.g. benzhexol, benztropine, orphenadrine, procyclidine) may be used in Parkinson's disease to reduce the relative excess of acetylcholine, and, as a result, reduce to some extent the tremor, rigidity and sialorrhoea. All are given in gradually increasing doses until an optimal balance of efficacy and side-effects is obtained (see Table 10.11).

The most common adverse reactions are dry mouth, constipation, blurred vision, tachycardia and dizziness. The antimuscarinics are contraindicated in urinary retention and glaucoma, and interactions may occur with antihistamines and tricyclic antidepressants. They can be useful for younger patients in the early stages when symptoms are mild. When treatment of mild symptoms is initiated with antimuscarinic drugs, levodopa is added or substituted as symptoms progress.

End-of-dose effects

The duration of the beneficial response to each dose of levodopa becomes progressively shorter and may be reduced from an initial 4–6 hours to as little as 30 minutes with a return of symptoms towards the end of each dose such as early morning immobility, dystonia and start hesitation. End-of-dose effects appear to be the result of failing levodopa plasma levels, as they can be abolished by levodopa infusions. This condition may respond to the administration of smaller

Table 10.11 Dosages of antimuscarinic drugs

Drug	Initial dose	Maintenance dose
Benzhexol	1 mg	5–15 mg
Benztropine	0.5–1 mg	1–4 mg
Orphenadrine	150 mg in divided doses	150–300 mg
Procyclidine	2.5 mg tds	10–20 mg

doses of levodopa at more frequent intervals with the first dose on waking and last dose at bedtime.

Adjunctive treatment may also be considered at this stage. Bromocriptine or selegiline are both useful in conjunction with levodopa for smoothing out the effects of end-of-dose deterioration. Controlled release preparations of Sinemet or Madopar can also be used.

'On–off' effects

'On–off' effects are sudden fluctuations in disability which can occur involving rapid and abrupt alterations between periods of good mobility and periods of hypokinesia, tremor and dyskinesia. This may last for only a few seconds or up to several minutes, or even hours, before normal function returns. Apomorphine has been used to overcome this effect. There is also some evidence that dietary manipulation may improve 'On-off' effects since there is competition for transport across the blood–brain barrier between levodopa and certain dietary amino acids.

Drug-induced parkinsonism

The features of drug-induced parkinsonism are the same as those of the idiopathic disease. There may be tremor, rigidity, bradykinesia, expressionless face, dysphagia and drooling. This occurs to some degree in all patients treated with antipsychotic drugs, although there is a wide variation between patients. The following have a high propensity for causing extrapyramidal effects:

- Piperazine phenothiazines – e.g. fluphenazine, trifluoperazine
- Butyrophenones – e.g. haloperidol, droperidol
- Diphenylbutylpiperidines – e.g. pimozide, fluspirilene

Chlorpromazine and thioridazine have a lower propensity. Metoclopramide blocks dopamine receptors and also enhances the action of acetylcholine.

Drug-induced parkinsonism does not always require treatment and it is reversible on dose reduction or drug withdrawal. Severe cases may require treatment with antimuscarinics, but the routine use of these drugs should be avoided as they add to the antimuscarinic side-effects of antipsychotic drugs and may increase the risk of tardive dyskinesia. Because of the tendency of antipsychotics to accumulate, side-effects may be very prolonged, lasting days or weeks after the drug has been withdrawn.

Care of the patient with Parkinson's disease

The symptoms of Parkinson's disease are fairly familiar to the general public. It follows therefore that when a diagnosis is made, the patient will be concerned, and so those involved must give every encouragement to the patient and those who are close to him.

Education of the patient and participation in treatment are important from the outset since treatment is likely to be prolonged and eventually problematic. Plans and objectives should be formulated in conjunction with the patient. Physiotherapy can assist in posture and walking, and regular exercise is important to maintain mobility. Occupational therapists can offer a wide range of helpful appliances. Constipation may be a concern for sufferers, but a high-fibre diet usually controls symptoms. In the United Kingdom The Parkinson's Disease Society is recommended as a source of support.

FURTHER READING

Andrews P, Whitehead S 1993 How to manage nausea and vomiting. Prescriber 4(6): 37–64
Baldwin D 1991 Drugs used in psychoses and related disorders. Prescriber 2: 25–41

Betts A 1993 Sleep insomnia and hypnotic drugs. Practice Nursing June/July: 8–10
Bushnell T G, Justins D M 1993 Choosing the right analgesic. Drugs 46(3): 394–408

Culshaw M 1989 Epilepsy and its treatment. Pharmaceutical Journal 242: 138–140

Farmer A E, Blewett A 1993 Drug treatment of resistant schizophrenia. Drugs 45(2): 374–383

Hassanyeh F, Edwards C 1992 Antidepressants. Pharmaceutical Journal 248: 117–119

MacGregor E A 1992 Migraine and its treatment. Pharmaceutical Journal 248: 285–288

Montastruc J L, Rascol O, Senard J M 1993 Current status of dopamine agonists in Parkinson's disease management. Drugs 46(3): 384–393

Moon C A L 1991 Insomnia: advice on managing this all-too-common complaint. Care of the Elderly 3(8): 361–366

Peet M, Pratt J P 1993 Lithium. Current status in psychiatric disorders. Drugs 46(1): 7–17

Rudorfer M V, Potter W Z 1989 Antidepressants. A comparative review of the clinical pharmacology and therapeutic use of the newer versus the older drugs. Drugs 37: 713–738

Stewart D A, Macphee G J A 1992 Parkinson's disease: current therapeutic strategies. Update 44(5): 3–11

11

Drug treatment of infections

INTRODUCTION

The discovery of sulphonamides in the 1930s, followed by penicillin in the 1940s, heralded a new era in the treatment of infections. Since then a large number of drugs has been produced which either kill or inhibit the growth of bacteria, fungi or viruses. These drugs, in tandem with the patient's natural immunity, have cured many infectious diseases which previously often proved fatal. It should be noted that where immunity is impaired due to prolonged illness, old age or the use of cytotoxic drugs, infections are more difficult to eradicate. As organisms become resistant to chemotherapy, a continuing search is necessary for new drugs and modifications of those already in use.

CLASSIFICATION OF BACTERIA

Bacteria can be broadly classified according to cell shape (Fig. 11.1), that is:

cocci   spherical
bacilli   straight rods
vibrios   curved rods
spirochaetes   spiral, flexible filaments
spirilla   spiral, non-flexible filaments

Subdivision of these categories is based on the Gram stain. This staining technique was developed by Christian Gram in 1884. A heat-fixed smear of bacteria is stained successively with a solution of crystal violet (or related dye) and iodine. This is then treated with an organic

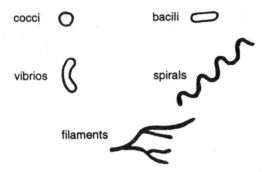

Figure 11.1   Bacteria – examples of cell shapes.

solvent such as acetone. The cells of some bacteria, termed Gram-negative bacteria, are rapidly decolorised. The treatment with organic solvent is normally followed by counterstaining with, for example, fuchsin or safranin. Gram-positive cells retain the deep purple conferred on them by the initial staining with crystal violet and iodine, whereas Gram-negative cells, which had been decolorised, exhibit the red colour of the counterstain. As a result, Gram-positive and Gram-negative cells can be readily distinguished under the microscope.

Microorganisms are also classified as aerobes – those that can live and grow in the presence of oxygen – or as anaerobes, those that can live and grow without oxygen. These three factors:

- cell structure
- reaction to Gram stain
- aerobe/anaerobe

can be used in the classification of infectious bacteria (Table 11.1).

MICROBIOLOGY

Most serious infections can be life-threatening, and decisions require to be made on the most appropriate antibiotic therapy often before a precise bacteriological diagnosis is available. The initial therapy will usually be broad-spectrum to cover as many microbiological causes (see Table 11.2) as possible, although treatment may be modified later depending on clinical developments and the results of microbiological tests. Some of the factors affecting the choice of antibiotics are as follows:

- known or suspected microorganism
- resistance patterns in hospital
- known allergies or hypersensitivities of the patient
- site of infection
- renal and hepatic function
- toxicity of chosen antibiotic
- route of administration
- cost

It is essential to obtain specimens for microbiological investigation before antimicrobial therapy is initiated so that the antibiotic therapy can be reassessed if an organism is identified. Conventional laboratory techniques for identification require at least 18 hours of incubation in appro-

Table 11.1   Classification of infectious bacteria

Gram-positive aerobes		Gram-negative aerobes	
Cocci, e.g.	Bacilli, e.g.	Cocci, e.g.	Bacilli e.g.
Staphylococcus aureus	*Corynebacterium diphtheriae*	*Neisseria meningitidis*	*Haemophilus influenzae*
Staphylococcus epidermidis	*Listeria monocytogenes*	*Neisseria gonorrhoeae*	*Klebsiella pneumoniae*
Streptococcus pneumoniae			*Escherichia coli*
Viridans streptococci			*Enterobacter* species
			Proteus species
			Pseudomonas aeruginosa
			Legionella species
			Campylobacter species
Gram-positive anaerobes		Gram-negative anaerobes	
Cocci, e.g.	Bacilli, e.g.	Cocci, e.g.	Bacilli, e.g.
Peptococcus	*Clostridium tetani*	*Veillonella* species	*Bacteroides* species
	Clostridium perfringens		*Fusobacterium* species

Table 11.2 Causative pathogens in some common bacterial infections

Respiratory infections	
Exacerbation of chronic bronchitis	*Haemophilus influenzae*
	Streptococcus pneumoniae
Pneumonia	*Streptococcus pneumoniae*
	Staphyloccus aureus
	Haemophilus influenzae
Urinary tract	*E. coli*
	Proteus spp
	Klebsiella spp
	Streptococcus faecalis
	Pseudomonas
Venereal disease	
Gonorrhoea	*Neisseria gonorrhoeae*
Non-specific urethritis	*Chlamydia*
Skin/soft tissue	
Intravenous catheter site	*Staphylococcus aureus*
	Staphylococcus epidermidis
Surgical wound	*Staphylococcus aureus*
	Gram-negative rods
Furuncle	*Staphylococcus aureus*
Endocarditis	
Acute	*Staphylococcus aureus*
	Streptococcus pyogenes
	Gram-negative bacilli
Subacute	*Streptococcus* spp
	Staphylococcus epidermidis
	Gram-negative bacilli
Septicaemia	*Staphylococcus aureus*
	Streptococcus pneumoniae
	Coliforms
	Enterobacter spp
Meningitis (adults)	*Streptococcus pneumoniae*
(Many organisms may cause meningitis in neonates)	*Neisseria meningitidis*
Food poisoning	Salmonellae
	Clostridium perfringens

priate media to allow detectable numbers of bacteria to grow. However, more rapid techniques help in diagnosis before culture results are available. The most valuable is a Gram-stained smear of blood or aspirate from the site of infection.

An identification of organisms from culture is followed by sensitivity tests. Filter paper discs impregnated with known concentrations of antibiotic are placed onto an agar culture plate containing the individual strain of organism isolated in the culture process. The degree of sensitivity of the organism to the antibiotic is assessed by the size of inhibition zones around the discs after further incubation. Results are reported back to the prescriber indicating antibiotics effective in treatment.

ANTIBACTERIAL DRUGS

Antibacterial drugs act by a number of mechanisms (Fig. 11.2). They can be either bactericidal (kill bacteria) or bacteriostatic (arrest the growth of bacteria) (Box 11.1). Bacteriostatic agents, since they do not kill bacteria, rely upon the host's immune and cell defence mechanisms to clear the bacteria. If these defence mechanisms are compromised, a bactericidal drug may be preferable.

Box 11.1 Some bactericidal and bacteriostatic drugs

Bactericidal drugs	Bacteriostatic drugs
Penicillins	Chloramphenicol
Cephalosporins	Erythromycin
Aminoglycosides	Tetracyclines
	Trimethoprim

MINIMUM INHIBITORY CONCENTRATION (MIC) OF ANTIBIOTICS

As a guide to the sensitivity of a specific microorganism to an antibiotic, the MIC is utilised. This is the lowest concentration of antibiotic which will inhibit the growth of a given strain of microorganism under controlled conditions. The lower the concentration, the more potent the antibiotic. However, the MIC is determined in a homogenous culture system in vitro. In vivo, the drug may have to pass from the plasma into infected tissue to destroy bacteria. The penetration of antibiotics into abscess cavities may be poor and surgical drainage is often necessary. In either case, higher doses would be required in vivo to achieve the MIC compared with in vitro.

Minimum bactericidal concentration (MBC) is the lowest concentration of antibiotic which will kill a given strain of microorganism under controlled conditions.

BACTERIUM

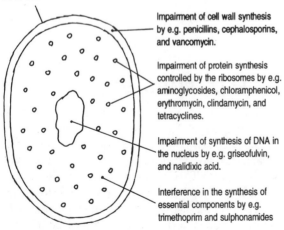

Impairment of cell wall synthesis by e.g. penicillins, cephalosporins, and vancomycin.

Impairment of protein synthesis controlled by the ribosomes by e.g. aminoglycosides, chloramphenicol, erythromycin, clindamycin, and tetracyclines.

Impairment of synthesis of DNA in the nucleus by e.g. griseofulvin, and nalidixic acid.

Interference in the synthesis of essential components by e.g. trimethoprim and sulphonamides.

Figure 11.2 Actions of antibacterial drugs.

BACTERIAL RESISTANCE TO ANTIBIOTICS

The resistance of bacteria to antibiotics is a problem that has continued to grow in parallel with the development of new antibiotics. Bacterial resistance reflects antibiotic use and is more of a problem where controls on antibiotic use are lax. The sensible use of antibiotics guards against this. There are several mechanisms by which resistance may emerge.

Selection

An antibiotic will eliminate the sensitive organisms within a bacterial population, and the resistant forms will proliferate.

Mutation

Resistance to an antibiotic may develop as a result of the spontaneous appearance of mutants during the process of cell division. These mutants will then proliferate.

Transferred resistance

Resistance may be acquired by the transfer of genetic material which confers antibiotic resistance from one organism to another. This may be achieved by (i) *transduction*, involving the transfer of genes contained within bacteriophages (viruses which infect bacteria); (ii) *conjugation*, involving the transfer of genes contained within plasmids. Transfer of plasmids is not confined to the same species and they can be passed from, for example, *E. coli* to *Salmonella*. Either way, new DNA enters the bacterium and codes for a mechanism which confers resistance. Such mechanisms involve:

- Enzymatic inactivation of the antibiotic. The bacterium produces enzymes that inactivate the antibiotic by altering its chemical structure. For example, the enzymes responsible for destroying penicillins and cephalosporins are called β-lactamases; these enzymes are found in Gram-negative bacteria such as *Escherichia coli*, *Salmonella* spp and

Pseudomonas spp and in Gram-positive bacteria, e.g. staphylococci. These enzymes open up the β-lactam ring of the penicillin which is the portion responsible for antimicrobial activity. Aminoglycoside resistance is often due to a similar mechanism where bacteria produce enzymes that alter the chemical structure of the aminoglycoside.

- Altered permeability of the bacterium to the drug. Some bacteria reduce the permeability of their cell membrane to antibiotics such as aminoglycosides or tetracycline so that less antibiotic is able to enter and bind to its target.
- Formation of alternative metabolic pathway. Sulphonamides and trimethoprim act by inhibiting the folate metabolic pathways within bacteria. However, where bacterial enzymes are produced that are much less inhibited by these two agents, resistance occurs.

The general spread of antibiotic resistance is most likely to occur in an environment in which there is a significant use of antibiotics and the opportunity to move from one host to another exists. In an environment where little use is made of antibiotics there will be no selective advantage for the resistant bacteria. Where antibiotics are used in low dose there will be greater opportunity for resistance to develop and spread since strains will survive at low dose which would have been eliminated at a higher dose. An example of this is the huge increase in the level of resistance in *Salmonella* due to the use of low-dose antibiotics as growth-enhancers in farm animals.

The cost of resistance is measured not only in terms of failure of therapy but also in the increased costs of more expensive drugs needed to combat the resistant bacteria.

CONTROL OF ANTIBIOTIC USAGE

Since the rates of resistance are proportional to antibiotic use, the unnecessary use of antibiotics contributes to the spread of resistance. Many hospitals have adopted antibiotic policies and guidelines which are aimed at reducing the induction of resistance through controlling the range and use of anti-infective agents. Good antibiotic prescribing requires information about the probable cause and the antibiotic susceptibility of the infective agent. This can be obtained by taking appropriate specimens for culture and prescribing according to the results.

General principles

The objective of drug therapy in the treatment of infectious disease is to assist the body in overcoming the infecting organism. This is accomplished by the use of an anti-infective agent which is toxic to the causative organism while the normal biochemical functions of the patient are not seriously impaired.

When selecting the anti-infective agent, consideration must be given to the dose, route and frequency of administration. The dosage regimen for antibiotics excreted primarily by the kidneys will be decided according to the type of infection to be treated and the toxicity of the drug. The dose of antibiotics with a narrow therapeutic spectrum, such as the aminoglycosides, requires to be titrated according to the serum concentration. This is in order to maintain an effective therapeutic level but avoid toxic effects due to too high a level. Where renal dysfunction is present which results in a longer half-life, dosage schedules should be lowered accordingly to prevent toxicity.

ROUTE OF ADMINISTRATION

If the infection is severe, the general condition of the patient may be poor. Oral absorption may therefore be poor due to nausea, vomiting or gastric stasis. In these instances, antibiotics are commonly administered by the parenteral route. After the infection is under control appropriate concentrations will be maintained by the oral route and this is more cost-effective.

Many antibiotic injections are presented as a sterile powder requiring reconstitution prior to administration. The nurse should refer to the manufacturer's product insert and to local policies in order to reconstitute the drug with correct diluent and the correct volume. Strict aseptic technique should be followed. It is advisable to discard any remaining solution after the initial dose has been withdrawn to avoid possible contamination or deterioration of the remaining solution.

ROUTINE PROPHYLAXIS

Routine antibiotic prophylaxis in surgical patients is only needed for procedures associated with a high risk of postoperative infection (e.g. vaginal or colorectal surgery) or prosthetic insertions. Normally, prophylactic antibiotic treatment should not be extended beyond 48 hours following surgery and should be given parenterally. Intravenous administration during induction, or intramuscular administration 30 minutes before surgery, usually ensures effective blood levels of antibiotic at the time when anticipated bacteraemia is likely to be highest. When gastrointestinal function is unimpaired during the postoperative period, oral administration of antibiotics provides an optimum non-invasive approach.

ALLERGIC RESPONSES

An accurate history of previous allergies is essential before antibiotics are administered. This applies particularly to penicillins with which anaphylactic shock occasionally occurs. Patients with a history of asthma, hayfever and eczema are more likely to experience severe reactions to penicillins. Some patients allergic to penicillins will also be allergic to cephalosporins. If patients are not allergic to penicillins, they are safe drugs with a high therapeutic index.

MONITORING THE PATIENT'S RESPONSE

The patient's response to antibiotic therapy is monitored with regard to (i) controlling the infection, and (ii) adverse effects.

Specific toxic effects of antibiotics should be noted, for example, hearing or renal impairment in patients receiving aminoglycosides. Phlebitis can occur on intravenous administration, and the nurse should monitor the patient's veins carefully for evidence of redness, swelling or pain

and report these to the doctor. Where blood samples are taken, the doctor should ensure that times are recorded accurately so that maximum and minimum drug concentrations during the dosing interval can be accurately estimated.

SUPERINFECTION

Superinfection may occur as a result of:

- proliferation of a resistant microorganism in place of the original sensitive microorganism at the site of infection.
- proliferation of a resistant microorganism in the alimentary tract due to suppression of the normal flora by antibiotic therapy. The broader the spectrum, the greater is the possibility of superinfection developing. Tetracyclines and ampicillin and its derivatives are examples. Pseudomembranous colitis results as an overgrowth of *Clostridium difficile* in the bowel presenting as watery diarrhoea, abdominal cramping, fever and leukocytosis. The most common treatment is oral vancomycin.
- drugs interfering with the immune response of the body, for example, corticosteroids and other immunosuppressive agents. Oral candidiasis, caused by *Candida albicans*, is the commonest example. This can be treated effectively with nystatin suspension.

THE PENICILLINS

The penicillins are bactericidal and interfere with cell wall synthesis in growing and dividing bacteria. Lysis and cell death result from weakening of the cell wall. Penicillins are excreted in the urine in therapeutic concentrations. Probenecid blocks renal tubular excretion producing higher and more prolonged concentrations.

The most significant and adverse effect of the penicillins is hypersensitivity which manifests as rashes and, on occasion, anaphylaxis. Allergy to one penicillin indicates allergy to them all since the hypersensitivity is related to the basic penicillin structure.

Two problems arise as a result of excessively high serum levels due either to very high doses or to renal failure in patients given normal doses.

The first problem is encephalopathy, a rare but serious toxic effect due to cerebral irritation. Patients should not be given an intrathecal injection as this can cause encephalopathy which may be fatal. The second problem is accumulation of electrolyte, since most injectable penicillins contain either sodium or potassium.

Diarrhoea often occurs during oral penicillin therapy.

Benzylpenicillin and phenoxymethylpenicillin

Benzylpenicillin (penicillin G) is readily inactivated by gastric acid juice and is best given by injection. It diffuses into most of the body tissues but does not pass the blood–brain barrier unless the meninges are inflamed, neither does it penetrate well into the pleural cavity nor into the synovial or ocular fluids. It is inactivated by bacterial penicillinases. Penicillinases are enzymes which inactivate penicillin by attacking part of the penicillin known as the β-lactam ring. This structure is an essential part of penicillins and cephalosporins, and the family of enzymes involved is known as the β-lactamases. Notable producers of penicillinase are staphylococci.

Benzylpenicillin may be combined with procaine or benzathine to produce the salts procaine penicillin and benzathine penicillin which have low solubility, resulting in delayed absorption and prolonged action. These are administered only by the intramuscular route.

Benzylpenicillin is effective in a wide range of infections, including those shown in Box 11.2.

Box 11.2 Infections for which benzylpenicillin is effective	
Organism	*Disease*
β-Haemolytic streptococci	Septicaemia, tonsillitis
Viridans streptococci	Subacute bacterial endocarditis
Streptococcus pneumoniae	Pneumonia
Neisseria meningitidis	Meningococcal meningitis
Clostridium tetani	Tetanus
Clostridium perfringens	Gas-gangrene
Treponema pallidum	Syphillis
Neisseria gonorrhoeae	Gonorrhoea
Borrelia burghdorferi	Lyme disease

Phenoxymethylpenicillin (penicillin V) has a similar but less active antibacterial spectrum. It is indicated principally for respiratory infections in children, streptococcal tonsillitis and continued treatment following benzylpenicillin injection. It is used as a prophylactic against re-infection after recovery from rheumatic fever. Phenoxymethylpenicillin is not destroyed in the stomach and is quickly but unpredictably absorbed from the small intestine. Absorption is superior when administered on an empty stomach. Phenoxymethylpenicillin is not suitable for the treatment of severe conditions where high blood levels of penicillin are necessary.

The dose range and side-effects of benzylpenicillin and phenoxymethylpenicillin are shown in Table 11.3.

Table 11.3 Benzylpenicillin and phenoxymethylpenicillin

Drug	Adult dose range	Onset of peak serum levels	Side-effects
Benzylpenicillin	By intramuscular or slow intravenous injection or by infusion, 1.2 g–2.4 g daily in 4 divided doses. Bacterial endocarditis – slow intravenous injection or by infusion 7.2 g daily in divided doses. Meningitis – slow intravenous injection or by infusion, 2.4 g every 4–6 hours.	15–30 minutes	Sensitivity reactions including urticaria, fever, joint pains, anaphylactic shock, diarrhoea after oral administration
Procaine penicillin (available as a combination product)	Procaine penicillin 300 mg benzylpenicillin 60 mg by intramuscular injection every 12–24 hours.	Biphasic	As for benzylpenicillin. It should be noted that *it is not for intravenous administration.*
Phenoxymethyl-penicillin	250–500 mg every 6 hours half an hour before food.	30–60 minutes	As for benzylpenicillin

Table 11.4 The penicillinase-resistant penicillins

Drug	Adult dose range	Notes
Cloxacillin	Oral: 500 mg 6-hourly at least 30 minutes before food. Intramuscular: 250 mg 4–6 hourly. Slow intravenous injection or infusion 500 mg every 4–6 hours.	Side-effects as for benzylpenicillin. Doses can be doubled in severe infections.
Flucloxacillin	Oral: 250 mg 6-hourly at least 30 minutes before food. Intramuscular: 250 mg 6-hourly. Slow intravenous injection or infusion 0.25–1 g every 6 hours.	As for cloxacillin.
Temocillin	Intramuscular, slow intravenous injection or infusion 1–2 g every 2 hours.	Side-effects as for benzylpenicillin.

Penicillinase-resistant penicillins

Some organisms are resistant to penicillin because of their ability to produce the enzyme penicillinase, which destroys penicillin. A range of penicillinase-resistant penicillins is available for treatment of staphylococcal infections where resistant organisms are particularly common (see Table 11.4). This is the sole indication for their use. The two in common use are cloxacillin and flucloxacillin, available in oral as well as injectable form since they are acid-stable. Flucloxacillin is preferred for oral therapy due to better absorption. Temocillin is a new penicillin active against Gram-negative bacteria except *Pseudomonas aeruginosa*.

Broad-spectrum penicillins

This group includes ampicillin and amoxycillin. Also included are pro-drugs bacampicillin and pivampicillin which are hydrolysed in the intestinal mucosa and portal system to form ampicillin. The main difference between ampicillin and amoxycillin is in absorption from the gut. Less than half the dose of ampicillin is absorbed from the gut and this is decreased by the presence of food. About 40% passes into the large bowel and diarrhoea, a common side-effect, is thought to be caused by a disturbance of the large bowel flora. Amoxycillin is better absorbed, producing higher plasma and tissue concentrations, absorption not being affected by the presence of food in the stomach. Both these drugs are inactivated by penicillinases, including those produced by almost all staphylococci, 50% of *E. coli* strains and 15% of *Haemophilus influenzae* strains. They should not be used for hospital patients without checking sensitivity.

Co-amoxyclav is a combination of amoxycillin and a β-lactamase inhibitor, clavulanic acid. The

Table 11.5 Broad-spectrum penicillins

Drug	Indications	Adult dose	Side-effects
Ampicillin	Urinary-tract infections, otitis media, sinusitis, chronic bronchitis, gonorrhoea.	Oral: 0.25–1 g every 6 hours at least 30 minutes before food. Intramuscular, intravenous 500 mg every 4–6 hours.	Nausea, diarrhoea, rashes.
Amoxycillin	As for ampicillin, plus typhoid fever and endocarditis prophylaxis.	Oral: 250–500 mg every 8 hours. Intramuscular: 500 mg every 8 hours. Intravenous: 500 mg every 8 hours, increased to 1 g every 6 hours.	As for ampicillin.
Co-amoxyclav	As for amoxycillin, but also effective against penicillinase-resistant *Staph. aureus*, *E. coli* and *Haemophilus influenzae* as well as *Bacteroides* and *Klebsiella* spp.	Expressed as amoxycillin 250–500 mg every 8 hours. Intravenous injection or infusion 1 g every 8 hours.	As for ampicillin.

clavulanate molecules penetrate the bacterial cell and combine with the β-lactamase molecules. This inactivates the β-lactamases, leaving the amoxycillin free to exert a full bactericidal effect. This makes the combination active against penicillinase-producing bacteria that are resistant to amoxycillin – *Staphylococcus aureus*, *E. coli* and *Haemophilus influenzae* as well as many *Bacteroides* and *Klebsiella* species.

The broad-spectrum penicillins are summarised in Table 11.5.

Antipseudomonal penicillins

Carbenicillin was the first antipseudomonal penicillin to be developed. Its antibacterial spectrum was similar to ampicillin but had in addition activity against *Pseudomonas*. However, high doses were required which tended to produce sodium overload and resistant bacteria also developed. It has largely been replaced by newer antibiotics, for example, by ticarcillin, which is more active against *Pseudomonas aeruginosa*, *Proteus* spp and *Bacteroides fragilis*. Timentin, a combination of ticarcillin and clavulanic acid, is active against penicillinase-producing bacteria resistant to ticarcillin.

The ureidopenicillins, azlocillin and piperacillin, have a broad spectrum and are both more active than ticarcillin against *Pseudomonas aeruginosa*. These drugs are used in pseudomonal septicaemias. In those life-threatening conditions it is preferable to give them in combination with an aminoglycoside such as gentamicin as this combination is synergistic.

The antipseudomonal penicillins are summarised in Table 11.6.

Mecillinams

Mecillinam and its pro-drug pivmecillinam are members of a class of penicillins called the amideno-penicillins. They are highly active against Gram-negative organisms, including salmonellae but excluding *Pseudomonas aeruginosa*. Indications and dose are given in Box 11.3.

Box 11.3 Mecillinams: indications and dose	
Indications	*Dose*
Uncomplicated cystitis	400 mg initially then 200 mg 8-hourly for 3 days
Chronic or recurrent bacteriuria	400 mg every 6–8 hours
Salmonellosis	1.2–2.4 g daily for 14 days

CEPHALOSPORINS AND CEPHAMYCINS

The cephalosporins were first obtained from a mould cultured from the sea near a Sardinian sewage outfall in 1945. The cephalosporins are related to the penicillins – both have a β-lactam ring which confers on them a similar mode of action. They act, like the penicillins, by inhibiting bacterial cell-wall synthesis.

The cephalosporins are broad-spectrum antibiotics and they are active against most Gram-positive and some Gram-negative organisms. All

Table 11.6 The antipseudomonal penicillins

Drug	Adult dose range	Side-effects
Azlocillin	Intravenous injection 2 g every 8 hours. Serious infections by intravenous infusion 5 g every 8 hours.	As for benzylpenicillin.
Carbenicillin	Intravenous injection or infusion 5 g every 4–6 hours. Intramuscular for urinary-tract infection 2 g every 6 hours.	As for benzylpenicillin.
Piperacillin	Intramuscular, intravenous injection and infusion 100–150 mg/kg daily in divided doses doubled for serious infections.	As for benzylpenicillin.
Ticarcillin	Intravenous injection or infusion 15–20 g daily in divided doses.	As for benzylpenicillin.

have a similar antibacterial spectrum, although individual agents have differing activity against certain organisms. Although cephalosporins are resistant to the penicillinase β-lactamases, cross-resistance between penicillinase-resistant penicillins and cephalosporins occurs.

The principal side-effect of the cephalosporins is hypersensitivity, and about 10% of penicillin-sensitive patients will be allergic to cephalosporins. Allergic reactions include rashes, pruritus, urticaria, fever and anaphylaxis. Other side-effects include diarrhoea, nausea, vomiting, erythema multiforme, eosinophilia and transient hepatitis.

Oral cephalosporins

Six oral cephalosporins are listed in Table 11.7.

Cefaclor, cephalexin and cephradine are acid-stable and are well absorbed from the gastro-intestinal tract, although the presence of food delays absorption but does not affect the total amount absorbed. They are excreted unchanged in the urine, and the dose or frequency of administration must be modified in response to the degree of renal impairment.

Cefaclor, cephalexin and cephradine are also very similar in antibacterial activity; all are active against staphylococci and streptococci (not enterococci, which are uniformly resistant to all cephalosporins) but less active against Gram-negative bacilli. Their principal use is in treating urinary-tract infections which do not respond to other drugs or which occur in pregnancy.

Table 11.7 Oral cephalosporins

Drug	Adult dose
Cefaclor	250–500 mg every 8 hours
Cefadroxil	0.5–1 g twice daily
Cefixime	200–400 mg daily as a single dose or in two divided doses
Cefuroxime axetil	250 mg twice daily
Cephalexin	250 mg every 6 hours; 1–1.5 g every 6 or 8 hours for severe infections
Cephradine	250–500 mg every 6 hours

Cefadroxil and cefixime both have longer serum half-lives, allowing a reduced frequency of dose. Cefixime also has good activity against *Haemophilus influenzae*. Cefuroxime axetil is an ester of the parent compound cefuroxime. Although it has high activity against Gram-negative bacilli, absorption is poor and variable.

Parenteral cephalosporins

In general, cephradine and cephazolin have been replaced by newer cephalosporins. Cefuroxime and cephamandole are less susceptible than first-generation cephalosporins to inactivation by penicillinase and have greater activity against *Haemophilus influenzae* and *Neisseria gonorrhoeae*.

Cefoxitin, a cephamycin antibioitic, is not susceptible to penicillinase produced by Gram-negative organisms. It is active against *E. coli* and anaerobes, including *Bacteroides fragilis*, and has been used peri-operatively to reduce the incidence of infections in patients undergoing large-bowel surgery. Cefoxitin is recommended for abdominal sepsis such as peritonitis.

Cefotaxime, ceftazidime, ceftizoxime, ceftriaxone and cefodizime are third-generation cephalosporins. They have a markedly increased resistance to Gram-negative penicillinase and thus possess a broader spectrum of activity against Gram-negative organisms. Cefsulodin and ceftazidime possess good activity against *Pseudomonas*. Cefsulodin has a very narrow spectrum of activity and should be used only for pseudomonal infections. The third-generation cephalosporins lack activity against Gram-positive bacteria, notably *Staphylococcus aureus*, and superinfection may occur with resistant bacteria. A recent introduction, ceftriaxone has potent bactericidal activity against a wide spectrum of Gram-positive and particularly Gram-negative organisms. The spectrum of activity includes both aerobic and some anaerobic species. It has considerable stability against degradation by most bacterial lactamases.

Parenteral cephalosporins are summarised in Table 11.8, and some other β-lactam antibiotics are given in Table 11.9.

Table 11.8 Parenteral cephalosporins

Drug	Indications	Dose
Cefodizime	Lower respiratory-tract infection, including pneumonia and bronchopneumonia. Upper and lower urinary-tract infections.	1 g every 12 hours. 1 g every 12 hours.
Cefotaxime	Infections due to sensitive Gram-positive and Gram-negative organisms	1 g every 8 hours. Increased for life-threatening infections.
Cefoxitin	See cefotaxime. Surgical prophylaxis, more active against Gram-negative organisms.	1–2 g every 6–8 hours, increased to maximum 12 g daily.
Cefsulodin sodium	Infections due to sensitive strains of *Pseudomonas aeruginosa*, surgical prophylaxis.	1–4 g daily in divided doses. Increased in severe infections.
Ceftazidime	See cefotaxime. Active against *Pseudomonas aeruginosa*.	1 g every 8 hours. Increased in severe infections.
Ceftizoxime	See cefotaxime. Gonorrhoea.	1–2 g every 8–12 hours. Increased in severe infections. 1 g intramuscularly as single dose.
Cefuroxime	See cefotaxime. Surgical prophylaxis More active against *H. influenzae* and *N. gonorrhoeae*	750 mg every 6–8 hours. Increased in severe infections. 1.5 g intravenously at induction followed by 750 mg 8 and 16 hours later (orthopaedic). Gonorrhoea 1.5 g intramuscularly as single dose.
Cephamandole	See cefotaxime. Surgical prophylaxis.	0.5–2 g every 4–8 hours. 1–2 g 30–60 minutes before surgery and then 1–2 g 6-hourly for up to 3 days.
Cephazolin	See cefotaxime. Surgical prophylaxis.	0.5–1 g every 6–12 hours.
Cephradine	See cefotaxime. Surgical prophylaxis.	0.5–1 g every 6 hours. Increased in severe infections.
Ceftriaxone	See cefuroxime.	1 g daily by deep intramuscular injection, slow intravenous injection or slow intravenous infusion. Severe injections 2–4 g. Gonorrhoea: 250 mg as a single dose. Once-daily dosing facilitates a single dose in surgical prophylaxis.

TETRACYCLINES

The most commonly used members of the tetracycline family are chlortetracycline, demeclocycline, doxycycline, minocycline, oxytetracycline and tetracycline.

Mode of action of tetracyclines

The tetracyclines are generally bacteriostatic rather than bactericidal in action. They inhibit protein synthesis in bacterial ribosomes in susceptible organisms thus preventing production of polypeptides.

Table 11.9 Other beta-lactam antibiotics

Drug	Indications	Side-effects	Dose
Aztreonam	Gram-negative infections, including *Pseudomonas aeruginosa*, *Haemophilus influenzae*, *Neisseria meningitidis*, *Neisseria gonorrhoeae*.	Nausea, vomiting, diarrhoea, abdominal cramps, mouth ulcers, urticaria and rashes.	1 g every 8 hours or 2 g every 12 hours.
Imipenem with cilastatin (Cilastatin inhibits inactivation of imipenem by kidney enzymes.)	Aerobic and anaerobic Gram-positive and Gram-negative infections, surgical prophylaxis.	Nausea, vomiting, diarrhoea, fever, anaphylactic reactions, allergic reactions, blood disorders.	Intramuscular 500–750 mg every 12 hours. Intravenous infusion, 1–2 g daily in divided doses.

Uses

Tetracyclines have a broad antimicrobial spectrum and demonstrate activity against most Gram-positive organisms that are sensitive to the penicillins and also against some Gram-negative organisms that are not susceptible to the penicillins. Table 11.10 lists some of the infectious diseases for which tetracyclines may be indicated. They are also used for the treatment of exacerbations of chronic bronchitis because of their activity against *Haemophilus influenzae*. Microbiologically there is little to choose between the various tetracyclines. Minocycline is an exception since it has a broader spectrum of activity, is active against *Neisseria meningitidis* and has been used in the prevention of meningococcal meningitis as an alternative to rifampicin. Tetracyclines may also be used in the treatment of acne vulgaris.

Pharmacokinetics

The tetracyclines in general are reasonably well absorbed (about 70%), minocycline and doxycycline being absorbed to a greater extent (about 90%). The concomitant administration of milk, agents such as antacids containing aluminium, magnesium or calcium, and iron salts reduces absorption from the gastrointestinal tract because of the formation of insoluble chelates. The tetracyclines are widely distributed to body tissues and are taken up in teeth and bone, especially growing bone and teeth during the early stages of calcification. This can cause both discolouration and enamel hypoplasia in teeth and decreased growth of long bones. They should not therefore be given in pregnancy or to children under 12 years of age.

Approximately 50% of most tetracyclines are excreted in the urine unchanged. Renal failure causes decreased clearance and accumulation resulting in toxicity. Minocycline and doxycycline are exceptions, being mainly metabolised in the liver, and doxycycline is the tetracycline of choice in compromised renal function.

Adverse effects

Tetracyclines commonly produce gastrointestinal adverse effects, e.g. nausea, vomiting and diarrhoea. A rarely occurring condition is superinfection with *Clostridium difficile*, resulting in pseudomembranous colitis. Oral superinfection with *Candida albicans* may result in thrush. Overgrowth in the bowel may cause diarrhoea. Treatment consists of stopping the administration of tetracycline and, in severe cases, treatment with nystatin. Minocycline in addition can cause dizziness, vertigo and severe exfoliative rashes.

Dosage

The dosages of the tetracyclines (see Table 11.11) vary, and this is partly accountable to different half-lives, e.g. chlortetracycline, oxytetracycline, tetracycline 8 hours, demeclocycline 14 hours, minocycline and doxycycline 18 hours.

Table 11.10 Main indications for the use of tetracyclines

Disease	Organism
Infections caused by chlamydia	
psittacosis	*Chlamydia psittaci*
lymphogranuloma venereum	LGV Chlamydiae
trachoma	*Chlamydia trachomatis*
non-specific urethritis	*Chlamydia* and *Ureaplasma* spp
Q fever	*Coxiella burnetii*
Typhus diseases	*Rickettsia* spp
Mycoplasma pneumonia	*Mycoplasma pneumoniae*
Brucellosis	*Brucella abortus*
(doxycycline with rifampicin)	
Lyme disease	*Borrelia burghdorferi*

Table 11.11 Dosages of tetracyclines

Drug	Dose
Chlortetracycline	250–500 mg every 6 hours
Demeclocyline	150 mg every 6 hours
Doxycycline	200 mg initially then 100 mg daily
Minocycline	100 mg twice daily
Oxytetracycline	250–500 mg 6-hourly
Tetracycline	Oral: 250–500 mg 6-hourly
	Intramuscular: 100–200 mg 6–8-hourly
	Intravenous infusion: 500 mg 12-hourly

AMINOGLYCOSIDES

This group of drugs includes amikacin, gentamicin, kanamycin, neomycin, netilmicin, streptomycin and tobramycin.

Mode of action

The aminoglycosides are bactericidal. The mechanism is not fully understood but they inhibit the synthesis of bacterial protein by binding to ribosomes within the pathogen.

Uses

The aminoglycosides are active against some Gram-positive and many Gram-negative organisms. Examples of bacteria which are sensitive to the aminoglycosides are given in Table 11.12.

Gentamicin is the most important aminoglycoside and is widely used for the treatment of serious infections. The main indication for amikacin is the treatment of serious infections caused by Gram-negative bacilli resistant to gentamicin. Neomycin is not significantly absorbed following oral administration and is used for bowel sterilisation prior to bowel surgery. It is also used to treat hepatic encephalopathy, reducing ammonia-producing bacteria in the gut. The aminoglycosides are effective agents for the local treatment of infections of the external ear and conjunctiva. Neomycin, which is too toxic for parenteral administration, framycetin and gentamicin are commonly used. Neomycin is also used, in combination with chlorhexidine, for attempted eradication of staphylococci in the nasal passage.

Pharmacokinetics

The aminoglycosides are poorly absorbed from the gastrointestinal tract and must be given by injection for systemic infections. They have a narrow therapeutic spectrum and plasma concentration monitoring ensures that optimal therapeutic levels are maintained thus preventing toxicity and ensuring efficacy. Plasma concentrations should be measured approximately 1 hour after injection (peak level) and just before the next dose (trough level). Trough and peak levels of gentamicin and kanamycin are shown in Table 11.13.

Parenterally administered aminoglycosides are excreted almost entirely by the kidneys. Care should be taken with dosage and, where possible, treatment should not exceed 7 days in order to minimise side-effects. Doses should be reduced in renal failure.

Adverse effects

The important side-effects are ototoxicity and, to a lesser degree, nephrotoxicity. These occur most commonly in the elderly and in patients with renal failure due to elevated serum levels, i.e. trough levels greater than 2 μg/ml and peak levels greater than 12 μg/ml. Long duration of treatment is also a causative factor. Gentamicin tends to cause vertigo and ataxia while neomycin and kanamycin cause deafness. Neomycin is too toxic for systemic use. Aminoglycosides should be avoided in pregnancy as they cross the placenta and cause damage to the eighth nerve of the fetus. Aminoglycosides may impair neuro-

Table 11.12 Examples of bacteria which are sensitive to aminoglycosides

Bacteria	Disease	Aminoglycoside
Gram-positive cocci	Streptococcal endocarditis	Gentamicin in combination with penicillin G
Gram-negative bacilli	Infections due to Escherichia coli Klebsiella pneumoniae Proteus Pseudomonas	Amikacin, gentamicin, tobramycin
Mycobacteria	Tuberculosis	Streptomycin

Table 11.13 Trough and peak levels of gentamicin and kanamycin

	Trough level	Peak level
Gentamicin	Less than 2 μg/ml	Less than 12 μg/ml
Kanamycin	Less than 10 μg/ml	Less than 40 μg/ml

muscular transmission and should not be given to patients with myasthenia gravis.

Interactions

Aminoglycosides should not be given with frusemide or ethacrynic acid as these may potentiate the ototoxic and nephrotoxic effects.

Dosages

The dosages of aminoglycosides are summarised in Table 11.14.

MACROLIDES

This group of drugs includes erythromycin, azithromycin, clarithromycin and spiramycin.

Mode of action

Erythromycin is classified as a bacteriostatic drug but it may be bactericidal in high concentrations or against highly susceptible organisms. Erythromycin inhibits protein synthesis in susceptible organisms by binding to ribosomes and inhibiting polypeptide synthesis. Resistance is rarely observed during successful short-term treatment.

Uses

Erythromycin has a similar antibacterial spectrum to benzylpenicillin and is used for infections in which benzylpenicillin would be the treatment of choice but where the patient is sensitive to penicillin. Erythromycin is indicated for respiratory infections, whooping cough, legionnaire's disease (*Legionella pneumophila*), chlamydia and mycoplasmas.

Azithromycin has greater activity than erythromycin against some Gram-negative bacteria.

Pharmacokinetics

Erythromycin may be administered orally or by injection. Oral formulations containing the erythromycin base must be enteric-coated as the base is decomposed by gastric acid. The enteric coating breaks down in the higher pH of the duodenum and the erythromycin is absorbed. The stearate, ethylsuccinate and estolate forms of erythromycin are not acid-labile. They dissociate in the duodenum, liberating active erythromycin which is absorbed. Following absorption erythromycin is widely distributed in the tissues. It penetrates the meninges only when they are inflamed. The drug is excreted primarily in the bile. Erythromycin may be given intravenously as the lactobionate.

Adverse effects

Erythromycin is one of the safest and least toxic of the antibiotics. The most common side-effects of the oral erythromycins are gastrointestinal and are dose-related. These include nausea, vomiting, diarrhoea and abdominal discomfort after large doses. Azithromycin and clarithromycin cause fewer gastrointestinal side-effects than erythromycin. The intravenous injection of erythromycin causes venous irritation and thrombophlebitis, particularly in high doses. It is recommended that the drug be well diluted and infused slowly over 20 to 60 minutes to minimise these effects.

Dosage

250–1000 mg four times daily, orally or intravenously.

Table 11.14 Dosages of aminoglycosides

Drug	Dose
Gentamicin	Intramuscular, slow intravenous injection or intravenous infusion 2.5 mg/kg daily in divided doses 8-hourly. (Monitor serum level, and creatinine clearance in renal impairment.)
Amikacin	Intramuscular, slow intravenous injection or intravenous infusion 15 mg/kg daily in 2 divided doses.
Kanamycin	Intramuscular 250 mg 6-hourly. Intravenous infusion 15–30 mg/kg daily in divided doses every 8–12 hours.
Neomycin	1 g every 4 hours for bowel sterilisation.

CLINDAMYCIN

Clindamycin acts by inhibiting bacterial protein synthesis. It has restricted use due to the significant side-effects, in particular, pseudomembranous colitis, which may be fatal. The drug should be immediately discontinued if diarrhoea or colitis develop.

Clindamycin is active against Gram-positive cocci (streptococci, penicillin-resistant staphylococci), Gram-negative bacilli (*Bacteroides*) and Gram-positive bacilli (*Clostridium* spp). Because of the adverse effects, clindamycin is generally reserved for staphylococcal bone and joint infections, peritonitis and endocarditis prophylaxis, and topically for severe acne.

Adverse effects

Adverse effects due to clindamycin include abdominal discomfort, nausea, vomiting, diarrhoea and pseudomembranous colitis, jaundice and blood dyscrasias. It may cause thrombophlebitis following an intravenous injection.

Dosage

Oral therapy, 150–450 mg every 6 hours. Deep intramuscular or intravenous infusion 0.6–4.8 g daily in 2–4 divided doses. Single dose above 600 mg by intravenous infusion only.

OTHER ANTIBIOTICS

A number of other antibiotics are described in Table 11.15.

SULPHONAMIDES AND TRIMETHOPRIM

The first of the sulphonamides was used in the treatment of infections in the 1930s. However, the importance of sulphonamides in this role has decreased in recent years as a result of increasing bacterial resistance and replacement by more effective and less toxic antibiotics.

A combination of trimethoprim one part and sulphamethoxazole five parts (cotrimoxazole)

has been used because of the synergistic activity of these drugs. Indications for this include urinary-tract infections caused by susceptible bacteria, including *Escherichia coli*, *Klebsiella* and *Enterobacter*, prostatitis, chronic bronchitis caused by *Streptococcus pneumoniae* and *Haemophilus influenzae*, and enteric fever due to *Salmonella*. High doses of cotrimoxazole are used for *Pneumocystis carinii* infections.

Apart from pneumocystis, trimethoprim is now usually used alone for the treatment of the above indications due to bacterial resistance to, and adverse effects of, sulphamethoxazole.

Mode of action

The sulphonamides are bacteriostatic and act by preventing the conversion of para-aminobenzoic acid to folic acid. Trimethoprim blocks bacterial folic acid synthesis at the stage immediately following that blocked by the sulphonamides, as shown in Box 11.4.

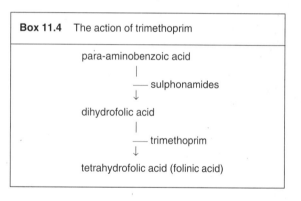

Box 11.4   The action of trimethoprim

para-aminobenzoic acid
|
—— sulphonamides
↓
dihydrofolic acid
|
—— trimethoprim
↓
tetrahydrofolic acid (folinic acid)

Pharmacokinetics

Individual sulphonamides differ markedly in their absorption, distribution and excretion. Sulphamethoxazole, sulphadiazine and sulphadimidine are generally well absorbed. Metabolism is very variable, the major route being acetylation in the liver. Variability is due to the fact that the population can be divided into two groups – those which acetylate the drug rapidly and those which acetylate slowly. This characteristic is genetically determined. The acetylated

Table 11.15　Other antibiotics

Indications	Pharmacokinetics	Adverse reactions	Dose
Chloramphenicol Only for life-threatening infections because of toxicity, e.g. meningitis due to *Haemophilus influenzae*, typhoid fever. Eye drops useful for bacterial conjunctivitis.	Well absorbed from GI tract.	Blood disorders, including aplastic anaemia, nausea, vomiting, diarrhoea. 'Grey syndrome' in neonates.	50 mg/kg daily in 4 divided doses.
Sodium fusidate Infections due to penicillin-resistant staphylococci, particularly osteomyelitis, often in conjunction with a second antistaphylococcal antibiotic to prevent resistance, e.g. flucloxacillin.	Well absorbed, widely distributed in body tissues, including bone. Metabolised in liver and excreted in bile.	Nausea, vomiting, skin rashes.	Oral: 0.5–1 g every 8 hours. Intravenous infusion 0.5 g over 6 hours 3 times daily.
Spectinomycin Treatment of *Neisseria gonorrhoeae* resistant to penicillin, or in penicillin-allergic patient.	Not absorbed from GI tract.	Nausea, dizziness, urticaria, fever.	Deep intramuscular 2–4 g.
Vancomycin Bactericidal activity against aerobic and anaerobic Gram-positive bacteria. Drug of choice in antibiotic related pseudo-membranous colitis (*Clostridium difficile*). Alternative to penicillins in infective endocarditis.	Very poorly absorbed from the gastrointestinal tract. Widely distributed in body tissues following intravenous infusion. Almost completely eliminated unchanged in the urine. It has a long duration of action and can be given every 12 hours. Accumulates in renal failure, necessitating a modified dosage schedule and serum concentration monitoring (below 30 µg/ml). Dose should be reduced in the elderly.	Ototoxic and nephrotoxic which are dose related. Extravasation causes necrosis and thrombophlebitis. After parenteral administration may get nausea, chills, fever, urticaria, rashes, tinnitus (discontinue use).	Oral: 125 mg 6-hourly. Intravenous infusion 500 mg every 6 hours.
Teicoplanin Bactericidal against most Gram-positive organisms. Serious Gram-positive infections, including endocarditis, treatment of staphylococcal infections of bone and joint.	Longer half-life than vancomycin and requires only once-daily dosing. Available as intramuscular and intravenous injection, low nephrotoxic, ototoxic and allergenic potential – routine serum monitoring not required.	No significant enhanced renal toxicity when used with aminoglycosides. Nausea, vomiting, diarrhoea, rash, fever, anaphylaxis, blood disorders, tinnitus, local thrombophlebitis.	Intravenous injection or infusion 400 mg initially, 200–400 mg daily.
Colistin Bactericidal in action, it is active against Gram-negative organisms, including *Escherichia coli*, *Klebsiella* spp, and *Pseudomonas aeruginosa*.	Not absorbed from the gastrointestinal tract so must be given intramuscularly or intravenously for treatment of systemic infections. However, it is toxic and seldom used systemically.	Nephrotoxicity is the most serious adverse effect. Allergic manifestations, paraesthesia, vertigo, apnoea and muscle weakness occur less frequently.	Oral for bowel sterilisation: 1.5–3 million units every 8 hours. Intramuscular, intravenous injection or infusion 2 million units every 8 hours.

drug, which is excreted in the urine, has a low solubility and there is a danger that it will precipitate in the urine (crystalluria). Renal damage may occur due to precipitation in the renal tubules. Crystalluria may cause pain and haematuria. Anuria can occur if the renal pelvis or the ureters become completely occluded. A high intake of fluid helps to minimise this side-effect.

Trimethoprim is rapidly absorbed. It is excreted mainly in the urine, and dosages should be reduced in renal failure. Crystalluria does not occur.

Adverse effects

Allergic reactions are common, their incidence increasing with increased dosage. These include maculopapular skin rashes, drug fever and photodermatitis. Occasionally blood dyscrasias may occur including thrombocytopenia, agranulocytosis, leucopenia. Crystalluria, which was a problem with the older, less soluble sulphonamides, does not occur with sulphamethoxazole. Nausea, vomiting and diarrhoea may occur. Special care should be taken where folate may be deficient, e.g. the elderly, chronic sick and those on prolonged treatment or high doses. Because of the possibility of jaundice and kernicterus (deposition of bilirubin in the brains of neonates), sulphonamides should not be given to pregnant women in the third trimester nor to newborn or premature infants. Side-effects which may occur with trimethoprim include nausea, vomiting, pruritus and rashes.

The dosages of sulphonamides and trimethoprim are summarised in Table 11.16.

Table 11.16 Dosages of sulphonamides and trimethoprim

Drug	Dose
Cotrimoxazole	1 tablet twice daily Intramuscular or intravenous infusion, 960 mg every 12 hours
Sulfametopyrazine	2 g once weekly
Trimethoprim	Oral: 200 mg twice daily; slow intravenous injection or infusion 150–250 mg every 12 hours

TUBERCULOSIS

Tuberculosis is a bacterial infection caused by the bacterium *Mycobacterium tuberculosis*. In humans, the lung is the most common site of infection, although numerous other areas (meninges, bones, joints, peritoneum, genitourinary tract, skin) may also become infected.

Tuberculosis is spread by airborne droplets, from coughing and sneezing, which contain viable bacilli. These are inhaled and lodge in the alveoli where the bacilli rapidly multiply. On primary infection the bacilli multiply rapidly in the lungs and spread to the lymph nodes and to the bloodstream. The organism is thus distributed throughout the body where it can remain viable but dormant for many years, particularly in the lungs, bones, lymphatic system and kidneys.

Primary infection is usually controlled by the host's immune system. The bacteria become engulfed by macrophages which coalesce to form a mass of cells – a tubercle or granuloma. The bacilli contained in the granuloma may survive and remain dormant for many years. The granuloma may break down in later years, leading to pulmonary or extrapulmonary clinical disease.

Widespread disease following primary infection is rare, although susceptible groups such as young infants, the immunocompromised, or malnourished and debilitated patients may be at risk.

Signs and symptoms

Primary tuberculosis is usually a mild asymptomatic illness which resolves spontaneously without problems. The onset of postprimary disease is slow. When symptoms occur they include chronic cough, sometimes with blood-streaked sputum (haemoptysis), malaise, weight loss, fever, night sweats, anorexia, anxiety and depression.

Diagnostic tests

The discovery of *Mycobacterium tuberculosis* by either microscopy of sputum smears or by culture is diagnostic of active tuberculosis. Tuberculin testing is an adjunct to diagnosis. The two tests used are as follows.

Mantoux test

This consists of the intradermal injection of between 1 and 100 units of tuberculin PPD (purified protein derivative) in 0.1 ml. (Five units is the normal dose.) The reaction is read 48–72 hours after injection, and a positive reaction indicating the presence of antibodies is demonstrated by an induration of 10 mm or more in diameter.

Heaf (multiple puncture) test

A syringe gun with six needles arranged in a circle is used to puncture the skin to which a drop of tuberculin PPD, 2 mg/ml, has been applied. The reaction is read 3–10 days later and a positive result is indicated by a solid induration of at least 5 mm.

Drug treatment of tuberculosis
(Table 11.17)

The treatment of tuberculosis has two phases – an initial phase using at least three drugs, and a continuation phase with two drugs. Recom-

Table 11.17 Drugs used in the treatment of tuberculosis

Drug	Adult dosage	Adverse effects/interactions	Comments
Isoniazid	300 mg daily	Peripheral neuropathy, particularly where diabetes, alcoholism, renal failure or malnutrition are present in which case 10 mg of pyridoxine should be given daily. Some epileptic patients treated with phenytoin experience symptoms of phenytoin toxicity when given isoniazid and rifampicin. Appears to be related to inhibition of metabolism in slow acetylators of isoniazid.	Elimination by acetylation in the liver.
Rifampicin	Under 50 kg – 450 mg daily; over 50 kg – 600 mg daily.	Anorexia and nausea may occur. Hepatotoxicity is a serious side-effect and alcoholics, the elderly and patients with pre-existing liver disease are at risk. Concurrent administration of rifampicin with oral contraceptives increases the metabolism of oestrogen and progestogen, which may result in contraceptive failure. Alternative contraceptive methods should be used. Anticoagulant effects of warfarin are reduced by concurrent administration of rifampicin due to increased metabolism of the anticoagulant.	Monitor liver function tests. Caution in pregnancy. Patients should be advised that rifampicin colours the urine, stools and tears. Soft contact lenses may become permanently discoloured.
Pyrazinamide	Under 50 kg – 1.5 g daily; over 50 kg – 2 g daily.	Liver damage, hyperuricaemia.	Monitor liver function tests. Readily absorbed and penetrates well into CSF, making it particularly useful in tuberculous meningitis. Should not be given to patients with gout.
Ethambutol	15 mg/kg daily.	Optic neuritis, colour blindness and restriction of visual fields. These are related to plasma levels and are more common where excessive dosage is used. Therapy should be discontinued where these adverse effects are experienced.	Reduce dosage in renal failure. Patients should be advised to seek medical advice if they experience visual disturbance.

mended regimens of the Joint Tuberculosis Committee of the British Thoracic Society for the treatment of tuberculosis in the United Kingdom are given below.

Initial phase

In order to reduce the population of viable bacteria rapidly and to prevent emergence of resistant bacteria, at least three drugs are given concurrently in the initial phase. This involves the daily use of isoniazid, rifampicin and pyrazinamide. Ethambutol is added where drug resistance is a possibility. This regimen should be continued for at least 8 weeks.

Continuation phase

This follows the initial phase and treatment with isoniazid and rifampicin is continued for a further 4 months.

METRONIDAZOLE AND TINIDAZOLE

Metronidazole has been used since 1959 to treat protozoal infections due to *Trichomonas vaginalis* and also amoebiasis. Since then the drug's activity against obligate anaerobes, including *Bacteroides fragilis*, has been recognised. Tinidazole is similar to metronidazole but has a longer duration of action.

Metronidazole

Data relating to metronidazole are given in Table 11.18.

4-QUINOLONES

The original quinolone antibiotic is nalidixic acid, which has been available for 30 years. More recently, molecular changes have produced fluorinated quinolones with a broader antibacterial spectrum and better pharmacokinetics.

Table 11.18   Metronidazole

Mode of action	Uses/dosage	Pharmacokinetics	Important adverse effects and interactions
Has high activity against anaerobic bacteria and protozoa. It is reduced to active metabolites which interfere with nucleic acid function.	*Anaerobic infections* Oral – treated for 7 days 800 mg initially then 400 mg every 8 hours. By rectum – 1 g every 8 hours for 3 days then 1 g every 12 hours. Intravenous infusion – 500 mg every 8 hours. *Bacterial vaginosis* Oral – 400 mg twice daily for 7 days or 2 g as a single dose. *Giardiasis* 2 g daily for 3 days. *Amoebiasis* Oral – 400–800 mg three times daily for 5–10 days. *Acute ulcerative gingivitis* Oral – 200 mg every 8 hours for 3 days. *Pseudomembranous colitis* Oral – 400 mg three times daily. *Surgical prophylaxis* Oral – 400 mg every 8 hours, started 24 hours before surgery then continued postoperatively by intravenous infusion or by rectum. Used topically to reduce the odour produced by anaerobic bacteria in fungating tumours.	Well absorbed after oral and rectal administration. Effective serum concentrations are reached in 1–3 hours and maintained for 8–10 hours. Excreted mainly in the urine. Crosses placental barrier and appears in the milk of nursing mothers.	The most common reactions to metronidazole therapy are rash, pruritus, urticaria, nausea, furry tongue, dry mouth, metallic taste in the mouth, headache and dizziness. Patients are advised to avoid taking alcohol when receiving metronidazole as the combination may produce abdominal cramps, nausea, vomiting, headaches and flushing. Caution in pregnancy and breast-feeding.

Mode of action

The quinolone antibiotics are bactericidal. They act by inhibiting the enzyme DNA gyrase required by the bacterial DNA.

Uses

The spectrum of microbiological activity of the 4-quinolone antibiotics is one of high activity against Gram-negative bacteria, slightly less activity against Gram-positive bacteria and little or no activity against anaerobes. Examples of the 4-quinolones are summarised in Table 11.19.

Pharmacokinetics

The 4-quinolones are well absorbed following oral administration. Antacids decrease their absorption. They are eliminated in three ways:

- secreted into the gut lumen and excreted in the faeces
- metabolised by the liver
- excreted as unchanged drug via the kidneys.

No differences have been found in serum half-lives in the elderly. Patients taking ciprofloxacin should ensure adequate fluid intake to minimise the risk of crystalluria.

Adverse drug reactions

Side-effects of the 4-quinolones commonly involve the central nervous system – headache, dizziness, sleep disorders and less frequently restlessness, hallucinations, confusion. Patients should be advised of this since performance of skilled tasks, e.g. driving, may be impaired. Because of these adverse reactions, the drugs should be used with caution in patients with a history of epilepsy. They may induce convulsions in patients with or without a history of convulsions and taking NSAIDs concurrently may potentiate this. Gastrointestinal side-effects including nausea, vomiting, abdominal pain and diarrhoea may occur. Allergic reactions to the 4-quinolones include rash and anaphylaxis. Photosensitivity reactions consisting of erythema on exposed skin surfaces may occur. Blood disorders including eosinophilia, leucopenia and thrombocytopenia have been noted. Other side-effects include an increase in blood urea and creatinine, arthralgia and myalgia.

Since weight-bearing joints of juvenile animals have suffered cartilage damage when quinolones were administered, caution should be exercised in children and adolescents. Care should be taken where hepatic or renal impairment exist and also in pregnancy and breast-feeding.

Table 11.19 The 4-quinolones

Drug	Indications	Dose
Acrosoxacin	*N. gonorrhoeae* where patient is allergic to penicillins or where strain is resistant to penicillins.	300 mg as single dose on an empty stomach.
Cinoxacin	Uncomplicated urinary-tract infection.	500 mg every 12 hours. Prophylaxis – 500 mg at night.
Ciprofloxacin	Particularly active against Gram-negative bacteria including *Campylobacter, Neisseria, Pseudomonas, Salmonella, Shigella*. Less activity against Gram-positive bacteria such as *Strep. pneumoniae* and *Strep. faecalis*. Used for infections of the respiratory tract (but not pneumococcal pneumonia), urinary tract, gastrointestinal system, gonorrhoea and septicaemia.	Oral – 250–750 mg twice daily. Gonorrhoea – 250 mg as a single dose. Available as intravenous infusion.
Nalidixic acid	Uncomplicated urinary-tract infections.	500 mg–1 g every 6 hours.
Norfloxacin	Uncomplicated urinary-tract infections.	400 mg twice daily.
Ofloxacin	Infections of urinary tract, lower respiratory tract, gonorrhoea.	200–400 mg daily. Gonorrhoea – 400 mg as a single dose. Available as an intravenous infusion.

URINARY-TRACT INFECTIONS

Explanation of terms

Bacteriuria. Bacteria cultured from urine. Asymptomatic bacteriuria exists if colony counts exceed 10^5/ml in a patient without urinary-tract infection (UTI) symptoms.

Pyelonephritis. Inflammation of the kidney with pain, tenderness, bacteriuria, pyuria and fever.

Pyuria. White blood cells in the urine.

Urethritis. Inflammation of the urethra with dysuria.

Prostatitis. Inflammation of the prostate.

Bladder urine is normally sterile, although transient small numbers of bacteria may be present after micturition or sexual intercourse. This occurs because of retrograde flow up the urethra. It is far more likely to happen with women because of the length of the urethra and the increased number of organisms resident on the surfaces surrounding the orifice. The first step in the development of UTI is colonisation of the peri-urethral mucosa, commonly by *Escherichia coli* from faeces.

To initiate infection, bacteria present in the urine must adhere to the urothelial cells on the bladder surface. One of the more important host defence mechanisms is the continual renewal of the surface by shedding cells together with attached bacteria and mucus. Urine does not normally support the growth of bacteria because of the large variation in pH, osmolality and the antibacterial substances present.

In managing patients with urinary-tract infection, the infection is often classified as simple (uncomplicated) or complicated. One way to define a complicated UTI is one that fails to respond to a short course of antibiotics. Symptoms commonly associated with lower UTIs (e.g. cystitis) include:

- urgency
- frequency
- pain or burning on micturition (dysuria)
- cloudy or malodorous urine
- suprapubic pain.

Patients with acute pyelonephritis may also present with loin pain, tenderness, fever, chills, nausea and haematuria.

UTI is predominantly a disease of females from the age of 1 until about the age of 50, most neonatal cases of UTI occurring in males. UTIs again become a problem for males after the age of 50 when prostatic obstruction, urethral instrumentation and surgery influence the infection rate. In general, 10–20% of the elderly living at home have bacteriuria, and up to 40% in long-stay hospitals. The reasons for higher UTI rates in older people include the high prevalence of prostatitis in males, poor bladder emptying and faecal incontinence.

Causes

Most organisms involved are bowel commensals, the commonest being *Escherichia coli*. Less common causes include *Proteus* and *Klebsiella* spp. *Staphylococcus epidermidis*, *Pseudomonas aeruginosa* and *Enterococcus faecalis* infection may occur following catheterisation or instrumentation.

Treatment

Table 11.20 outlines the drugs used according to the degree of infection being treated.

NITROFURANTOIN

Nitrofurantoin is bacteriostatic. It acts by inhibiting a number of bacterial enzymes essential for bacterial function.

Pharmacokinetics

Nitrofurantoin is rapidly and well absorbed following oral administration at a dosage of 50 mg four times daily. About 40% of the dose appears unchanged in the urine.

Adverse reactions

Nausea and vomiting are common, but this can be reduced by administering with food and lowering the dose. Mild allergic reactions may occur. Long-term therapy occasionally results in peripheral

Table 11.20   Treatment of urinary-tract infections*

Condition	Uncomplicated infection	Serious infection (pending culture results or in primary treatment failure)	Notes
Cystitis	Trimethoprim, cephradine, nalidixic acid, nitrofurantoin for 5–7 days.	Ciprofloxacin, augmentin	
(in pregnancy)	Cephradine, amoxycillin	Nitrofurantoin	
Acute pyelonephritis		Cefotaxime, ciprofloxacin, augmentin, gentamicin, cefuroxime	Best treated initially by injection, especially if the patient is vomiting or severely ill.
Prostatitis	Trimethoprim	Ciprofloxacin, cefotaxime	Can be difficult to cure and requires treatment for several weeks with an antibiotic which penetrates prostatic tissue.

* Apart from nitrofurantoin, details of the drugs in this table have appeared in earlier pages.

neuropathy, which is dose-related. It occurs as a result of renal failure, and patients with this condition should not be given nitrofurantoin. Other adverse effects include arthralgia, agranulocytosis, thrombocytopenia and aplastic anaemia.

FUNGAL INFECTIONS

Two general types of fungal infections exist:

- topical infections affecting the skin and mucous membranes
- systemic infections.

The patient's underlying condition may predispose to fungal infection, for example (i) a severely immunocompromised patient, (ii) a patient receiving antibiotic therapy that eliminates normal flora, (iii) a patient who wears dentures.

Topical infections are more common and include candidiasis and infections by dermatophytes. The causative organism in candidiasis is usually *Candida albicans*, a yeast which may be found in up to 50% of healthy mouths and about one-third of adult vaginas. Infection caused by this organism is usually superficial, for example, invasion of the superficial layers of the epidermis of the mouth or vagina, or very occasionally skin which has become damp and macerated, as in the nappy area. This condition is commonly referred to as thrush. Vaginal thrush is an opportunistic infection which affects women predomi-

nantly of child-bearing age because *Candida* enjoys the low pH and abundant glycogen present in the urine at this time. The initially harmless *Candida* is transformed into a pathogen either by local changes in the vagina or by lowered immune resistance. Pregnancy and diabetes are two predisposing factors.

Vulval pruritus and vaginal discharge are the usual presenting symptoms. Dysuria may be severe, especially when there is local excoriation and maceration due to scratching. Painful intercourse (dyspareunia) may occur and may be severe. When present, the discharge is usually thick and white or creamy.

Oral candidiasis presents in different forms, denture stomatitis being the most common. Acute pseudomembranous candidiasis is the form commonly referred to as oral thrush. The infected epithelium proliferates rapidly, producing the characteristic soft, creamy yellow plaques and can occur on any mucosal surface of the mouth. Steroid inhalers are a common cause of thrush by thinning the oral mucosa and suppressing inflammatory reaction. Patients should be advised to rinse out the mouth following administration to help prevent this.

Dermatophytes cause many common infections which are named according to the affected part of the body:

- Tinea pedis – athlete's foot

Table 11.21   Drugs used to treat fungal infections

Mode of action	Pharmacokinetics	Indications	Dose	Adverse effects
POLYENE ANTIFUNGAL DRUGS				
Nystatin				
Alters permeability of cell membranes resulting in loss of essential cell constituents.	Not absorbed after oral or topical administration. Too toxic for parenteral use.	Principally used for *Candida albicans* infections of GI tract, skin, vagina and respiratory tract.	Oral – intestinal candidiasis, 500 000 units every 6 hours; oral or peri-oral candidiasis – 100 000 units four times daily after food.	Usually unimportant – may experience nausea, vomiting and diarrhoea at higher doses.
Amphotericin				
As for nystatin.	Poorly absorbed from GI tract. May be administered orally as suspension, tablets or lozenges for treatment of superficial candida infections. Administered parenterally to treat systemic infections.	Active against most fungi and yeasts (*Aspergillus*, *Candida* spp, *Cryptococcus*, *Coccidioides*, *Histoplasma*).	Intestinal candidiasis 100–200 mg every 6 hours. Lozenges given four times daily are used to treat oral candidiasis. Intravenous infusion in glucose – 250 µg – 1 mg/kg daily. (It is precipitated from solutions containing cations such as sodium or potassium.)	When given parenterally toxicity is common and close supervision is necessary. Renal impairment occurs due to renal vasoconstriction and a direct effect on the tubules resulting in diminished renal plasma flow giving rise to acidosis and hypokalaemia. Other adverse reactions include nausea, vomiting, febrile reactions, headache, anaemia, blood disorders, rash, anaphylactoid reactions. Fever is common and may be reduced by intravenous hydrocortisone at start of treatment.
TRIAZOLE ANTIFUNGAL DRUGS				
Fluconazole				
Alters cell membrane permeability.	Absorbed by mouth. Effective parenterally.	Mucosal and systemic candidiasis; cryptococcal infections including meningitis.	Oral – single dose of 150 mg for vaginal candidiasis. 50–100 mg daily in oropharyngeal candidiasis. 200–400 mg daily orally or by intravenous infusion for systemic candidiasis or cryptococcal meningitis.	GI side-effects. Caution in pregnancy, breast-feeding and renal impairment.
Itraconazole				
As for fluconazole	As for fluconazole	Mucosal candidiasis and dermatophyte infections.	Oral preparation only. Oral candidiasis – 100 mg daily – 15 days. Vaginal candidiasis – 200 mg twice daily for one day. Tinea pedis and corporis – 100 mg daily.	GI side-effects. Caution in pregnancy and breast-feeding.
IMIDAZOLE ANTIFUNGAL DRUGS				
Ketoconazole				
Increases membrane permeability. Also inhibits cellular enzymes.	Poorly absorbed after local application. Widely distributed parenterally.	Systemic mycoses, serious candidiasis, resistant dermatophyte infections of skin and finger nails.	200–400 mg orally once daily with food until at least 1 week after symptoms have cleared.	GI side-effects, rashes, pruritus. Contraindicated in hepatic impairment. Avoid in pregnancy and porphyria. Monitor liver function.

Table 11.21 *Cont'd*

Mode of action	Pharmacokinetics	Indications	Dose	Adverse effects
Miconazole As for ketoconazole.	As for ketoconazole.	Oral, intestinal and systemic fungal infections.	250 mg every 6 hours. Continue for 2 days after symptoms clear. Intravenous infusion for systemic fungal infection – 600 mg every 8 hours.	Nausea, vomiting, pruritus, rashes. Change infusion site to avoid phlebitis. Avoid in prophyria.
OTHER ANTIFUNGAL DRUGS **Flucytosine** Penetrates certain fungal cells where it is converted to fluorouracil and alters protein synthesis.	Well absorbed and widely distributed. Undergoes little metabolism.	Systemic yeast infections.	Orally or by intravenous infusion – 200 mg/kg daily in 4 divided doses. Reduce dose in renal impairment.	GI reactions, rashes, thrombocytopenia, leucopenia. Caution in pregnancy and breast-feeding.
Griseofulvin Binds to keratin and makes it resistant to fungal infection. Must be continued until all infected tissue has been shed and replaced.	Absorption variable. It is improved if given after food.	Dermatophyte infection of the skin, nails and hair where topical therapy is ineffective.	0.5 –1 g daily for up to a year depending on site of infection.	Well tolerated. Headache, GI effects or hypersensitivity may occur. Caution in breast-feeding.
Terbinafine Interferes with fungal sterol biosynthesis, at an early stage. This leads to deficiency in ergosterol and to intracellular accumulation of squalene resulting in fungal cell death.	Well absorbed orally. Rapidly diffuses through dermis and concentrates in the stratum corneum . Distributed into nail plate within first few weeks of commencing therapy. Metabolites excreted predominantly in urine.	Dermatophyte infection of the nails. Ringworm infection.	250 mg daily up to 3 months or longer, depending on site of infection.	GI effects, headache, rash, arthralgia, myalgia.

- Tinea capitis – scalp ringworm
- Tinea corporis – body ringworm
- Tinea unguium – nail infection (onychomycosis)

Tinea versicolor is a fungal infection of the horny layer of the skin which shows as oval, light brown patches in fair-skinned people.

Treatment

The treatment of fungal infections is outlined in Table 11.21.

Clotrimazole, econazole, ketoconazole and miconazole are applied topically to treat fungal skin infections. Treatment should continue for 10–14 days after the lesions have healed.

VIRUSES

Viruses are much smaller than bacteria, consisting essentially of a core of nucleic acid in a protective protein envelope. They possess only one of the two classes of nucleic acids as carriers of their genetic information, either ribonucleic acid (RNA) or deoxyribonucleic acid (DNA). These organisms have no enzymes of their own such as are necessary for internal metabolism. It is for this reason that they are resistant to antibi-

Table 11.22   Drugs used to treat viral infections

Mode of action	Use	Pharmacokinetics	Adverse effects	Dose
Acyclovir				
Acyclovir enters all cells. It is changed by a virus-specific enzyme, thymidine kinase, to the active derivative acyclovir triphosphate. This then inhibits DNA polymerase, an enzyme necessary for viral growth, and disrupts viral replication.	Active against herpes virus if started early. It is used intravenously for the treatment of systemic infections of herpes simplex and varicella-zoster; topically for treating herpes infections of the skin and mucous membranes (including genital herpes); as an eye ointment in herpes simplex eye infections.	15–30% absorbed orally, but this results in therapeutic serum concentration levels. Widely distributed throughout the body. There are a number of metabolites formed either in the liver or in cells infected by the herpes virus; the active acyclovir triphosphate is formed in the latter. The half-life increases as renal function deteriorates and dosage needs to be adjusted in patients with renal impairment.	Headache can occur with oral administration as can GI reactions such as nausea, vomiting and diarrhoea. Local reactions at the injection site particularly with inadvertent extravasation can occur. These include irritation, phlebitis, inflammation and pain.	Must be started at the onset of infection to be effective. Viral herpes simplex treatment 200–400 mg five times daily. Herpes zoster (shingles) 800 mg five times daily for 7 days. By intravenous infusion over 1 hour, 5–10 mg/kg every 8 hours. Cream or eye ointment to be applied every 4 hours.
Idoxuridine				
Idoxuridine is similar in structure to thymidine. It inhibits an enzyme involved in DNA synthesis, thus inhibiting growth and replication of DNA viruses. Since it is not specific to viral DNA but also affects DNA in human cells, it produces bone marrow depression and leucopenia, and cannot therefore be given systemically. It is therefore used only locally.	Local treatment of herpes simplex infections.	Used only topically. Idoxuridine 5% in dimethylsulphoxide (DMSO) is used less frequently for herpetic infections of the skin since acyclovir is more effective.	Idoxuridine in dimethyl-sulphoxide may sting on application. It should be applied for 3–4 days or the skin may become macerated. Must not be applied to the eye or mucous membranes. Contraindicated in pregnancy.	Apply eye ointment every 4 hours. Idoxuridine in DMSO – 4 times daily for 3–4 days.
Amantadine				
Not viricidal at normal concentrations. Interferes with the penetration of the virus into susceptible cells.	Has been used orally for herpes simplex but effectiveness not established. Has also been used for prophylaxis of influenza A virus – should be commenced immediately influenza A is known to be epidemic.	Effective only during the period of its administration. Available as an oral preparation.	May produce amphetamine-like side-effects such as nervousness, difficulty in concentration, dizziness, insomnia, drowsiness, slurred speech. Atropine-like side-effects such as blurred vision, dry mouth and palpitations may occur. It may affect the performance of skilled tasks such as driving.	Herpes zoster – 100 mg twice daily for 14–28 days. Influenza A – 100 mg twice daily.

otics which act by blocking some stage of microbial metabolism.

Viruses can be regarded as intracellular parasites. Since new proteins, not present in the normal cell, are synthesised in virus infected cells, this offers the possibility of selective inhibition of viral replication by chemical agents.

ANTIVIRAL AGENTS

The only therapeutic approach to viral illness until recently was prevention by immunisation. Examples of vaccines include those against rubella, poliomyelitis and yellow fever. There are now a small number of therapeutic agents available to treat certain viral infections (Table 11.22).

Inosine pranobex has been used orally for herpes simplex infections but its effectiveness has not been established. The dose is 1g four times daily for 7–14 days. It does not act directly on the viruses but is mainly of value as an immunostimulant by increasing the proliferation of T and B cells, which is depressed during viral infections. Inosine pranobex is well tolerated but care is necessary in gout and renal impairment as it increases uric acid levels.

HUMAN IMMUNODEFICIENCY VIRUS (HIV)

HIV-related diseases are caused by the HIV virus binding, entering and damaging the host cells that have a CD4 receptor on their cell surface. These cells are predominantly T helper cells and macrophages. T cells are critical in the development of all cell-mediated immune reaction, controlling and modulating the development of the immune response to infection. Depletion of T helper cells by HIV produces immunosuppression, which predisposes the host to infection, tumour and neurological disease.

In addition to depression of the person's immunity (and subsequent development of opportunistic infections), significant haematological abnormalities including bone marrow dysplasia, thrombocytopenia, anaemia and leucopenia are also associated with HIV infection, its treatment and the treatment of associated problems. Reduction of CD4 T helper cells causes depression of the functions of:

- other types of T cell
- B cells (and therefore antibody production)
- macrophages
- natural killer cells
- granulocytes
- interleukins
- cytokines (for example, tumour necrosis factor and interferon).

If the CD4 T helper cells count falls below 200 per mm^3 from an average of about 800–1000 per mm^3, the risk of infection is significantly increased.

Drugs used in HIV-positive persons

Zidovudine (AZT, 3'-azido-3'-deoxythymidine)

Action Zidovudine interferes with RNA-dependent DNA polymerase (reverse transcriptase) and elongation of the viral chain. It was originally used in patients with advanced disease. Results from the large Anglo-French 'Concorde' study indicate that there is no significant clinical benefit from starting therapy early, before symptoms appear. The immediate short-term benefits include prolonged survival, a decrease in frequency and severity of opportunistic infections, improved neurological and performances status, weight gain and increases in CD4 T cells. However, at least 6 weeks' treatment is required for improvements in outcome to be fully realised. Initial benefits generally persist for the first 9–14 months. After this time it is not uncommon to note progressive HIV disease and increased zidovudine toxicity.

Pharmacokinetics Zidovudine is absorbed from the GI tract and gives a peak concentration in about 0.5–1.5 hours (65% bioavailability).

Adverse reactions Adverse reactions to zidovudine are quite common. During the first few weeks zidovudine can lead to confusion, headache, insomnia, nausea, vomiting, abdominal discomfort, diarrhoea, malaise, myalgias, fever and rash. Headache and nausea are the most common adverse reactions. Symptoms will generally subside after several weeks of therapy. The most serious adverse reactions are haematological. These include anaemia (often requiring transfusions), neutropenia, leucopenia and thrombocytopenia. Blood tests should be carried out at least every 2 weeks for the first 3 months and then at least once a month. Zidovudine should be avoided in breast-feeding.

Dose Doses vary from patient to patient depending on tolerance and severity of disease. Zidovudine should be commenced in symptomatic patients with CD4 T cell counts less than 500 per mm^3 at 200 mg three times daily. The dose may require adjustment in the event of anaemia or myelosuppression. Patients temporarily unable to take zidovudine orally may receive an intravenous infusion – 2.5 mg/kg every 4 hours.

Didanosine (DDI, dideoxyinosine)

Action Once in the cell, the DDI is converted to its active metabolite, dideoxyadenosine triphosphate (DDATP). DDATP inhibits the viral enzyme reverse transcriptase, so inhibiting viral nucleic acid replication.

Pharmacokinetics DDI is active orally. However, it is acid-labile so that oral preparations must be given with an antacid buffer to prevent inactivation by stomach acids. It is rapidly absorbed after oral administration, maximum concentrations occurring within an hour of administration. Although the half-life is 1.4 hours, active metabolites of DDI remain within the cell for much longer, so that twice daily dosing is sufficient. Taking food with DDI reduces the absorption by as much as 50%, so it should be given on an empty stomach.

Adverse effects The most serious adverse effects are pancreatitis and peripheral neuropathy. Other side-effects include nausea, vomiting, chills, fever, headache, pain, rash, asthma and seizures.

Dose 250 mg twice a day on an empty stomach.

Zalcitabine (DDC/dideoxycytidine)

Like didanosine, zalcitabine is a dideoxynucleoside. It inhibits the action of reverse transcriptase. Peripheral neuropathy and arthralgia are common side-effects. Patients may also experience numbness, pain or burning sensations in their feet or hands, and painful mouth ulcers.

The use of antivirals as single agents is associated with several problems, including dose-limiting drug toxicities and viral resistance. Researchers are now investigating the use of combined or alternating regimens. It is hoped that combination therapy will overcome the problems posed by the tendency of HIV to mutate in the presence of antiretroviral drugs. To achieve immunity to a multidrug regimen the virus would need to undergo several mutations simultaneously.

Drugs used in opportunistic infections (HIV-positive patients)

Pneumocystis pneumonia

Pneumonia caused by *Pneumocystis carinii* occurs in immunosuppressed or severely debilitated patients. It is the commonest cause of pneumonia in AIDS. Cotrimoxazole (see p. 165) in high dosage is the drug of choice for the treatment of pneumocystis pneumonia.

Pentamidine isethionate is an alternative to cotrimoxazole and is particularly indicated for patients with a history of adverse reactions or who have not responded to cotrimoxazole. It can be given by intravenous injection or by nebulisation. Prophylaxis is given by nebulisation: 150–300 mg every 2–4 weeks. Pretreatment with bronchodilators such as salbutamol is given to reduce the incidence of cough and bronchoconstriction caused by pentamidine. Treatment comprises 600 mg daily for 3 weeks or by intravenous infusion 4 mg/kg daily for at least 14 days.

Side-effects include metallic taste and pneumothorax. With intravenous therapy side-effects also include severe hypotension, hypoglycaemia, pancreatitis, cardiac arrhythmias, leucopenia, thrombocytopenia, acute renal failure, hypoglycaemia and muscle necrosis at the injection site.

Fungal infections

Nystatin mouthwash is used for local treatment. In systemic infections, fluconazole is active against *Candida* and *Cryptococcus*, and doses of up to 400 mg daily are required for prolonged periods.

Cryptosporidia diarrhoea

This is a prolonged infection, and the illness is usually self-limiting. In the immunocompromised it becomes chronic, severe and life-threatening. The diarrhoea may be caused by a toxin. No uniformly effective specific anticryptosporidial therapy is available. Spiramycin (a macrolide) and paromomycin (an aminoglycoside) have been tried but patient responses are often only temporary. Octreotide is a long-acting analogue of the hypothalamic release-inhibiting hormone somatostatin. It is used in cryptosporicidal diarrhoea to inhibit the secretion of peptides in the gastroenteropancreatic system to alleviate severe secretory diarrhoea. It is given by injection, usually 50 mg subcutaneously three times daily. Side-effects include anorexia, nausea, vomiting, abdominal pain and flatulence. Symptoms can be reduced by injecting between meals or at bedtime. Pain and irritation can occur at injection but this can be controlled by rotating sites.

Herpes simplex and zoster

This can be controlled by acyclovir (see p. 175)

Cytomegalovirus (CMV)

Ganciclovir is related to acyclovir but has a greater activity against CMV. It is indicated only for sight- or life-threatening cytomegalovirus infections in immunocompromised patients since it is much more toxic than acyclovir. It can cause leucopenia and thrombocytopenia and is also a potential carcinogen. It is contraindicated in pregnancy and breast-feeding. Ganciclovir causes profound myelosuppression when given with zidovudine. Foscarnet is also active against CMV and is indicated for cytomegalovirus retinitis in patients with AIDS in whom ganciclovir is contraindicated or inappropriate. Foscarnet is toxic and can cause renal impairment in up to 50% of patients.

MALARIA

There are four malaria parasites that infect man, by far the most hazardous being *Plasmodium falciparum*, which causes malignant malaria; this can rapidly progress from an acute fever to severe multi-organ disease, leading eventually to cerebral malaria with coma and death. Falciparum malaria usually presents within 3 months of acquiring the infection and once successfully treated it does not relapse.

Infection with *Plasmodium vivax*, benign malaria, can present many months after exposure and may relapse for years after the initial infection. It is a less severe illness than that caused by *P. falciparum*. Benign malaria is caused less commonly by *P. ovale* and *P. malariae*.

Most of Africa south of the Sahara is highly malarious, the risk decreasing in southern Africa. Many popular tourist destinations in South-East Asia are low-risk. However, Vietnam, Cambodia and the Thai–Cambodian border are high-risk areas where multidrug-resistant falciparum malaria is transmitted. Melanesia and parts of South America are also malarious.

Protection

It is important to reduce the chance of an infective bite as much as possible, e.g. travellers should sleep in screened accommodation and use aerosols or vaporisers to eliminate mosquitoes.

Chemoprophylaxis

Drug regimens should be started at least 1 week before departure and continued without interruption for 4 weeks after return. This ensures therapeutic blood concentrations before travelling and enables unwanted effects to be dealt with before departure. The continued use of drugs after returning home will deal with infection contracted at the end of the trip. The drugs used in prophylaxis are chloroquine, proguanil and pyrimethamine, either alone or in combinations depending on the risk factor and the emergence of resistant strains. Mefloquine used alone for short-term travellers is also an option for certain areas of the world.

Treatment

In the treatment of falciparum malaria, quinine, mefloquine or halofantrine can be given by mouth, or quinine can be given by intravenous infusion if the patient is seriously ill or unable to take tablets. Quinine is the drug of choice in pregnant women with falciparum malaria. *P. falciparum* is now resistant to chloroquine, but this is still the drug of choice for the treatment of benign malaria.

The drugs used in the treatment of malaria are outlined in Table 11.23.

THREADWORMS (*Enterobius vermicularis*, PINWORMS)

Anthelmintics are effective in threadworm infections, and their use should be combined with hygienic measures to break the cycle of auto-infection. All members of the family require treatment.

Adult threadworms do not live longer than 6 weeks, and, for development of fresh worms, ova must be swallowed and exposed to the action of digestive juices in the upper intestinal tract. Adult female worms lay ova on the peri-anal skin and cause pruritus. Scratching the area then leads to ova being transmitted on fingers to the mouth, often via food eaten with unwashed hands. Washing the hands and fingers with the aid of a nail brush before each meal and after each visit to the toilet is essential. A bath taken immediately after rising will remove ova laid during the night.

Treatment

Mebendazole is the choice drug for patients over 2 years; a 100 mg single dose is repeated after 2–3 weeks. Alternatively, 15 ml of piperizine elixir (750 mg/5 ml) is taken daily for 7 days.

Table 11.23 Treatment of malaria

Drug	Indications	Adverse effects	Dose
Chloroquine	Malarial prophylaxis and treatment of benign malaria.	Mild headaches, nausea and vomiting, pruritus and skin rashes may occur. Can cause irreversible retinal damage, corneal opacities and depigmentation of hair and skin. Avoid in pregnancy because of risk of ototoxicity in the fetus. May cause haemolysis in patients with glucose 6-phosphate dehydrogenase deficiency.	300 mg weekly alone or in combination with proguanil 200 mg daily.
Halofantrine	Treatment of uncomplicated chloroquine resistant falciparum malaria.	Diarrhoea, nausea, vomiting and abdominal pain. Contraindicated in pregnancy.	500 mg – 3 doses 6 hours apart, repeated 1 week later.
Mefloquine	Chemoprophylaxis and treatment of chloroquine resistant falciparum malaria.	GI side-effects, dizziness, headache, rash, paraesthesia. Contraindicated in pregnancy, breast-feeding and psychiatric disorders.	250 mg each week.
Proguanil	Chemoprophylaxis of malaria.	Mild gastric intolerance.	200 mg daily.
Quinine	Falciparum malaria.	Tinnitus, headache, nausea, abdominal pain, rashes, visual disturbances, blood disorders and hypoglycaemia.	Oral – 600 mg every 8 hours for 7 days. Intravenous infusion – 20 mg/kg over 4 hours, then 10 mg/kg over 8–12 hours until patient can swallow tablets.

FURTHER READING

Behrens R 1993 Prevention of malaria. Practitioner 237: 714–716

Lockie C 1993 The new macrolides. Practitioner 237: 527–529

Maskell R 1993 Urinary tract infections. Practitioner 237: 57–62

Nathwani D, Wood M J 1993 Penicillins. A current review of their pharmacology and therapeutic use. Drugs 45(6): 866–894

Roig J, Carreres A, Domingo C 1993 Treatment of Legionnaires' disease. Drugs 46(1): 63–79

Turnridge J, Lindsay Grayson M 1993 Optimum treatment of staphylococcal infections. Drugs 45(2): 353–366

Walters J 1993 How antibiotics work. Professional Nurse 8(12): 788–791

Wilde M I, Langtry H D 1993 Zidovudine. An update on its pharmacodynamic and pharmacokinetic properties and therapeutic efficacy. Drugs 46(3): 515–578

Wolfson J S, Hooper D C 1989 Fluoroquinolone antimicrobial agents. Clinical Microbiology Reviews October: 378–424

12

Drug treatment of endocrine disorders

The endocrine system regulates the inner environment of the body, adjusting and correlating the activities of the various body systems. This regulation is possible through chemical agents which act as messenger substances: **hormones**. Hormones are secreted by endocrine or ductless glands which are situated in various parts of the body (see Fig. 12.1). They are released directly into the blood which carries them, some attached to a transport protein, to their target organ or tissue where they act upon specific receptor mechanisms on the surface of the cell or in the cell cytoplasm, producing their characteristic effects, such as the stimulation or inhibition of enzymatic processes.

Some hormones, e.g. **adrenalin** and **aldosterone**, are released in response to internal or external stimulation. Others, e.g. the **corticosteroids**, follow a 24 hour (circadian) rhythm or an even longer rhythm such as the **female sex hormones** (menstrual cycle). In the case of **thyroxine** a constant blood level is maintained.

HORMONAL REGULATION

Although each ductless gland produces a hormone with specific functions in health, there is an integrated relationship between the activities of the several ductless glands.

The hypothalamus and the pituitary gland together form the central control unit for the production and secretion of many hormones. The hypothalamus produces 'releasing' and 'inhibiting' hormones which influence the

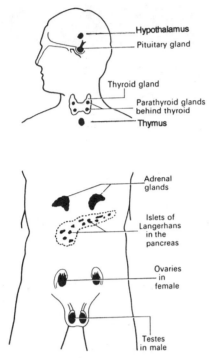

Figure 12.1 The endocrine glands. (Adapted from Ross & Wilson 1990 Anatomy and physiology in health and illness, 7th edn. Churchill Livingstone.)

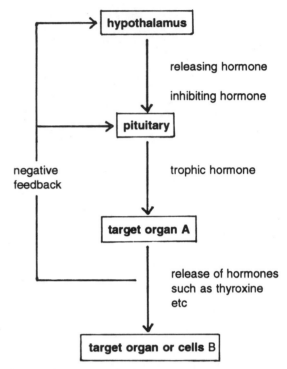

Figure 12.2 Negative feedback mechanism.

anterior lobe of the pituitary gland to release corresponding hormones, the **trophic** hormones, some of which, e.g. **somatotrophin**, affect target cells in the body directly while others, e.g. **thyrotrophin (TSH)** do so through the intermediary of a second endocrine organ such as the thyroid, the adrenal cortex and the gonads. The second endocrine organ, in turn, produces a third specific hormone such as **thyroxine, corticosteroids** or **sex hormones**, which influence various other body functions.

Chemoreceptors in the hypothalamus register the blood hormone level and react accordingly by either increasing or decreasing hormone production. If the blood hormone level is low, more hormone is secreted; if the blood hormone level is high, hormone production is reduced (negative feedback) (see Fig. 12.2). An example of a positive feedback is the stimulation of luteinizing hormone secretion by oestrogens and progestogens, which is important for ovulation.

Not all hormonal activities follow the above mechanism. An example of a much simpler mechanism is the release of insulin from the islets of Langerhans, which depends directly on the blood glucose level.

HYPOTHALAMUS AND PITUITARY GLAND

The hypothalamus forms the base of the diencephalon (the base of the brain). It is responsible for the coordination of nervous and endocrine systems and therefore many basic life functions such as cardiovascular, respiratory and alimentary functions, sexual behaviour and reproduction. It is connected to the pituitary gland, a small endocrine gland of great importance, by the hypophyseal stalk or infundibulum. The pituitary gland lies almost completely surrounded by bone in the base of the skull. It consists of three parts, the **adenohypophysis** (anterior lobe), the **median eminence** and the **neurohypophysis** (posterior lobe).

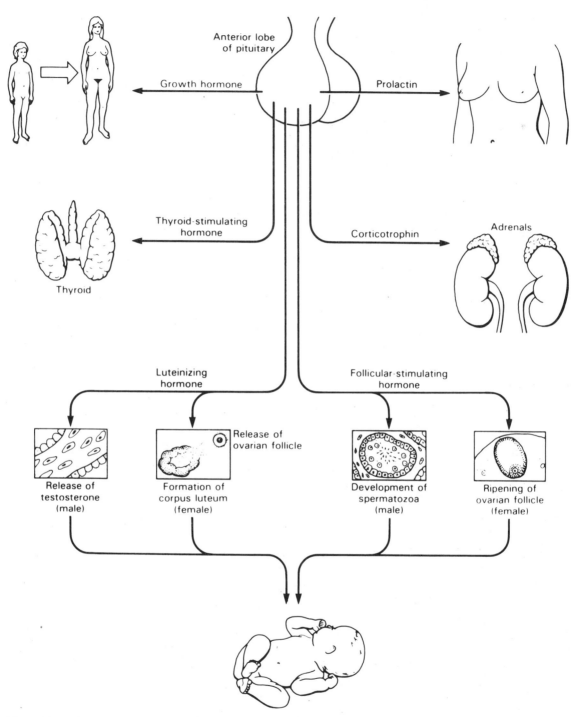

Figure 12.3 Hormones released by anterior pituitary. (From Trounce 1994 Clinical pharmacology for nurses, 14th edn. Churchill Livingstone.)

The **adenohypophysis** (see Fig. 12.3) synthesises and releases seven known trophic hormones. These are *somatotrophin (STH)*, which is involved in prepubertal body growth; *prolactin* which stimulates the growth and secretory activity of the female breasts during pregnancy; *melanocyte stimulating hormone* which causes an increase in cutaneous pigmentation; *adrenocorticotrophic hormone (ACTH)* which governs the secretions of some of the hormones by the adrenal cortex; *thyrotrophin (TSH)* which stimulates thyroid activity; *follicle stimulating hormone (FSH)* or *human menopausal gonadotrophin*, which stimulates growth of ovarian follicles and secretion of oestrogen in the female and spermato-genesis in the male; and *luteinizing hormone (LH)*, which stimulates the production of progesterone in the corpus luteum of the follicle (female) and activates androgen secretion by the Leydig cells of the testis (male).

The **neurohypophysis** (see Fig. 12.4) hormones *vasopressin (antidiuretic hormone ADH)* and *oxytocin* are produced in the hypothalamus and secreted (neurosecretion) directly into the blood stream of the infundibulum and posterior lobe of the pituitary gland from where they can be released into the body.

Vasopressin controls the re-absorption of water by the kidney tubules. In large doses it causes vasoconstriction of the smooth muscles with a concomitant rise in blood pressure. It also causes muscle contraction in the gastrointestinal tract and uterus.

Oxytocin causes the contraction of the uterine muscle towards the end of pregnancy and at parturition and contraction of the mammary smooth muscle which stimulates the release of milk into the ducts. The secretion of *oxytocin* from the pituitary gland is stimulated by the baby sucking at the mother's breast.

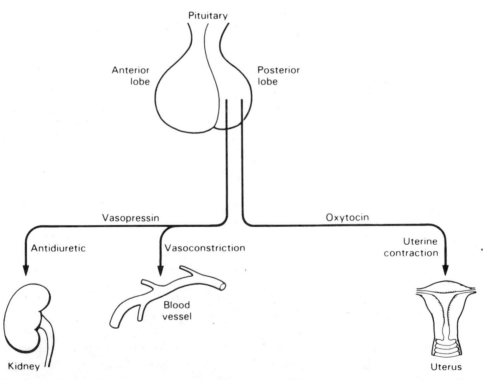

Figure 12.4 Hormones released by posterior pituitary. (From Trounce 1994 Clinical pharmacology for nurses, 14th edn. Churchill Livingstone.)

COMMON DISORDERS OF THE PITUITARY GLAND

Hypopituitarism

Reduced secretion of pituitary hormones caused by tumour, trauma, etc. often results in a progressive loss of function of organs stimulated by trophic hormones, starting with *growth hormone deficiency* in children, then gonadotrophin deficiency, which causes amenorrhoea and anovulatory infertility in women and impotence and reduced spermatogenesis in men. At a later stage, levels of **ACTH** and eventually **TSH** decrease, resulting in hypothyroidism (see p. 189) and Addison's disease (see p. 195).

Hypersecretion of pituitary hormones

Acromegaly and gigantism

The excessive secretion of growth hormone (somatotrophin) leads to *gigantism (excessive growth of the whole body)* in prepubertal children and *acromegaly* in adults (increased size of tongue, lips and organs such as the heart and liver); both conditions are usually caused by a pituitary adenoma, and patients tend to have other problems associated with abnormal function of the pituitary gland such as Cushing's syndrome caused by hypersecretion of **ACTH**.

Hyperprolactinaemia may be due to a variety of causes such as prolactinoma (prolactin secreting tumour), trauma and drugs. Hyperprolactinaemia causes infertility in women and impotence in men. Treatment usually consists of a combination of surgery, radiotherapy and drug treatment depending on the size of the tumour.

Diabetes insipidus occurs either when there is failure of secretion of **ADH** from the neurohypophysis (cranial diabetes insipidus) or when **ADH** secretion is adequate but the kidney fails to respond (nephrogenic diabetes insipidus). This causes a reduced re-absorption of water in the kidney tubules and an increased output of very diluted urine (up to 40 1/day). The loss of water has to be replaced by increased drinking (polydipsia).

MAIN DRUG GROUPS

- Anterior pituitary hormones, antioestrogens and hypothalamic hormones
- Posterior pituitary hormones
- Dopamine agonists

Anterior pituitary hormones, anti-oestrogens and hypothalamic hormones

Corticotrophins (tetracosactrin)

Tetracosactrin is a synthetic anterior pituitary hormone and has the same physiological properties as **ACTH** but a shorter duration of action. It stimulates the biosynthesis of glucocorticosteroids, mineralocorticosteroids and androgens in the adrenal cortex.

Use Synacthen depot, a slow-release formulation of tetracosactrin with a prolonged duration of action of 12–24 hours, is used as a short-term alternative to corticosteroids in acute cases of, e.g. ulcerative colitis and juvenile rheumatoid arthritis or in patients who do not tolerate oral corticosteroids.

Tetracosactrin and its slow-release form are both used for diagnostic purposes to investigate adrenocortical insufficiency. **Tetracosactrin** is used for a short 30-minute test based on the measurement of plasma cortisol concentration immediately before and 30 minutes after injection. The depot preparation is used for a 5-hour test based on the same principle in cases where the 30-minute test has been inconclusive or the functional reserve of the adrenal cortex is being tested.

Administration and dose As a polypeptide, **tetracosactrin** is inactivated in the stomach and therefore has to be given as an intravenous or intramuscular injection. The depot preparation is given by intramuscular injection only.

For diagnostic use, a single 0.25 mg injection of **tetracosactrin** or 1 mg **tetracosactrin depot** is given.

For therapeutic use, 1 mg Synacthen depot is given in acute cases followed by 1 mg every 2–3 days, and in patients who respond well the dose may be reduced to 0.5 mg every 2–3 days or 1 mg weekly.

Contraindications and adverse effects As a polypeptide, **tetracosactrin** may cause allergic reactions, and in severe cases anaphylactic shock (see p. 37). It should not be used in patients with known hypersensitivity to tetracosactrin, for the treatment of asthma and allergic disorders, in Cushing's syndrome, patients with peptic ulcers, or adrenocortical insufficiency. Over-treatment can result in Cushing's syndrome, hyperglycaemia and hypokalaemia.

Anti-oestrogens

Anti-oestrogens act as antagonists to oestrogens at the relevant chemoreceptors in the hypothalamus, preventing the inhibitory effects of oestrogens on the gonadotrophin releasing hormone **gonadorelin**. This causes an increased release of gonadotrophins from the pituitary gland and, by stimulating the ovaries, ovulation in women with anovulatory cycles.

Use Anti-oestrogens are used in the treatment of anovulatory infertility attributed to dysfunction of the hypothalamo-pituitary ovarian axis or when the cause is unknown. Before considering treatment with an anti-oestrogen other causes of infertility should be excluded. Appropriate treatment should first be given to other treatable endocrine disorders, such as hyperprolactinaemia and pituitary tumours. To make a successful outcome of the treatment more likely, the patient should also have an adequate level of endogenous oestrogens. Some anti-oestrogens such as **tamoxifen** are used in breast cancer (see p. 248).

Drugs used in this group

- clomiphene
- cyclofenil

Administration and dose Both drugs are available as tablets: **clomiphene** as 50 mg tablets, and **cyclofenil** as 100 mg tablets.

Clomiphene is given generally as a dose of 50 mg/day for 5 days (**cyclofenil** 200 mg twice daily for 10 days) starting on the fifth day (third day for **cyclofenil**) of the cycle and any time in women who are not menstruating. If there is no ovulation after the first course the dose may be increased to 100 mg/day for 5 days starting 30 days after the first course. If no ovulation has occurred after the third course treatment should be stopped and a new evaluation of the cause of infertility should take place.

Contraindications and adverse effects Liver disease, abnormal uterine bleeding and pregnancy are contraindications for treatment with anti-oestrogens. To exclude pregnancy careful monitoring of basal temperature throughout the cycle is necessary. Adverse effects are usually dose-related and include hot flushing, rashes, breast discomfort and weight gain. If visual side effects and ovarian hyperstimulation occur treatment should be withdrawn immediately.

Important points Multiple pregnancy, mostly twins, occurs in about 8% of successful pregnancies induced with anti-oestrogen treatment. Patients have to be made aware of this possibility and the risks associated with multiple pregnancies.

Gonadotrophins and gonadorelin

There are three known human gonadotrophins, two of which, follicle stimulating hormone (FSH) and luteinizing hormone (LH), are secreted by the pituitary gland, whereas human chorionic gonadotrophin (HCG) is secreted by the placenta and has LH-like properties. HCG for therapeutic use is obtained from the urine of pregnant women, and FSH and LH are extracted from the urine of menopausal women (HMG = human menopausal hormone).

Gonadorelin is the gonadotrophin-releasing hormone secreted by the hypothalamus. Gonadotrophins and gonadorelin are used in the treatment of secondary female infertility after a negative response to anti-oestrogens and exclusion of any other causes.

Use The uses are outlined below:

- amenorrhoea and infertility due to abnormal release of endogenous gonadorelin
- diagnostic purposes for the assessment of pituitary functions in patients with suspected pituitary impairment (gonadorelin)

- secondary female infertility due to the absence of follicle-ripening or ovulation (FSH and LH followed by HCG)
- women undergoing superovulation for in vitro fertilisation (FSH and LH or in conjunction with HCG)
- male infertility due to deficient spermatogenesis associated with hypopituitarism (FSH, LH and HCG)
- delayed puberty in men due to hypogonadotrophic hypogonadism (FSH, LH and HCG)
- cryptorchidism (HCG)

Drugs used in this group

- **gonadorelin**
- **human chorionic gonadotrophin (HCG)**
- **menotrophin** contains HMG, a mixture of 75 units of FSH, and 75 units of LH extracted from the urine of menopausal women
- **urofollitrophin** contains HMG with 75 units of FSH but no LH

Administration and dose (i) *Gonadorelin*. For the treatment of infertility, **gonadorelin** is administered as a pulsatile subcutaneous infusion (using an ambulatory pump system), initially 10–20 µg over 1 minute, repeated every 90 minutes for a period of a maximum of 6 months. For the assessment of pituitary function, 100 µg of **gonadorelin** is administered by rapid intravenous infusion, followed by measurement of LH and FSH serum levels. (ii) *Gonadotrophins*. As glycoproteins, which would be destroyed in the digestive system, gonadotrophins must be given parenterally and are generally given intramuscularly. They are available as powder for reconstitution with Water for Injections. The dose depends on the indication and the individual circumstances, e.g. responsiveness of the ovaries to exogenous gonadotrophins; therefore, it is impossible to set a uniform dosage scheme.

Examples for dose regimens are: female infertility: daily administration of 75 or 150 iu HMG increasing gradually until oestrogen levels start to rise then reach pre-ovulatory oestrogen levels, followed by a single dose of HCG (5000 iu intra-muscularly) 2 days later; cryptorchidism: HCG 500–4000 iu intramuscularly three times a week.

Contraindications and adverse effects Gonadotrophins are contraindicated in ovarian, pituitary and testicular tumours.

- HCG can cause precocious puberty when used in cryptorchidism
- HCG can cause fluid retention and therefore careful monitoring is advised in patients with cardiac failure, migraine, renal dysfunction, hypertension and epilepsy
- HCG can also cause gynaecomastia, ovarian hyperstimulation with multiple ovulations, ovarian enlargement and even rupture
- HMG (FSH and LH) can cause ovarian hyperstimulation with an increased risk of multiple pregnancies, fluid retention and oliguria

Side-effects after treatment with **gonadorelin** are very rare and include nausea, abdominal pain and increased menstrual bleeding.

Somatotrophin

Somatotrophin, a biosynthetic human growth hormone has replaced growth hormone of human origin.

Use Growth hormone is used in the treatment of short stature in children with hypopituitarism whose epiphyses have not yet fused, and in short stature associated with Turner syndrome.

Administration and dose Like other peptides, **somatotrophin** must be given parenterally by subcutaneous or intramuscular injection. It is available as powder for reconstitution with Water for Injections (2; 3; 4; 12; 24 unit vials).

The dosage of **somatotrophin** is individual. Generally, a dose of 0.5–0.7 units/kg/week divided into six or seven daily injections is recommended.

Contraindications and adverse effects These are as follows:

- use of somatotrophin is contraindicated in patients with fused epiphyses
- lipo-atrophy at the injection site may occur; it can be prevented by varying the injection site

- somatotrophin may influence glucose tolerance, and patients with diabetes mellitus might have to change the dosage of their hypoglycaemic drugs.

Posterior pituitary hormones

Vasopressin

The use of vasopressin, a peptide with antidiuretic and vasoconstrictor properties, has declined considerably since the development of its more selective semi-synthetic analogues **desmopressin** and **terlipressin**. Desmopressin has no vasoconstrictor effect but it has an increased antidiuretic activity and a longer duration of action than vasopressin or lypressin (synthetic porcine vasopressin); terlipressin is used for its vasoconstrictor effects.

Use The uses are as follows:

- treatment of cranial diabetes insipidus (desmopressin, lypressin and vasopressin); for long-term treatment desmopressin is usually used
- diagnosis of diabetes insipidus (desmopressin)
- primary nocturnal enuresis in adults and children (desmopressin)
- treatment of bleeding oesophageal varices (vasopressin, terlipressin).

Administration and dose (i) *Cranial diabetes insipidus*. In acute cases, such as after a head injury, vasopressin or desmopressin are used as intramuscular or subcutaneous injection; because of its much longer duration of action desmopressin has to be given only once a day (1–2 µg). For long-term maintenance treatment desmopressin is available as nasal spray (10 µg/metered dose) or nasal solution (100 µg/ml); lypressin is also available as nasal spray but is used much less because of its shorter duration of action. The average maintenance dose for the treatment of diabetes insipidus is 10–20 µg once or twice a day. (ii) *Oesophageal varices*. For the initial treatment of bleeding oesophageal varices vasopressin is given as an intravenous infusion (20 units diluted in 100 ml glucose 5% w/v).

Terlipressin is given as a single intravenous dose of 2 mg, which can be repeated every 4–6 hours.

Contraindications and adverse effects These are outlined as follows:

- Despite its reduced vasopressor effects, desmopressin, like all vasopressins, has to be used with extreme caution in patients with cardiovascular problems.
- Water retention and water intoxication may occur in large doses.
- In low doses, nausea, abdominal cramps, rise in blood pressure, etc. may occur.
- Nasal preparations may cause nasal congestion and local ulceration.

Important points Patients on nasal preparations have to be instructed thoroughly in the proper use of the device. Improper use will result in unsatisfactory response to treatment.

Oxytocin

Oxytocin is used in obstetrics (see p. 184).

Dopamine agonists

Bromocriptine is structurally related to ergotamine and is a stimulant for dopamine receptors in the brain (see also Parkinson's disease). It also inhibits the release of prolactin and growth hormone from the pituitary.

Use The uses are outlined as follows:

- treatment of prolactin-secreting tumours of the pituitary gland (prolactinoma) and acromegaly alone or in conjunction with surgery and radiotherapy
- galactorrhoea, hyperprolactinaemic infertility
- suppression of lactation after childbirth
- in the treatment of idiopathic Parkinson's disease
- cyclical breast pain and cyclical menstrual disorders.

Dose and administration Bromocriptine is available as 1 mg and 2.5 mg tablets and 5 mg and 10 mg capsules. There is a great difference in the dosage range depending on the condition treated and the individual response to treatment.

In most indications, apart from suppression and prevention of lactation, the optimum dosage is achieved by gradual introduction of bromocriptine. In this way optimum response and minimum side-effects can be properly balanced.

Contraindications and adverse effects Bromocriptine is contraindicated in hypertension after childbirth, toxaemia of pregnancy and known hypersensitivity reactions to bromocriptine or other ergot alkaloids. Adverse effects are numerous and dose-related, and can usually be reduced by dose adjustment:

- gastrointestinal disturbance
- hypotensive reactions at the beginning of the treatment
- ovulation in hyperprolactinaemic women; this effect may be desired as in the treatment of hyperprolactinaemic women; if the effect is undesired patients should be advised on the use of contraception
- dry mouth, leg cramps, cardiac arrhythmias
- peptic ulceration in acromegaly patients.

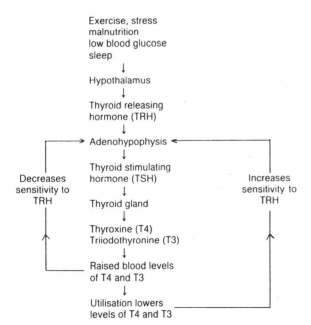

Figure 12.5   Production and regulation of thyroid hormones.

THYROID GLAND

The thyroid gland is situated anteriorly in the lower part of the neck. It consists of two side lobes connected by a narrow region, the **isthmus**. The gland is made up of two types of secretory cell: the **thyroid follicles** secreting the hormones **tri-iodothyronine (T3)** and **thyroxine or tetra-iodothyronine (T4)**, and **the parafollicular cells**, which secrete t**hyrocalcitonin (calcium-lowering hormone)**. Tri-iodothyronine and thyroxine are derivatives of the amino acid *tyrosine*. They are formed in the thyroid follicles by incorporating circulating iodine, stored and transported in the plasma almost entirely bound to **thyroxine-binding globulin (TBG)**. After secretion, the minute unbound (free) hormone fraction diffuses into tissues and exerts its hormonal activity after conversion of thyroxine into the more effective tri-iodothyronine.

Production of T3 and T4 is stimulated by thyrotrophin (thyroid stimulating hormone TSH), which is released from the pituitary gland in response to hypothalamic thyrotrophin-releasing hormone (TRH). The production is regulated by negative feedback through circulating concentrations of free T4 (see Fig. 12.5).

Tri-iodothyronine and thyroxine increase the oxygen consumption of almost all metabolically active tissues; this means an increase in metabolic rate of the whole organism. They also affect growth and maturation, especially brain and skeletal development.

COMMON DISORDERS OF THE THYROID GLAND

Hypothyroidism (thyroid deficiency) Hypothyroidism results from a reduced secretion of thyroxine (T4) and tri-iodothyronine (T3) by the thyroid gland, irrespective of the cause. The most common causes of primary hypothyroidism are thyroid failure following radioactive iodine-131 (^{131}I) therapy and surgical treatment; thyroid failure associated with Hashimoto's thyroiditis or an autoimmune disease; and congenital thyroid failure (congenital hypothyroidism or cretinism).

Hypothyroidism due to pituitary failure (secondary hypothyroidism) is much less common.

Hypothyroidism causes a reduction in the basal metabolic rate and affects most systems in the body. Symptoms vary in range and severity. They may include goitre, bradycardia, depression, iron deficiency anaemia, infertility, constipation, dermatological symptoms.

In children with hypothyroidism the dominant features are reduction in growth and arrest of pubertal development.

Severe hypothyroidism in the adult is called **myxoedema** and is marked by a thickening and swelling of the skin. **Myxoedema coma** is the severest form of thyroid deficiency and a medical emergency. The patient has a reduced level of consciousness and a body temperature which may be as low as 25°C.

Hyperthyroidism Hyperthyroidism (thyrotoxicosis) results from exposure of the body tissues to excess circulating levels of free thyroxine (T4) and/or free tri-iodothyronine. It is a common disorder which affects about 20 in 1000 women but five times fewer men.

Hyperthyroidism is not a sufficient diagnosis and it is very important to establish the correct cause to be able to provide adequate treatment. The most common causes are:

- Grave's disease
- toxic multinodular goitre
- toxic solitary nodule (autonomous thyroid hormone secreting adenoma).

Hyperthyroidism causes an increase in the basal metabolic rate and affects almost every system in the body. It presents with a wide variety of symptoms and severity. Symptoms include:

- an increase in body temperature
- tachycardia
- restlessness
- vomiting and diarrhoea
- loss of libido and infertility
- pruritus
- ocular symptoms such as exophthalmos in Grave's disease
- goitre.

Thyrotoxic crisis ('thyroid storm') is a life-threatening increase in the severity of the clinical features of thyrotoxicosis and requires immediate treatment. It is very unusual but may occur after subtotal thyroidectomy or within a few days after ^{131}I therapy or it may be precipitated by infection in a patient inadequately controlled on antithyroid drugs.

Non-toxic goitre Non-toxic diffuse goitre may be caused by iodine deficiency, drugs such as lithium carbonate, Hashimoto's thyroiditis or Grave's disease. It is usually easy to make the right diagnosis and provide adequate treatment. The simple goitre is of unknown aetiology and usually requires no treatment.

Drugs and thyroid function

Drugs can influence thyroid function in different ways. Some drugs alter thyroid function tests, e.g. androgens, oestrogens, salicylates. Some drugs may induce thyroid disease. Those which induce hypothyroidism: antithyroid drugs, lithium, sulphonylureas (chlorpropamide, tolbutamide); those which induce hyperthyroidism: amiodarone, iodides, thyroxine.

Thyroid disease can alter the distribution, metabolism and elimination of some drugs such as digoxin.

Thyroid disease may also alter the pharmacodynamic effects of some drugs such as cardiac glycosides and warfarin.

MAIN DRUG GROUPS

- **thyroid hormones**
- **antithyroid drugs**

Thyroid hormones

Thyroxine (T4) and tri-iodothyronine (T3) are the naturally occurring thyroid hormones. Tri-iodothyronine with a half-life of 1–2 days has a much faster onset of action than thyroxine with a half-life of 7 days. Thyroxine reaches its maximum effect after about 10 days. The difference in the onset of action is important for the therapeutic use of thyroid hormones.

Use Because of its rapid and more potent

effect, **tri-iodothyronine** is used in the treatment of severe and acute hypothyroid states. In the treatment of myxoedema coma, **tri-iodothyronine** as injection is the treatment of choice, usually in conjunction with other measures such as intravenous corticosteroids, intravenous fluids, slow re-warming using blankets and foil, broad-spectrum antibiotics and oxygen.

Thyroxine is normally the drug of choice for routine replacement therapy in hypothyroidism of any cause. In congenital hypothyroidism treatment has to begin as soon as possible after birth to prevent irreversible brain damage.

Thyroid hormones are also used to suppress the release of thyroid-stimulating hormone from the pituitary gland in the treatment of non-toxic diffuse goitre, Hashimoto's thyroiditis and thyroid carcinoma, and in combination with antithyroid drugs to prevent the development of a goitre in hyperthyroid patients.

Dose and administration 20 μg of T3 is equivalent to 100 μg of T4. Dosage for replacement therapy is individual and is usually started slowly with a dose of 50 μg of thyroxine and then increased to a dose of 100–200 μg daily. In the elderly, and patients with ischaemic heart disease, the initial dose should be 25 μg/day.

When first treating severe hypothyroidism, tri-iodothyronine is used as an initial dose of 5 μg, increased to 60 μg in weekly intervals. When a dose of 60 μg is reached treatment should switch to low-dose thyroxine increased by 50 μg in 4-week intervals up to 200 μg if required.

The dose can be monitored by the clinical response of the patient, but serum T4 and TSH levels should be measured at intervals. The correct dose of T4 is that which restores serum TSH concentration to normal.

For the treatment of myxoedema coma, 5–20 μg of tri-iodothyronine are given by slow intravenous injection, repeated at 12-hour intervals or more frequently if necessary.

Contraindications, cautions and adverse effects These are as follows:

- Thyroid hormones should be used with caution in patients with cardiovascular problems, prolonged myxoedema or adrenal failure in the elderly.
- Adverse effects are dose-related and usually disappear on reduction of dosage or withdrawal of treatment. Especially in the early stages of treatment patients may suffer from anginal pain, cardiac arrhythmias or myocardial infarction. Patients with a pre-existing heart condition are especially at risk.
- Other side-effects include gastrointestinal disturbance, tremors, restlessness, excessive loss of weight and muscular weakness.

Interactions Thyroxine increases the effects of anticoagulants, phenytoin, digoxin and adrenoceptor agonists such as salbutamol, and it accelerates the response to tricyclic antidepressants and also raises blood sugar levels – the dosage of antidiabetic agents in diabetics may therefore have to be adjusted.

Important points Patients on replacement therapy should be advised that treatment has to continue for life and follow-up is important, and that tablets should be taken regularly to ensure an adequate level of serum T4 and TSH.

Antithyroid drugs

Antithyroid drugs suppress the production or the release of thyroid hormones. Drugs used in this group are:

- **carbimazole and propylthiouracil**
- **iodine and iodide**

Carbimazole and propylthiouracil prevent the conversion of iodide into iodine, the incorporation of iodine into the pre-hormonal stages and therefore the production of thyroid hormones. Propylthiouracil also inhibits the conversion of T4 to the active T3 in the plasma.

Use Carbimazole and propylthiouracil are used in:

- the long-term management of hyperthyroidism
- the preparation for thyroidectomy in hyperthyroidism
- the preparation for, and as concomitant therapy with, radio-iodine treatment
- in combination with thyroxine as a blocking-

replacement therapy to prevent the development of goitre and hypothyroidism.

Dose and administration Carbimazole and propylthiouracil are both available as tablets only. The initial dose of **carbimazole** is 20–60 mg (propylthiouracil 300–600 mg) daily in two or three divided doses. **Carbimazole** is not effective until 10–14 days after the beginning of treatment because the thyroid is still releasing its existing hormone reserves for a period of time. After about 3–4 weeks the patient is usually clinically and biochemically euthyroid. The dose might then be reduced progressively to a maintenance dose of between 5 and 15 mg (propylthiouracil 50–150 mg) daily as a single dose. The dose should be determined by clinical status and ideally by the measurement of plasma thyroid hormone levels. Treatment should continue for 12–18 months. If a relapse occurs after discontinuation of treatment further measures may have to be considered (see Management of hyperthyroidism).

Adverse reactions, side-effects and cautions The most serious adverse effect of **carbimazole and propylthiouracil** is bone marrow depression which can lead to *agranulocytosis*. This is almost always reversible following withdrawal of the drug. Since there is usually no cross-sensitivity between the antithyroid drugs, carbimazole may be successfully substituted by propylthiouracil and vice versa.

Common side-effects are skin rashes and pruritus, which are usually self-limiting and do not require withdrawal of the drug.

Both drugs may be used in pregnancy as long as the dose is in the standard range and the patient is monitored regularly.

Both drugs are secreted in breast milk, and the patient should not breast-feed while taking the drug.

Important points Patients should be advised to report sore throats, mouth ulcers, fever or rashes immediately, since these might be early signs of bone marrow depression, and to keep follow-up appointments, especially in the initial stages.

Iodine and iodide

Iodine and iodide act by inhibiting the release of T3 and T4 from the thyroid into the plasma; it therefore reduces thyroid function very rapidly.

Use Iodine and iodide are used (i) in the treatment of *thyrotoxic crisis (thyroid storm)* in conjunction with a beta-adrenoceptor agonist (usually propranolol), high doses of antithyroid drugs and corticosteroids to inhibit the peripheral conversion of T4 to T3, and (ii) to prepare a patient for thyroidectomy by reducing vascularity and friability of the thyroid, and therefore lessening the risk of haemorrhage during surgery.

Dose and administration Iodine and iodide are available as Lugol's solution (aqueous iodine oral solution) which contains 5% iodine and 10% potassium iodide.

In the treatment of thyrotoxic crisis the dose is 2–3 ml daily.

Pre-operative Lugol's solution has to be given for 10 –14 days in a dose of 0.1–0.3 ml three times daily.

Long-term treatment with iodine and iodide is not recommended because its antithyroid action diminishes in time.

Contraindications, adverse reactions and side-effects Iodine is contraindicated in breast-feeding mothers because it might cause goitre in the infant. Iodine might cause hypersensitivity reactions, conjunctivitis, pain in salivary glands, bronchitis, gastroenteritis, insomnia and depression.

Management of hyperthyroidism (i) *Short-term treatment*. Beta-adrenoceptor blocking agents, usually propranolol, are used to relieve acute symptoms such as tachycardia, tremor and anxiety in the latent period before antithyroid drugs become effective and in conjunction with Lugol's solution for the preparation of patients with mild to moderate hyperthyroidism for surgery. (ii) *Long-term treatment* involves three options: (a) antithyroid drugs for 12–18 months; (b) radioactive iodine (^{131}I) for those cases in which drug therapy fails; or (c) surgery in recurrent hyperthyroidism, a large goitre or a single adenoma.

PARATHYROID GLANDS

The parathyroids consist of four small endocrine glands which are situated at the back of the thyroid gland. They produce **parathormone (PTH)**, which is essential for life. Parathormone regulates the metabolism of calcium and phosphorus in the body by action on the kidney, gut and bone (in a dual control mechanism with thyrocalcitonin). It also stimulates the formation of 1,25-hydroxycholecalciferol (vitamin D$_3$), which plays an important part in the mineralisation of bone. The release of PTH from the parathyroid glands depends directly on the blood calcium level.

COMMON DISORDERS OF THE PARATHYROID GLANDS

Hypoparathyroidism is a deficiency in parathormone which may be caused by surgical damage to the parathyroids after total or partial thyroidectomy. It results in a decrease of the blood calcium level (hypocalcaemia) and an increase in blood phosphorus (hyperphosphataemia). Hypocalcaemia causes a condition known as *tetany* which is characterised by increased tone of skeletal muscles with spasms of the hands, feet and larynx, and generalised convulsions.

Hyperparathyroidism (primary) is an increased release of parathormone, usually due to a parathyroid adenoma. The presenting features are due mainly to the raised blood calcium level (hypercalcaemia). They include fatigue, weakness, polydipsia and polyuria, renal stones, nephrocalcinosis, bone changes (osteitis fibrosa), duodenal ulceration and chronic pancreatitis.

Hypercalcaemia. The most common causes of hypercalcaemia are malignant disease and primary hyperparathyroidism, vitamin D intoxication, immobilisation (paraplegia in the young and Paget's disease in the elderly). Some drugs such as the **thiazides and lithium** can also cause hypercalcaemia. Main symptoms are fatigue, weakness, polydipsia, and polyuria. *Severe hypercalcaemia* is an emergency and requires urgent treatment.

MAIN DRUG GROUPS

- **calcitonin and analogues**
- **bisphosphonates**
- **plicamycin in hypercalcaemia** associated with malignancy (see p. 249).
- **other drugs affecting bone metabolism** such as vitamin D, calcium, phosphorus and oestrogens in postmenopausal osteoporosis.

Calcitonin

Calcitonin (thyrocalcitonin) lowers the blood calcium level by reducing the renal tubular reabsorption of calcium and increasing its deposition in the bone. By reducing the blood calcium level it also relieves bone pain. Calcitonin is available as porcine and the more potent synthetic calcitonin (salcatonin). Salmon calcitonin is more suitable for long-term treatment because the formation of neutralising antibodies is much less likely than with porcine calcitonin. Calcitonin is used for the treatment of:

- hypercalcaemia due to a raised bone turnover such as in Paget's disease of bone and malignancies with bone metastases
- primary hyperthyroidism
- vitamin D intoxication
- postmenopausal osteoporosis (salcatonin)

Dose and administration As a peptide, calcitonin would be destroyed in the stomach and can therefore be given only as an injection (subcutaneous or intramuscular). The dose depends on the condition treated and its severity. Dose adjustments should be made according to the patient's clinical and biochemical response. Dose regimens may range from 50 international units of salmon calcitonin three times a week to 100 international units daily in Paget's disease of bone and may be as high as 400 international units every 6–8 hours in severe hypercalcaemia. Fifty international units of salmon calcitonin equal 80 units of porcine calcitonin.

Adverse effects and caution Adverse effects of calcitonin include nausea, vomiting, diarrhoea, flushing, paraesthesia and an unpleasant taste in the mouth. There does not seem to be other serious toxicity. However, calcitonin should be used with caution in pregnancy and lactation.

Patients with a history of allergies should undergo a scratch test before the onset of treatment.

Bisphosphonates

Bisphosphonates reduce bone turnover by inhibiting the growth and dissolution of hydroxyapatite crystals and retarding bone resorption and formation. Drugs used in this group:

- **disodium etidronate**
- **disodium pamidronate**
- **disodium clodronate**

Use Bisphosphonates are used in the treatment of:

- Paget's disease of bone
- hypercalcaemia due to malignancies
- established vertebral osteoporosis as a combination preparation of disodium etidronate and calcium carbonate

Dose and administration Bisphosphonates are available as oral and parenteral preparations. For the treatment of hypercalcaemia due to malignancies, pamidronate is given in a single slow infusion of 15–60 mg on 3 successive days (must not exceed 30 mg in 2 hours). Adequate hydration should be ensured. For the treatment of Paget's disease of bone 5 mg/kg bodyweight of etidronate is given in a single daily oral dose for up to 6 months and then withdrawn. Improvements after drug therapy generally persist for 3 months to 2 years.

Contraindications and cautions Bisphosphonates are contraindicated in patients with known hypersensitivities to etidronate, pamidronate or clodronate. Since bisphosphonates are excreted by the kidney they should be used with caution in patients with renal impairment. In higher doses etidronate causes demineralisation of bone, which might lead to spontaneous fractures. Patients might also experience increased bone pain during the first month of treatment. The adverse effects of bisphosphonates are nausea and diarrhoea and a metallic taste.

Important points Patients should avoid food for 2 hours before and after oral treatment. Tablets should not be taken with milk.

EMERGENCY TREATMENT OF SEVERE HYPERCALCAEMIA

Whatever the cause of hypercalcaemia the initial treatment consists of intravenous fluid replacement with sodium chloride 0.9% solution and added potassium chloride. The administration of 3–4 litres of fluid daily will be needed in the first few days. Once the patient has been rehydrated adequately, intravenous frusemide which has a calciuretic effect may be added. If these measures are sufficient a bisphosphonate, calcitonin or plicamycin, may be used to lower the blood calcium level further.

ADRENAL GLAND

Corticosteroids are secreted from the outer section of the adrenal gland known as the cortex. It is regarded as a separate endocrine gland from the inner section, which is called the medulla. The cortex is divided into three different zones, each of which secretes different hormones as shown in Box 12.1.

Box 12.1 Hormones secreted by the cortex of the adrenal gland

Outer zone (zona glomerulosa) mineralocorticoids
Middle zone (zona fasciculata) glucocorticoids
Inner zone (zona reticularis) glucocorticoids, sex hormones

Mineralocorticoids

These hormones play an important part in regulating mineral salt (electrolyte) metabolism. The hormone with the most physiological importance is aldosterone. The release of aldosterone from the adrenal cortex is controlled by angiotensin, which is formed by renin. Renin is an enzyme released by the kidneys whenever the blood pressure in the afferent arterioles decreases to a certain level. Aldosterone facilitates the reabsorption of sodium by the kidney tubules. When there is an increase in the amount of aldosterone secreted there is retention of sodium chloride and hence water, leading to oedema.

Glucocorticoids

The main glucocorticoids are cortisol, also known as hydrocortisone, and corticosterone, which are essential to life. Glucocorticoids have a number of vital functions. They:

- accelerate the breakdown of cellular proteins to amino acids; the amino acids in turn circulate to the liver where they are converted to glucose, a process referred to as gluconeogenesis
- accelerate the mobilisation and breakdown of fats; fat metabolism therefore tends to take over from the usual carbohydrate metabolism
- are essential for maintenance of the blood pressure
- increase their secretion in times of physical or emotional stress
- in high concentration, reduce the number of eosinophils and cause the lymphatic tissues to atrophy, reducing the number of lymphocytes and plasma cells
- in conjunction with noradrenalin, they have anti-inflammatory properties.

Corticosteroids, like other hormones, are used in both replacement therapy and in the treatment of a wide range of conditions, such as inflammatory bowel disease, asthma, malignant diseases and skin diseases, both orally and topically. For topical use of corticosteroids see page 312. The main properties of corticosteroids are summarised in Table 12.1.

Clinical indications for the use of glucocorticoids (other than replacement therapy)

The use of corticosteroids (glucocorticoids) in certain conditions is dealt with as follows:

Table 12.1 Properties of corticosteroids

Corticosteroids	Main properties/actions
Mineralocorticoids Fludrocortisone acetate (Florinef)	Fludrocortisone has only minimal anti-inflammatory action and is used solely for its mineralocorticoid activity in Addison's disease. The daily dosage range is 50–300 micrograms (μg) per day. If glucocorticoid activity is required cortisone or hydrocortisone is given concurrently, especially at times of stress and severe illness. Adverse effects are broadly similar to those occurring with glucocorticoids but, as would be expected from the physiology, major problems are oedema, weight gain, hypertension and electrolyte disturbances. Biochemical monitoring is advised.
Glucocorticoids Betamethasone Cortisone Dexamethasone Hydrocortisone Methylprednisolone Prednisolone The above glucocorticoids have varying potencies in terms of the anti-inflammatory effects, e.g. 5 mg of prednisolone is equivalent to 20 mg hydrocortisone. Although all the above drugs have broadly similar properties, differences between them influence the choice of drug in particular conditions.	*Beneficial properties* Anti-inflammatory action Euphoria* Stimulation of appetite* Protect the body from effects of acute hypersensitivity reactions (see p. 39). Immunosuppression *Adverse effects* Diabetes Osteoporosis Mental disturbances Retardation of growth in children Muscle wasting Moonface, striae and acne in Cushing's syndrome Gastric irritation/peptic ulceration

* In certain situations these properties may cause problems in the management of patients.

INSTRUCTIONS

1- DO NOT STOP taking the steroid drug except on medical advice. Always have a supply in reserve.
2- In case of feverish illness, accident, operation (emergency or otherwise), diarrhoea or vomiting the steroid treatment MUST be continued. Your doctor may wish you to have a LARGER DOSE or an INJECTION at such time.
3- If the tablets cause indigestion consult your doctor AT ONCE.
4- Always carry this card while receiving steroid treatment and show it to any doctor, dentist, nurse or midwife whom you may consult.
5- After your treatment has finished you must still tell any new doctor, dentist, nurse or midwife that you have steroid treatment.

I AM A PATIENT ON -

STEROID
TREATMENT

WHICH MUST NOT BE STOPPED ABRUPTLY

and in the case of intercurrent illness may have to be increased

full details are available from the hospital or general practitioners shown overleaf ➤

	Name and address	Tel. No.	Treatment was commenced on		
			DRUG	DATE	DOSE
Patient					
General Practitioner					
Hospital					
Consultant or Specialist		Hospital No.			

Figure 12.6 Steroid treatment card.

- emergency treatment (see p. 39)
- eye diseases (see p. 300)
- diseases of the gastrointestinal tract (Treatment of inflammatory bowel disease see p. 64)
- malignant disease (see p. 247)
- palliative care (see p. 334)
- diseases of the respiratory tract (see p. 116)
- skin diseases (topically) (see p. 312)
- renal disease (see p. 213)
- rheumatic disease (see p. 290)

The choice of glucocorticoid for use in a particular condition will depend on many factors, notably the side-effect profile of the drug. The main properties of the commonly used glucocorticoid drugs are summarised in Table 12.2. *All glucocorticoids should be used with care*; all exhibit the adverse effects listed in Table 12.1 to a greater or lesser extent. Patient education is an important aspect of clinical management. Patients taking corticosteroids on a regular basis should be provided with a 'steroid card' (Fig. 12.6).

Sex hormones

In both sexes, the adrenal cortex secretes significant amounts of both oestrogens (female hormones) and androgens (male hormones). In the female, the ovaries produce oestrogens and progesterone: oestrogen from the graafian follicles and progesterone from a temporary structure known as the corpus luteum. In the male, testosterone is secreted by the testes. The functions of the sex hormones are described on page 184.

Treatment using sex hormones

Sex hormones are used in replacement therapy, when natural secretions are deficient and for the treatment of certain hormone dependent tumours (see p. 249). Long-term therapy with oestrogens requires the addition of a progestogen to reduce the risk of endometrial cancer. The main uses of sex hormones are summarised in Table 12.3.

THE PANCREAS

In addition to its predominantly exocrine function, the pancreas has two types of cell – alpha cells and beta cells – which make up the remaining endocrine part of the gland, known as

Table 12.2 The glucocorticoids

Drug	Dose range*/route	Properties
Betamethasone	Oral 0.5–5 mg daily. Parenteral intramuscular or intravenous 4–20 mg 6-hourly.	High glucocorticoid activity. Low mineralocorticoid activity.
Cortisone	Oral 25–37.5 mg daily in divided doses.	Has significant mineralocorticoid activity. Not suitable for long-term therapy. Useful for replacement therapy.
Dexamethasone	Oral 0.5–9 mg daily. Parenteral in cerebral oedema. 10 mg initially then 4 mg intramuscular every 6 hours.	As betamethasone.
Hydrocortisone	Oral 20–30 mg per day in divided doses. Parenteral intramuscular or intravenous 100–500 mg 3–4 times daily. Rectal foam 125 mg.	Hydrocortisone is produced by conversion of cortisone in the liver. Hydrocortisone is the active agent and is therefore often preferred to cortisone. Other properties similar to cortisone.
Prednisolone	Oral 10–20 mg daily. Parenteral intramuscular 25–100 mg weekly. Rectal foam 20 mg.	Prednisolone is a derivative of hydrocortisone and has predominant hydrocorticoid activity. It is the most commonly used oral glucocorticoid.

* Wide variation of dosage will be seen depending on the condition treated.

Table 12.3 Main uses of sex hormones		
Drug group	**Mode of action**	**Dosage/clinical indications/side-effects/precautions**
OESTROGENS **Ethinyloestradiol** **Mestranol** is available . as a composite pack with norethisterone. The tablets are graded in dose and are taken in a specific sequence **Oestradiol**	See Physiology, above.	In the treatment of menopausal symptoms 10–20 μg per day for 21 days orally (Ethinyloestradiol). Oestrogens must not be given to patients with oestrogen-dependent cancer. The risk of thromboembolic disorders precludes the use of oestrogens in patients with a history of active thrombophlebitis. Nausea, vomiting, weight gain, withdrawal bleeding, oedema and sodium retention may be troublesome. Available both in tablet and transdermal form. An implant is also available. Oestradiol is used in hormone replacement therapy (HRT) and in the prophylaxis of osteoporosis. Dosage regimens vary according to form of drug used and condition being treated, e.g. implantation 25–100 mg every 6 months; orally 1–2 mg daily; transdermally in menopausal symptoms, 50 μg/24 hours, change the patch twice weekly with a course of progestogen 12 days a month for patients with an intact uterus. The dose can be adjusted as necessary to control the symptoms.
TIBOLONE **(Livial)**	This compound has both oestrogenic and progestogenic properties and some weak androgenic activity.	Used to treat menopausal symptoms.
PROGESTERONE (the naturally occurring hormone). A wide range of compounds with progestogen activity is available including: dydrogesterone, hydroxyprogesterone, medroxyprogesterone, norethisterone.	See Physiology, above.	Since progesterones act on tissues sensitised by oestrogens the drugs are often administered on a cyclical basis with an oestrogen. Dosage regimes vary according to the condition being treated, e.g. dydrogesterone orally in dysmenorrhoea 10 mg twice daily for 5th–25th day of cycle, norethisterone orally in endometriosis 10 mg on 5th day of cycle increasing if spotting occurs. Injectable preparations are available. Progesterones can cause acne, urticaria, oedema, gastrointestinal problems and effects on the menstrual cycle.
MALE SEX **HORMONES** **Testosterone** is available in a number of forms for use orally or by slow intramuscular injection.	See Physiology, above.	In deficiency states 120–160 mg daily by mouth as the undecanoate compound. Testosterone enanthate is given intramuscularly 250 mg every 2–3 weeks. In breast cancer 250 mg intramuscularly every 2–3 weeks. Side-effects are as would be expected from the physiology, e.g. virilism in women and precocious sexual development in men. Caution must be exercised in patients suffering from candida, renal or hepatic impairment. Fertility is not enhanced by testosterone administration.
Androgenic steroids	Related to androgens but have less virilising effects.	These drugs have limited use in medicine in osteoporosis and aplastic anaemia. Illegal use by athletes has been well documented. Side-effects are similar to those seen with testosterone.

the islets of Langerhans. The alpha cells secrete the hormone glucagon; the beta cells secrete the hormone insulin. In health, insulin and glucagon work in harmony with each other, insulin decreasing the blood glucose level and glucagon increasing it.

When an excess of carbohydrate has been taken in, insulin promotes storage of glucose by accelerating the transport of glucose through the cell membrane. Insulin also converts glucose to glycogen, which is stored in the liver and muscles. It also has the capacity to synthesise protein and to convert glucose to fat. The secretion of insulin is stimulated by a rise in blood glucose reaching the islet cells.

When the blood glucose level is low due to an insufficient intake of carbohydrate or to an excessive amount of exercise having been taken, glucagon acts by mobilising the glycogen stores in the liver, converting them into glucose and thus raising the blood glucose level. Glucagon also has the capacity to convert amino acids to glucose in the liver and to increase the conversion of fat to glucose.

Diabetes mellitus

Diabetes mellitus is a syndrome in which there is an elevation of the blood glucose with consequent glycosuria resulting from an absolute or relative deficiency of insulin. The factors which predispose to the condition are:

- genetic
- coxsackie virus
- autoimmunity
- pregnancy
- endocrine disorders
- pancreatic disease
- stress
- obesity
- drugs, e.g. corticosteroids, thiazide diuretics.

There are two types of diabetes: (i) type I, juvenile-onset diabetes or insulin-dependent diabetes mellitus (IDDM), and (ii) type II, maturity-onset diabetes or non-insulin-dependent diabetes mellitus (NIDDM).

Diabetes mellitus is a major challenge to all those involved in the care of patients in the hospital or community. It is a serious multi-system disease which, if not properly controlled, can cause serious renal, neurological, ophthalmological, vascular, metabolic and biochemical disorders. Some of these disorders can be very dangerous. Diabetes mellitus in children and in pregnancy presents particularly difficult management problems. Diabetic patients facing major surgery also need special care.

Diabetes mellitus is characterised by hyperglycaemia and glycosuria. Glycosuria occurs when the glucose concentration in the blood exceeds the capacity of the renal tubules to re-absorb it. The presence of glucose in the glomerular filtrate increases the osmolality which prevents the re-absorption of water. This considerably increases the volume of urine produced, leading to polyuria. Loss of water and minerals leads to thirst and polydipsia. If the fluid and mineral (electrolyte) loss is not corrected significant complications can ensue. Poor utilisation of glucose triggers the compensatory mechanisms of glycogenolysis (breakdown of glycogen) and gluconeogenesis (breakdown of protein). Lipolysis (breakdown of fats) also occurs leading to a raised fasting plasma concentration of non-esterified fatty acid (NEFA). In severe insulin deficiency, high levels of NEFA lead to the accumulation of ketone bodies leading to the dangerous condition of ketoacidosis. The chain of events leading to ketoacidosis is summarised below:

- Lipolysis → plasma concentration of NEFA rises.
- Fatty acids are normally broken down in the liver to give acetylcoenzyme A.
- Levels of acetylcoenzyme A exceed the body's ability to clear it.
- Acetylcoenzyme A forms acetoacetic acid.
- Acetoacetic acid is converted into acetone (ketone bodies).
- Normally the ketone bodies are metabolised but in diabetes mellitus levels accumulate causing a fall in the pH of body fluids.
- The fall in pH is countered to some extent by bicarbonate.
- Bicarbonate levels fall and ketoacidosis results.
- Hydrogen ion concentration increases, as does pCO_2.
- Clinically, this may be seen as hyperpnoea.

Diagnosis of diabetes mellitus

Although diabetes mellitus is characterised by an elevated blood glucose and glycosuria, it is essential to differentiate it from other conditions such as renal glycosuria caused by a low renal threshold for glucose. Estimation of the fasting blood glucose concentration and random blood glucose concentrations will normally be sufficient to confirm the diagnosis of diabetes mellitus.

The oral glucose tolerance test (OGTT) is occasionally used in the diagnosis of diabetes mellitus if there is doubt about diagnosis. The glucose level of capillary plasma is measured after the patient has been fasting overnight. The patient is then given a 75 g glucose drink called a glucose load. Capillary plasma glucose levels are then checked half-hourly for 2 hours (see Fig. 12.7). Urine is also tested half-hourly for glucose to assess the renal threshold. To prevent an increase in metabolism and consequently an increase in glucose absorption, the patient should be advised not to smoke and to remain seated or lying down for the duration of the test. The results are as follows:

- *Fasting plasma glucose.* Should be less than or equal to 7.8 mmol/litre. If greater than 9 mmol/litre the patient has diabetes mellitus. (This figure may vary slightly from one health authority to another.)

- *2 hours after glucose load.* If the capillary plasma glucose level is between 8.9 and 12.2 mmol/litre the patient has an impaired glucose tolerance. If the capillary plasma glucose level is greater than 12.2 mmol/litre the patient has diabetes mellitus.

Aims of treatment

The overall aims of treatment can be summarised as follows:

- to enable the patient to lead a normal life
- to achieve and maintain a normal metabolic state
- to avoid the complications of the disease, especially vascular disorders
- to avoid acute episodes, e.g. ketoacidosis
- to involve the patient fully in the management programme.

With the generally increasing life expectancy, complications are of particular concern in the older patient since ischaemic changes may lead to serious morbidity, e.g. diabetic gangrene. Apart from drug treatment, particular attention must be paid to diet, personal hygiene (especially the feet), exercise and other aspects of life styles.

Major complications

- ketoacidosis (see above)
- renal damage – diabetic glomerulosclerosis
- diabetic retinopathy – a common condition which can cause blindness due to damage to the retinal veins, haemorrhages and exudates in the retina
- diabetic neuropathy – which may affect the CNS to varying degrees
- lowered resistance to infection.

Treatment of NIDDM

Oral antidiabetic drugs are widely used in the treatment of this condition, especially in older, obese patients. Treatment has to be supplemented by careful attention to diet. Younger patients or patients with brittle diabetes cannot

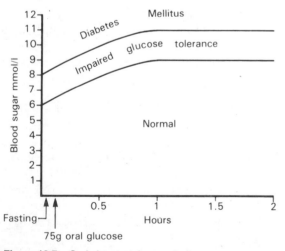

Figure 12.7 Oral glucose tolerance test.

be treated with oral agents. The range of drugs available is described in Table 12.4.

Many patients with NIDDM may not exhibit any overt symptoms but their hyperglycaemia may be causing vascular damage without the awareness of either doctor or patient. Particular attention needs to be paid to patients with a family history of ischaemic heart disease and blood lipid abnormalities. Hypertension is another major risk factor as is smoking. Regular screening and well managed therapy can help patients (especially older patients) achieve a better quality of life with reduced incidence of morbidity.

Treatment of IDDM

Patients suffering from IDDM must be treated by injections of insulin. Parenteral routes must be used as insulin (a protein) is destroyed by the gastric acid and enzymes. For many years, efforts have been made to produce an insulin product utilising more convenient routes of administration, e.g. intranasal insulin. It appears that the parenteral route will remain the mainstay of therapy for the immediate future.

Aims

The aims of treatment of IDDM are essentially the same as the aims discussed in the treatment of NIDDM. However, owing to the more brittle and serious nature of this condition more sophisticated dosage regimes and monitoring are often required. Specialist clinics and shared care protocols help to ensure the continuity of care that is vital if the serious complications of diabetes mellitus are to be avoided. The role of the dia-

Table 12.4 Drugs used in the treatment of NIDDM

Drug groups	Mode of action	Dose/notes

Sulphonylureas
  chlorpropamide
 	
  glibenclamide
	These compounds stimulate the synthesis and release of insulin and have other beneficial effects such as increasing the sensitivity of receptors to insulin. It is clear that to achieve benefit these drugs depend on endogenous insulin and a functioning pancreas.	These drugs have a prolonged action and may cause problems in older patients who are prone to hypoglycaemia. Other drugs are now preferred.
		All dosages of these agents must be adjusted in response to the patient's condition. The doses given below may vary from patient to patient.

tolbutamide
  gliclazide
  glipizide
		500 mg–1.5 g daily in divided doses.
		40–80 mg daily up to 160 mg as a single dose.
		Normally 2.5–5 mg daily. Up to 15 mg may be given as a single dose before breakfast. Maximum daily dose 40 mg. The use of all oral hypoglycaemic agents should be carefully managed. Patients with hepatic or renal insufficiency are at risk of hypoglycaemia. The short-acting tolbutamide may be used if there is renal impairment. Blood disorders have been reported and weight gain may occur.

Biguanides metformin	Acts by decreasing gluconeogenesis and by increasing peripheral utilisation of glucose. As with the sulphonylureas it is effective only where there is endogenous insulin.	500 mg every 8 hours or 850 mg every 12 hours with food. Avoid in patients with renal problems and a tendency to lactic acidosis; cardiac problems; trauma; infection; and pregnancy. Gastrointestinal problems are common at higher doses.
Alpha-glucosidase *inhibitors* (especially active against the enzyme sucrase) acarbose	Reduce post-prandial blood glucose peaks by inhibiting intestinal alpha-glucosidases. This has the effect of delaying the digestion of starch and sucrose into absorbable monosaccharides. The blood glucose profile is smoothed and fluctuations in blood glucose levels are reduced. These compounds have no stimulatory action on the pancreas. Fasting blood glucose levels are also reduced.	50 mg three times daily adjusting if necessary to 100 mg three times daily taken with food. Due to the action of acarbose, dietary carbohydrate is digested in the large bowel. This can lead to gastrointestinal problems such as flatulence, abdominal distension and diarrhoea. Attention to diet may help to alleviate these symptoms.

betes care sister both in hospital and community practice is seen as being of key, and increasing, importance.

Insulins

Great progress has been made with the development of sophisticated insulins designed to help physicians achieve good control of blood glucose levels. Insulin can be obtained from the pancreatic tissue of slaughtered animals (bovine or porcine insulins) but insulin with a structure corresponding exactly with that of human insulin is now available routinely. Human insulin is prepared by recombinant DNA technology or other biological technique, e.g. enzymatic modification of porcine insulin. Many patients do well on insulin obtained from animal tissue and the need to change established patterns to human insulin should be carefully evaluated.

A wide range of insulins is available, each product being formulated to achieve a specific profile in terms of speed of onset and length of action. In practice a combination of insulins is used, designed to achieve optimal control for the particular patient. The ideal is to achieve a control of blood glucose level corresponding as nearly as is possible to the non-diabetic physiological profile. Insulin is secreted in the non-diabetic in two ways. About half of the insulin secreted is in response to an intake of food; the remainder is secreted to cover basal requirements (Fig. 12.8).

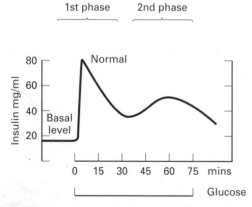

Figure 12.8 Insulin secretion in non-diabetic.

Insulin formulations

Insulin is available as a simple solution which has a rapid onset and short duration of action. The onset, duration and peak effects depend on the route of administration. Combined with protamine or a zinc salt, longer-acting preparations of insulin have been developed. The combined use of short-acting and long-acting insulins is the preferred approach to treatment of diabetes mellitus other than in acute conditions such as ketoacidosis where the soluble, rapid acting form of insulin must be used. The main preparations of insulin are described in Table 12.5. In view of the wide range of preparations available it follows that great care must be taken in selecting the correct product for the particular patient.

All insulin formulations must be stored between 2 and 8°C. Freezing or exposure to excessive heat will destroy the product. If refrigeration is not available, storage at room temperature for one month is acceptable.

A range of biphasic insulins is available containing differing proportions of isophane and soluble insulins ranging from 10% soluble insulin and 90% isophane insulin to 40% soluble insulin and 60% isophane insulin.

All insulins are 100 units per 1 ml, and, since the packaging is a multidose vial, suitable preservatives are added at a formulation stage. The mixture of soluble and long-acting insulin is designed for twice-daily administration but dosage levels are always determined in response to the patient's needs. If a ready-mixed preparation of insulin is unsuitable for the patient's needs certain insulins may be mixed in the syringe. The shorter-acting insulin must be drawn into the syringe first to avoid contaminating the longer-acting preparation. Increased dosage levels may be needed during illness or emotional disturbances.

Administration of insulin

In many cases subcutaneous administration using a disposable insulin syringe will meet the patient's needs. The use of a pen injector system

Table 12.5 Insulin preparations

Type of preparation/route of administration	Approximate* duration of action (hours) of subcutaneous injection		
	Onset	Duration	Peak
Soluble insulin (neutral) s.c., i.m., i.v. and i.v. infusion (short-acting insulin)	0.5–1	8	2–4
	(Human insulin has a more rapid onset and shorter duration of action.) When given intravenously its effect lasts about 0.5 hour.		
Insulin zinc suspension mixed (IZS Lente) (long-acting insulin)	2.5	up to 24	4–16
Insulin zinc suspension amorphous (intermediate acting insulin)	1.5	1.5–16	5–10
Insulin zinc suspension crystalline (long-acting insulin)	3	20–24	6–14
Protamine zinc insulin (PZI) (long-acting insulin)	4–6	24–36	10–20
Isophane insulin (intermediate acting insulin)	1.5	up to 24	4–12
Biphasic insulins (these insulins consist of a suspension of a longer-acting insulin in a solution of insulin)	0.5	0.5–22	4–12

* There are some variations between the onset of action, duration and peak depending on the type of insulin–human, bovine or porcine.

and a cartridge presentation of insulin may be an advantage for some patients. (Fig. 12.9).

Pen injection systems have the advantage of portability, greater social acceptability and flexibility of lifestyle since meal times can be varied. Disadvantages of this means of administration are, however, significant. Patients may be lulled into a false sense of security due to the ease of use. This may lead to poor control of diet. Patients need to understand the adjustment of dosage, taking into account blood glucose levels. Cartridges of mixed insulins may not always be appropriate especially for younger diabetics.

The constant quest to achieve control of blood glucose levels corresponding to those of a well non-diabetic continues to challenge manufacturers and clinicians. Four to six injections daily of a small dose of soluble insulin is an option that would achieve good control but this is clearly not practicable. Controlled continuous subcutaneous infusion of insulin may be administered using a pump system. Additional doses can be administered to cover meals by the activation of a mechanism incorporated into the pump. An implantable device which releases insulin in response to blood glucose level fluctuations remains an objective for the researchers.

Some problems of insulin therapy

Hypoglycaemia is always a potential problem. Change of preparation can create problems. Changing from insulin of animal origin to human insulin has been reported to cause hypoglycaemic reactions which were not always easy for the patient to anticipate. Insulin requirements may be increased due to illness or emotional upset. Conditions where insulin requirements are reduced include diseases of the adrenal, pituitary or thyroid gland. Reduced doses are also required where there is renal or hepatic

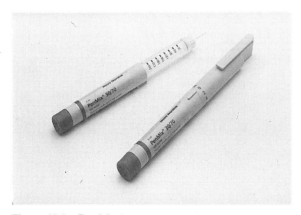

Figure 12.9 Pen injector.

impairment, or by the concurrent administration of drugs which have a hypoglycaemic action.

Local side-effects of insulin therapy include local hypersensitivity reactions, lipodystrophy and insulin resistance. Reactions to human insulin are claimed to be less than with insulins of animal origin.

Treatment of hypoglycaemia

A hypoglycaemic patient is pale and may appear slower than usual, stupid, aggressive or intoxicated. Beads of sweat appear on the brow or upper lip. Hypoglycaemic attacks are more likely to occur before the mid-day meal and at night. If hypoglycaemia does occur, due to whatever cause, prompt action is required. Diabetics are taught to recognise the onset of hypoglycaemia and to take glucose appropriately. If the patient is conscious, oral glucose is used, in the form of a drink e.g. Lucozade, Coca-Cola, or in the form of sugar lumps or Dextrosol tablets. In hospital, the nurse should prepare a glucose drink using glucose monohydrate 25 g thoroughly dissolved in warm water and carefully assist the patient to drink the solution at once. A record should be kept of the amount of glucose required and the time taken by the patient to return to normal.

Hypostop is a gel containing 40% glucose monohydrate (equivalent to 32% glucose anhydrous). It is used orally for the treatment of hypoglycaemia. The gel formulation is claimed to help to achieve a more rapid absorption than an aqueous solution.

Alternatively, glucagon injection may be given i.m. or s.c. if prescribed. This is a valuable method for those patients troubled by recurrent hypoglycaemia for whom a trained family member can give the injection. If the patient does not respond to oral glucose or to glucagon, or if the patient is discovered unconscious, intravenous glucose 50% 20–50 ml should be given. The assistance of the nurse is desirable since glucose is highly irritant to the tissues and must be directed carefully into the vein. The dose may have to be repeated. The nurse should remain with the patient and be ready to provide reassurance and support as he regains consciousness.

Blood glucose testing

Whenever possible self-monitoring of the blood glucose in diabetics is to be encouraged to allow the patient to be independent and to reduce the risk of blood-borne infection. Admission to hospital provides an opportunity for the nurse to check the patient's technique, especially where there is some concern over diabetic control. Some hospital patients are of course not well enough to perform this procedure and so the responsibility temporarily falls to the nurse.

The sample of capillary blood may be obtained from the pinna of the ear or from the side of the thumb nail, the former being the more vascular.

Box 12.2 Blood glucose testing

Documentation
  diabetic prescription sheet
The medicine
  e.g. BM-Test 1– 44 strips in container with colour scale
  strips fit for use
The environment
  no special requirements
The nurse and patient
  patient given explanation of what is involved
  patient's ear/hand washed with soap and water and dried thoroughly
  patient seated if not in bed (with hand resting comfortably if appropriate)
Technique
  nurse attends to own hand hygiene and dons gloves
  strip placed on clean surface
  pinna or side of thumb sharply pricked using lancet or Glucolet if available
  part gently squeezed to obtain large suspended drop of blood
  blood allowed to drop so as to cover test area of strip
  blood carefully and firmly wiped off strip using clean piece of cotton wool after exactly one minute; strip gently wiped twice more using clean part of cotton wool
  after further whole minute, colours of the two test zones compared with colour scale on container
  if, after two minutes, the blood glucose value is in excess of 13 mmol, another minute is allowed to elapse before making comparison again
  careful disposal of lancet, test strip and wool
Hazards
  infection
  inaccurate blood glucose reading

Apart from reasons of cleanliness, the patient's ear/hand should be washed with soap and warm water and dried before carrying out the blood test so as to improve the circulation and allow blood to be more easily obtained. An alcohol swab is not used to clean the skin as the spirit contained in the swab reacts with the blood and may cause a false reading. Since the maintenance of an optimum blood glucose level is highly dependent on the use of reagents, it is essential to follow the manufacturer's instructions implicitly. It should be noted, for example, that the comparison colours on the container label are specific to each pack of strips and so it is important to compare the reaction colour with the colour scale on the container of test strips used.

Reagent strips used for measuring plasma glucose levels may be read against a colour chart or by using a meter specially designed to

Table 12.6 Areas to cover in a teaching programme for new diabetics

Subject area	Detail

Anatomy and physiology	A clear understanding of
	    the pancreas, the blood and the tissues
	    carbohydrate metabolism

The disorder itself	What has gone wrong with the pancreas and why treatment is essential

Controlling the blood glucose level	Administration of insulin or oral antidiabetic agent as appropriate
	    prescriptions
	    supplies
	    storage (especially insulin)
	    equipment
	    aids to administration
	    dosages
	    timing
	    frequency
	    sites of administration
	    technique

Controlling the diet	An understanding of the different classes of food and the need to avoid pure sugars Knowledge of dietary exchanges The need to eat regularly, including snacks between meals and before bedtime Importance of trying to eat, even if feeling unwell

Monitoring the disorder	The importance of keeping careful records of
	    blood glucose readings
	    urinalysis
	    insulin administered
	    hypoglycaemic episodes and action taken

The patient's care of himself	How to recognise hypoglycaemic reactions
	The importance of meticulous care of the feet
	The importance of attending clinics as arranged
	    diabetic clinic
	    dietetic clinic
	    eye clinic
	    chiropody
	Encouragement of healthy lifestyle with adequate sleep, minimisation of stress and reduced exposure to infections where possible
	Advice and encouragement to allow the continuation of normal activities such as schooling, work, sport, travel
	The benefits of carrying some indication that he is diabetic e.g. card, medical pendant/bracelet
	What to do when feeling unwell
	Sources of help
	    medical
	    nursing
	    dietetic
	    financial

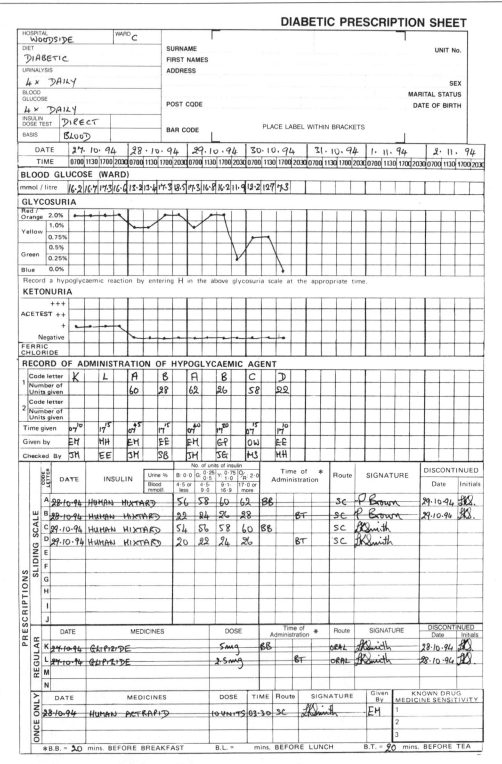

Figure 12.10 Diabetic prescription sheet.

accurately record the result. Since colour vision is not infrequently impaired in diabetics, the glucometer is a considerable advantage for self-monitoring where it can be used. There are several different kinds of glucometer. Each type has its own reagent strip.

Blood glucose testing is outlined in Box 12.2.

Future developments in the treatment of IDDM

It seems likely that continual improvements will be made both in insulin formulations and delivery systems. Since some forms of IDDM may have autoimmunity as a causal factor, immunosuppressants such as cyclosporin may be useful.

Role of the nurse in diabetes mellitus

Nurses play a vital role at all stages in the management of diabetes. The routine screening of patients attending any clinic is performed with a view to identifying previously undiagnosed diabetes. Assisting in the assessment and diagnosis of suspected diabetes including carrying out the oral glucose tolerance test, for example, is another important part of the nurse's role. Once diabetes is diagnosed and treatment agreed, the day-to-day management of the condition and the education of the patient (and his family) are largely left in the hands of the nurse. On no other occasion are the nurse's teaching skills more greatly drawn upon than during the period between confirmation of the diagnosis and discharge from hospital. The challenge for the nurse is to have a patient who is both competent and confident in managing his condition. Such an opportunity lends itself to a planned programme of teaching using different teaching methods including explaining, demonstrating (possibly also with videotapes), supervising practice and providing suitable written information. Subject areas to be covered are detailed in Table 12.6.

In any clinical setting at any time, the nurse may be involved with the diabetic patient and so it is essential that nurses in all disciplines have a grasp of the condition and an understanding of the aims of treatment. Nurses in accident and emergency departments and acute medical wards will from time to time have to care for the acutely ill diabetic patient. Especially with the insulin-dependent diabetic, the need to be observant, adhere to correct procedure, maintain high standards of hygiene and keep meticulous records cannot be overemphasised. Diabetic prescribing and recording sheets should reflect an accurate diabetic 'picture' (Fig. 12.10). Nurses also have an important coordinating role with other relevant health professionals.

The aim for nurses in primary care is to maximise quality of life for the diabetic, prevent long-term diabetic complications and increase longevity. Increasingly, health authorities are utilising the skills of nurses specialising in care for diabetics. The importance of close liaison between diabetic clinic and general practitioner cannot be over-stressed. Similarly, good communication between nurses and doctors is paramount.

In summary the nurse plays an especially full part in the diagnosis, treatment and care of the diabetic patient. It is however in her teaching role that there is greatest potential to contribute to maximum independence and otherwise good health for diabetics.

FURTHER READING

Betts A 1993 Diabetes mellitus. Practice Nursing
    18–31 May: 21–22
Diabetes update 1993 Nursing 93 August: 59–61
Marshall S M 1993 Hyperglycaemic emergencies. Care of the
    Critically Ill 9(5): 220–223

Murphy C, Hall G 1993 Diabetes facilitators in general
    practice. Diabetes Care 2(1): 4–5
Thompson A, Gibbon C 1993 Setting standards in diabetes
    education. Nursing Standard 7: 25–28

13

Drug treatment of renal and urinary-tract disorders

ANATOMY

The major excretory function of the production of urine is performed by a structure consisting of secretory organs (two kidneys), and a system which conveys the urine (two ureters) to a collection and temporary storage organ (the bladder). Urine is discharged from the bladder via the urethra (see Fig. 13.1).

A longitudinal section of the kidney (see Fig. 13.2) indicates the structures visible to the naked eye. At the microscopic level the kidney is made up of nephrons which, in health, are responsible for maintaining the fluid and electrolyte balance.

AN OUTLINE OF RENAL PHYSIOLOGY

In health, the intake and output of fluids and electrolytes are maintained in a state of balance by the kidneys. The kidneys also excrete the products of metabolism, urea, creatinine and uric acid. Many drugs are also excreted by the kidneys in the urine. Renal function is subject to a number of control mechanisms, such as the production of antidiuretic hormone produced by the pituitary gland. The adrenal cortex produces aldosterone, which also influences renal activity.

PRODUCTION OF URINE

Urine is produced in the kidney within the nephron of which there are about 1 million in each kidney. Each nephron is a functional unit

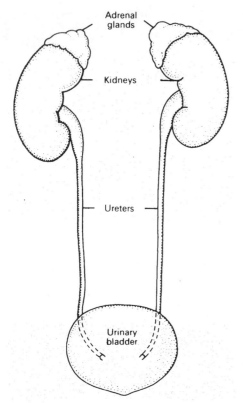

Figure 13.1 The urinary system. (From Ross & Wilson 1990 Anatomy and physiology in health and illness, 7th edn. Churchill Livingstone.)

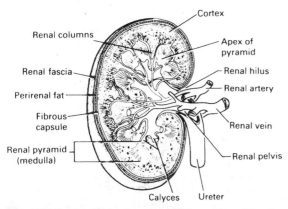

Figure 13.2 Longitudinal section of kidney. (From Chandler 1991 Tabbner's nursing care: theory and practice, 2nd edn. Churchill Livingstone.)

which consists of a cup-shaped capsule and a tortuous tubule and ends as a reservoir for the urine (Fig. 13.3). The tubule walls are one epithelial cell thick and at certain points are flattened to allow them greater permeability. Lying within each capsule in close proximity to the capsule wall is a cluster of intertwining arterial capillaries known as the glomerulus. Arterial blood enters the glomerulus via the afferent arteriole and leaves via the efferent arteriole. The autonomic nervous system provides the nerve supply. Essentially there are three phases in urine production.

Glomerular filtration

Water and most small molecules filter through the semi-permeable walls of the glomerulus and the glomerular capsule because the blood pressure in the glomerulus is greater than the pressure of the filtrate within the glomerular capsule. Large molecules and large cells (e.g. erythrocytes) and plasma proteins remain in the capillaries.

Tubular re-absorption

Constituents which have filtered through the glomerulus into the tubules but which the body still requires are re-absorbed. This process ensures fluid and electrolyte balances are maintained and blood pH is maintained. Selective re-absorption is regularised by both the autonomic nervous system and by hormones. Water re-absorption is regulated by the antidiuretic hormone on the distal part of the tubule, the parathyroid hormone and calcitonin regulate the re-absorption of calcium and phosphate. Aldosterone influences the re-absorption of sodium and the excretion of potassium.

Tubular secretion

Substances which were not given sufficient time to filter through the glomerular wall are cleared from the body by secretion into the convoluted tubules. Some drugs are excreted in this way.

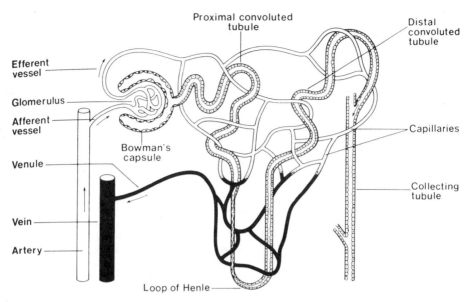

Figure 13.3   Structure of nephron. (From Chandler 1991 Tabbner's nursing care: theory and practice, 2nd edn. Churchill Livingstone.)

EXCRETION OF URINE

From the collecting tubule the urine is received into the renal pelvis before passing into the ureter and thence to the bladder. The smooth muscle of the bladder wall comes under the influence of the autonomic nervous system. The external urethral sphincter is under voluntary control and only when it is released will micturition occur. Depending on fluid intake and other factors, a healthy adult will pass 1–2.5 litres of urine daily.

WATER BALANCE

The amount of water excreted in the urine is influenced by the antidiuretic hormone and the level of waste material to be removed from the blood. Antidiuretic hormone is released as part of a feedback mechanism involving the hypothalamus and the posterior pituitary.

ELECTROLYTE BALANCE

Sodium, potassium, calcium and magnesium ions exist in body fluids. For the body to maintain a constant internal environment the concentration of each electrolyte in the body fluids must be maintained (see p. 213). Changes in concentration of electrolytes may result from changes in the amount of water or electrolytes. The amount of sodium and potassium in the urine is regulated by a feedback mechanism dependent on the blood flow through the kidneys (see Fig. 13.4).

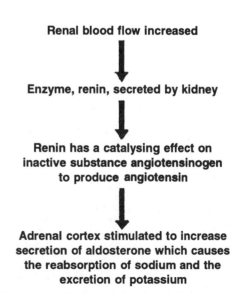

Renal blood flow increased

↓

Enzyme, renin, secreted by kidney

↓

Renin has a catalysing effect on inactive substance angiotensinogen to produce angiotensin

↓

Adrenal cortex stimulated to increase secretion of aldosterone which causes the reabsorption of sodium and the excretion of potassium

Figure 13.4   Regulation of sodium and potassium.

Table 13.1   Major diseases of the kidney

Condition	Main features/causes	Treatment
Glomerulonephritis (acute)	Inflammation of glomeruli (bilateral). Caused by an immune response to bacterial toxins, especially streptococci. Viral infection may also cause the disease. Histological examination is needed to differentiate various forms of the disease. The main signs are haematuria, hypertension, proteinuria and oedema.	Bed rest, low-sodium diet, fluid restriction. Penicillin for streptococcal infection. Most younger patients recover well from the disease. The prognosis is less favourable in the older (+40 years) patients.
Glomerulonephritis (chronic)	Chronic glomerulonephritis leads to chronic renal failure. As renal failure develops the levels of body fluids and electrolytes become abnormal. Acid-base balance is disturbed and nitrogenous waste products normally excreted in the urine accumulate. Platelet dysfunction results in bleeding episodes. The hypertension that accompanies the condition may cause retinopathy.	Unless this disease is treated either by dialysis or transplantation the prognosis is grave. Treatment is based on dietary control, low protein, high carbohydrate and fat. Fluid intake is not restricted since it is important to achieve a large urinary volume to aid the excretion of the end products of metabolism. Cardiac failure is a contraindication to a large fluid intake as is salt intake. Acidosis is treated by an appropriate regime, depending on blood chemistry results. An infusion of sodium bicarbonate may be required. Any infection must be treated, but care is needed with dosage levels since excretion of the antibiotic may be impaired. Gastrointestinal symptoms must be treated, and bone pain may respond to vitamin D. Hypertension must be carefully managed so as not to cause a fall in renal blood flow. Dialysis and renal transplantation will not be considered. However, these are life-saving methods of dealing with renal failure.
Infections (see also Ch. 11)	It may be difficult to determine the extent of an infection of the urinary tract. Any infection of the urinary tract has the potential to involve the kidneys. However, most urinary tract infections are capable of being treated in such a way that the spread of the infection is contained.	The antimicrobial treatment of urinary-tract infections (UTI) is described in Chapter 11. Approach to treatment depends on a number of factors. Owing to differing anatomical and other features the approach to the treatment of UTI depends on the sex and age of the patient. Particular care must be taken to prevent kidney damage in children due to vesico-ureteric reflux. Careful assessment of the patient is essential, a full history is required, e.g. in men it is important to exclude prostatic malignancy. In pregnant women pyelonephritis must be considered. Advice on prevention, e.g. passing urine after intercourse and vulval hygiene, are important.
Pyelonephritis (acute)	Acute inflammation of the parenchyma and pelvis of the kidney. The condition may affect one or both kidneys. Many of the infections are due to *E. coli*, but there are other causative organisms, e.g. *proteus* species. There is a greater degree of prevalence in women than men, due to the anatomical differences. Fever, pain, frequency and dysuria are seen.	Antimicrobial therapy (see p. 153). Antimicrobial agent should not be delayed until the organism causing the infection has been identified. Treatment should be continued until bacteriological tests are negative. Surgical treatment may be required if the root cause of the infection is a physical obstruction.

Table 13.1 *Cont'd*		
Condition	**Main features/causes**	**Treatment**
Pyelonephritis (chronic)	The condition may present with a combination of symptoms, e.g. tiredness, general ill-health and urinary symptoms such as frequency, dysuria and lumbar pain. Careful checks should be made for any mechanical obstruction.	Removal of any obstruction and long-term antimicrobial treatment. Suitable changes in antimicrobial therapy should be considered to avoid the possibility of resistance developing.
Renal failure (acute)	Renal failure arises from a variety of causes. Disease or drugs, circulatory failure, obstruction and acute renal ischaemia.	Water and electrolyte balance must be restored and dietary control exercised (low protein). Acidosis must be treated and hyperkalaemia corrected. Great care must be taken with drug therapy (see p. 24). Haemodialysis or peritoneal dialysis must be considered since acute renal failure is life-threatening. Discussion of these techniques is beyond the scope of this book.
Nephrotic syndrome	Several kidney diseases are characterised by hypoproteinaemic oedema and proteinurea. The term 'nephrotic syndrome' is used to describe this chemical state.	Treatment includes diuretics, corticosteroids, restriction of salt in diet, spironolactone is indicated in hypokalaemia.

OTHER FUNCTIONS OF THE KIDNEY

In addition to the important functions of fluid and electrolyte control the kidneys are responsible for the production of erythropoietin (see p. 270) and dihydroxycholecalciferol (a form of vitamin D). Prostaglandins are also produced in the kidneys.

DISEASES OF THE KIDNEYS

In view of the vital functions performed by the kidneys it is evident that any disturbance of renal function will be of major significance for the patient. Any suspected failure of renal function must be investigated by a range of tests including cystoscopy, radiological examination, the use of radioisotopes and scanning techniques. A full chemical examination of the urine is required for the presence of glucose, protein, blood and microorganisms. Chemical analysis of the blood is undertaken to determine the concentration of metabolites such as urea and creatinine. Metabolic acidosis can arise in certain kidney conditions when the excretion of hydrogen ions is diminished. Determination of arterial pH will give an indication of the extent of the acidosis. A detailed discussion of the major diseases of the kidneys is beyond the scope of this book. Table 13.1 gives an outline of the major kidney diseases together with an outline of treatment regimes.

FLUID AND ELECTROLYTES
Fluid and electrolyte deficiency

Disorders of fluid balance are almost always accompanied by changes in the concentration of plasma sodium, potassium, other electrolytes and urea. Changes in fluid balance also have an effect on electrolyte levels. Such changes may have profound implications for the patient and must therefore be corrected by the administration of both water and electrolytes. The volume and chemical content of the fluid, and route of administration depend on the condition being treated and biochemical status of the patient as determined by laboratory tests and clinical findings. The physiological significance of the main electrolytes is summarised in Table 13.2.

In order to enhance understanding of the terms used in the text a series of definitions are given in Table 13.3.

ABNORMALITIES OF ELECTROLYTE LEVELS AND FLUID BALANCE

The main abnormalities of electrolyte levels are closely linked with changes in fluid balance. For

Table 13.2 Physiological significance of the main electrolytes

Electrolyte/normal range	Physiological significance/metabolism
Sodium (Na^+): 137–144 mmol per litre in plasma	Sodium is the most important extracellular cation, making up more than 90% of the total extracellular cations. Sodium accounts for a substantial proportion of the extracellular osmotic pressure. The cell membrane is not readily permeable to sodium ions. However, sodium diffuses slowly into the intracellular compartment according to the concentration gradient. The 'sodium pump' in the cell membrane transports sodium out of the cell. This movement of sodium is important in the establishment and maintenance of the electrical potential of the cell membrane and in the transmission of nerve impulses. A complex process is responsible for the maintenance of the sodium concentration in the body. Intake is normally dietary. Excretion in the urine in controlled by aldosterone and the antidiuretic hormone (ADH).
Potassium (K^+): 3.5–4.9 mmol per litre in plasma (intracellular concentration is of the order of 150 mmol/litre)	Potassium is the most important and abundant intracellular cation. It is present in low concentrations in the extracellular fluid. Potassium is responsible for a major portion of the intracellular fluid's osmotic pressure. Potassium plays a vital role in neuromuscular contraction and cardiac rhythm. Potassium is also important in aspects of carbohydrate metabolism and the synthesis of protein. As with sodium, intake is normally dietary and excretion is in the urine and to a lesser extent in the faeces.
Calcium (Ca^{2+}): 2.2–2.6 mmol per litre (total body calcium greatly exceeds the amount present in the extracellular fluid)	Calcium is found in the bones and teeth in combination with phosphate to give strength and rigidity. Most of the calcium in the body is in deposits, with only a small proportion present in plasma (extracellular fluid). Calcium is important in blood coagulation processes, neuromuscular functions and cardiac activity. Intake is mainly dietary (especially dairy products) and excretion is mainly in the faeces. Small amounts are excreted in the urine. Vitamin D and gastric pH influence the absorption of calcium. Regulation of calcium metabolism is by parathyroid hormone, vitamin D and calcitonin.
Magnesium (Mg^{2+}): 0.7–1.2 mmol per litre (total body magnesium greatly exceeds the content of the plasma)	Magnesium is present mainly in the bony skeleton, the remainder is found in the intracellular fluid especially in the heart, liver and skeletal muscles. Magnesium is important in enzyme activity – especially in the metabolism of glucose to provide energy. Magnesium also plays a part in the synthesis of protein. The functioning of nervous tissue depends on the presence of magnesium ions. The control mechanisms for magnesium are poorly understood, but aldosterone is known to influence renal excretion. Other control mechanisms may be parathyroid hormone and vitamin D. Magnesium is in plentiful supply in a normal diet and the kidney reabsorbs most of the magnesium from the glomerular filtrate.
Chloride (Cl^-): 100–106 mmol per litre	Chloride is the most abundant extracellular anion. Low concentrations are present in the intracellular fluid. Chloride plays a key role in the maintenance of the osmotic pressure of the extracellular fluid. Changes in the acid–base balance may influence chloride concentration. Chloride regulation is fundamentally linked with the regulation of the major cations (e.g. sodium) since electrical neutrality must always be maintained. It follows that chloride regulation is influenced by aldosterone, which enhances the tubular re-absorption of chloride and sodium. Intake is mainly dietary (as table salt NaCl). Apart from excretion in the urine some chloride is lost in the sweat and gastrointestinal secretions.
Phosphate (PO_4^{2-}): 0.7–1.2 mmol per litre	Phosphate occurs mainly in the intracellular fluid and in combination with calcium is a vital constituent of bones and teeth. Phosphate also helps to maintain acid–base balance by providing a buffer system. Phosphates are vitally important in a number of metabolic processes especially carbohydrate metabolism. Phospholipids are important structural components of cell membranes. Phosphate regulation is linked closely with calcium metabolism. Parathyroid hormone liberates phosphate and vitamin D probably enhances renal excretion of phosphate. An increase in serum phosphate is associated with a decrease in plasma calcium and vice versa. Phosphate is widely present in foodstuffs, especially milk and other dairy products. Excretion is via the urine and faeces.

Table 13.3 Definitions

Term	Definition
Acid–base balance	In health there is a balance between the carbonic acid and bicarbonate (base) content of plasma. Other basic (alkaline) substances in plasma are phosphates and protein.
Acidosis (metabolic)	Acidosis has developed when the plasma level of bicarbonate falls to 15 mmol/litre. In severe acidosis the bicarbonate level may fall below 10 mmol/litre.
Alkalosis (metabolic)	Alkalosis has developed when the plasma bicarbonate is elevated to 35 mmol/litre. The pH of blood also rises.
Anion	Negatively charged ion, e.g. Cl^- or HCO_3^-.
Buffering effect	Blood has the property to adjust to the pressure of acids produced by metabolic processes. Hydrogen ions are removed by the carbonic acid/bicarbonate buffer system so that the pH of plasma remains within the normal range 7.37–7.45.
Cation	Positively charged ion, e.g. Na^+ or K^+.
Electrolyte	A chemical substance that dissociates in water to yield ions (charged particles) e.g. sodium chloride (NaCl) dissociates to yield Na^+ and Cl^-.
Isotonic	An isotonic solution has the same osmotic pressure as the comparison solution. The osmotic pressure of plasma is the accepted standard in medicine. A 0.9% w/v solution of sodium chloride is isotonic with plasma. Solutions with a lower osmotic pressure than plasma are hypotonic. Solutions with a higher osmotic pressure are hypertonic.
Milliequivalent	Is 1/1000 of the equivalent weight of a substance. This term has been replaced by the millimole.
Millimole (mmol)	A mole is the molecular weight of a substance expressed in grams. A millimole is 1/1000 of the molecular weight.
Osmolality	A measure of osmotic activity in terms of the concentration of solute particles in a unit of *weight* of solvent.
Osmolarity	Is also a measure of osmotic activity of a solution but is expressed in terms of the concentration of solute particles in a given *volume* of solvent.
Osmosis	When two solutions of differing concentration of dissolved solids (solute) are separated by a semi-permeable membrane (e.g. cell membrane) water flows to the side of the membrane with the higher concentration of solute. Water flow ceases when the concentrations become equal.
Osmotic pressure	Is the pressure created by the flow of water due to osmosis.
pH (hydrogen ion concentration)	Is a measure of the degree of acidity or alkalinity of a solution. A pH below 7 indicates an acidic pH whereas a pH above 7 indicates an alkaline solution. pH 7.0 is neutral.

example, hypernatraemia is associated with fluid retention, loss of sodium is associated with a reduction in water content of the body. In many cases abnormalities in electrolyte and fluid balance must be urgently treated by the parenteral (usually i.v.) route. In milder, chronic cases the oral route may be practicable and is always preferred where it can be used. The importance of accurate diagnosis, choice of fluid and concentration of electrolytes cannot be overstated. Accurate monitoring of the changes in plasma and other electrolyte levels achieved by the therapy is a prerequisite. In order to obtain a complete picture of losses of electrolytes from the body it may be necessary to examine faeces, vomitus and aspirations in addition to the blood and urine.

Hyponatraemia (lowered plasma sodium levels)

The main causes of hyponatraemia are:

- excessive sweating in hostile environments, e.g. tropical countries
- loss of sodium in the urine due to renal disease or poor hormonal control (Addison's disease)
- uncontrolled diabetes mellitus
- chronic uraemia

- over-use of diuretics
- gastrointestinal problems, e.g. diarrhoea, vomiting and intestinal fistula
- loss of fluid due to trauma, e.g. extensive burns.

Patients with hyponatraemia may experience nausea, weakness, headache and drowsiness. The degree and nature of the symptoms depend on the level of sodium in the plasma. Concentrations in the range 120 mmol/litre give rise to weakness, at 90–105 mmol/litre neurological signs and symptoms develop.

Treatment of hyponatraemia in milder, chronic forms is by the oral administration of sodium, usually as chloride in the form of a slow-release tablet. The choice of sodium compound administered depends on the acid–base status of the patient. In acidotic patients sodium bicarbonate is required, whereas in the alkalotic patient sodium chloride is required. In more severe hyponatraemia treatment by parenteral administration of a fluid containing a sodium compound is required. This will also help to correct the fluid loss that almost always accompanies sodium depletion. The administration of sodium parenterally is not without risk. Hypertension and fluid overload must be avoided. Plasma sodium levels must be monitored, and physical signs such as pulse rate and blood pressure give a good indication of the patient's response to the therapy. Fluids commonly used to correct hyponatraemia (and other electrolyte deficiencies) are summarised in Table 13.4.

Hypernatraemia (increased plasma sodium levels)

Just as hyponatraemia is associated with fluid loss, hypernatraemia is accompanied by water retention. Hypernatraemia results from inadequate renal excretion. The main causes of hypernatraemia are:

- hypoproteinaemia (as in the nephrotic syndrome)
- primary heart failure
- inability to excrete salt and water due to glomerulonephritis

- certain drugs, e.g. corticosteroids, androgens, oral contraceptives
- hepatic cirrhosis.

Treatment of hypernatraemia

The treatment is based on a combination of measures. Underlying disease must be treated, e.g. heart failure by digoxin therapy and by administration of plasma proteins in glomerulonephritis. Restriction of dietary intake of salt and water is always required. Diuretics promote the excretion of salt and water, and are the most important drugs used in the treatment of hypernatraemia.

Diuretic therapy (see p. 80)

Alterations in potassium levels

Potassium depletion (hypokalaemia)

Lowered potassium levels occur due to an excessive loss of potassium from the body in the urine or from the gastrointestinal tract. Losses from the gastrointestinal tract result from acute or chronic diarrhoea. Loss from a fistula or gastric aspiration may also be significant.

Use of laxatives and diuretics may cause potassium depletion. It is important to take a full drug history to eliminate the possibility of laxative abuse.

Renal loss of potassium is due to a complex range of factors. Primary aldosteronism, Cushing's syndrome and corticosteroid therapy may be implicated. Metabolic or respiratory acidosis is associated with loss of potassium in the urine. Certain renal diseases can cause potassium loss in the urine. A poor diet may also result in mild potassium depletion.

The clinical features of potassium depletion (less than 3.5 mmol/litre) include apathy, weakness and mental disturbances. Polyuria and thirst may be seen, and cardiac arrhythmias may occur. Potassium depletion increases the sensitivity of cardiac tissue to digoxin and this may result in toxic reactions. Chloride depletion and metabolic alkalosis are often associated with hypokalaemia.

Table 13.4   Fluids used to correct hyponatraemia and other electrolyte deficiencies

Solution/strength	Content (mmol/litre)	Main indications/contraindications
Sodium bicarbonate intravenous infusion 4.2% w/v and 8.4%. Other strengths are available. The 1.26% w/v solution is used as a continuous infusion.	150 mmol each of Na^+ and HCO_3^- per litre.	Corrections of severe metabolic acidosis. May cause thrombophlebitis at site of infusion. This is a common problem with all long-term intravenous infusion sites.
Sodium chloride intravenous infusion 0.45% w/v (hypotonic), 0.9% w/v (isotonic). The term 'normal saline' should not be used as it could be confused with a chemically normal solution, which is much stronger.	75 mmol/litre Na^+, 75 mmol/litre Cl^-, 150 mmol/litre Na^+, 150 mmol/litre Cl^-.	To correct fluid balance and as a source of sodium and chloride. Must be used with care in patients with reduced ability to handle sodium (e.g. organic heart disease).
Sodium chloride and glucose intravenous infusions. Sterile solutions containing a range of combinations of sodium chloride and glucose are available, e.g. 0.18% w/v sodium chloride and 4% w/v glucose; 0.18% w/v sodium chloride and 10% w/v glucose; 0.9% w/v sodium chloride and 5% w/v glucose.		These solutions are a source of sodium, chloride, water and energy. As with all these intravenous infusions the choice of solution, rate of administration, and period of treatment depends on the condition being treated. Combinations of sodium chloride and glucose help to achieve rehydration of both the body cells and the extracellular space.
Compound sodium chloride intravenous infusion. Contains in each litre: sodium chloride 8.6 g, calcium chloride dihydrate 330 mg, potassium chloride 300 mg.	Sodium 147.5 mmol/litre, potassium 4 mmol/litre, calcium 2 mmol/litre, chloride 150 mmol/litre.	Source of water and electrolytes in cases of fluid and electrolyte depletion due to vomiting, diarrhoea, fistula drainage and diabetic acidosis. Prolonged administration may cause metabolic acidosis due to an excess of chloride ions.
Sodium lactate intravenous infusions. A number of different formulations containing sodium lactate are available.	Sodium lactate m/6 intravenous infusion contains: 167 mmol/litre sodium, 167 mmol/litre lactate. Compound sodium lactate intravenous infusion contains in mmol/litre: sodium 131, potassium 5, calcium 2, chloride 111, lactate 29.	Sodium lactate intravenous infusion m/6 has been used to correct metabolic acidosis and as a source of water and electrolytes. All lactate-containing solutions are contraindicated in patients with impairment of lactate utilisation. Also known as Hartmann's solution compound. Sodium lactate intravenous infusion is a source of water and electrolytes. It restores diminished alkali reserves by the slow conversion of lactate into bicarbonate. Sodium lactate infusions are not now advocated in metabolic acidosis owing to the risks of the patient developing lactic acidosis.
Potassium chloride and sodium chloride intravenous infusion: 0.15% potassium chloride, 0.9% sodium chloride. A wide range of strengths are available.		Fluid replacement and prevention treatment of potassium deficiency. Care must be taken to avoid cardiotoxicity.
Potassium chloride is also available in combination with glucose.		The indications are similar to potassium chloride and sodium chloride intravenous infusion. The glucose content provides a source of energy.
Darrow's intravenous infusion.	Sodium 121 mmol/litre, potassium 35 mmol/litre, chloride 103 mmol/litre, lactate 53 mmol/litre.	This solution is used to correct mild and moderate potassium deficiency. As with all potassium-containing solutions this infusion is contraindicated in renal disease and where lactate utilisation is impaired.

Treatment of potassium depletion (hypokalaemia) As with sodium replacement therapy, the oral route is preferred since it is less likely to cause hyperkalaemia. Potassium chloride is highly irritant to the gastric mucosa. A slow-release tablet formulation or soluble (effervescent) tablet or liquid preparation is often preferred. The dosage will depend on the extent of potassium depletion. A range of potassium-containing solutions is available for intravenous infusion. These are summarised in Table 13.4.

Potassium chloride is available as a concentrated solution for addition to infusion fluids. Great care must be taken with the dosage levels so as to reduce the risk of toxic hyperkalaemia. Wherever possible ready-prepared sterile solutions containing potassium should be used so as to avoid the possible hazards of adding strong potassium solutions (10% and 15%) to infusion fluids. All drug additives to infusion fluids must be carefully checked to avoid chemical incompatibility and care must be taken to ensure adequate mixing. Intravenous infusions of potassium-containing substances are best managed using an infusion pump with adequate controls.

Hyperkalaemia

The commonest cause of this potentially dangerous condition is severe oliguria or anuria. Acute renal failure results in hyperkalaemia. Diabetic ketoacidosis may cause hyperkalaemia. Consequences of hyperkalaemia include muscular weakness, abdominal distension and cardiac disturbances. Pulse irregularities are accompanied by heart block, and other irregularities of cardiac function. Hyperkalaemia is a serious condition because of the dangers of cardiac arrest. Levels of 7.5 mmol/litre are very dangerous.

Treatment of hyperkalaemia Glucose and insulin given together intravenously encourages migration of potassium into cells. The administration of alkali in the form of sodium bicarbonate isotonic solution may also be helpful. The cardiotoxicity of potassium may be reduced by the i.v. administration of calcium gluconate in the form of a 10% solution. Sodium and water deficits must also be corrected. Dietary restriction is necessary and the oral (or rectal) administration of an ion-exchange resin may be required.

The choice of the particular ion-exchange resin to use depends on the patient's condition. A sodium resin should not be used where there is hypernatraemia since the resin liberates sodium as potassium is taken up. Similarly a calcium resin must not be used where the patient's calcium levels are already too high.

If the above measures fail to control the hyperkalaemia, consideration must be given to peritoneal dialysis or haemodialysis.

Rehydration therapy

Oral

As previously stated, the oral route is always preferred when it is necessary to replace losses of both water and electrolytes. The BNF describes a wide range of preparations available for oral rehydration therapy (ORT). This approach to rehydration is especially important in countries where diarrhoea is a major health problem. Products available for ORT contain glucose (to enhance absorption of electrolytes) and the three main electrolytes: sodium, potassium and chloride. The choice and dose of formulation depend on the patient's age, severity of the condition and other factors. The WHO formulation has significant differences from the formulations normally used in the United Kingdom.

Parenteral

If the parenteral route (i.v.) has to be used, a wide range of solutions is available. Since dehydration is almost always accompanied by loss of electrolytes a fluid containing the necessary electrolytes, often in combination with glucose, will be selected. Where there is no significant loss of electrolytes a simple solution of glucose in water is used. Between 2 and 10 litres per day may be required to make good the deficit.

DRUG TREATMENT OF DISORDERS OF THE GENITOURINARY TRACT

Major disorders of the genitourinary tract

It is important to note that while drug treatment plays an important role in treating disorders of the genitourinary tract, a combination of treatment strategies may be required. Surgery and/or the use of various appliances may be required in addition to drug therapy. The skills of specialist nurses are becoming increasingly valued in the care of patients with urinary problems. Patients with the following conditions may derive benefit from drug therapy:

- enuresis and incontinence
- impotence
- infections (usually bacterial)
- malignancy
- pain
- urinary frequency
- urinary retention.

Products used following surgical procedures on the genitourinary tract and other irrigations are included for ease of reference (see Table 13.5).

Enuresis and incontinence (see also drugs used to treat urinary frequency)

Imipramine is used to treat nocturnal enuresis in children. A bedtime dose of 25–75 mg is given depending on the age and body weight of the child. Treatment should be for a period of 3 months, including gradual withdrawal as the condition is controlled. Further courses of treatment should not be undertaken without a full physical examination of the child.

Amitriptyline may also be used to treat nocturnal enuresis in children, the dose range being 20–50 mg, depending on the age and weight of the child.

Table 13.5 Sterile solutions used in bladder irrigation

Active ingredient	Strength (all percentages given are w/v)	Pack or presentation	Uses, indications and precautions
Amphotericin	100 µg/ml	50 mg vial (powder) made up before use into a solution.	Fungal infections
Chlorhexidine	1 in 5000 (0.02%)	100 ml 'Uro-Tainer' 500 ml bottle	Used for its mechanical effect. Also has a bacteriostatic action on organisms commonly found in the urinary tract. Inactive against *Pseudomonas* species.
Glycine	1.5%	3 l plastic bag	Used in transurethral resection of the prostate gland. Non-haemolytic, weakly ionised. Any glycine absorbed is metabolised, ammonia may be produced which has toxic effects. Cases of hyponatraemia have been reported, but these are rare.
Mandelic acid	1%	100 ml 'Uro-Tainer'	Used if resistance to chlorhexidine is encountered. Effective against *Pseudomonas* and *Proteus* species.
Sodium chloride	0.9%	A variety of presentations, e.g. 500 ml bottle or 3 l plastic bag.	Used for its mechanical effect. It is also used as a vehicle for certain drugs instilled into the bladder.
Sodium citrate	3%	500 ml bottle	Used primarily for the dissolution of blood clots.
Solution R	6% citric acid, 0.6% gluconolactone, 2.8% magnesium carbonate, 0.1% disodium edetate.	100 ml 'Uro-Tainer'	Used to dissolve existing encrustations. Use between twice and four times a week for 2 weeks, before reverting to Solution G. Should not be used for a period of 10–14 days following prostatic surgery due to absorption of salts leading to electrolyte imbalance.
Solution G (Suby G)	3.23% citric acid	100 ml 'Uro-Tainer'	Use between twice daily and twice weekly to prevent the formation of encrustations. Should not be used for a period of 10–14 days following prostatic surgery due to absorption of salts leading to electrolyte imbalance.
Streptokinase–Streptodornase	100 000 units streptokinase with streptodornase 25 000 units	Rubber-capped vial	Used to dissolve blood clots in bladder or urinary catheter. Must not be used where there is active haemorrhage or known sensitivity to the enzymes.

Desmopressin is an analogue of the natural antidiuretic hormone vasopressin. It is administered as a nasal spray in the treatment of nocturnal enuresis.

Impotence

The injection of papaverine into the corpus cavernosum has been found to be an effective treatment. The initial dose is 7.5 mg, increasing up to 60 mg. Phentolamine can be added if papaverine alone is inadequate. Careful physical examination must be undertaken before this treatment is initiated, since the side-effects are a cause of concern, especially in patients with cardiovascular disease.

Infections

Most infections of the genitourinary tract are treated with systemic antibiotics (see p. 170). In certain conditions local instillation of antimicrobial agents may be used. Table 13.5 shows the range of products available. Bladder instillations (irrigations or washouts) are of some value but risks of cross infection, poor antimicrobial action and local irritancy limit their use. Wherever possible systemic therapy, based on the results of microbial sensitivity tests, is preferable.

Malignancy

Instillation of locally acting cytotoxic drugs may be indicated in the treatment of superficial bladder tumours. Doxorubicin, epirubicin, mitomycin and thiotepa are used made up in sterile water or sodium chloride solution. Any evidence of absorption must be taken into account in selecting the 'dose' and period of treatment (see p. 228).

Pain

Pain in the urinary tract may be due to a number of conditions. The acute pain of ureteric colic is treated with pethidine or diclofenac (see p. 288). Lignocaine in the form of a 1% or 2% gel may be useful for urethral pain and prior to catheterisation. Discomfort caused by cystitis may be relieved by alkalisation of the urine using potassium citrate or sodium bicarbonate. Hyperkalaemia and hypernatraemia are possible side-effects of this treatment (see p. 215). Pain due to metabolites of the cytotoxic drug cyclophosphamide can be relieved using mesna (see p. 242).

Urinary frequency

Flavoxate is a selective urinary-tract antispasmodic. In an oral dose of 200 mg three times daily, it is used in the treatment of dysuria, urgency, nocturia and the incontinence that may result from cystitis and prostatitis. Side-effects include gastrointestinal problems, vertigo, tachycardia and palpitations. Since the drug is an antispasmodic it must be used with caution in patients with suspected glaucoma (see p. 296).

Flavoxate must not be used in patients with obstructive conditions of the gastrointestinal tract since the antispasmodic action would cause a worsening of the condition (see p. 50). Oxybutynin given orally is used to treat urinary frequency and incontinence in adults (up to 5 mg four times daily) and nocturnal enuresis in children over 7 years (up to 5 mg three times

Table 13.6 Parasympathomimetics used in the treatment of urinary retention

Drug	Dose/route	Notes/precautions/side-effects
Bethanechol	10–25 mg three or four times daily, orally, *before* food.	If given after food, nausea and vomiting may be caused. Avoid in asthmatic patients, and patients with gastrointestinal obstruction. Due to the effect on the eye, blurred vision may occur.
Carbachol	2 mg three times daily, orally, *before* food. May also be given by s.c. injection for post-operative urinary retention, in a dose of 250 μg.	Similar side-effects and precautions, but likely to be more accurate than with bethanechol. Carbachol (and bethanechol) must be used with great caution in older patients.

daily). Dosage levels must be carefully adjusted especially in the older patient. Side-effects are typical of drugs of this type as are the contra-indications.

Urinary retention

Given that the treatment of urinary frequency involves the use of antispasmodic (atropine-like) drugs it follows that the treatment of urinary retention is based on the use of parasympatho-mimetics for their muscarinic effects (see p. 50). Acute retention of urine requires catheterisation to relieve pain and reduce the likelihood of infection and renal damage. Parasympathomimetics used include carbachol and bethanechol. (see Table 13.6). These drugs have potentially dangerous side-effects such as bradycardia and intestinal colic. Patients with asthma or susceptibility to asthmatic attacks must not be treated with parasympathomimetic drugs owing to the danger of precipitating an acute episode of bronchoconstriction.

Another parasympathomimetic is distigmine which is given orally (5 mg half an hour before breakfast) or by i.m. injection 500 µg 12 hours after surgery to prevent urinary retention. This drug acts by inhibiting the breakdown of acetylcholine (see p. 48) (anticholinesterase). Distigmine is a long-acting drug and should be used with care, especially after surgery, particularly where bowel anastomosis has been carried out.

14

Drug treatment of malignant disease

INTRODUCTION

In spite of the fact that survival rates for many cancers have considerably improved over the past decades, malignant disease remains a major cause of morbidity and mortality. Cancer has existed for thousands of years. It can occur in infants but is more commonly associated with increasing age. Certain cancers show an increased incidence in lower socio-economic groups and different cancers can affect different populations. Cancer is not one disease; indeed, over 100 different cancers have been identified.

CAUSATION

There is no known single cause of cancer, although a number of predisposing factors have been incriminated.

These include:

- chemical factors, e.g. tars in tobacco, asbestos
- physical factors, e.g. sunlight, radiation, chronic trauma/infection
- viruses, e.g. herpes simplex virus
- genetic factors, e.g. increased incidence in Down's syndrome; Philadelphia chromosome found in chronic myelocytic leukaemia
- familial factors, e.g. polyposis coli in families leading to colonic cancer
- geographical factors, e.g. Japanese women who go to the USA to live go from a low risk of developing breast cancer to high risk and have as great a chance of developing it as American women; bowel cancer is almost

Table 14.1 Classification of tumours according to tissue of origin

Tissue of origin	Type of tumour
Epithelial tissue	Carcinoma, e.g. of breast, of lung
Connective tissue	Sarcoma, e.g. of bone, of muscle
Lymphatic tissue	Malignant lymphoma, e.g. Hodgkin's disease, non-Hodgkin's lymphoma
Bone marrow	Leukaemia, e.g. myeloblastic leukaemia
Pigment cells	Malignant melanoma

unknown on the African continent, probably due to dietary factors.

CLASSIFICATION OF CANCERS

Cancers may be classified in different ways. They may be considered as solid tumours, e.g. lung, liver, or 'liquid' tumours, i.e. of the blood or lymph. Alternatively, they may be classified according to their tissue of origin (Table 14.1).

SPREAD OF CANCER

Cancer spreads either by direct infiltration of adjacent tissues or by cells from the primary tumour being transported to another often distant site (or sites) in the body where they settle down and grow. These secondary deposits are known as metastases. The pathways taken by the metastasising cells include the lymphatic system, the blood, serous cavities and CSF pathways. Different primary tumours tend to show preference for particular secondary sites – see, for example, Box 14.1.

Box 14.1 Spread of some primary tumours

bronchus	→	brain
breast	→	bone
testis	→	lung
colon	→	liver

Some patients develop a second primary tumour.

PRESENTATION

A malignancy may be an incidental finding when some other condition is being investigated or at a routine check. It otherwise presents in many different ways ranging from bleeding, swelling and loss of function to anaemia and general malaise depending on the type of tumour and its location.

DIAGNOSIS

The diagnosis of cancer is arrived at through careful history-taking, physical examination, cytological and pathological examination, radiological examination, and ultrasonic and radioisotope scanning.

TREATMENT

Treatment mainly takes the form of surgery, radiotherapy or chemotherapy or any combination of these. Increasingly a multi-modal approach is taken. Much will depend on the stage the cancer has reached, the condition and wishes of the patient, and the sensitivity of the tumour.

CELL BIOLOGY

In order to appreciate how cancer chemotherapy affects cellular function, it is necessary to have a basic understanding of cell biology. Present in the nucleus of every cell is deoxyribonucleic acid (DNA) which provides the blueprint or template for the chromosomes which carry our genetic characteristics in the form of genes. Also in the nucleus is another acid, ribonucleic acid (RNA) which transmits genetic instructions from the nucleus to the cytoplasm. A cell is stimulated to reproduce in response to the death of another cell. It does this by means of the cell cycle.

Cell cycle

The cell cycle is a continuous process during which some cells are replicating while others are

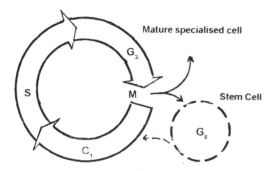

Figure 14.1   Cell life-cycle.

resting. The cycle comprises four discrete phases of activity resulting in the production of two identical daughter cells (Fig. 14.1).

G_1 = RNA synthesis occurs in preparation for DNA synthesis

S = DNA synthesis occurs in preparation for supplying two new cells

G_2 = RNA synthesis occurs in preparation for cell division

·M = Cell mitosis occurs, i.e. production of two new cells

G_0 = Resting phase

The synthesis (S) and mitosis (M) phases are the main points of activity. The G_1 and G_2 phases occupy the gaps between these phases and allow nutrients to be gathered in to supply energy for the immediately following S and M phases respectively.

Once the two new cells have been formed, one will mature and differentiate to become a specialised cell while the other remains a stem cell which will go into a resting (only from replication) phase known as the G_0 phase. There it will remain until it is stimulated to undergo cell division.

Some cells therefore are 'cycling' and some are resting. Of those 'cycling', at any point in time the cells of any given tissue may be at any stage of the cycle. The time taken for the completion of the cycle varies, depending on the type of tissue. Although malignant cells replicate in exactly the same way as normal cells their cell cycle time is often shorter.

CHARACTERISTICS OF CANCER

Cancer is a problem of abnormal cell growth resulting from an interaction between the causal factor and DNA in a normal cell. The result is that normal control mechanisms are lost and the cancer cells reproduce uncontrollably, invading the surrounding tissues eventually metastasising to sites distant from the primary tumour.

Malignant cells are therefore not new cells. They are just an alteration of existing cells – a change which may have taken place as many as 15 years previously as the result of some insult or combination of effects on the body. The malignant cell behaves in a delinquent way, with no respect for the normal patterns of cell differentiation, growth and control. It is a parasite to the body and as such harms the host, ultimately leading to death if untreated.

CANCER CHEMOTHERAPY

Cancer chemotherapy is directed towards controlling abnormal cell growth and reducing the number of actively dividing cells. Cytotoxic drugs are used to kill cancer cells but they kill healthy cells as well. All cells, whether they are normal or malignant, are in different stages of the cell cycle at any time or they may be resting (G_0 phase). Chemotherapy drugs are described as being either phase-specific, i.e. they are more powerful, acting in one specific phase of the cycle, or cycle-specific, i.e. they work equally well killing cells in any or all phases of the cycle. Chemotherapy drugs will not kill cells in the G_0 phase. They are also more effective when the number of cancer cells is small. It is for this reason that chemotherapy is used as adjuvant therapy, i.e. following surgery and/or radiotherapy. High individual doses of chemotherapy will kill a high percentage of cancer cells. Although healthy cells will be destroyed they will repair themselves quickly and regrow to normal numbers far more quickly than cancer cells following chemotherapy (Fig. 14.2). Intervals between doses are needed to allow normal cells to recover. Repeat doses at intervals are needed to kill those cells which were in the

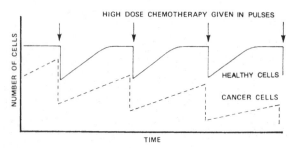

Figure 14.2   Effect of chemotherapy on normal and cancer cells.

resting phase and therefore protected from chemotherapy. By combining different chemotherapy drugs, e.g. in some cases using four drugs together, remission rates in many situations are hugely increased. Cancer chemotherapy is therefore at its most effective when used:

- where the tumour is small, has been surgically removed or reduced in size with radiotherapy
- in high doses
- intermittently
- in conjunction with other cytotoxic drugs.

The timing of each pulse of treatment is critical for achieving success in eradicating the malignant cells. However, it must always be borne in mind that the patient's normal cells, especially the rapidly dividing ones, are also being damaged. To ensure that the patient can withstand the treatment, regular haematological monitoring is essential. The tissues that are most chemosensitive are the:

- bone marrow
- epithelial lining of the gastrointestinal tract
- skin and hair
- ovaries and testes.

ROUTES OF ADMINISTRATION
Oral

Although cytotoxic drug therapy is very often given parenterally, there are nevertheless quite a number of oral cytotoxic preparations. These formulations are no less toxic in tablet or capsule form and the same attention to care in their administration is required. Where nausea and vomiting are known side-effects an anti-emetic may need to be given in advance. Patients who are to take cytotoxic drugs while at home should be given clear written instructions in their use.

Subcutaneous and intramuscular

Because of the risk of damage to the tissues, only a few cytotoxic drugs are administered by these routes. Care should be taken to select an area with adequate subcutaneous/muscle tissue and to give the injection with a fresh needle of the smallest possible calibre.

Intravenous

Absorption is more reliable by the intravenous route and, hence, it is the one most commonly used. Drugs with vesicant properties must always be given intravenously. The need for strict asepsis is even greater than normal since many chemotherapy patients will have some degree of immunosuppression.

A central venous catheter (e.g. Hickman catheter) may be used to provide long-term access to the patient's circulatory system, thus obviating the need for repeated venepuncture and injections. Under general anaesthetic, an incision is made just below the right clavicle and the cephalic vein isolated. A skin tunnel is then formed starting at a point between the nipple and the sternum. The catheter is drawn through the tunnel under X-ray control and inserted into the subclavian vein before reaching the cephalic vein and the superior vena cava where it is positioned at the entrance to the right atrium. Both veins are sutured. A Dacron cuff plugs the tunnel in the subcutaneous tissues which gradually become fibrosed, thus reducing the risk of ascending infection from the catheter exit point. A dressing is applied and a cap placed on the protruding end. The patient and/or his family are taught to heparinise the line every second day to keep it patent. A daily shower or bath is encouraged. The patient should be encouraged to report any signs of discharge, pain or redness round the catheter or any movement of the catheter. The wound should be dressed and the cap renewed on a weekly basis and a bacterial swab taken if indicated.

CYTOTOXIC DRUG GROUPS

Cytotoxic drugs fall into four main categories (i) alkylating agents, (ii) antimetabolites, (iii) cytotoxic antibiotics and (iv) vinca alkaloids.

Alkylating agents

- Phase-specific (M phase)
- Cause breaks in and cross-linking of the strands of DNA, resulting in inhibition of or inaccurate replication and finally cell death

Examples of alkylating agents include busulphan, carmustine, chlorambucil, cyclophosphamide, estramustine, ifosfamide, lomustine and melphalan.

Antimetabolites

- Cycle-specific.
- Substances which substitute for or compete with intracellular metabolites and become incorporated into the nucleic acids, DNA and RNA, preventing DNA synthesis and leading to cell death.

Examples of antimetabolites include cytarabine, fluorouracil, mercaptopurine, methotrexate and thioguanine.

Cytotoxic antibiotics

- Phase-specific (S phase).
- Act by binding to the DNA helix, inhibiting its synthesis and replication, and disrupting RNA synthesis.

Examples of cytotoxic antibiotics include aclarubicin, bleomycin, dactinomycin, doxorubicin, epirubicin, idarubicin and mitomycin.

Vinca alkaloids

- Phase-specific (M phase).
- Bind to the microtubular proteins which are needed for formation of the mitotic spindle. Because the cell is unable to divide, it dies.

Examples of vinca alkaloids include vinblastine, vincristine and vindesine.

KEY ELEMENTS OF THE TREATMENT OF MALIGNANT DISEASE WITH CYTOTOXIC DRUGS

The treatment of malignant disease with cytotoxic drugs presents many challenges for clinicians, nurses and pharmacists. In order to achieve the best outcome for the patient, and protect the staff involved, it is vitally important that all those involved in providing anti-cancer treatment work together within the following framework.

- The importance of discussing the full implications of the treatment with the patient and/or the patient's relatives cannot be overstated.
- Only clinicians having specialised experience and access to full back-up laboratory and other services should initiate and control cytotoxic therapy.
- Where treatment is provided on a shared-care basis with the patient's GP, communications and flow of information must be well managed and clearly understood by all involved.
- All personnel involved in providing the drug therapy must observe the regulations designed to prevent chronic exposure to cytotoxic drugs. These regulations are intended to minimise the risk to handlers of cytotoxic drugs from the known hazards, e.g. teratogenicity.
- Particular attention must be paid to all aspects of drug management such as drug selection, dosage determination, calculation, prescribing, presentation of the drug, route of administration and timing of the

administration of individual doses within a course of therapy.

- Every effort must be made to reduce the impact on the patient of forseeable adverse effects of the therapy.

DRUG MANAGEMENT IN CYTOTOXIC DRUG THERAPY

The general principles of drug management are discussed in detail in Chapter 26. However, in view of the special importance of drug management in cytotoxic drug therapy the following additional guidance is offered. All the factors listed are not of equal 'weight' but nevertheless must be given full consideration in patients' particular circumstances. Factors in drug selection include:

- condition being treated, stages of disease and prognosis
- regime to be followed–single or combination therapy
- cost-benefits of the therapy
- back-up resources available locally
- general condition of the patient–any previous exposure to cytotoxic drugs and/or radiotherapy
- current 'state of the art'
- any co-existing condition that could affect treatment and/or cause complications for the patient
- reproductive status of the patient
- possibility of drug interactions

Dose determination

Many factors are involved in dosage determination, and it is the responsibility of the clinician to take all factors into account in arriving at the actual dosage and frequency of administration. All the above factors will be considered along with the following:

- patient's age, sex, body weight and other physical parameters, e.g. body surface area
- full haematological 'picture'
- renal and hepatic function
- neurological status
- pharmacokinetics of the drug

Doses are determined according to generally well-defined regimes, being modified according to the factors outlined above. The main approaches are based on two parameters, body weight and surface area.

Dosage determination based on body weight

Many examples are given in the following pages. To take just one example – melphalan – the dosage range in multiple myeloma is 150–300 µg per kg body weight daily, by mouth, for 4–6 days. The course is repeated after 4–8 weeks. Given that the patient has some degree of renal impairment, it may be decided to begin the course of therapy at the lower end of the dosage range. Blood counts will enable the effect of this dose to be monitored.

For a patient of body weight 68 kg the dose would be 150×68 µg per day for, say, 5 days: i.e. 10 200 µg, i.e. 10 200/1000 mg $\simeq$ 10 mg.

The number of 5 mg tablets to be administered each day is $10/5 = 2$ tablets per day.

It is important to realise that the patient's 'true' body weight must be taken into account. In a patient suffering from fluid retention or obesity the actual weight on the scales should be treated with some caution since this is not generally a good indication of the patient's ability to metabolise the drug. Reference to standard height/ weight tables may be required. The main factor to take into account is the patient's lean body mass.

Dosage determination based on body surface area (BSA)

This parameter is felt to be a more accurate indicator of the patient's ability to 'handle' the drug than body weight. The patient's surface area is derived from tables. Given the patient's height (in cm) and body weight (in kg) the patient's body surface area can be determined from a nomogram (Fig. 14.3). Nomograms are available for both adults and children.

Body surface area for a man, height 175 cm and weighing 80 kg, is obtained by joining the height column with a line to the weight column.

Nomogram for determination of body surface from height and mass¹

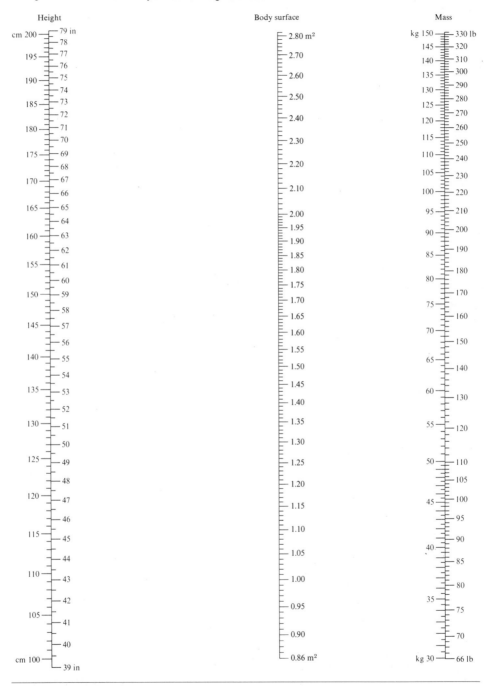

¹ From the formula of Du Bois and Du Bois, *Arch. intern. Med.*, **17**, 863 (1916): $S = M^{0.425} \times H^{0.725} \times 71.84$, or $\log S = \log M \times 0.425 + \log H \times 0.725 + 1.8564$ (S: body surface in cm², M: mass in kg, H: height in cm).

Figure 14.3 Nomogram (adult).

CYTOTOXIC MEDICINES PRESCRIPTION SHEET

REGULAR MEDICINES

DATE PRESC.	MEDICINES (Block Letters)	DOSE	ROUTE OF ADMIN.	TIMES OF ADMINISTRATION 6am 8am 10am 12md 2pm 6pm 10pm 12mn	DURATION OF THERAPY IN DAYS	PRESCRIBED BY	FOR PHARMACY USE
							DISCONTINUED DATE / INITIALS / AMOUNT DISPENSED / DISPENSED DATE / INITIALS
R							
S							
T							
U							
V							
W							
X							
Y							
Z							

REPEAT MEDICINES

DATE	MEDICINES (Block Letters)	ROUTE	PRESCRIBED BY	DATE	DOSE	TIME OF ADMIN.	GIVEN BY	DATE	DOSE	TIME OF ADMIN.	GIVEN BY	DATE	DOSE	TIME OF ADMIN.	GIVEN BY

ONCE ONLY MEDICINES

DATE	MEDICINES (Block Letters)	DOSE	ROUTE	TIME OF ADMIN. ✱	PRESCRIBED BY	GIVEN BY	TIME IF DIFF. ✱	COMMENTS

WARD	HOSPITAL	SURNAME	FORENAME	AGE	UNIT NUMBER	CONSULTANT	KNOWN DRUG/MEDICINE SENSITIVITY

DATE	HT.	WT.	SURFACE AREA

DATE	WBC	Hb	PLATELETS

1

2

Figure 14.4 Cytotoxic medicines prescription sheet. **A.** Front.

CYTOTOXIC MEDICINES PRESCRIPTION SHEET

REGULAR MEDICINES FOR OUT-PATIENTS

DATE	MEDICINES (Block Letters)	DOSE	ROUTE OF ADMIN.	TIMES OF ADMINISTRATION 6am 8am 10am 12md 2pm 6pm 10pm 12mn	DURATION OF THERAPY IN DAYS	PRESCRIBED BY	DISCONTINUED DATE	INITIALS	FOR PHARMACY USE AMOUNT DISPENSED	DISPENSED DATE	INITIALS

WARD	HOSPITAL	SURNAME	FORENAME	AGE	UNIT NUMBER	CONSULTANT	KNOWN DRUG/MEDICINE SENSITIVITY
							1 2

Figure 14.4 B Reverse.

Where the line crosses the BSA line indicates the surface area, which is 1.95 m².

Example: A dose of cisplatin as a single agent is 50–120 mg/m² as a single intravenous dose. The dose for a patient with a body surface area of 1.95 m² using a dose of 100 mg/m² would therefore be 1.95 × 100 mg = 195 mg. A further calculation would be needed to obtain this quantity from the vials available.

Prescribing

Prescribing cytotoxic drug therapy is more complex than the prescribing of more routine therapy. Great care must be taken to ensure that all the personnel involved in the management of the patient have all the necessary information. Special prescription forms have been developed since it is not possible to provide all the necessary information on the standard format (Fig. 14.4).

The special prescription sheet provides the opportunity to indicate the exact timing of the intervals of administration of the drug(s).

Presentation

In view of the well recognised hazards of manipulating cytotoxic drugs it is essential to ensure that the drugs are prepared for use in a specially designated area within the pharmacy. This helps to ensure protection of staff, accuracy of compounding/reconstitution, and best presentation in a ready-to-use form, preferably in a syringe fully labelled with all the necessary details. Particular care is required in the labelling of the vinca alkaloid drugs which must carry a warning that the drug is not for intrathecal use (see p. 428). The Data Sheet Compendium gives a quite specific instruction on this matter.

Administration

Very careful attention must be paid to the route of administration. While the use of an inappropriate route of administration is always potentially hazardous, the consequences of using an incorrect route of administration for cytotoxic drugs can be catastrophic. Most cytotoxic drugs are highly irritant to the tissues and, if extravasation occurs, local tissue damage and/or necrosis can occur. Most parenteral cytotoxic drugs are given intravenously either as a bolus into a freely running solution, or as an infusion. As with all parenteral administration the diluent used must be selected carefully and all expiry dates and storage instructions of reconstituted solutions observed. It is also important to ensure that the time taken to inject or infuse the drug is in accordance with defined practice.

SAFE MANAGEMENT OF CYTOTOXIC DRUGS

The widespread use of cancer chemotherapeutic agents has led to an increased number of employees being exposed to contamination by them. The dangers which may be encountered fall into two categories. Certain cytotoxic drugs produce a local irritant effect causing immediate damage to the skin and eyes. Others are in addition known to be mutagenic, carcinogenic and teratogenic agents. These long-term consequences resulting from absorption of substances via the skin, the lungs or the gastrointestinal tract warrant energetic implementation of policies by health authorities to reduce to the minimum, risks to their staff.

Personnel

Doctors, nurses and pharmacists involved in the handling of cytotoxic drugs should be instructed in the dangers, precautions, and techniques of their preparation and administration. Training may be given by a suitably experienced senior member of medical, nursing or pharmacy staff and *only* those so trained should be responsible for the handling of these drugs. All personnel involved in the handling of cytotoxic drugs should be familiar with the written guidelines on the handling of cytotoxic drugs and be given a personal copy. A departmental register of those staff involved in such procedures should be maintained. In the event of an accident involving cytotoxic drugs, staff must report to their Head of Department. Such measures comply with the Code of Practice for COSHH Regulations.

Members of staff of childbearing potential should not be involved in reconstituting parenteral cytotoxic drugs. These people are however not at risk if they are only involved in the administration of cytotoxic drugs provided that they adhere to the guidelines. While taking precautionary measures to protect staff from the hazards of cytotoxic drugs is of the utmost importance, in so doing care should be taken to avoid increasing apprehension among patients.

Location for reconstituting cytotoxic drugs

Ideally, the preparation of cytotoxic drugs should take place within the pharmacy department where a limited number of personnel working in this field are involved. In any event, all manipulations involving cytotoxic drugs should be undertaken only in areas specifically designated by local policy for the purpose. Such areas should be placed centrally as in a sideroom within an oncology ward or department. Wherever possible, operator protection during reconstitution of the drugs should be provided by a laminar-flow biological safety cabinet. This device creates constant recirculation of air and removes contaminants through its filters to produce clean conditions in a contained environment. When this facility is not available, the locally designated area must be one that is away from normal ward traffic and food areas. The windows and door should be kept closed but at the same time the room should be well ventilated. These areas should be equipped with a work top which has an impervious surface and intact edges. A sink and running water should be available in the room. A ready filled eye irrigation container should be available. Work should not be done at a position where draughts, mechanical ventilation or the air-conditioning system might convey aerosols or dusts to another occupied area. Drugs should be reconstituted over a foil tray to contain any spillage.

Protection against occupational exposure

Protection against exposure to cytotoxic drugs (or their metabolites) must be available for and utilised by all staff involved in the preparation of cytotoxic drugs. Protective clothing must be of the correct specification to ensure adequate protection of the skin and eyes, and to prevent inhalation of aerosolised drug particles. It should consist of:

- gown, trouser suit or white coat; these should have long sleeves – otherwise, disposable sleeves must be worn
- plastic apron; this should be worn in addition to the items mentioned above
- gloves; these should be latex rubber, disposable except when preparing mustine injections for which PVC gloves are required; they should provide a close fit with the sleeves; for long procedures, two pairs of gloves should be worn and should be changed every hour; gloves should be changed following spillage
- safety glasses; it is advisable to wear protective glasses or goggles complying with BS2092C which provide all-round protection, whether or not ordinary spectacles are worn; these should be washed thoroughly in soap and water after use
- face mask; in wards and clinical areas, a good-quality disposable surgical mask should be worn.

Every effort should be made to reduce aerosolisation. Ampoules, including those containing diluents, should be opened with care using a file if necessary and plastic ampoule breaker to avoid cuts and scratches. They should be held away from the face when being opened or drawn up from. Care should be taken when adding diluent to allow it to run slowly down the side of the ampoule. The exact volume of drug required should be drawn into a syringe and the remainder discarded or used immediately for another patient. Air from the syringe should be expelled into the empty ampoule over sterile cotton wool or a gauze swab. The guard should

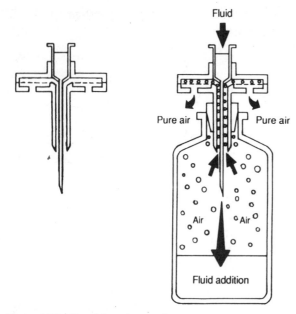

Figure 14.5 Special venting needle.

be placed over the needle before the final expulsion of air bubbles.

Drugs in powder form must be reconstituted with particular care as they may be released as a fine spray through the needle hole if excess pressure is produced in the vial. This may be avoided by removing an appropriate amount of air from the vial before injecting the diluting fluid or by the use of a special venting needle (Fig. 14.5).

Filled syringes should be suitably labelled and placed in a receiver ready for use. They should also carry a biohazard or cytotoxic drug warning label.

Disposal of surplus drugs and contaminated equipment

The use of disposable equipment is recommended whenever possible. Items of waste should be disposed of as follows:

- unused solution: seal ampoule or vial in a polythene bag and place bag in needleproof, leakproof disposable bin, e.g. Cinbin

- syringes, needles, empty ampoules, intermittent infusion sets: place in rigid disposable bin
- masks, gloves, apron, foil trays, towels, swabs: seal in polythene bag and place in yellow incinerator bag.

All these items are incinerated at 1000°C.

Safety glasses should be washed thoroughly in soap and water, dried and hung up. The hands must be thoroughly washed on completion of any procedure involving cytotoxic drugs. Time-expired cytotoxic drugs should be returned to pharmacy for disposal.

Parenteral administration of cytotoxic drugs

An assessment of the patient and a peripheral blood count are carried out prior to the administration of cytotoxic drugs to ensure that the patient is fit to withstand the treatment. Monitoring is also essential throughout the course of treatment. The patient's weight and height are measured in order to calculate the precise dose of drug(s) to be given.

All cytotoxic drugs must be prescribed by a doctor and the dosage agreed after consultation with a senior member of the medical staff. The calculation of the dose, volume and concentration should be checked and recorded.

Each syringe should be clearly labelled with the name and dose of the drug. The used vial or ampoule should be placed with the loaded syringe(s) in a receiver bearing the patient's name and/or prescription to allow a final check to be made.

Prior to administration of the drug, the prescription should be compared with the patient's name, the labelled syringes and the used ampoules/vials. When the person administering the drug is the one who prepared it, a check should be made by a second qualified person and recorded appropriately. For intramuscular and subcutaneous injections, two nurses must be involved, one of whom is registered and the checking procedure followed in the standard way.

Risks of contamination are still present during administration and therefore precautions should be continued. Protective clothing should be worn, although if there is a likelihood of the patient being unduly alarmed by the donor's 'spaceman image' some modification may have to be made. For example, protective goggles and face masks may have to be removed before taking the drugs to the patient. Close-fitting gloves, however, must be worn.

The area round the injection site should be protected by an absorbent, disposable towel. A 'butterfly' needle is convenient when drugs which require a dilution intravenous infusion are being given. If there is any doubt about the siting of the needle, whether for infusion or direct bolus administration, the procedure should be abandoned and begun elsewhere.

Once an infusion of cytotoxic drugs has been established, responsibility rests with the nurse to observe the patient and provide him with continuing physical and emotional support. The point of entry of the needle into the vein should be observed frequently and any comments from the patient about the comfort of the area heeded. Leakage of the drug into the surrounding tissues, known as extravasation, may have disastrous consequences because of its irritant nature. Any evidence of pain, burning or stinging at the injection site calls for an immediate assessment of the site. The doctor should be called at once and the infusion stopped. A ready-prepared pack for the first aid treatment of extravasation should be brought. The doctor will aspirate with the needle in place as much of the infiltrated drug as possible. Thereafter, frequent checking of the site will be required with careful documenting of progress until resolution occurs. Cytotoxic drugs which are known to be particularly damaging on extravasation are given in Box 14.2.

Vomitus, urine and faeces from treated patients may contain unchanged drug or active metabolites; therefore, skin contact should be avoided by wearing latex gloves, a face mask and a long-sleeved gown when disposing of excreta. Disposable utensils should always be used and care taken when placing them in the waste-disposal unit to avoid splashing the contents. Heavily soiled linen of patients receiving cytotoxic drugs should be dealt with as infected linen. It is the responsibility of the nurse in charge of the ward to advise all members of the nursing staff of those patients for whom these precautions must be taken.

Box 14.2   Cytotoxic drugs which are particularly damaging on extravasation

carmustine	epirubicin	mustine
dacarbazine	etoposide	plicamycin
dactinomycin	idarubicin	vinblastine
daunorubicin	melphalan	vincristine
doxorubicin	mitomycin C	vindesine

Procedure in the event of an accident

Spillage of a cytotoxic drug onto intact skin

If any cytotoxic drug apart from dacarbazine (DTIC) and melphalan (Alkeran) comes into contact with the skin, the affected area should be flushed with copious amounts of water.

If dacarbazine is spilled onto the skin, it should be washed off immediately with soap and water. In the case of melphalan, the contaminated skin should be treated with a *fresh* solution of sodium carbonate 3% w/v.

After skin contamination with methotrexate, if transient stinging occurs following washing with water, a bland cream, e.g. aqueous cream BP, should be applied to the affected area.

Spillage of a cytotoxic drug onto broken skin, into eyes or through needle penetration of the skin

If accidents involve cuts or needle penetration of the skin, the area should be washed with copious amounts of water.

If any cytotoxic drug enters the eye(s), the eye(s) should be irrigated thoroughly with sterile normal saline.

In all such cases, the doctor and person in charge of the ward, department or clinic should be notified. The normal accident reporting procedure should then be followed and a copy of the accident form sent to the Occupational Health Department.

Oral administration of cytotoxic drugs

Oral solid-dose forms of cytotoxic drugs constitute no risk to the handler if a few simple precautions are taken. If the patient has difficulty swallowing such preparations, advice should be sought from the pharmacy where crushing of tablets or preparation of an alternative formulation can be carried out safely. No attempt should be made to break coated tablets, crush a compressed tablet or open capsules. All tablets and capsules should be dispensed and administered using a non-touch technique, if necessary wearing disposable gloves. Disposable spoons and medicine measures should be used. A stainless steel triangle should be used when tablets require to be counted. It should be washed after use. In the event of contamination by free powder or the contents of a capsule, the same principles for dealing with spillage of parenteral drugs apply. To prevent inhalation of powder, it is essential to use a well-fitting face mask. For mopping up spilled powder, the disposable towel used should first be made damp. Disposal is by incineration.

Conclusion

Without causing unnecessary alarm among staff or patients, a respect for cytotoxic drugs should be engendered in much the same way as is required for radioactive materials. Provided that staff make themselves fully conversant with the guidelines laid down on the safe handling of these drugs and are seen to incorporate the practical measures into their day-to-day work, protection for the user, the patient and all other personnel working near treatment areas should be guaranteed.

THE ROLE OF THE NURSE IN CANCER CHEMOTHERAPY

Nowhere in drug management is the nurse required to be more vigilant than in the care of the patient receiving cytotoxic drug therapy. She must also have a clear grasp of the principles of cytotoxic drug therapy and the likely effects the main drug groups will have on the patient. In this way she will know how to advise the patient, what to look out for and what action to take if required. She must act calmly, be available at those times when she is most required by the patient and take on the roles of teacher and counsellor. Extreme care is required in correctly identifying the patient and maintaining accurate records.

Assessment of the patient

A full nursing assessment should be carried out since the relationship between the nurse and the chemotherapy patient may last a considerable length of time. Special attention should be paid to the patient's understanding of the treatment planned for him, his attitude towards the treatment and his thoughts about the longer term. Measurements of weight and height are taken for use in calculating cytotoxic drug dosages. A bone marrow aspiration or trephine biopsy will be carried out at intervals in patients with acute leukaemia or with multiple myeloma and call for particular support from the nurse.

With each pulse of treatment and at the start of a new course, there must be a willingness to reassess the patient's condition, checking up on the development of infection or any other new symptoms of note. A review of the patient's psychological condition is equally important.

Support and encouragement

Patients require a careful explanation of their course of chemotherapy, how it is to be given, how it will work and what effects it is likely to have. The challenge for the nurse is to pitch the information at a level the individual patient can cope with. The patient should be gently told that he is to receive powerful drugs which may make him feel less well before he starts to get better again. He should be discouraged from comparing himself with neighbouring patients as no two patients react in an identical way. Realistic goals should be set in consultation with the patient. For example, the patient may be very anxious to continue working as much as possible throughout the treatment and this may demand some degree of flexibility on both sides. Patients often need to have information repeated partly because they have a lot to assimilate and partly because they need the reassurance that treatment is progressing. They need to be reassured that someone will listen to their anxieties. Wherever possible, there should be continuity of nursing staff to ease communication and so that the patient can build up a feeling of trust.

Patients spend a lot of time waiting. Most patients, resigned to the fact that they need treatment, just want to get on with it. Waiting for blood results can be tedious. In some cases the treatment may have to be temporarily stopped because the white count is too low and this news can be received with disappointment and even anger. The nurse must allow for such reactions and provide the necessary encouragement for both the patient and his family.

The chemotherapy patient has a lot to contend with. He may still be coming to terms with his diagnosis at the same time as trying to cope with treatment. He may also be trying to protect his family from the full impact of his condition and the treatment. Although he may be attending as an out-patient he may not be feeling very well. There may be issues that he wants to discuss only with his carers in the expectation that they will understand. The ward or clinic becomes something of a 'haven' for him where, for example, hair loss and vomiting are accepted. Time must be found for the patient who needs to talk. As an active listener the nurse can gain much valuable information while at the same time help the patient to off-load. Keeping a special record of how the patient is feeling about his progress can be extremely helpful to all members of the health care team.

Management of side-effects

The commonest adverse effects of cytotoxic drugs fall into four main categories:

- bone marrow suppression
- damage to the gastrointestinal mucosa
- damage to the skin and hair
- altered sexuality and fertility.

These effects reflect the areas of the body where normal cell turnover is greatest. *The severity of side-effects will depend on the drug(s) used and the dose given.*

Bone marrow suppression

Lowered resistance to infection

Immunity to infection is provided by the white blood cells. Because of their very rapid rate of turnover, the white blood cells are the ones most readily damaged by cytotoxic drugs. As treatment progresses and the white count falls, the patient's ability to combat infection lessens. Frequent monitoring of the white cell count assists the clinician in deciding whether the patient has sufficient white cells to withstand the next dose of treatment and still combat an infective attack. A white blood count of less than 5×10^9 litre significantly increases the risk of infection. Care is directed to minimising the risk of infection. Chemotherapy is likely to be withheld when the leucocyte count is less than 4×10^9/litre.

Decisions sometimes have to be made as to where and how best to nurse in-patients receiving cytotoxic therapy. In the early stages of treating acute leukaemia, for example, when the white count is still at a reasonable level, the patient may be nursed alongside other patients and indeed this may be important to maintain his morale. As treatment progresses, increasing levels of protection may be necessary. A single room, a laminar air flow unit and protective isolation nursing measures may have to be introduced depending on the white cell count.

Staff caring for an immunosuppressed patient should be free from colds and sore throats, and must not be involved if they have been in contact with viruses such as measles or chickenpox. Personal hygiene must be of the highest standard, especially hand hygiene. A strictly aseptic technique must be employed while carrying out invasive procedures.

Recordings of the patient's temperature and pulse should be taken at least every 4 hours. Even a low-grade pyrexia must be reported. Regular inspection of the body for evidence of infection is essential. The commonest sites of local infection are the mouth, axillae, groins and perineum. Infections of lungs, gut and urinary tract produce signs and symptoms with which the nurse should be familiar. Observing, recording, reporting, taking laboratory samples and administering prescribed antibiotics are standard procedures. Fresh blood or a white cell transfusion may be ordered. Nursing care is directed towards keeping infection to an absolute minimum. An overwhelming infection can have fatal consequences.

Increased risk of bleeding

Platelets (thrombocytes) are essential for blood clotting. When the platelet level falls below 20×10^9/litre, the risk of spontaneous bleeding is significant. Although the patient's platelet count will be estimated at frequent intervals, it is also important for the nurse to observe for any signs of bleeding. This may range from overt bleeding, such as from an intravenous injection site or menorrhagia, to tiny petechial haemorrhages in the mouth or skin. More sinister is internal bleeding such as a subarachnoid haemorrhage or splenic bleed which may have fatal consequences. As a safeguard, chemotherapy is withheld when the platelet count falls below 100×10^9/litre.

Efforts must also be made to reduce the risk of bleeding. Injections should be kept to a minimum and restricted to the intravenous route. The risk of bleeding into a large and highly vascular area such as the buttock make intramuscular injections unacceptable. Mouthwashes are preferable to the trauma which a toothbrush may place on the gums. An electric razor should be used for shaving to reduce the risk of cuts to the skin.

Blood pressure recordings are not taken in thrombocytopenic patients because the pressure caused by an inflated sphygmomanometer cuff may be enough to cause internal bleeding in the upper arm. Finally, care should be taken when handling and moving such patients to reduce the likelihood of bruising.

Platelet transfusions are given when the platelet count falls below 10×10^9/litre.

Anaemia

When the number of red blood cells or the haemoglobin is reduced the patient becomes anaemic and will experience breathlessness on exertion, feel the cold and generally lack energy. Although anaemia is not life-threatening and can be effectively treated with blood transfusions, the patient does not feel at his best and may have less of a will to get better. Nursing care is directed towards providing comfort, assistance, reassurance and encouragement. Patients whose haemoglobin had dropped to 8 g/dl would be transfused.

Damage to gastrointestinal mucosa

Nausea and vomiting

The severity of the symptoms of anorexia, nausea and vomiting are dependent on the drug(s) used, dose, frequency, route and regimen, and patients need to be reassured of this. Not all chemotherapy patients are sick. In some cases, however, vomiting has been so distressing that the patient has refused to accept a subsequent course of treatment.

Care should be taken in placing the patient in a suitable part of the ward. A supply of disposable sickness basins, towels, paper tissues and disposal bags should be made ready. Where appropriate, a container for dentures should be provided. A mouthwash and/or supply of cold water for rinsing the mouth after a bout of sickness should always be available. A call bell must always be to hand. Many patients appreciate the support of a nurse when they are being sick. Privacy is also essential. The patient is alarmed at this time and may be hampered by an intravenous infusion at least. By placing a hand across the patient's forehead, the nurse can provide a resistance against which the patient can push reducing the strain on the patient. She can with the other hand help to support the sickness basin. Help is also often required to wipe the mouth and dispose of tissues. Sickness basins should be in plentiful supply so that the patient is not faced with a half-filled basin while waiting for the next wave of sickness to come. Used basins should be removed from the bedside immediately and measurements of volume recorded on a fluid balance chart. Repeated vomiting is exhausting for the patient and so whenever possible the patient should be given every assistance to try to sleep.

Patients troubled by nausea often find their own ways of minimising the problem. These include for example taking small amounts of food and fluid at frequent intervals and listening to relaxation tapes. There is some evidence to suggest that receiving chemotherapy sitting in a chair rather than lying in bed reduces the risk of vomiting. If the patient's condition permits, this is an option which can be offered to him. Care must be taken to ensure that the chair is comfortable and supportive, that the patient is not allowed to get cold and that the legs are supported if the patient is seated for prolonged periods. Acupressure wrist bands have proved a useful non-invasive method of controlling nausea and vomiting in some patients undergoing cytotoxic chemotherapy.

In some cases, past experience of vomiting following chemotherapy can lead to anticipatory nausea. The sight of the hospital, the ward, a particular doctor, or the arrival of equipment at the bedside can, in themselves, make the patient feel very sick and can even provoke an attack of vomiting.

Loss of appetite commonly accompanies treatment with cytotoxic drugs. In the short term, a reduced intake of food does no harm and so, if the patient declines a meal, he should not be badgered about it. Patients should however be encouraged to take some nourishment once the acute reaction has passed. Finding nourishing foods and liquids which appeal to the patient calls for some imagination on the part of the nurse. Involvement of the family is important here in providing the patient with his favourite (often home-made) tasty items of food. Flexibility is essential so that the patient may eat or drink at any time of the day or night as the fancy takes him. The involvement of the dietitian is of course vital in many cases so that the patient's nutritional status can be successfully monitored and maintained.

Breakdown of oral mucosa

Very strict attention to oral hygiene is of the utmost importance in patients receiving cancer chemotherapy, especially methotrexate and corticosteroids. Guidance on mouth care should be given to the patient at the outset and he should be encouraged to get into the habit of attending to this himself, wherever this is possible. He should be taught to inspect his mouth regularly and to report any changes without delay, and to rinse his mouth with an effective mouthwash such as chlorhexidine gluconate. Where this is not possible, oral hygiene must be carried out by the nurse. Any suspect lesions should be swabbed for 'culture and sensitivity'. Treatment for clinically obvious thrush will be begun before laboratory results are received. Mouth pain may be relieved by using benzydamine hydrochloride oral rinse. Liquids which sting the mouth and hard foods should be avoided. Some patients like to suck crushed ice, chilled pineapple cubes, and lemon and glycerine swabs.

Constipation

The neurotoxic effect of vincristine can lead to severe constipation and may result in paralytic ileus. Preventive measures should therefore be taken at the start of treatment. These will include increased fibre in the diet and plenty of fluids.

Diarrhoea

Fluorouracil and doxorubicin may cause diarrhoea, necessitating the use of codeine phosphate and the appropriate nursing measures.

Damage to the skin and hair

Extravasation

Certain cytotoxic drugs are especially vesicant and if allowed to leak from the vein into the surrounding tissues can cause burning and necrosis which in some cases have resulted in skin grafting and amputation. The nurse plays a vital role in explaining, observing for and reporting this phenomenon. The management of extravasation is described on p. (235).

Hair loss

Damage to the hair follicles reduces all hair growth on the body and makes the hair fall out. The term for this is alopecia or epilation. For both men and women this is a very distressing side-effect affecting body image, sexuality and self-confidence. Scalp-cooling techniques using gel packs may be used to reduce the concentration of drug in the capillaries of the scalp. The hair should always be groomed gently and, where it is clear that a wig will be required, arrangements should be made for it to be ordered while the colour, texture and style of the patient's hair are still apparent. The imaginative use of scarves and caps can help the patient through this period. Many patients however prefer to have no head covering at all and, particularly when at home, or in hospital where they feel safe, leave the head uncovered, especially when sleeping.

Altered sexuality and fertility

As well as alterations to body image in both males and females caused by chemotherapy, there may be a loss of sexual function and ability to reproduce. In the female, cytotoxic therapy may cause fibrosis of the ovary leading to amenorrhoea and sterility. The accompanying fall in oestrogen secretion may produce menopausal symptoms. In the male, there may be a total absence of sperm. Impotence and gynaeco-mastia may alter body image and reduce self-esteem. In both females and males, sterility may be temporary or permanent. Although women who have received chemotherapy have subsequently given birth to normal infants, genetic counselling should be given where pregnancy is desired by patients who have previously had chemotherapy because of the possible effects on the unborn child. For men who have received cancer chemotherapy, 'sperm banking' is a possibility. If nurses are to help patients to cope with sexual dysfunction caused by treatment, then they need to feel comfortable discussing the subject. Where this is not the case, the help of a trained counsellor may be required.

CYTOTOXIC DRUGS

The most commonly used cytotoxic drugs are detailed in Table 14.2.

Calcium leucovorin rescue for patients receiving methotrexate

Calcium leucovorin is chemically related to the essential coenzyme for nucleic acid synthesis. It is used to diminish the toxicity of folic acid antagonists such as methotrexate. The dose of calcium leucovorin will depend on the dose of methotrexate previously administered. As an example, 150 mg would be given in divided doses over 12–24 hours by intramuscular injection, intravenous bolus or intravenous infusion. Following the initial doses, 12–15 mg intramuscularly or 15 mg is given orally every 6 hours for the next 48 hours. Steps should be taken to increase the rate of excretion of the methotrexate, e.g. by alkalinisation of the urine and maintaining the urinary output at a high level. In advanced colorectal cancer combination therapy of calcium leucovorin and fluorouracil is used. Calcium leucovorin at a dose of 200 mg/m^2 is given by *slow* intravenous injection followed at once by fluorouracil 370 mg/m^2 by intravenous injection. The treatment is repeated for 5 consecutive days. Further courses can be given after 21–28 days. Each treatment course must be carefully monitored and any necessary dosage adjustments made.

Table 14.2	Cytotoxic drugs in common use		
Drug name(s)	Classification and mode of action	Main indications	Dose/route/side-effects/precautions
Aclarubicin	Cytotoxic antibiotic. Preferentially inhibits RNA synthesis.	Acute non-lymphocytic leukaemia in patients resistant to first-line chemotherapy.	175–300 mg/m² body surface area over 3–7 days. Intravenous via freely flowing peripheral line or central venous line. Side-effects: nausea and vomiting, bone marrow depression. Irritant to tissues. Monitor cardiac function; avoid extravasation.
Bleomycin	Cytotoxic antibiotic. Inhibits cell growth and DNA synthesis in tumour cells.	Squamous-cell carcinoma of mouth, nasopharynx, larynx, oesophagus, external genitalia or skin.	Wide dosage range depending on condition being treated. Intravenous or instillation into cavity. Total dose of 500 units should not be exceeded. Younger men with testicular teratoma may tolerate higher doses. Side-effects: fever, anorexia, nausea, local pain; interstitial pneumonia which may lead to a fatal pulmonary fibrosis (this condition is dose-related and rarely occurs on normal doses); local lesions, skin and mucosa. Chest X-rays carried out weekly. Not to be used in pregnant or breast-feeding women.
Busulphan (Myleran)	Alkylating agent. Binds to DNA. Selective action on granulocytopoiesis.	Palliative treatment of chronic granulocytic leukaemia.	60 µg/kg/day, initial maximum dose of 4 mg as a single daily dose, given orally. Treatment is continued until the leukocyte count has fallen to an acceptable level. Maintenance therapy 0.5–2 mg per day may be instituted following a break in treatment. Side-effects: bone marrow depression, especially thrombocytopenia; interstitial pulmonary fibrosis; skin hyperpigmentation; hepatotoxicity has been seen when used in combination with thioguanine; many other effects/toxicity reactions have been reported; myelosuppression/risk of irreversible bone marrow aplasia. Careful monitoring of blood counts essential. Avoid during pregnancy, especially in the first 3 months due to possible teratogenic effects.
Carmustine (BiCNU)	Alkylating agent.	Multiple myeloma, lymphoma and brain tumours.	200 mg/m² intravenous every 6 weeks as a single dose or divided into two doses of 100 mg/m² on 2 successive days. If given in combination therapy, dosage adjusted. Side-effects: myelosuppression – which may be delayed (this is dose-related) nausea and vomiting; pulmonary toxicity; renal damage. As with all cytotoxic agents, handle with care. Haematological monitoring essential.
Chlorambucil (Leukeran)	Alkylating agent.	Hodgkin's disease, non-Hodgkin's lymphomas, chronic lymphatic leukaemia, breast cancer, ovarian cancer.	Dosage will depend on condition being treated, e.g. Hodgkin's disease 0.2 mg/kg/day orally for 4–8 weeks. Often used in combination therapy. Side-effects: bone marrow suppression; gastrointestinal disturbances; nausea and vomiting, oral ulceration; hepatotoxicity and jaundice; lung damage has been reported. Haematological monitoring essential. Should not be given to patients who have recently undergone radiotherapy. Dose reduced in presence of hepatic dysfunction.

Table 14.2 *Cont'd*

Drug name(s)	Classification and mode of action	Main indications	Dose/route/side-effects/precautions
Cisplatin. Carboplatin has similar actions/ indications but is generally less toxic than cisplatin.	Antineoplastic drug with an alkylating action.	Testicular tumours, ovarian tumours.	Often used in combination therapy (with bleomycin and vinblastine). As a single agent 50–120 mg/m^2 body surface as a single intravenous dose every 3–4 weeks or 15–20 mg/m^2 intravenously daily for 5 days every 3 or 4 weeks. Lower doses used in combination therapy. Side-effects: severe nausea and vomiting; nephrotoxicity; myelosuppression; neurotoxicity/ototoxicity; hypersensitivity reactions; anaphylaxis. In view of nephrotoxicity, renal function should be measured prior to initiating therapy and prior to each subsequent course. Avoid in pregnancy and breast-feeding mothers. Ensure that means of dealing with anaphylactic reactions are to hand. Adverse effects are cumulative. Haematological monitoring is carried out.
Cyclophos-phamide (Endoxana)	Alkylating drug. Inert until activated in the body by microsomal enzymes in the liver.	Leukaemia, lymphomas, soft-tissue and osteogenic sarcoma, certain paediatric malignancies, breast and lung cancer.	Often used in combination with other drugs. Dose used will depend on condition being treated. Conventional dosage levels are 100–300 mg daily as a single intravenous or oral dose OR 500 mg–1 g as a single intravenous dose weekly. Higher dose regimes are 20–40 mg/kg as a single intravenous dose given at 10–20-day intervals. Side effects: produces toxic metabolites which can cause haemorrhagic cystitis. Concurrent use of mesna reduces local toxicity. Maintain high fluid intake. As with all cytotoxic drugs, special care must be taken in patients with co-existing disease. Monitoring of haematological and biochemical parameters essential.
Cytarabine (Alexan)	Antimetabolite. Inhibits DNA synthesis.	Acute myeloid leukaemia, acute nonlymphoblastic leukaemia, acute lymphoblastic leukaemia. Children show greater tolerance than adults to cytarabine therapy.	Dosage according to body surface area. Acute leukaemia 100–200 mg/m^2 per day or 3–6 mg/kg per day. Duration of therapy depends on clinical findings and bone marrow results. Remission maintenance therapy 75–100 mg/m^2 per day for 5 consecutive days once a month. Used intrathecally in CNS leukaemias. Side effects: mild nausea and vomiting; granulocytopenia; infection; haemorrhage due to thrombocytopenia; skin rashes. Avoid in pregnancy and lactation. Regular haematological monitoring essential. Renal and liver function monitored. CNS toxicity occurs with high-dosage regimens. Particular care to be taken in disposing of equipment used in administration (see p. 234).
Dacarbazine (DTIC–DOME)	Exact mechanism of action not known. May have some alkylating action.	Malignant melanoma, sarcoma, Hodgkin's disease. Used in combination therapy in the treatment of colon, ovary, breast and other cancers.	Various dosage schedules recommended, e.g. 2–4.5 mg/kg for 10 days repeated at 4 week intervals intravenously. Side-effects: anorexia, nausea and vomiting; haemopoietic depression; influenza like symptoms; alopecia; hepatotoxicity; irritant to tissues. Avoid extravasation. Full haematological monitoring. Nausea and vomiting can be reduced by restricting intake of food and drink 4–6 hours prior to therapy.

Table 14.2 *Cont'd*			
Drug name(s)	**Classification and mode of action**	**Main indications**	**Dose/route/side-effects/precautions**
Dactinomycin	Cytotoxic antibiotic. Inhibits cell proliferation by combining with DNA.	Paediatric cancer, e.g. Wilms' tumour, rhabdomyosarcoma, carcinoma of testis and uterus on sequential basis with methotrexate.	This is a very toxic drug. Dosage should not exceed 15 µg/kg or 400–600 µg/m^2 body surface area. Intravenously for maximum of 5 days. Dosage for children 15 µg/kg per day intravenously. Adult dosage 500 µg/day for 5 days intravenously. May be used in isolation – perfusion techniques. If seepage of drug into the general circulation can be prevented, higher 'doses' can be given than in systemic therapy. Side-effects: irritant to tissues; nausea and vomiting; possible anaphylaxis; severe haemopoietic depression; oral lesions; anaemia; alopecia. Avoid extravasation. Administer via rubber tube of freely running infusion solution. As with other cytotoxic drugs, may cause established mild infections to become fatal.
Doxorubicin	Cytotoxic antibiotic.	Acute leukaemia, lymphomas, soft-tissue and osteogenic sarcoma, paediatric malignancies, breast and lung cancer.	30–40 mg/m^2 when given in combination therapy. 60–75 mg/m^2 every 3 weeks when used alone. Intravenously via freely running intravenous infusion. On the basis of body weight, 1.2–2.4 mg/kg as a single dose every 3 weeks. A balance has to be achieved between dosage intervals and resulting toxicity. Dosage must be reduced if the patient has had previous therapy with other cytotoxic drugs. Can be given by intra-arterial or intravesical routes. Side-effects: haematological damage; cardiotoxicity – congestive cardiac failure; alopecia; GIT symptoms, nausea and vomiting; causes red colour in urine. Account must be taken of treatment with other cardiotoxic agents. ECG monitoring before and after treatment required.
Epirubicin	Cytotoxic antibiotic.	Breast, ovarian, gastric and colorectal cancer, lymphomas, leukaemia and multiple myeloma.	75–90 mg/m^2 repeated at 21-day intervals intravenously. Can also be given by intravesical administration in the treatment of bladder cancer. The side-effect profile and precautions are similar to those of doxorubicin.
Estramustine (Estracyt)	Alkylating agent. As a combination of oestradiol and normustine has oestrogenic action also.	Cases of prostatic cancer unresponsive to other therapy.	0.14–1.4 g daily in divided doses orally. With meals (avoid milk and milk products). Side-effects: gastrointestinal problems; gynaecomastia; thromboembolic disorders; bone marrow depression. Use with caution in patients with concurrent disease, e.g. diabetes, hypertension. Haematological monitoring needed.
Etoposide (Vepesid)	Mitotic inhibitor. Classed along with vinca alkaloids.	Small-cell lung cancer and resistant non-seminomatous testicular carcinoma. May be used in combination therapy.	60–120 mg/m^2 intravenously daily for 5 consecutive days repeated at not more than 21-day intervals. Twice the intravenous dose is given orally. Side-effects: myelosuppression; irritant to tissues; alopecia; nausea and vomiting; hypotension due to rapid infusion rate. Avoid extravasation. Haematological monitoring. Liver function monitoring.

Table 14.2 *Cont'd*

Drug name(s)	Classification and mode of action	Main indications	Dose/route/side-effects/precautions
Fluorouracil (as a 5% cream Efudix)	Antimetabolite. Inhibits cell division by interfering with DNA and RNA synthesis.	Colon and breast cancer, malignant skin lesions.	Intravenous infusion or injection. By infusion 15 mg/kg at a slow rate over 4 hours (not more than 1g in 500 ml of fluid) or infuse over 30–60 minutes. Continuous infusion over 24 hours may be preferred. Dose is repeated on successive days to a total of 12–15 g. Toxicity may cause treatment to be discontinued before the full 'course' is given. The dividing line between effective and toxic doses is very fine, so careful monitoring is essential. Side-effects: haematological damage; gastrointestinal haemorrhage; stomatitis (diarrhoea, nausea and vomiting). Discontinue therapy when signs of toxicity appear (leucopenia and thrombocytopenia). Fluorouracil may be used locally as a 5% cream for superficial pre-malignant or malignant skin lesions. Applied once or twice daily with occlusive dressing to enhance effect. Avoid contact with mucous membranes or the eyes.
Hydroxyurea (Hydrea)	Antineoplastic agent, acts by interfering with DNA synthesis.	Chronic myeloid leukaemia. In combination with radiotherapy in the treatment of cancer of the cervix.	20–30 mg/kg daily in single doses. Side-effects: anorexia, gastrointestinal symptoms; myelosuppression; anaemia; alopecia; skin rashes. Monitor renal and liver function. Blood parameters monitored before, during and after treatment. Correct severe anaemia with blood transfusions.
Idarubicin (Zavedos)	Cytotoxic antibiotic.	Acute non-lymphocytic leukaemia (ANLL) and acute lymphocytic leukaemia (ALL). May be used in combination therapy.	Dosage in ANLL 12 mg/m^2 intravenously daily for 3 days with cytarabine. Dosage in ALL as a single agent 12 mg/m^2 intravenously daily for 3 days. Children 10 mg/m^2 intravenously daily for 3 days. Side-effects: myelosuppression (leukocytes); cardiotoxicity, potentially fatal congestive heart failure; tissue irritancy; causes red colouration of urine. Cardiac function should be monitored. Renal and hepatic function should be monitored. Avoid extravasation.
Ifosfamide (Mitoxana)	Alkylating agent (similar to cyclophosphamide activated in the liver by microsomal enzymes).	Tumours of lung, ovary, cervix, breast, testis and soft-tissue carcinoma, carcinoma of pancreas, and head and neck tumours.	Used in combination therapy and with radiotherapy. Dosage varies according to condition and treatment regime. Total dose for a course is 8–10 g/m^2 as equal daily doses over 5 days. Courses are repeated at intervals of 2–4 weeks. Side-effects and precautions similar to those of cyclophosphamide. Give with mesna to protect against urethral toxicity. As with many cytotoxic agents particular attention should be given to mouth care.
Lomustine (CCNU)	Alkylating agent with enzyme-inhibiting properties.	Hodgkin's disease, brain tumours, lung tumours, malignant melanoma.	Used in combination therapy and with radiotherapy. 120–130 mg/m^2 as a single dose every 6–8 weeks. Side-effects: marrow depression – delayed; nausea and vomiting; loss of scalp hair (infrequent). Give prophylactic antinauseants, e.g. metoclopramide. Haematological monitoring.

Table 14.2 *Cont'd*			
Drug name(s)	**Classification and mode of action**	**Main indications**	**Dose/route/side-effects/precautions**
Melphalan (Alkeran)	Alkylating agent. Prevents cell replication by cross-linking with DNA strands.	Multiple myeloma, ovarian adenocarcinoma in combination therapy to treat breast cancer. Localised treatment of malignant melanoma.	Considerable variation in dosage regimes, e.g. in multiple myeloma 150 μg/kg body weight daily orally in divided doses for 4 days repeated at intervals of 6 weeks. Regional perfusion has been used in malignant melanoma. The drug is unstable in infusion fluids. It is preferable to inject slowly via the injection port of a freely running infusion system. Side-effects: bone marrow depression; nausea and vomiting especially with high dose intravenous therapy; skin rashes; diarrhoea. Haematological monitoring essential. Avoid in pregnancy and breast-feeding mothers.
Mercaptop-urine (Puri-Nethol)	Antimetabolite. Acts by interfering with synthesis of nucleic acid in proliferating cells.	Acute lymphoblastic leukaemia and acute myelogenous leukaemia.	Adults and children are given 2.5 mg/kg body weight orally. Dosage period of administration will depend on the condition being treated and if given with other drugs. Side-effects: myelosuppression – leucopenia and thrombocytopenia; hepatotoxic; hyperuricaemia due to cell lysis. Careful blood monitoring essential. Supportive action needed for patient who may develop a relative bone marrow aplasia. Liver function monitoring.
Methotrexate	Antimetabolite acts during 'S' phase of cell division. Inhibits certain enzyme functions which, in turn, interfere with DNA production. It is a folic acid antagonist.	A wide range of conditions: leukaemia, lymphoma, breast cancer, osteogenic sarcoma, lung cancer, head and neck cancer bladder cancer (has also been used in uncontrolled psoriasis).	Can be administered by all main routes, including intrathecal. This is a very important drug in the treatment of many malignant diseases. As a result, a wide range of dosage regimes and routes of administration are employed. Specialist literature should be consulted for details. Side-effects: nausea/abdominal distress; stomatitis; leukopenia; anaphylactic reactions (rare); rashes, photosensitivity; bone marrow depression; mucositis; hepatic toxicity; genitourinary toxicity; CNS symptoms – blurred vision; adverse effects of intrathecal administration are complex and may include headache, fever, paraplegia (transient), nerve palsies, convulsions and dementia. Use with great caution in patients with haematological impairment, inflammatory bowel disease and peptic ulcer. Possible dangers from drug interactions, e.g. with NSAIDs (see p. 44). Full laboratory monitoring of patients receiving methotrexate therapy is essential. See also *Calcium leucovorin rescue for patients receiving methotrexate.* (p. 240)
Mitomycin (Mitomycin C, Kyowa)	Cytotoxic antibiotic. In the tissues the drug has an alkylating action, forming a complex with DNA in cancer cells.	Breast, stomach, pancreatic, colonic, bladder, rectal and skin cancer.	60–150 μg/kg at 1–6-weekly intervals depending on any drug combination used and bone marrow condition. Also used as an instillation in bladder cancer. Side-effects: myelosuppression; nausea and vomiting; local ulceration due to extravasation; renal toxicity. Haematological monitoring. Avoid skin and eye contact. Avoid in pregnancy and breast-feeding.

Table 14.2 *Cont'd*

Drug name(s)	Classification and mode of action	Main indications	Dose/route/side-effects/precautions
Mitozantrone (Novantrone)	Cytotoxic antibiotic.	Advanced breast cancer, non-Hodgkin's lymphoma and acute non-lymphocytic leukaemia. May be useful in liver cancer that cannot be resected.	Dosage – consult specialist literature. Reduced dosage in combination therapy. The drug is very irritant and must be handled with care. Careful technique is essential when diluting the drug for intravenous infusion.
Mustine	Alkylating drug.	Hodgkin's disease.	Single dose of 0.4 mg/kg body weight or a course of 4 daily doses of 0.1 mg/kg intravenously. Side-effects: very toxic; irritant to tissues; nausea and vomiting; bone marrow depression – severe; peptic ulcers; thrombophlebitis and venous thrombosis. Blood counts are essential prior to each treatment.
Procarbazine (Natulan)	The mechanism of action is thought to be inhibition of protein, RNA and DNA synthesis.	Hodgkin's disease in combination with mustine, prednisolone and vincristine (MOPP).	50 mg daily orally increasing by 50 mg daily to 250–300 mg daily in divided dose. Maintenance dose 50–150 mg daily. Side-effects: nausea, vomiting; myelosuppression; hypersensitivity; rashes; fever chills; lethargy. As with all cytotoxic therapy, careful monitoring is required.
Thioguanine (Lanvis)	Antimetabolite, acts by inhibition of purine synthesis.	Acute leukaemia, especially acute myelogenous leukaemia and acute lymphoblastic leukaemia. Also chronic granulocytic leukaemia usually in combination therapy.	Dose dependent on combination treatment regime used. Adults for induction 100–200 mg/m² per day as a single or twice-daily regime over 5–20 days. Similar doses for children with reduction for smaller surface area of a child. Side-effects: gastrointestinal symptoms; stomatitis; hepatotoxicity; bone marrow suppression. Careful monitoring essential.
Thiotepa	Alkylating agent. Acts by alkylating DNA.	Malignant effusions and bladder cancer. Also in ovarian cancer, often in combination with other agents.	Dosage levels depend on white cell count. Intravenous, intramuscular and intrathecal routes are used. Also, instillation into a cavity, e.g. in bladder cancer. Used as a 1-in-2000 solution as eye drops following surgery to remove pterygium. Side-effects: myelosuppression; vomiting; headache. Careful blood monitoring is essential; if the white blood cell count falls below 3000 cells/mm³, the drug is not given.
Treosulfan	Alkylating agent.	Ovarian cancer.	Dosage schedules follow a number of regimens. A total dose of 21–28 g is given over an initial 8-week treatment period. Oral and intravenous administration is used. Side-effects: bone marrow depression; gastrointestinal upsets; nausea, vomiting and abdominal pain; alopecia; stomatitis (if capsules chewed). Regular blood counts essential. Avoid extravasation.
Vinblastine (Velbe)	Vinca alkaloid.	Hodgkin's disease, non-Hodgkin's lymphoma. Breast, renal cell and testicular cancer.	Adult dose 6 mg/m² at weekly intervals. Higher doses may be given in testicular cancer. The intravenous route is used. As with vincristine inadvertant intrathecal use results in fatality. Side-effects: gastrointestinal; haematological damage; nausea and vomiting; neurological, e.g. parasthesiae; cardiovascular, e.g. myocardial infarction. Avoid eye contamination. Granulocyte counts essential.

Table 14.2 *Cont'd*			
Drug name(s)	**Classification and mode of action**	**Main indications**	**Dose/route/side-effects/precautions**
Vincristine (Oncovin)	Vinca alkaloid.	Acute lymphocytic leukaemia, acute myelogenous leukaemia, malignant lymphomas, multiple myeloma, breast cancer and certain paediatric tumours, e.g. Wilms' disease.	This is a very potent drug. As with all cytotoxic drugs great care in calculating dosage levels. 1.4–1.5 mg /m^2 up to a maximum weekly dose of 2 mg. In children 2 mg/m^2 is the usual dose. Lower doses are used for children weighing less than 10 kg. Under no circumstances must this drug be given intrathecally; deaths have resulted from inadvertant intrathecal use. Side-effects: irritant to tissues; alopecia; neuromuscular reactions, neuritic pain, sensory loss, parasthesiae, difficulty in walking; granulocytopenia; bronchospasm. Avoid eye contamination. The appearance of neuromuscular adverse effects must be carefully watched for and doses reduced if side-effects occur.
Vindesine	Vinca alkaloid.	Acute lymphoblastic leukaemia in children, advanced carcinoma of the breast.	3 mg/m^2 for adults by intravenous bolus. In children 4 mg/m^2. Subsequently dose based on granulocyte count. If there is no granulocytopenia the dose can be carefully increased. Inadvertant intrathecal injection can be fatal. Side-effects: bronchospasm; nausea, vomiting and other gastrointestinal effects; paralytic ileus; neurological symptoms; granulocytopenia; alopecia. Daily blood counts. Side-effects can be reduced by appropriate treatment, e.g. reduction of fluid intake, cathartics to avoid ileus, administration of an anticonvulsant, since vindesine lowers blood levels of anticonvulsants. Cardiovascular monitoring.

Table 14.3 Other drugs used in malignant disease		
Drug(s)	**Mode of action**	**Dosage/clinical indications/ side-effects/precautions**
ANTIBACTERIAL AGENTS	See p. 153.	Immunosuppression associated with some types of malignant disease, and certain cytotoxic drugs may result in the need for antibiotic cover.
Corticosteroids especially prednisolone	See p. 195.	Wide variation in dosage. Acute lymphoblastic leukaemia. Hodgkin's disease. Breast cancer. Palliation in terminal conditions.
***Corynebacterium parvum* vaccine (Coparvax)**	Immunostimulant.	7–14 mg into pleural or peritoneal cavity. Used to alleviate malignant pleural effusions and malignant ascites. Side-effects depend on site of instillation. An intense fibrinous reaction may occur in pleural or peritoneal cavities. Fever, pain and discomfort have been reported. Should not be instilled into pleural cavity within 10 days of thoracotomy.

Table 14.3 *Cont'd*

Drug(s)	Mode of action	Dosage/clinical indications/side-effects/precautions
HORMONE ANTAGONISTS Aminoglutethimide (Orimeten)	Acts by inhibiting certain enzymes involved in the conversion in the body of androgens into oestrogens.	In advanced breast cancer a course of treatment commencing with 250 mg orally daily, increasing in weekly instalments to 1000 mg daily. The drug has a poorly understood action in advanced prostatic cancer. Usual dose: 750 mg daily. Since the drug interferes with hormone metabolism in the body it is necessary to administer corticosteroids concurrently. Side-effects are very variable but include CNS problems such as dizziness, somnolence and lethargy. Leucopenia, agranulocytosis and other blood dyscrasias may cause problems.
Cyproterone (Cyprostat)	An anti-androgen which competes with testosterone at prostatic receptors.	Given orally 100 mg three times daily. Adverse effects include impotence and gynaecomastia.
Formestane	This drug has been shown to be as effective as aminoglutethimide for the treatment of breast cancer in post-menopausal women resistant to tamoxifen treatment. The side-effect profile is better than aminoglutethimide and drug–drug interactions are less likely. Formestane acts by decreasing oestrogen levels. However, in pre-menopausal women with functioning ovaries oestrogen levels are largely unaffected.	By intramuscular injection 250 mg every 2 weeks. Higher doses have been used on a trial basis. Local reactions at injection site, CNS disturbances and gastrointestinal problems.
Gonadorelin-like substances (see p. 186): buserelin, goserelin.	Prostatic cancer cells require androgens for continued growth and development. Goserelin deprives the cancer cells of androgens by inhibition of pituitary LH secretion which causes a fall in serum testosterone.	Used in advanced prostatic cancer in the form of a biodegradable implant. A 4-weekly implant of 3.6 mg (depot) maintains the fall of testosterone levels to the castrate range. Patients at risk of developing ureteric obstruction or spinal cord compression. Should be monitored closely during the early stages of therapy. Side-effects include flushes, decrease in libido and a temporary increase in bone pain.
Tamoxifen (Nolvadex)	Some patients suffering from breast cancer have tumours that have receptors which are oestrogen-positive. Such patients are likely to respond to treatment with an oestrogen receptor antagonist.	Tamoxifen is a widely used oestrogen antagonist. The main indication for the use of this drug is in breast cancer both in post- and pre-menopausal women. The dose in breast cancer is 20–40 mg per day by mouth. Side-effects include hot flushes, vaginal bleeding, gastrointestinal disturbances and skin rashes. Dosage reduction may relieve the side-effects.
DRUGS USED TO TREAT HYPERCALCAEMIA (see p. 192).	Hypercalcaemia is a common complication of some cancers. The cause of this condition is thought to relate to the ectopic production of a peptide which has a parathyroid hormone-like action. Another cause of hypercalcaemia may be local breakdown of bone (osteolysis).	See p. 194.
Octreotide (Sandostatin)	The drug acts by inhibiting the release of growth hormone and other hormones in the	This drug has been used to treat hypercalcaemia resistant to the diphosphonates. Dosage levels

Table 14.3 *Cont'd*		
Drug(s)	**Mode of action**	**Dosage/clinical indications/ side-effects/precautions**
	GIT. Because of its diverse effects it has been found useful in patients with severe secretory diarrhoea that can occur in VIPomas.	vary but are of the order of 50 μg once or twice daily subcutaneously.
INTERFERONS (alpha, beta and gamma). The alpha form of interferon is normally used in treatment regimes.	The mode of action of the interferons is not well understood. They have complex effects on immunity and cell function. It has been suggested that interferons have a direct effect on malignant cells by binding to receptors on cell surface membranes.	Dosage levels vary according to the condition being treated. Examples are: hairy-cell leukaemia: 3 mega units (MU) intramuscularly or subcutaneously daily. Depending on response maintenance, doses may be given three times weekly. Interferons can be self-administered by subcutaneous injection. Renal cell carcinoma: 3 MU daily intramuscularly over 10–12 weeks. Kaposi's sarcoma: an escalating dosage schedule is used beginning with 3 MU daily, increasing to 36 MU daily if tolerated over a period of 84 days. Other conditions treated by interferons: multiple myeloma, chronic myelogenous leukaemia. (Interferon is also valuable in the treatment of chronic hepatitis B.) Side-effects include influenza-like symptoms, fever, chills, etc. CNS effects including depression, confusion, dizziness, drowsiness, somnolence or even coma. Effects on blood pressure and CVS have been reported. Anorexia, nausea, diarrhoea and vomiting. Reduction in white blood cell count and platelet count may result in the need to suspend treatment to allow the counts to recover to pre-treatment levels. Electrolyte disturbances may be associated with anorexia and dehydration. Skin reactions may occur at the site of injection and mild to moderate alopecia has been reported. As with other drugs used in the treatment of malignant disease, careful laboratory monitoring is needed during treatment, e.g. standard haematological tests, biochemical profile, urinalysis. Adequate hydration of the patient should be maintained.
INTERLEUKIN-2		This drug (also known as Aldesleukin) has been used in the treatment of metastatic renal cell carcinoma. It is a very toxic drug of doubtful value.
PLICAMYCIN	Cytotoxic antibiotic.	Although introduced as a cytotoxic antibiotic this drug is now mainly used to treat the hypercalcaemia of malignancy. This drug is very toxic to the bone marrow and its use is very limited as a result.
SEX HORMONES	Treatment with sex hormones or hormone antagonists plays an important part in the treatment of cancer affecting breast, prostate and endometrium. Hormones produce a temporary benefit to patients by suppressing the growth of cells which is, to some extent, hormone-dependent.	

Table 14.3 *Cont'd*		
Drug(s)	**Mode of action**	**Dosage/clinical indications/ side-effects/precautions**
Androgens	See p. 197.	Androgens hava a limited place in the treatment of metastatic breast cancer. Testosterone compounds in an oily vehicle may be administered by slow intramuscular injection 250 mg every 2 or 3 weeks. If hypercalcaemia develops treatment must be discontinued. As with all hormone therapy used in the treatment of cancer, the development of secondary sexual characteristics may be troublesome.
Oestrogens		Oestrogens such as stilboestrol have been used in the treatment of cancer of the prostate. Due to an unacceptable level of side-effects, e.g. gynaecomastia, fluid retention and risk of thrombosis, treatment with stilboestrol has largely been superceded. Other oestrogens that may be used in the treatment of prostatic cancer are fosfestrol (Honvan) and ethinyloestradiol.
Progestogens		Progestogens are used in the treatment of breast cancer and endometrial cancer. Megestrol is given orally in doses ranging from 160 mg/day to 320 mg/day. Side-effects include weight gain due to appetite stimulation and nausea. Deep-vein thrombosis and alopecia have been reported. Myelosuppression is not a problem. Medroxyprogesterone acetate is given orally or by deep intramuscular injection. The dose is 0.4–1.5 g daily by mouth or 250 mg–1 g by injection. Side-effects include insomnia, fatigue, depression and headache. Skin reactions, nausea and indigestion occur at higher doses.

Other drugs used in the treatment of malignant diseases

Malignant disease is treated by a range of drugs in addition to the cytotoxic drugs previously described. Table 14.3 lists the range together with a brief description of the mode of action, dosage levels and clinical indications, side-effects and precautions in use.

FURTHER READING

Barnet and Central Manchester Open Tech Project 1987 The nature of cancer. Continuing Nurse Education Programme. Open Learning for Nurses, London
Lee L 1993 The risks of handling cytotoxic therapy. Nursing Standards 7: 25–28

Power A, Anderson R W, Cortopassi R et al 1990 Update on safe handling of hazardous drugs: the advice of experts. American Journal of Hospital Pharmacy 47: 1050–1060
Valanis B G, Vollmer W M, Labuhn K T et al 1993 Acute symptoms associated with antineoplastic drug handling among nurses. Cancer Nursing 16(4): 288–295

15

Drugs affecting the immune response

THE IMMUNE SYSTEM

The immune system is the body's defence against potentially harmful substances and microorganisms. Specific and non-specific mechanisms take part in the immunological response. The blood and lymphatic systems, bone marrow, thymus gland, liver and spleen interact to make this system effective. The bone marrow is responsible for the production of lymphocytes which are primed in the thymus gland (T lymphocytes) and possibly the bone marrow itself (B lymphocytes). These immunologically competent cells together with phagocytes (macrophages) circulate in the blood and lymphatic systems, liver and spleen, ready to react to an invasion by foreign substances (antigens).

Specific immune response

When a foreign substance (antigen) enters the body two different types of immunological response may occur (see Fig. 15.1).

Humoral immune response (antibody mediated immunity)

On contact with the antigen, immunologically competent B lymphocytes change into plasma cells (effector cells). These plasma cells are capable of producing specific antibodies, the immunoglobulins. The antibody combines with the antigen (antigen–antibody reaction) and

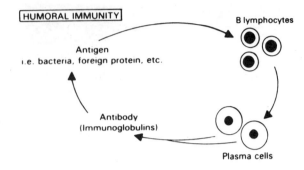

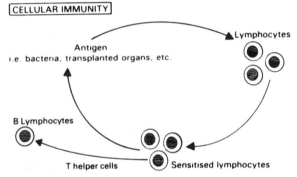

Figure 15.1 Humoral and cellular immunity. (From Trounce 1994 Clinical pharmacology for nurses, 14th edn. Churchill Livingstone.)

neutralises it, for example by coating bacteria to enhance their destruction by phagocytosis.

Another product of the primary contact of antigen with immunologically competent B lymphocytes are the memory cells. Memory cells are able to recognise the same antigen on a second contact which results in a more rapid and sometimes more intense response. Plasma cells are formed much faster which in turn results in a large amount of antibodies. The capability of the memory cells to recognise specific antigens sometimes years after the primary contact forms the basis of active immunisation against bacteria and their toxins.

Cellular immune response (cell-mediated immunity)

Depending on the physicochemical properties of the antigen and its way of entry into the body,

some antigens cause the production of sensitised lymphocytes, the T lymphocytes, which have antibody-like molecules on their surface (cell-bound antibody). The T lymphocytes are responsible for the specific cell-mediated immune response. On primary contact with the antigen they proliferate like the B lymphocytes and produce memory cells and effector cells. Unlike B lymphocytes, T lymphocytes produce different types of effector cells which directly take part in the immune reaction:

- cytotoxic effector cells (killer T cells) which can destroy other cells; this reaction to foreign cells is especially important in the rejection of transplanted organs
- T helper cells, which cooperate with the cytotoxic effector cells and also take part in the humoral immune response
- suppressor T cells, which can suppress the function of B lymphocytes and other T lymphocytes.

Non-specific immunity

Apart from the specific immune response, a number of non-specific antimicrobial mechanisms have been recognised. These non-specific factors often operate in conjunction with the specific immune response which greatly increases the overall effectiveness. These non-specific mechanisms include:

- bactericidal lysozyme, which is present in tears and saliva
- phagocytosis: some leucocytes are able to ingest and kill bacteria
- acute inflammatory response to a foreign substance: release of histamine from sensitised mast-cells
- the non-specific antiviral agent interferon, which is a lymphokine produced by T cells in response to viral infections; interferon inhibits the intracellular viral replication (it also acts on the immune system by increasing the cytotoxic activity of T lymphocytes and inhibits the mitosis of tumour cells).

IMMUNISATION

Immunity can be induced, either actively or passively, against a variety of bacterial and viral agents.

Active immunisation

The objective of vaccination is to provide protection against certain infections such as diphtheria, tetanus etc. Active immunity is induced by injection of antigen in the form of inactivated or attenuated live organisms or their products (toxins). This stimulates the production of antibodies and a population of primed cells, which can expand rapidly on renewed contact with the antigen and inactivate the invading organism or its toxins. This means prevention or at least minimisation of the disease. Established disease cannot be treated by this method.

Active immunisation is used for the routine vaccination of babies and children, opportunistic vaccination of previously non-immunised adults and children, for the vaccination of travellers going to contaminated areas and people at risk from infection through the nature of their work or their living conditions.

Types of vaccines used for active immunisation

Live attenuated vaccines such as **poliomyelitis (OPV), mumps, measles, rubella, tuberculosis (BCG), oral typhoid TY21, yellow fever and smallpox vaccines** contain strains of attenuated live organisms which, although harmless, are still capable of producing antibodies. Some live vaccines also contain small amounts of antibiotics such as kanamycin, neomycin, polymyxin. Live vaccines are listed in Table 15.3.

Inactivated vaccines (see Table 15.2) Bacterial and viral vaccines such as **whooping cough, typhoid, cholera and inactivated poliomyelitis (IPV) vaccines** contain heat-killed or chemically inactivated organisms. Human diploid cell vaccines (HDVC) such as **rabies and hepatitis A vaccines** contain organisms cultured on human diploid cells and chemically inactivated. **Haemophilus influenza B vaccine (HIB),** pneumococcal vaccine, influenza, hepatitis B and Vi polysaccharide typhoid vaccine contain immunising components of the organism.

Inactivated vaccines are listed in Table 15.4.

Toxoid vaccines such as **tetanus and diphtheria vaccine** contain toxins inactivated by formaldehyde, which are capable of acting as antigens.

Adsorbed vaccines such as **diphtheria/tetanus/pertussis (DTP), and hepatitis B vaccine** are inactivated vaccines adsorbed to an adjuvant such as aluminium phosphate or aluminium hydroxide. The adjuvant releases the antigen slowly and achieves a higher production of antibodies or antitoxins. Adsorbed vaccines are usually better tolerated by the patient.

Combined vaccines such as **mumps/measles/rubella (MMR), diphtheria/tetanus/pertussis (DTP), diphtheria/tetanus (DT) vaccines** are available to reduce the number of injections when immunising babies and children.

Duration of immunity

Injection with a vaccine does not provide immediate protection. There is usually an interval of a few days before the first antibodies appear. For **live attenuated vaccines**, with the exception of oral poliomyelitis vaccine (three doses), a single dose is sufficient to produce enough antibodies to achieve durable immunity. An important additional effect of OPV is the establishment of local immunity in the intestine. OPV boosters are also recommended for pre-school children and school leavers. Rubella immunisation is routinely given in girls at the age of 10–14 since there are no girls in this age group yet who had MMR vaccine when they were babies.

Inactivated vaccines produce a slow antibody or antitoxin response (primary response). Two injections may be needed to produce this effect. Further injections lead to an accelerated production of antibodies or antitoxins (secondary response) and therefore better protection. If the level of detectable antibody falls, a booster injection may be given to reinforce immunity. Immunity achieved in this way varies from months to years.

Routes of administration

Oral vaccines OPV (oral poliomyelitis vaccine) must never be injected; it should not be allowed to remain at room temperature as this may decrease its potency. Oral typhoid Ty 21a: one tablet has to be taken on alternate days for three doses; the vaccine is unstable at normal room temperature and has to be kept in the refrigerator.

Vaccines for injection With the exception of BCG and oral vaccines, all vaccines should be given by deep subcutaneous or intramuscular injection. In infants, the antero-lateral aspect of the thigh or upper arm is recommended. If the buttock is used, injection into the upper outer quadrant avoids the risk of sciatic nerve damage. Injection into fatty tissue of the buttock has been shown to reduce the efficacy of hepatitis B and rabies vaccine.

BCG vaccine is always given intradermally, except in infants and very young children; the percutaneous route by multiple puncture technique may be an acceptable alternative. In this case percutaneous BCG vaccine has to be used. For the intradermal administration of BCG a separate syringe and needle should be used for each patient. The operator should stretch the skin between the thumb and forefinger of one hand, and with the other slowly insert the needle (size 25G), bevel upwards, for about 2 mm into the superficial layers of the dermis, almost parallel with the surface. A raised, blanched bleb showing the tips of the hair follicles is a sign that the injection has been made correctly. If this is not felt, and it is suspected that the needle is too deep, it should be removed and reinstated before more vaccine is given. A bleb of 7 mm diameter is approximately equivalent to 0.1 ml injection.

Injection sites For BCG the site of injection is over the insertion of the left deltoid muscle; the tip of the shoulder must be avoided because of increased risk of keloid formations. For tuberculin sensitivity tests (Mantoux or Heaf), intradermal injections are given in the middle of the flexor surface of the forearm. This site should not be used for injecting vaccines. Rabies vaccine may be given intradermally if more than one person needs to be immunised or a rapid immunisation is required, e.g. staff caring for a patient with rabies. Subsequent doses of cholera and typhoid vaccines may also be given intradermally to minimise adverse reactions.

Contraindications

There are some contraindications which apply to most vaccines. However, manufacturers' leaflets should always be consulted before administration of a vaccine.

- Vaccination should be postponed if the patient suffers from an acute febrile illness; minor infections such as a cold are no reason to postpone immunisation.
- Severe local reactions, such as extensive redness and swelling, or general reactions, such as anaphylaxis, bronchospasm, general collapse, convulsions etc. to previous vaccination.
- Vomiting and diarrhoea for oral poliomyelitis vaccine (OPV).
- Hypersensitivity to egg (influenza vaccine); anaphylactic reactions to egg (yellow fever, MMR, influenza vaccine). Hypersensitivity to egg is not a contraindication for the use of yellow fever and MMR vaccine. These vaccines have been prepared on chicken embryos or egg, and the egg protein might cause a reaction in allergic patients. However, a personal or family history of allergy is not a contraindication for the use of live vaccines in general; neither is a stable neurological condition such as cerebral palsy.
- Live vaccines should not be given in pregnancy because of the theoretical possibility of harm to the fetus. After rubella injection pregnancy should be avoided for one month after immunisation. Polio and yellow fever vaccination may be given if the risk of infection outweighs the possible risk associated with the vaccine.
- Two live vaccines may be given at two different sites at the same time or 3 weeks apart; OPV should not be used at the same time as oral typhoid vaccine.

- Immunoglobulins and live vaccines should be given 3 months apart, because the antibodies in the immunoglobulin would inactivate the live vaccine; yellow fever vaccine may be given at the same time, because immunoglobulin prepared in the UK does not contain yellow fever antibodies (see passive immunisation).

Live vaccines must **not** be given to the following groups of patients:

- Patients on high-dose corticosteroids until 3 months after treatment has finished (children on lower dose corticosteroids may receive a live vaccine after 2 weeks; children on low-dose alternate-day treatment may receive live vaccines; corticosteroid replacement therapy is not a contraindication.)
- Immunocompromised patients either through illness or drug treatment; IPV (inactivated poliomyelitis vaccine) should be used instead of OPV in household contacts of immunocompromised children because the vaccine could cause the disease in these children. After exposure to measles or chickenpox these patients should receive the appropriate immunoglobulin (see passive immunisation).
- Malignant conditions such as lymphoma, leukaemia, Hodgkins' disease.

Adverse reactions

Adverse reactions to vaccines are usually mild, and severe reactions are very rare. Since vaccines have become safer the risk associated with immunisation, particularly in children, is very much smaller than the risk of complications of the disease.

Most vaccines may produce mild local or systemic reactions such as redness and swelling at the injection site, raised temperature and screaming. Some vaccines such as measles vaccine may cause a mild form of the disease. Parents should be informed about possible adverse effects and advised on fever management after routine immunisation of their children.

Severe site reactions after BCG administration, such as large ulcers, abscesses and keloid formations, are due largely to the wrong immunisation technique (see routes of administration).

After poliomyelitis immunisation there is a very rare occurrence of vaccine-related polio. Since the vaccine is excreted in the stool for up to 6 weeks after the immunisation the need for strict personal hygiene has to be stressed to household contacts of the vaccinee, e.g. the importance of washing their hands after changing their babies' nappies.

Despite the rarity of severe adverse reactions, doctors and nurses always have to be prepared for an anaphylactic reaction after vaccination and must be familiar with the management of anaphylactic shock (see Ch. 8).

All severe reactions should be reported to the Committee on Safety of Medicines.

Tuberculosis: BCG (Bacille Calmette–Guérin) immunisation

Vaccination against tuberculosis needs to be discussed in greater detail because of the special tests and immunisation technique involved.

The incidence of tuberculosis and the mortality rate have declined rapidly since the introduction of the BCG vaccine, national immunisation programmes and effective chemotherapy.

Recommendations for immunisation

The following groups are recommended for immunisation with BCG, provided successful BCG immunisation has not previously been carried out, and the tuberculin test is negative and there are no other contraindications:

- routine immunisation for all children between the ages of 10 and 13, all students and persons requesting immunisation for themselves or their children
- high-risk groups such as health care staff, veterinary staff, contacts of cases with active respiratory tuberculosis
- immigrants from countries with a high prevalence of tuberculosis, their children and infants

- those intending to stay in Asia, Africa, Central or South America for more than a month.

For information on immunisation technique, contraindications and adverse reactions see p. 255.

Immunisation reaction

Normally a local reaction develops at the injection site within 2–6 weeks; this consists of a small papule increasing in size for a few weeks up to 7 mm in width with scaling, crusting and occasional bruising. Occasionally a shallow ulcer develops; this should be exposed to the air. The lesion slowly subsides over a period of several months, leaving a small scar.

Use of BCG in bladder cancer

Intravesical BCG has been shown in numerous studies to be highly successful in the treatment of superficial bladder cancer. The mechanism of action by which BCG inhibits tumour growth is at present unknown (see malignant diseases Ch. 14).

The tuberculin test

Before BCG immunisation a tuberculin skin test has to be carried out, except on babies under 3 months of age. A positive test implies immunity through past infection or immunisation. Therefore, test-positive people should not receive BCG. Those with a strongly positive test may have active disease and have to be referred.

Mantoux and Heaf tests are the only recommended techniques for tuberculin testing. Both tests use purified protein derivative (PPD), which is available in several strengths, as shown in Table 15.1.

The Mantoux test

The solution is injected intradermally on the upper third of the flexor surface of the forearm. The results should be read 48–72 and up to 96 hours later. A positive result consists of a

Table 15.1 Tuberculin PPD

Strength (units/ml)	Dilution of PPD	Units in dose of 0.1 ml	Main use
100 000	–	10 000	Heaf (multiple puncture) test only
1 000	1 in 100	100	For special diagnostic purposes only
100	1 in 1 000	10	Mantoux test (routine)
10	1 in 10 000	1	Mantoux test (special), TB suspects or hypersensitive to tuberculin

transverse induration of at least 5 mm diameter; 0–4 mm induration is negative; 5–14 mm is equivalent to a Heaf grade 2, and 15 mm or more, strongly positive (Heaf grade 3 or 4).

The multiple puncture test (Heaf test)

The Heaf test is carried out with a **disposable head apparatus** which does not require any disinfection as the standard re-usable Heaf gun does. The use of the disposable head apparatus avoids the transfer of blood-borne infections such as hepatitis B and HIV and is now the preferred method of Heaf testing.

The disposable heads attach by a magnet to a handle. Six standard steel needles are retained in a plastic base which is enclosed in an outer plastic case with holes corresponding to the needles. The needles protrude only after actuation and then remain protruding so that it is easy to detect and discard ones which have been fired. The heads are prepacked and sterile. There are three versions of the disposable head:

- white standard version for tuberculin testing in adults and children 2 years and over; the needles protrude 2 mm on firing
- blue for tuberculin testing of children under 2 years; needles protrude 1 mm
- red, containing 18 needles; it is used for giving BCG by the percutaneous multiple puncture technique and must never be used for Heaf testing.

Performing the Heaf test The recommended site for testing is on the flexor surface of the left forearm at the junction of the upper third with the lower two-thirds, avoiding any eczematous skin. The correct disposable head has to be attached to the gun; tuberculin solution should be dropped from a syringe directly onto the skin at the testing site. The solution is then dispersed by the head of the gun, the gun pressed to the skin and fired. Excess tuberculin should be wiped off the skin, and six puncture marks observed. If the puncture marks are not present the test has not been carried out adequately. The results should be read ideally at 7 days, but can be read between 3 and 10 days.

The reaction is graded 0–4 according to the degree of induration produced:

Grade 0: no induration at the puncture sites
Grade 1: discrete induration at 4 or more needle sites
Grade 2: induration around each needle site merging with the next, forming a ring of induration but with a clear centre
Grade 3: the centre of the reaction becomes filled with induration to form one uniform circle of induration 5–10 mm wide
Grade 4: solid induration over 10 mm wide; vesiculation or ulceration may also occur.

Grades 0 and 1 are regarded as negative, and previously non-immunised individuals should receive BCG.
Grade 2 is positive, and no further immunisation is required.
Grades 3 and 4 are strongly positive and should be referred for further investigation.

Factors affecting the tuberculin test

The reaction to tuberculin protein may be suppressed by the following factors:

- glandular fever
- viral infections in general
- live viral vaccines
- Hodgkins' disease
- sarcoidosis
- corticosteroid therapy
- immunosuppressing diseases, including HIV.

Other factors which also affect the consistency of tuberculin testing include patient's age, skin thickness, tuberculin adsorption onto the surface of the syringe and tester/reader variation.

Immunisation of children

The immunisation of babies and children against infectious diseases such as **diphtheria, pertussis, tetanus, measles, mumps, rubella and poliomyelitis** has greatly reduced infant mortality and permanent physical and mental handicap caused by the illness. The introduction of the *Haemophilus influenzae* **type B (Hib) vaccine** should prevent another 65 deaths and 150 cases of brain damage caused by Hib meningitis each year in the United Kingdom.

The aim of the vaccination programme is to eliminate these diseases as far as possible from the population. For example, by giving rubella vaccine to young children it is intended to interrupt the circulation of rubella and thereby remove the risk of infection to non-immune pregnant women. Rubella immunisation of girls between the ages of 10 and 14 who previously have not received MMR vaccine, and non-immune women, continues to reduce the considerable risk to unborn babies. To achieve this aim a high uptake in child vaccinations is required. For this reason a more accelerated schedule (see Table 15.2) has been adopted following recognition that one of the most frequent reasons for low vaccine uptake was the mobility of young families who move out of districts before their children have completed their primary course.

Risk groups

The risk groups are: HIV-positive, children with special conditions, people living in institutions such as old people's homes, occupational risk groups and travellers.

Table 15.2 Immunisation schedule for children

Vaccine	Age		Notes
D/T/P and polio Hib	1st dose 2nd dose 3rd dose	2 months 3 months 4 months	Primary course
Measles/mumps/ rubella (MMR)	12–18 months		Can be given at any age over 12 months
Booster D/T and polio MMR (if not previously given)	4 – 5 years		
Rubella	10–14 years		Girls only
BCG	10 –14 years or infancy		Interval of 3 weeks between BCG and rubella
Booster tetanus and polio	15–18 years		

HIV-positive

HIV-positive patients are at increased risk from infectious diseases. Symptomatic and asymptomatic HIV-positive individuals should therefore receive **measles, mumps, rubella, polio (live or inactivated), whooping cough, diphtheria, tetanus, typhoid, cholera, hepatitis B** and **Hib vaccines** as appropriate.

In HIV-positive individuals, polio virus may be excreted for longer periods than is the case in normal persons. Contacts of recently immunised HIV-positive individuals should be advised to follow strict personal hygiene, especially after changing an immunised child's nappy.

HIV-positive patients should *not* receive BCG and yellow fever vaccines. Travellers intending to visit infected areas where a valid immunisation certificate is required should obtain a letter of exemption from their medical practitioner.

Vaccine efficacy may be reduced in HIV-positive individuals, and consideration should be given to the use of normal immunoglobulin after exposure to measles.

Children and adults with special conditions

Some conditions, such as HIV (see above), asthma, chronic lung and congenital heart diseases, Down's syndrome, small-for-dates and prematurity, increase the risk from infectious diseases. Children with such conditions should be immunised as a matter of priority. Small-for-dates and premature babies should be immunised according to the recommended schedule like any other children. Apart from routine immunisations, children and adults at risk should also be immunised against **influenza and pneumococcal infections**.

Hepatitis B immunisation is recommended for haemophiliacs on regular blood transfusions and patients with renal failure, drug abusers, and babies born to hepatitis B carrier mothers.

Children with neurological problems

In the 1960s and 70s there was considerable public and professional anxiety on the safety of pertussis vaccine. The development of severe neurological illness in children, in some cases resulting in permanent brain damage and death, was attributed to the vaccine. Between 1976 and 1979 a major study (the National Childhood Encephalopathy study) was carried out. Only 39 out of 1182 children with serious acute neurological illnesses had received pertussis vaccine recently, and in these cases the association of the neurological illness with immunisation could have occurred by chance. The number of cases was too small to show conclusively whether or not the vaccine can cause permanent brain damage if such damage occurs at all.

Immunisation of children against whooping cough is recommended when they have established neurological problems such as cerebral palsy. In doubtful cases advice should be sought from a consultant paediatrician.

Children with a personal or family history of febrile convulsions and epilepsy should also receive the pertussis vaccine.

Children and adults living in institutions

Children in residential care, including those in nurseries and playgroups, are at special risk from **measles** and should be immunised.

Residents of nursing homes, old people's homes and other long-stay facilities where

Table 15.3 Live vaccines

Live vaccine	Indication	Route	Dose	Intervals	Boosters	Specific contraindications	Comments
BCG	Contacts, active TB	intradermal	0.1 ml	Single	–	Generalised septic skin conditions	–
	Health care staff	intradermal	0.1 ml	Single	–	Generalised septic skin conditions	–
	All students	intradermal	0.1 ml	Single	–	Generalised septic skin conditions	–
	Children 10–14 years	intradermal	0.1 ml	Single	–	Generalised septic skin conditions	–
	Vet staff	intradermal	0.1 ml	Single	–	Generalised septic skin conditions	–
	Travellers	Intradermal	0.1 ml	Single	–	Generalised septic skin conditions	–
Measles/mumps/rubella	Routine immunisation children 12–15 months	SC/IM	0.5 ml	Single	–	Allergy to egg	–
	Risk group children	SC/IM	0.5 ml	Single	–	Allergy to egg	–
Oral poliomyelitis (OPV)	Routine immunisation of children	Oral	3 drops × 3	At intervals of 4 weeks	School entry, school leaving	–	Not with oral typhoid
	Travellers	Oral	3 drops × 3	At intervals of 4 weeks	10 years	–	Not with oral typhoid
	Health workers	Oral	3 drops × 3	At intervals of 4 weeks	10 years	–	Not with oral typhoid
Oral typhoid	Laboratory workers	Oral	1 cap × 3	Alternate days	Non-endemic areas, 3 doses annually	–	Keep vaccine in fridge
	Travellers >6 years	Oral	1 cap × 3	Alternate days	Non-endemic areas, 3 doses anually	–	Keep vaccine in fridge
Rubella	Routine immunisation girls 10–14 years	SC/IM	0.5 ml	Single	–	–	–
	Non-immunised women	SC/IM	0.5 ml	Single	–	–	Avoid in early pregnancy
Smallpox	Only laboratory workers who handle virus		See BNF				1979 last case of smallpox – routine immunisation unnecessary
Yellow fever	Laboratory workers	SC	0.5 ml	Single	10 years	Allergy to egg	–
	Travellers >9 months	SC	0.5 ml	Single	10 years	Allergy to egg	Children <9 months risk of encephalitis

Table 15.4 Inactivated vaccines

Inactivated vaccine	Indication	Route	Dose	Intervals	Boosters	Specific contraindications	Comments
Cholera	Travellers to areas where border guards ask unofficially for certificate	SC/IM	0.5 ml × 2 (adult)	One week to one month	Six months after last injection	Hypersensitivity to previous dose	No legal requirement for travel. No role in outbreak of disease
Diphtheria	Routine immunisation of children	SC/IM	0.5 ml × 3	At intervals of four weeks	School entry	–	Usually as DT or DPT
	Contacts of diphtheria cases – immunised	SC/IM	0.5 ml	Single	–	–	–
	– unimmunised	SC/IM	0.5 ml × 3	At monthly intervals	–	–	–
Diphtheria, tetanus and pertussis (DTP triple vaccine). A diphtheria and tetanus vaccine (DT) is available for use when immunisation against whooping cough is contraindicated	Routine immunisation of children	SC/IM	0.5 ml × 3	First dose at age 2 months followed by second dose after 4 weeks and third dose after another 4 weeks	A dose of DT is recommended at school entry at least 3 years from last dose of DPT	Where immunisation against whooping cough is contraindicated	Oral poliomyelitis vaccine may be given at the same time
Hepatitis A	Travellers	IM (deltoid)	1 ml × 2	Two weeks to one month	6–12 months	–	Should not be given to children
	Occupational risk	IM (deltoid)	1 ml × 2	Two weeks to one month	6–12 months	–	–
Hepatitis B	Occupational risk	IM (deltoid)	1 ml × 3 (adult)	One month and 6 months	–	–	–
	Cases or carrier contact	IM (deltoid) anterolateral thigh in infants	1 ml × 3 / 0.5 ml × 3 (0–12 years)	One month and 6 months	–	–	–
	Lifestyle e.g. parenteral drug abuser	IM (deltoid)	1 ml × 3 (adult)	One month and 6 months	–	–	–
Hib	Primary immunisation of children up to 13 months	SC/IM	0.5 ml × 3	At monthly intervals	–	–	–
	Children 13–48 months	SC/IM	0.5 ml	Single	–	–	–
Influenza	Special risk conditions and/or environments	SC/IM	0.5 ml	Single (adult)	–	Allergy to egg; Pregnancy	–
	Special risk conditions and/or environments	SC/IM	0.5 ml × 2	4–5 weeks (Children 4–13 years)	–	Allergy to egg	–

Table 15.4 Cont'd

Inactivated vaccine	Indication	Route	Dose	Intervals	Boosters	Specific contraindications	Comments
Meningococcal	Contacts of cases (groups A, C meningitis)	SC/IM	0.5 ml	Single	–	–	No vaccine available for group B meningitis
	Travellers (e.g. meningitis belt in Africa)	SC/IM	0.5 ml	Single			–
Pertussis	Routine immunisation of children						See DTP vaccine
Pneumococcal	Special risk conditions	SC/IM	0.5 ml	Single	5–10 years in individuals with declined antibody level	Pregnancy	Should not be given to children under 2 years
Rabies	Occupational risk Staff caring for a patient with rabies	SC/IM intradermal	1 ml × 3 0.1 ml into each limb (0.4 ml total)	Day 0,7,28 Single	– –	– –	– –
	Travellers to remote areas	intradermal	0.1 ml × 3	Day 0,7,28			–
	Post-exposure (not immunised)	SC/IM	1 ml × 6	Day 0,3,7, 14,30,90	–	–	Post-exposure treatment (not immunised) in combination with immunoglobulin
	Post-exposure (immunised)	IM	1 ml × 2	Day 0 and 3–7	–		–
Tetanus	Primary immunisation	SC/IM	0.5 ml × 3	At intervals of 4 weeks	School entry, school leaving Injury 10 years after primary course	–	see DPT, DT
	Unimmunised adults	SC/IM	0.5 ml × 3	At intervals of 4 weeks		–	–
Typhoid	Occupational risk	SC/IM	0.5 ml × 2	4–6 weeks	3 years	Hypersensitivity to previous dose	–
	Travellers to areas with poor hygiene	SC/IM	0.5 ml × 2	4–6 weeks	3 years	Hypersensitivity to previous dose	–
	Travellers to areas with poor hygiene	SC/IM	0.25 ml (child >1 year)	Single	1 year	Hypersensitivity to previous dose	–

rapid spread after introduction of the infection may occur should be immunised against **influenza**.

Hepatitis B immunisation is recommended for staff and clients in residential accommodation for the mentally handicapped and inmates of custodial institutions.

Occupational risk groups

Health care staff such as doctors and nurses, veterinary staff, customs officers, prison staff etc. may be at increased risk from infectious diseases such as hepatitis B, tuberculosis and rabies etc. due to the nature of their work; they should be immunised.

Travellers

Travellers to areas where the risk of contracting an infectious disease is especially high, or the nature of travel presents a special risk, or a valid immunisation certificate such as for yellow fever and meningococcal meningitis is required, should get immunised. Advice on which immunisation is necessary for which country and on other measures for the prevention of diseases should be obtained from general medical practitioners well before travelling.

Apart from immunisation, the main measure for preventing diseases such as typhoid, cholera and hepatitis A in areas of poor hygiene and sanitation is strict personal, food and drink hygiene. Immunisation against cholera is not recommended any more since it does not provide adequate protection and does not prevent the spread of disease.

Hepatitis A vaccine is an alternative to immunoglobulin for those who need longer term protection or who travel frequently to endemic areas. Immunoglobulin for protection against hepatitis A and strict personal, drink and food hygiene are still recommended for short-term and single holiday trips.

For many countries malaria chemoprophylaxis is strongly advisable.

Storage and disposal of vaccines

Most vaccines have to be stored and transported under refrigeration at the recommended temperature. This means a cold chain should be maintained at all times by using insulated cooled containers for the transport of vaccines from one refrigerator to another. The potency of vaccines can be guaranteed only if they have been kept at the recommended temperatures. (Manufacturers' leaflets should be consulted.) For most vaccines, with the exception of OPV (0–4°C Wellcome and 2–6°C Smith Kline and French), the recommended storage temperature is 2–8°C. However there is a 48-hour period built into the shelf life of live vaccines (except OPV) and 72 hours for inactivated vaccines during which the vaccine may be out of refrigeration. OPV deteriorates very quickly and should not be allowed to remain at room temperature. At room temperature the potency of OPV is maintained for 2 weeks (SKF) and 1 week (Wellcome). If vaccines are sent by post, the date and time of despatch must be marked clearly on the parcel. If more than 48 hours have elapsed since posting, the vaccine should not be accepted. Vaccines should not be kept at temperatures below 0°C as freezing can cause deterioration of the vaccine and breakage of the container.

Reconstituted vaccines must be used within the recommended period of time, usually between 1 and 4 hours, and discarded after an immunisation session.

Opened multidose containers of any vaccine have to be discarded after 1 hour for non-preservative and 3 hours for preservative-containing vaccines, including OPV. Single-dose containers should be used where possible.

Unused vaccine and spent or partly spent vials should be discarded, preferably by heat inactivation or incineration.

Spillage and contaminated waste should be dealt with by heat sterilisation, incineration or chemical disinfection.

Passive immunisation

In this method of immunisation the appropriate

antibody or antitoxin against the invading organism or toxin is injected. The antibodies are retrieved from immunised animals (antisera), e.g. **diphtheria antitoxin**, which is prepared in horses, or from immunised humans (immunoglobulins). The use of antisera has been widely replaced by the use of human immunoglobulins because of the serious side-effects associated with antisera, such as serum sickness and other allergic-type reactions. Reactions to human immunoglobulins are very rare.

Types of human immunoglobulins

Non-specific polyvalent human immunoglobulin (human normal immunoglobulin) is produced from pooled plasma of a large group of donors, which contains antibodies currently prevalent in the population. Human normal immunoglubin is used for:

- the protection of immunosuppressed children exposed to measles
- children under 12 months in whom there is a particular reason to avoid measles; immunisation with MMR vaccine should follow after a 3-month interval
- prophylaxis of infections following bone marrow transplantation
- protection of individuals against hepatitis A.

Human normal immunoglobulin is *not* recommended for the protection of previously non-immunised pregnant women exposed to *rubella*. If termination of pregnancy is not acceptable it may be given to reduce the likelihood of a clinical attack which may possibly reduce the risk for the fetus.

Immunisation with human normal immunoglobulin produces immediate protection which lasts for 4–6 weeks.

Specific immunoglobulin such as **tetanus, hepatitis B, rabies and varicella/zoster immunoglobulin** is produced from pooled blood of convalescent patients or recently immunised donors or donors who have a sufficient antibody titre.

Specific immunoglobulin is used for postexposure treatment of previously unimmunised patients usually in combination with the appropriate vaccine. Previously immunised patients need only a booster injection of the appropriate vaccine. Since varicella/zoster vaccine has no licence in the UK yet and is available only on a named basis for immunocompromised individuals, postexposure treatment for individuals at risk, such as pregnant chickenpox contacts and infants whose mothers develop chickenpox 1–4 weeks after the birth, receive only the immunoglobulin.

Treatment of the established disease with specific immunoglobulins is effective only if a high proliferation of the invading organism, especially viruses, or the bonding of toxins to body structure has not taken place yet. For example, in clinical tetanus a decrease of symptoms is only sometimes possible.

Anti-D (Rh0) immunoglobulin is used to prevent a rhesus-negative mother forming antibodies to fetal rhesus-positive cells. It should be injected within 72 hours of birth or abortion to protect any subsequent child from haemolytic disease of the newborn.

Administration

Human immunoglobulins are administered intramuscularly because of the danger of aggregation and anaphylactic reactions if given intravenously. To produce intravenous preparations the immunoglobulin has to undergo specific treatment. Intravenous preparations, e.g. **tetanus immunoglobulin for intravenous use**, is indicated if a large amount of antibody or a quick rise of antibody titre is necessary, as in the case of clinical tetanus.

CONDITIONS TREATED WITH DRUGS AFFECTING THE IMMUNE SYSTEM

Intervention into this most important defence mechanism is justified only in certain circumstances. Risks and benefits of drug treatment have to be weighed up carefully. Treatment should be initiated only in a specialist unit under the supervision of an experienced physician. Drug treatment is indicated in the following conditions.

Organ transplantations

The immune system enables the body to distinguish between 'self' and 'non-self'. This causes the rejection of transplanted organs which are recognised as 'non-self' by the immune system of the recipient. Drugs which act by suppressing the immune response are vitally important in helping to prolong the life of a transplanted organ.

Autoimmune diseases

Sometimes the body's mechanism for preventing the recognition of 'self' components as antigen is disturbed and the system turns against itself: autoantibodies are produced. All diseases associated with the formation of autoantibodies are called autoimmune diseases. Major examples are:

systemic lupus erythematosus
scleroderma
rheumatoid arthritis
ulcerative colitis
myasthenia gravis
active chronic hepatitis
chronic glomerulonephritis.

Some cancers

Examples include hairy-cell leukaemia, certain lymphomas and solid tumours and Kaposi's sarcoma associated with AIDS (acquired immune deficiency syndrome). The treatment of these and other cancers is dealt with in more detail in Chapter 14. It is very important to recognise that treatment with immunosuppressive drugs greatly weakens the patient's defence mechanism. This fact must be taken into account when providing nursing care and planning treatment, e.g. every effort must be made to reduce the risk of infection to a minimum.

MAIN DRUG GROUPS

Immunosuppressants

Cytotoxic immunosuppressants
Corticosteroids
Cyclosporin

Immunostimulants
Interferons
IMMUNOSUPPRESSANTS
Cytotoxic immunosuppressants

Azathioprine, the most commonly used drug in this group, is metabolised to 6-mercaptopurine, which suppresses cell-mediated immune reactions by preventing lymphocyte proliferation and function.

Usage

Azathioprine is used either alone or, more commonly, in combination with corticosteroids and/or other immunosuppressive agents in the management of renal and other organ transplantations, and autoimmune diseases, e.g. autoimmune haemolytic anaemia. The therapeutic effect may be evident only after a few weeks and may be corticosteroid-sparing, thereby reducing side-effects associated with high dosage and prolonged use of systemic corticosteroids.

Dosage and administration

Azathioprine is available as tablets and injection. Wherever possible oral administration is the preferred route of administration. The standard dose range in transplant rejection therapy is 1–4 mg/kg daily and 1–2.5 mg/kg daily for the treatment of autoimmune diseases. When the therapeutic effect is evident, doses should be reduced to the lowest effective level and should be maintained indefinitely in transplant patients because of the risk of organ rejection.

Elderly patients and patients with renal or hepatic impairment should receive doses at the lower end of the range.

Side-effects and cautions

Cytotoxic immunosuppressants are potentially dangerous drugs and have numerous side-effects. Careful monitoring and regular blood counts are required with dose adjustments if necessary. The most important side-effects are:

- marrow toxicity, which is dose-related and reversible
- hair loss, usually more significant in transplant patients
- increased susceptibility to viral, fungal and bacterial infections, usually more significant in transplant patients
- increased risk of neoplasia, particularly lymphomas
- gastrointestinal disturbances
- cholestatic hepatotoxicity, which requires an immediate withdrawal of the drug.

Azathioprine should be used with caution in patients with severe bone marrow depression; it should not be started in pregnancy owing to possible teratogenic effects. The decision to continue therapy in pregnancy must be very carefully considered.

Interactions

Allopurinol inhibits the metabolism of azathioprine, thereby increasing its toxicity.

Important points

Azathioprine tablets should be taken after food to avoid gastrointestinal disturbances. The handling of azathioprine injections should follow the guidelines on the 'handling of cytotoxic drugs' (see p. 232). The contents of the vial should be reconstituted with Water for Injections to 15 ml. The solution is stable for 24 hours at room temperature (15–25°C). Any remaining solution should be discarded. Note and report any signs of infection, abnormal bleeding, jaundice, dark urine, clay-coloured stools. Advise patients on the importance of regular blood counts.

Corticosteroids

Corticosteroids (e.g. hydrocortisone and prednisolone) have multiple pharmacological properties (see Ch. 12). Corticosteroids are powerful immunosuppressants. They suppress the immune function of lymphocytes and interfere with both humoral and cell-mediated immune reactions. They are used to prevent organ transplant rejection, commonly in conjunction with other immunosuppressants. In autoimmune diseases they are used for their immunosuppressive and their anti-inflammatory effects.

Cyclosporin

Cyclosporin is a cyclical polypeptide (a complex protein-like substance, derived from a soil fungus). It mainly suppresses cell-mediated immune reactions by inhibition of T lymphocyte proliferation. Since the use of cyclosporin the number of successful organ transplantations has increased significantly. It is virtually non-myelotoxic and can therefore be used for bone marrow transplantations as well. It has no cytotoxic actions. Oral cyclosporin is also used for the treatment of severe psoriasis which is unresponsive to other forms of treatment.

Dosage and administration

Cyclosporin is available as an oral and parenteral preparation. Concentrate for infusion is used for initiation of therapy in organ and bone marrow transplantations usually one day before the operation and in the immediate follow-up period. Oral treatment should commence as soon as possible, depending on the patient's condition. The dosage for organ transplantations is initially 14–17.5 mg/kg daily, reduced over a period of months to a maintenance dose of 6–8 mg/kg daily. If corticosteroids are used at the same time, lower maintenance doses (5 mg/kg/day) can be used.

The dosage for bone marrow transplantations is initially 3–5 mg/kg daily by infusion followed by 12.5 mg/kg daily orally, which is slowly reduced after 6 months to zero or to a very low maintenance dose. Dosage levels may be adjusted with the aid of blood-level determinations.

Side-effects

The most important dose-related side-effect is its nephrotoxicity. Other side-effects are abnormalities in liver function, gum hypertrophy and gastric disturbances. Fluid retention, convulsions and hypertension occur more often in children than adults.

Interactions

Cyclosporin should not be given in conjunction with other potentially nephrotoxic drugs such as aminoglycosides. Ketoconazole can increase the plasma concentration of cyclosporin.

Important points

The total daily dose may be given as a single dose or in two divided doses. Oral solutions may be taken with milk, fruit juice or chocolate drink to mask the taste.

IMMUNOSTIMULANTS

The immunostimulant *Corynebacterium parvum* **vaccine** is used for the alleviation of malignant pleural effusions and malignant ascites. It is administered by intrapleural or intra-abdominal injection. Treatment should not be initiated in the first 10 days after thoracotomy and lung resection because of the possibility of systemic absorption.

INTERFERONS

Interferons (alpha, beta and gamma) are naturally occurring glycoproteins which have complex effects on the immune system.

Alpha interferons are used in the treatment of hairy-cell leukaemia, chronic myelogenous leukaemia, AIDS-related Kaposi's sarcoma and chronic active hepatitis B.

Interferons have become more readily available in recent years due to improved production methods involving biological 'engineering' techniques.

Administration

Interferons are available only as injections to be administered subcutaneously, intramuscularly or directly into the lesions of Kaposi's sarcoma.

Side-effects and cautions

The most frequently occurring side-effects are 'flu-like symptoms' which can be successfully treated with paracetamol. Alpha-interferons also have a suppressive effect on the bone marrow which can lead to leuco- and thrombocytopenia. Safety has not been established in children and therefore interferons are usually not recommended for use under the age of 18.

FURTHER READING

Bedford H 1993 Immunisation: facts and fiction. Health Visitor 66 (9): 314–316

Department of Health, Welsh Office, Scottish Office Home and Health Department, DHSS (Northern Ireland) 1992 Immunisation against infectious disease

16

Drug treatment of anaemias

ANATOMY AND PHYSIOLOGY

Blood consists of a pale yellow fluid called plasma in which red cells, white cells and platelets are suspended. These cellular components all develop in the bone marrow. The blood fulfils a multitude of purposes, the chief functions being the transport of oxygen and nutritional materials to all the cells of the body and the removal of carbon dioxide and waste materials. Oxygen is carried by haemoglobin contained in the red cells, while carbon dioxide is transported partly in the plasma and partly in the red cells.

The main control mechanism ensuring the maintenance of a constant circulating red cell mass is provided by erythropoietin, which is produced by the kidney in response to anoxia and acts on the bone marrow to increase the rate of cell division, cell maturation and haemoglobin synthesis. Abnormality of any of these factors may give rise to anaemia. Excessive blood loss or destruction of blood cells may also lead to anaemia. Anaemia may therefore be defined as a reduction in the normal amount of red cells or haemoglobin or both.

THE ANAEMIAS

The types of anaemia most often encountered are iron-deficiency anaemia and megaloblastic anaemia.

Other conditions of the blood include anaemia associated with chronic renal failure, iron overload, aplastic anaemia and haemolytic anaemia.

IRON-DEFICIENCY ANAEMIA

Iron is an essential constituent of haemoglobin. When red cells break down the iron is retained by the body and utilised in the formation of further haemoglobin. In health, the loss of iron from the body is 1–2 mg, which is replaced by absorption from a dietary intake of 10–20 mg. The main causes of iron-deficiency anaemia are:

- chronic blood loss
      profuse menstruation
      disease of the gastrointestinal tract – ulceration, carcinoma, hiatus hernia, bleeding haemorrhoids
      drug-induced – aspirin, non-steroidal anti-inflammatory drugs
- increased requirements
      pregnancy
      breast-feeding
- malabsorption
- dietary deficiency.

Iron is absorbed as the ferrous salt in the duodenum and upper small intestine. It is carried to the bone marrow for the synthesis of haemoglobin. About 70% of the total body iron is present in erythrocyte haemoglobin. The remainder is stored in the liver, spleen and bone marrow. The absorption of iron is carefully regulated so that just enough is absorbed to make good any deficiency.

Oral iron

Iron is usually given orally to correct a deficiency. The following formulations are available:

- ferrous salts in liquid and solid oral dose, including controlled release preparations
- formulations containing both ferrous sulphate and folic acid for use in pregnancy
- formulations containing vitamins and minerals in addition to ferrous sulphate.

The daily dose of elemental iron should be 150–300 mg. The choice is dependent on efficacy, side-effects and cost.

Efficacy

Absorption of a soluble ferrous salt occurs in the upper part of the small intestine where the pH is lower; at higher pH levels, ferrous phosphates form which are not suitable. The efficacy of an iron preparation depends on how much of its iron content is released in this part of the gastrointestinal tract. Fluids and solid oral dose preparations are preferable to controlled-release preparations since the latter may release only a proportion of iron in the area where absorption takes place. Some inhibition of iron absorption can occur if it is taken with milk, tea or eggs.

Side-effects

Patient acceptability may be influenced by adverse effects. Gastrointestinal disturbances, including nausea, abdominal discomfort, diarrhoea or constipation may occur. The nausea may be reduced by taking the iron preparation after food. Patients should be advised of the possibility of these side-effects and also that iron causes discolouration of the stool.

Cost

Controlled release and liquid preparations are more expensive than simple tablet and capsule forms. Ferrous sulphate 200 mg ($\equiv$ 60 mg elemental iron) three times daily provides an effective dose which is relatively inexpensive.

Where gastrointestinal disturbances cause difficulties, the dose may be reduced or a change to ferrous gluconate or ferrous fumarate may help. In the prevention of iron deficiency in pregnancy, a formulation containing folic acid as well as ferrous sulphate acts as a prophylactic against megaloblastic anaemia of pregnancy.

Treatment of iron deficiency should be continued for 3 months after the blood haemoglobin has returned to normal in order to replace depleted iron stores. Extra encouragement may have to be given to ensure that the patient completes the course of treatment.

Interactions

Iron salts should not be given with tetracyclines as the absorption of both drugs is impaired. Antacids and penicillin can also impair the absorption of iron.

Parenteral iron therapy

When oral iron cannot be tolerated in any form, or there is malabsorption of iron, it may be necessary to give the iron by injection. Iron injections by-pass the mechanism which controls the degree of iron absorption and the dose must be based on the actual iron deficiency as calculated from laboratory test results. Iron sorbitol injection and iron dextran injection are given by *deep* intramuscular injection using the Z-track technique to prevent leakage along the needle track and subsequent staining of the skin. Iron dextran injection may also be administered by slow intravenous infusion over 6–8 hours. As a severe allergic reaction can take place, a test dose is essential prior to giving the infusion. The patient should be kept under close observation for the duration of the infusion and for 1 hour after completion. A nurse should stay at the bedside during this time to observe the patient, make frequent recordings of the pulse rate and summon medical assistance if indicated. It is important to try not to create undue alarm in so doing. There is no significant difference in the rate of haemoglobin response to injectable iron compared with oral iron, i.e. a rapid cure of anaemia cannot be effected by use of the injectable route.

MEGALOBLASTIC ANAEMIA

Both vitamin B_{12} and folate are necessary for the production of mature red blood cells. A deficiency of either will result in megaloblastic anaemia. The main causes are:

- vitamin B_{12} deficiency
    malabsorption
        pernicious anaemia
        gastrectomy
    inadequate intake of vitamin B_{12}
        veganism
- folate deficiency
    malabsorption
        coeliac disease
    increased demands
        pregnancy and lactation
        malignancy and chronic inflammatory diseases
        haemolytic diseases
    drugs
        anticonvulsants, including phenytoin and phenobarbitone
        dihydroxyfolate reductase inhibitors, e.g. methotrexate, triamterene, trimethoprim, pyrimethamine
    inadequate intake of folate
        dietary deficiency.

Pernicious anaemia

A deficiency of vitamin B_{12} results in a condition termed pernicious anaemia in which the mature red cells are irregular in shape and size, and reduced in number. The cause of pernicious anaemia is a deficiency in the production of the so-called intrinsic factor, a protein normally secreted by the stomach, and essential for the satisfactory absorption of vitamin B_{12} in the terminal ileum. In addition to the megaloblastic anaemia, a deficiency of vitamin B_{12} leads to degenerative changes in the nervous system which, if untreated, ultimately render the patient immobile.

The diagnosis of pernicious anaemia is confirmed by the Schilling test, a dual isotope test which confirms malabsorption of vitamin B_{12}. The test involves fasting the patient overnight, asking him to empty his bladder in the morning and discarding the urine. Two capsules of radioactive vitamin B_{12} are given to the patient to swallow with as little water as possible and the patient fasts for a further 2 hours. Hydroxocobalamin 1 mg is then given intramuscularly. A 24-hour urine collection is obtained from the time the capsules were taken. It is essential that the collection is complete. In health, radioactive vitamin B_{12} would be absorbed into the gut and excess to requirements (15–40%) would be excreted in the urine. In pernicious anaemia, radioactive vitamin B_{12} is *not* absorbed and therefore passes in the stools instead of the urine (less than 3%).

Hydroxocobalamin is the form of vitamin B_{12} which is now used. Initial treatment is 1 mg by intramuscular injection repeated at intervals of 2–3 days until a total dose of 5 mg has been given. A course of oral iron may be required to supply the increased number of mature red cells. Thereafter the maintenance dose of hydroxocobalamin is 1 mg every 3 months. Unless it is caused by dietary insufficiency, the lack of vitamin B_{12} in pernicious anaemia is permanent, and therefore replacement therapy must be parenteral and for life. Consequently, education of the patient/relative is important.

Folate deficiency

Most causes of folate deficiency will yield to a course of treatment comprising 5 mg by mouth daily for 4 months. A daily dose of 10 or 15 mg may be necessary where malabsorption occurs. Where megaloblastic anaemia is due to dihydroxyfolate reductase inhibitors, the conversion of folic acid to its active metabolites is inhibited. Folic acid will therefore not be effective; folinic acid may be used, 15 mg orally once daily.

Folate deficiency may occur in pregnancy, and prophylactic folic acid/iron combinations can be given. The level of folic acid in these preparations is insufficient to treat megaloblastic anaemia.

ANAEMIA ASSOCIATED WITH CHRONIC RENAL FAILURE

Erythropoietin is used for the management of severe anaemia associated with chronic renal failure. It can be administered by subcutaneous or intravenous injection. Careful monitoring of ferritin levels and blood pressure is required. If there is a deficiency of iron or folate this should be corrected.

IRON OVERLOAD

Iron overload may occur as a result of repeated blood transfusions to treat haemolytic anaemias. Desferrioxamine is used to reduce the iron level. It is a powerful iron-chelating agent which is given by subcutaneous infusions (20–40 mg/kg) or through the infusion line at the time of blood transfusion. Desferrioxamine is also used to treat acute toxicity usually seen in children who have swallowed iron tablets in mistake for sweets. The result of the ingestion of large quantities of iron tablets is severe necrotising gastritis with vomiting, haemorrhage and diarrhoea followed by circulatory collapse.

APLASTIC AND HAEMOLYTIC ANAEMIAS

Aplastic or hypoplastic anaemia is caused by depression of the bone marrow. This may affect the formation and development of the red cells, leucocytes or platelets. Anabolic steroids such as oxymetholone have been used to treat aplastic anaemia, but their effectiveness is unclear although they appear to benefit certain patients. A dose of 2–3 mg/kg is given daily for at least 3–6 months. Virilising effects are seen in females and in children.

Anaemias caused by excessive destruction of red blood cells are termed haemolytic anaemias. They are due either to the breakdown of red blood cells which are defective or to the effects of poisons or infection. Corticosteroids have an important place in the management of autoimmune haemolytic anaemia.

17

Nutrition and vitamins

BACKGROUND

Since the late 1970s there has been an increasing awareness of the requirements for nutritional support. The King's Fund report, *A Positive Approach to Nutrition as Treatment* (1992), is a comprehensive and helpful document which highlights current deficiencies in care and outlines the rationale and standards for both parenteral and enteral nutritional support. It is now well established that people who are ill can greatly benefit from well-managed nutritional support. Team working is the key to the success of this aspect of patient care. Within the nutritional support team, medical, surgical, nursing, dietetic and pharmaceutical skills must be available if patients are to receive high-standard, cost-effective therapy.

PHYSIOLOGY

The body has only limited reserves of immediately available energy and nitrogen sources. In the absence of adequate food ingestion, energy is derived from stores of glycogen in the liver, from muscle protein, and from fat in adipose tissue. However, glycogen stores are limited and are exhausted within the first 24 hours of starvation. Over the next few days muscle protein is broken down to provide glucose. In more prolonged starvation, fat is used to provide the energy source, and the brain adapts to utilise ketone bodies. When the fat stores have been utilised, accelerated protein breakdown resumes and leads eventually to death.

NUTRITIONAL SUPPORT

The aim of nutritional support is to arrest catabolism due to these losses and to restore the patient to a positive nitrogen balance. This can be accomplished by administering calories, nitrogen, fluid, electrolytes, vitamins and trace elements. Increasingly, the place of nutritional support is being recognised. Advances in the management of severe illness and trauma have meant that more patients survive the initial phase of their illness and require continuing supportive treatment. This involves the administration of appropriate fluids, electrolytes and nutritional requirements.

Protein

If nutrition is deficient, not only does the patient lose weight by the loss of skeletal muscle, but also tissue repair and immune mechanisms are significantly inhibited as these processes require active cell turnover and therefore new protein formation. Amino acids are building blocks of protein. They can be divided into two groups: essential amino acids and non-essential amino acids. It is necessary that nutrition solutions contain a balanced content of essential amino acids and a broad spectrum of non-essential amino acids.

Energy

Energy is provided as carbohydrate or fat.

Electrolytes and trace elements

Sufficient quantities of electrolytes and trace elements must be given, not only for maintenance, but also to replace any significant losses. The action of each is summarised below:

sodium
    predominant cation in extracellular fluid
    maintains integrity of cell membrane along with potassium
potassium
    major intracellular cation
    required for transport of glucose across cell membrane

calcium
    continuous supply necessary to form and maintain skeleton, and to maintain homeostasis in nerve and muscle tissue
magnesium
    important factor in many enzyme reactions
iron
    required for haemoglobin synthesis
copper
    involved in release of iron from liver
zinc
    essential for many enzyme reactions
cobalt
    essential constituent of vitamin B_{12}
manganese
    involved in calcium and phosphorus metabolism
iodine
    required in synthesis of thyroid hormones
fluoride
    required for maintenance of skeleton
chromium
    deficiency leads to glucose intolerance.

Vitamins

All vitamins can be supplied by parenteral and enteral feeding regimens.

NUTRITIONAL ASSESSMENT

Nutritional support must be designed to suit the particular metabolic and nutritional needs of each individual. Careful assessment of the patient's nutritional state is required before the decision to use a particular product is made. This is normally carried out by the dietitian who will obtain information from a variety of sources, including the patient, relatives, doctor and nursing staff. Close liaison between dietetic, medical and nursing staff is important.

Methods for building up a profile of the nutritional status of a patient include the following:

- clinical examination
- body weight and height – particularly recent changes in body weight

- dietary history
    social, economic factors
    eating habits
    diminished food intake
    changes due to recent disease or ill health
- measurement of skinfold thickness
- biochemical assessment.

Nursing responsibility will encompass the measuring of height and weight, collection of urine samples, making specific enquiry about recent weight loss and current dietary intake, and visually assessing the patient. Where there is a nutritional team, they may undertake other anthropometric measurements and collection of blood samples.

NUTRITIONAL THERAPY

Once the nutritional status of the patient has been assessed, it is necessary to decide what nutritional support, if any, should be given. Nutrition that is introduced directly into the gastrointestinal tract is known as enteral nutrition. The administration of nutrients by a route other than through the gastrointestinal tract is referred to as parenteral nutrition. The usual method of administration, in this case, is intravenously. However, a patient unable to tolerate a normal diet does not necessarily require parenteral nutrition. Where there is a functioning small bowel, nutritional requirements can be met by the enteral route either by:

- manipulating the diet, or
- supplementing the diet, e.g. with supplementary drinks, sip feeds, with the aid of specialised tube feeds, given via a fine-bore nasogastric tube, gastrostomy or jejunostomy feeding tube.

Enteral nutrition is preferable to parenteral nutrition as it is more physiological, is safer, and is more cost-effective, but it is not always possible to administer enteral nutrition safely. Where the small bowel is not functioning adequately parenteral nutrition may be considered.

ENTERAL TUBE FEEDING

Administration of enteral nutrition via a tube is commonly used in the nutritional management of the critically ill, the debilitated, and in those who are unable to swallow but who have a functioning small intestine. Tube feeding may be carried out using the nasogastric, nasoduodenal, gastrostomy or jejunostomy routes. Liquid feeds can be introduced directly into the stomach or intestine via the tube. Many manufacturers have now designed comfortable, durable tubes which are compatible with the present enteral feed administration systems.

Nasogastric tube feeding

This has been the most widely used approach. In the past it was standard practice to pass a Ryle's tube into the stomach. However, this tube was poorly tolerated and the incidence of side-effects was high. When used for feeding, these tubes increase the risk of gastric reflux and aspiration. Pharyngitis, otitis, and nasal, pharyngeal, oesophageal and gastric mucosal erosions may occur. The fine-bore nasogastric tube has reduced these problems. However, since there is now such a wide range of systems available, it is advisable to seek the advice of the dietitian and nutrition nurse specialist.

The importance of ensuring correct positioning of a nasogastric tube cannot be over-emphasised. Confirmation that the tube is not kinked and is in the stomach rather than in the oesophagus or lung must be made before starting a feed, using one of the following methods:

- aspirating the stomach contents and testing with pH indicating paper
- syringing a small amount of air down the tube and at the same time listening over the epigastrium with a stethoscope.

X-ray confirmation is time-consuming and costly, and so it is now used only for certain categories of patient, for example, the unconscious, or where neither gastric position nor misplacement has been confirmed by the above two tests. In the comatosed, drowsy or restless patient the tube position should be checked more frequently, according to local hospital policy. In the event of the tube becoming partially withdrawn, no attempt should be made to push it back down as there is a danger of the tube becoming kinked or entering the lungs. The tube should be completely removed and a fresh tube passed.

In the acutely ill or unconscious patient it is important to establish that the stomach is emptying. This is an important precaution to take and can prevent potential hazards such as vomiting or gastric reflux which may lead to aspiration pneumonia. It is also important that the volume of feed given is increased gradually, particularly in patients who have received nothing via their gut for several days, in order to prevent gastrointestinal side-effects.

Regular aspiration of gastric contents is especially important for patients receiving intensive care, for the unconscious and for those on drug therapy which may interfere with absorption. Absorption can be assumed if there is little or no aspirate, abdominal distension or nausea, and where bowel sounds are normal. Gastric emptying can be enhanced and gastric reflux minimised by raising the head of the bed while feeding.

The availability of nutritional preparations, diverse in composition and nutrient ratios, permits the selection of a feed to meet the specific requirements of the patient. Manufactured polymeric feeds generally suit most tube-fed patients. Compared to hospital made feeds, they are sterile until opened, their composition is known and constant, and they are more convenient.

To reduce the risk of bacterial contamination correct preparation and storage of feeds are necessary. All individually prepared feeds should be refrigerated at 4°C until required for use. The feeds must be clearly labelled to indicate the date and time by which they must be used. To minimise the risk of growth of microorganisms, hospital-made feeds should be administered within 4–6 hours of hanging, and aseptically administered sterile feeds within 12–24 hours. Reservoirs and administration sets should be renewed once every 24 hours. Regular bacteriological testing of the feeds should also be carried out, i.e. quality control procedures should be introduced both in the diet kitchen and at ward level.

Tube feed regimen

Nausea and abdominal distension may be induced if the feed is administered too quickly. Continuous administration can minimise this problem, using either gravity drip or pump-assisted feeding. Continuous drip administration also minimises the risk of diarrhoea which may result from administering bolus feeds, particularly if the feed is hyperosmolar. Pump-assisted feeding will help patients who have some impairment of gastrointestinal function, as the flow rate can be controlled to meet their absorptive capacity.

Whatever method of feeding is used, accurate entries should be made on the patient's fluid balance chart and a record kept of the patient's tolerance of the feed. 'Today's feed tolerance will influence tomorrow's feeding regimen.' Doctors and nurses require access to details of the daily regimen, which has been worked out for each patient, including:

- a breakdown of energy, protein, electrolyte values, vitamins and minerals
- the total volume
- instructions regarding the volume of feed to be given per hour and how many hours in a 24-hour period the feed is to be administered.

The nurse has a considerable contribution to make to the care of the patient fed by tube. She is involved in:

- assisting in the assessment of the patient's nutritional state
- communicating with dietetic and medical staff
- storing feeds appropriately
- initiating and supervising the feed
- observing the patient, for example, respiratory difficulty, tolerance of the feed

- providing the patient with encouragement
- keeping accurate records.

Administration of medicines via enteral feeding tube

Enteral feeding tubes may be used as an alternative route for the administration of medicines. When prescribed by this route, medicines are administered in the form of a solution, suspension or emulsion. If the drug is not normally available in a liquid form the pharmacist should be consulted for advice and assistance. It may be possible for a liquid form of the drug to be prepared in the pharmacy using a suitable formulation that takes account of the properties of the drug, such as stability in an aqueous form.

Crushing of tablets into the necessary fine powder cannot be achieved satisfactorily on the ward. If tablets are insufficiently powdered there is a risk of the tube being blocked with consequent risk of under-dosage. It should be borne in mind that some solid-dose forms cannot be crushed, even to give a coarse powder. In some cases the crushing of a tablet may destroy the essential properties of the product.

Apart from using an oral liquid it may be acceptable to administer the injectable form of the drug via the enteral feeding tube. If this procedure is adopted, clear instruction must be given by the prescriber on the patient's drug prescription sheet. The pharmacist must first be consulted to ensure that the procedure is satisfactory and that there is no suitable alternative.

Adding a medicine to a feed is not recommended as chemical or physical interaction may adversely affect the drug, the feed or both. An unknown quantity of the drug may be lost if the food is altered or some is lost due to spillage or leakage from the delivery system.

The standard procedure for checking the position of the tube must be followed before administering medicines via the tube. Prior to and following the administration of each medication, a volume of water (20–30 ml) should be instilled. This will minimise the risk of tube blockage, and ensure that the medicine has passed through the tube and into the stomach.

Administration of continuous nasogastric feeding using a fine-bore tube

This is outlined in Box 17.1.

Box 17.1 Administration of continuous nasogastric feeding using a fine-bore tube	
Documentation	Feed prescription sheet
The medicine	Feed in feed container
The environment	Patient seated or in bed; warmth, comfort, privacy (if preferred)
The nurse and the patient	Patient identified; explanation given to patient
Technique	Nurse ensures that hands are thoroughly washed before and after feed; feeding set connected to feed; feed run through to expel air; correct position of tube confirmed by: auscultation aspiration of stomach contents (turns blue litmus paper pink) tube flushed with 20 – 30 ml water; feeding set connected to tube; flow and volume of feed regulated as per feed prescription; feed recorded
Hazards	Aspiration pneumonia

Throughout the ongoing administration of the feed the nurse's responsibilities are as follows:

Checking the position of the tube
Prior to commencing each feed the position of the tube should be checked.
If the patient is restless or comatose, it is recommended that the tube position be checked more frequently.

(If the tube starts to protrude, even as little as 1 cm, it should be removed and a fresh one passed. A partially removed tube must NEVER be pushed back down.)
Maintaining the flow of the feed
The flow rate should be checked hourly or more frequently as instructed.
If the rate of flow becomes sluggish, the tube and feed set should be checked to ensure they are functioning properly:
If the fault is in the tube, it can be flushed through with luke-warm water.

If the fault is in the administration set, it should be disconnected and replaced.

Keeping the tube patent

20–30 ml water should be instilled through the feeding tube between each feed container change, and before and after each dose of medication to reduce the risk of occlusion caused by feed or build up of drug deposits.

When the feed is stopped (e.g. X-ray visit) and on completion of a feed, the tube must be flushed with 20–30 ml of water and plugged/capped. This will trap a column of water in the tube, reducing risk of blockage.

Minimising risk of infection

The feed container and feeding set should be changed at least once every 24 hours.

Keeping accurate records

The following records must be maintained:

    feed prescription
    fluid balance chart
    nursing care plan and progress notes

Providing nursing care as required

    Assisting with the activities of living
    Special attention to oral hygiene

Reporting abnormalities

Gastrostomy/jejunostomy tube feeding

Gastrostomy and jejunostomy also give access to the gastrointestinal tract as routes for long-term feeding or for those patients with upper gastrointestinal dysfunction but who have a functioning small bowel.

PARENTERAL NUTRITION

This method of nutritional support should be used only to prevent or correct malnutrition when no other route for the administration of nutrients is available. The intravenous route is the one referred to in this text.

Indications

The indications for parenteral nutrition are:

- postoperative – when complications prevent a return to oral intake, e.g. prolonged postoperative ileus, sepsis or fistulae
- extensive burns where nutritional requirements cannot be met enterally
- where there is impairment of intestinal mobility and/or absorption of nutrients, e.g. chronic gastrointestinal tract disease – Crohn's disease, pancreatitis, short bowel syndrome
- premature infants – where functional immaturity causes intestinal failure or difficulty in establishing oral or tube feeding.

Intravenous (i.v.) nutrition solutions

Protein is supplied by solutions of crystalline amino acids.

Glucose, which provides 16.8 kj (4 kcal) per gram, is the best carbohydrate for intravenous use, but glucose solutions of high calorific value are hypertonic and must be infused via a central vein to provide rapid dilution. This minimises the risk of vein thrombosis which can occur if these hypertonic solutions are infused peripherally. Where glucose intolerance occurs insulin may be required and blood glucose levels should be monitored.

Fat emulsion in the form of a lipid solution of, for example, Intralipid or Lipofundin, may also be used as an energy source, providing 37.8 kj (9 kcal) per gram. Lipid is also used as a source of essential fatty acids and a medium for giving fat-soluble vitamins. Lipid should not be used as the sole caloric source. The fat emulsion is hypotonic and can be infused by peripheral vein. In neonates the nutrients can be continuously infused along with fat emulsion via a peripheral vein. Peripheral vein feeding can be carried out in adults where fat emulsions are incorporated using the 3-litre bag, commonly named the 'Big Bag' system.

Electrolyte levels in intravenous solutions vary according to the individual requirements of the patient. Sodium, potassium, calcium, magnesium and phosphate are added to the nutrient solutions. Sodium acetate, a bicarbonate precursor, is incorporated to regulate the acid–base balance. It is necessary to incorporate trace elements into the intravenous admixture.

All vitamins can be supplied intravenously. Fat-soluble vitamins A, D, E and K are available in commercial preparations. Commercial water-soluble vitamin preparations for addition to intravenous nutrition solutions contain some or all of the following: ascorbic acid, thiamine, riboflavine, niacin, pyridoxine, pantothenic acid, vitamin B_{12}, folic acid and biotin.

Preparation of intravenous nutrition solutions

Standard total parenteral nutrition formulations may be acceptable for many patients because of the kidney's ability to maintain homeostasis. No single parenteral regimen would be ideal for all patients because of the wide variety of pathology and differing age groups, or for the same patient throughout. The composition of the solution requires to be determined from day to day by clinical and chemical monitoring. Figure 17.1 shows an example of an intravenous nutrition prescription sheet. The patient's details are filled in by the prescriber along with the date, day of prescription, duration of prescription, volume of amino acids and glucose solutions, quantities of electrolytes and other additives.

The advantages of using a system where the i.v. nutrition is provided in a 3-litre bag are:

- risk of contamination by frequent bottle changes and the use of airways and connections is minimised
- requires changing only once in 24 hours and therefore staff time is saved
- amino acids and calorie source are delivered simultaneously, thus spreading the dextrose load over 24 hours so that the incidence of glycosuria is reduced.

The intravenous admixtures should be prepared in the pharmacy, as pharmaceutical calculations, drug stability incompatabilities, solubility and sterility are important factors. The ward preparation room is an unsuitable location for aseptic procedures, which are better carried out in the aseptic suite within the pharmacy department.

Regular checks of airborne contamination by particle counts and settle plates must be carried out. The operations must follow a set procedure for scrubbing up and donning clean room clothing.

The solutions and equipment should be assembled on a tray in a preparation room and then passed through a hatch into the aseptic suite. Double doors on the hatch maintain the integrity of the aseptic suite. The manipulations should be carried out under a laminar flow hood in which a constant supply of filtered air passes over and around the assembled items.

Admixtures should be carried out in the centre of the screen, well inside the outer edge of the work surface. Interruptions to air flow should be guarded against.

The amino acids and glucose solutions are run into a 3-litre ethyl vinyl acetate pack. Additions of vitamins, electrolytes and other small volume components are made by injecting through an additive port. The lipid source is run in last.

Incompatibilities

It is essential that potential incompatibilities or the degradation rate of certain additive drugs in the presence of others are taken into consideration. Incompatibilities can usually be avoided or corrected. For example:

- insulin is unstable in the presence of bicarbonate
- insoluble carbonates may form if bicarbonate is added to calcium or magnesium; it is simpler to use a bicarbonate precursor such as sodium acetate
- vitamins are unstable in hypertonic intravenous solutions, especially in the presence of light.

The reaction can be slowed by using a freshly prepared solution and protecting it from bright light. It is essential that the solution be examined prior to setting up, and during the infusion, as precipitate may appear after a few hours. Pharmacists are aware that the fat emulsion may 'crack', especially if there are high levels of electrolytes, in particular calcium and magne-

CONSULTANT Dr. Smith	PATIENT'S NAME JANE BROWN	UNIT NO. 342907
HOSPITAL VICTORIA WARD 7	DATE OF BIRTH 9.9.32	WEIGHT 54 kg

Date _____ Day _____ of Intravenous Nutrition

Infusion Rate ___100___ ml per hr   over ___20___ hours   & then _____ mls for _____ hours

Solution Requested	Volume Requested
Amino Acids Vamin 9 Glucose	1000 ml.
Glucose 20 %w/v	500 ml.
Fat Emulsion 20 %w/v	500 ml.
Basic Volume before Additives =	2000 ml.

Solution Supplied	Volume Supplied
Amino Acids V9G	1000 ml.
Glucose 20 %w/v	500 ml.
Fat Emulsion 20 %w/v	500 ml.
Basic Volume before Additives =	2000 ml.

Ionic Requirement

Ion	m.mol., 24 hrs.	In form of	Vol. Added	Prep. Added
Acetate	42.5	Sodium Acetate	10.6 ml	4 mmol/ml
Sodium	100	Sodium Chloride	/	
Phosphate	10	Addiphos	5 ml	Addiphos
Potassium	70	Potassium Chloride	15.9 ml	20%
Calcium	7.5	Calcium Gluconate	22.4 ml	10%
Magnesium	6	Magnesium Sulphate	11 ml	10%
Zinc	0.1	Zinc Sulphate	/	
Chloride	From fluid & electrolytes = 97.5 mmol.

NUTRITIONAL INFORMATION

Nitrogen (g) =	9.4
Protein Equivalent (g) =	59
Non Protein Calories =	1800
Total Calories =	2050

...1... vials Solivito N	1 vial	
...10... ml. Trace Element	10 ml	Additrace
...10... ml. Vitlipid N Adult	10 ml	
7500u Heparin	1.5 ml	5000u/ml
....		

Total Volume Supplied 2086 ml.

Prescribed by:- G. Wilson

(Consultant/Snr Registrar)

001.013

Figure 17.1   Intravenous nutrition prescription sheet.

sium, in the bag. If calcium and phosphate are present above a certain level, a precipitate of calcium phosphate may form, particularly if the solution has been stored in the refrigerator.

Intravenous nutrition and the administration system should not be used as a means of administering drugs. In addition to the risk of contamination, many chemical changes can occur. For example, penicillins are rapidly degraded in amino acid solutions, and tetracyclines from insoluble complexes with calcium and magnesium.

Administration of intravenous nutrition

Insertion of a central line

Intravenous nutrition is normally administered through a central vein, preferably the superior vena cava. The vein may be approached via the subclavian vein, the jugular vein, the upper cephalic vein or the antecubital fossa-basilic vein. The central venous line (CVL) should be inserted by a doctor experienced in the technique. The CVL is inserted using full aseptic surgical technique and under local or general anaesthetic, preferably in theatre.

Assistance is required to position the patient optimally, that is, lying flat with a rolled-up towel between the scapulae and with the patient's head turned away from the proposed insertion site.

The skin is prepared by cleansing with chlorhexidine 0.5% in spirit or by povidone-iodine. The administration set is primed using sodium chloride 0.9% w/v. An intravenous infusion pump is made available.

The CVL should be taken through a subcutaneous tunnel, about 10–12 cm (4–5 inches) across the chest wall. A skin tunnel separates the skin entry site from the venepuncture site, enabling the skin site dressing to remain more intact and thus minimise the incidence of sepsis. Once the CVL is sited, patency is maintained by either:

- 'heplocking', i.e. instilling 5 ml of heparinised saline and capping the line, or

- connecting the administration set and allowing the clear infusion solution to infuse slowly.

A suitable occlusive dressing is then applied to the skin site.

The position of the CVL tip is always confirmed by a chest X-ray, which should also be examined for a pneumothorax.

Peripheral intravenous nutrition

Peripheral intravenous nutrition is suitable for patients requiring up to 7 days' intravenous nutrition. The peripheral cannula must also be inserted following strict skin cleansing and an aseptic insertion technique.

The care of both the central venous and the peripheral venous line used with i.v. nutrition should be meticulous. Responsibility for the care of the line is a combined one between medical and trained nursing staff, the overall aim being that no harm should come to the patient. The nurse's role is to explain to the patient what is involved and to try to reassure him. It is essential therefore that the nurse is fully conversant with the procedure and associated care.

Complications of intravenous nutrition

The major complications associated with i.v. nutrition include:

- complications at line insertion
- sepsis
- CVL blockage
- air embolism
- phlebitis
- thrombosis
- metabolic complications associated with the nutrients
- mechanical problems
- psychological problems.

It is therefore important that protocols and procedures are designed to minimise the risk of such complications. Key factors in the prevention of complications are:

- meticulous aseptic handwashing
- strict attention to aseptic procedures
- adherence to hospital protocol for care
- staff who are:
    knowledgeable
    competent.

Care of the patient receiving intravenous nutrition

Patients receiving i.v. nutrition should be closely observed for the early detection of complications. Urinalysis should be performed every 4–6 hours to note the presence of glucose or ketone bodies. A 24-hour urine collection for measurement of urea level is used to estimate the nitrogen balance. The patient should be weighed regularly (e.g. twice weekly). Four-hourly recordings of temperature and pulse are made, and the character of the respirations observed. Accurate recordings of the intake and output of fluid must be kept. Care must be taken to maintain accuracy of fluid recordings, especially on completion of one chart and the commencement of the next (e.g. at midnight). Regular checks should be made to ensure that the prescribed rate of infusion is being maintained and that sufficient volume of feed remains in the infusion pack.

Transparent dressings allow for easy visualisation of the CVL insertion site; any evidence of swelling, discolouration or pain should be reported at once.

No medications should be added to any part of the system nor should it be used for blood sampling or central venous pressure monitoring.

A special cover can be obtained for placing over the 3-litre bag to protect the feed from strong sunlight. Administration sets made of ultraviolet absorbent material are also available.

The nurse has a vital role, not only in minimising the entry of microorganisms, but also in vigilant monitoring of the rate of the infusion. Three-litre bags must be used in conjunction with some form of infusion pump. This is not a substitute for frequent checking and, if necessary, making minor adjustments to the infusion rate. No attempt should be made to 'catch up' if the infusion is behind time.

The patient receiving nutritional support may be malnourished and/or debilitated to some degree. This patient requires much encouragement. General physical care increases in importance, including skin care, mouth care and exercise within the limitations of the infusion system and/or his clinical condition. Bowel activity, which may be reduced, should be carefully noted.

Changing the infusion pack

Accurate identification of the patient is essential. Details on the pack must be compared carefully with the prescription. The infusion solution should be checked to ensure that it is not out of date, that the solution is free from precipitate and that there is no evidence of the bag having been damaged, rendering it unsterile.

Care is needed to connect up the new infusion bag as an aseptic procedure. This can be achieved by thorough handwashing and careful introduction of the administration set into the infusion pack. Utmost care should be taken to avoid perforating the bag. The administration set must be free of air bubbles before setting the rate controller and starting the infusion. A record of the new pack, batch number, and starting time is made and initialled by the nurse(s) involved. The volume of solution which has been administered is recorded on the patient's fluid balance chart.

Changing the administration set

The intravenous infusion tubing should be changed to the level of the hub of the CVL every 24 hours at the time the infusion pack is changed in order to minimise the growth of microorganisms. This aseptic procedure is performed by a doctor assisted by a nurse or, in most centres, by a specially trained nurse. For all tubing changes, meticulous aseptic technique is required. All connections of the intravenous system should be made secure to prevent air embolism.

The site dressing

Transparent dressings need be removed only if there is local redness, swelling or other evidence of infection, or if the dressing starts to detach itself from the skin. Otherwise these dressings are normally changed once a week. If an extension piece is in use, this should be changed weekly along with the dressing.

Conventional dressings should be changed approximately every second day, and this may be carried out at the same time as the tubing is changed. A standard surgical dressing technique is used, but extra precautions are required in respect of skin care. The skin area is cleansed using sodium chloride solution 0.9%, then disinfected using, e.g. chlorhexidine 0.5% in spirit. The CVL should also be swabbed from skin site to hub with chlorhexidine 0.5% in spirit. The site is allowed to 'air dry'. An airtight dressing is applied, with the patient's head turned away and the arm abducted to allow movement to be unrestricted and the dressing to adhere firmly to the skin.

Removal of the central venous line

Central venous line removal carries with it the risk of air embolism and sepsis. The procedure is carried out by a doctor assisted by a nurse, or, specially trained nurse. The patient should be in the recumbent position. The CVL is shut off by means of the control clip (with the intravenous system always left connected) or by capping the end.

The site is cleaned with isopropyl alcohol or chlorhexidine 0.5% in spirit. The suture securing the CVL is cut and while the patient performs the Valsalva manoeuvre, the CVL is removed with care. (The Valsalva manoeuvre is used to increase thoracic pressure so that venous return to the heart is momentarily reduced, and is achieved by a forced expiration with the mouth and nose closed.)

Care should be taken to ensure that the entire length of the CVL has been removed. The puncture site should be covered immediately with a sterile airtight dressing and pressure applied. The area should be kept covered for 12–24 hours. The tip of the CVL is cut off using sterile scissors and sent to the microbiology department for culture studies.

Intravenous nutrition at home

An increasing number of patients who have had, e.g. small-bowel resection with resulting short bowel syndrome, require long-term intravenous nutrition. This may be carried out at home, if it is anticipated that more than 3 months' i.v. nutrition will be required. Thorough training is given to the patient and spouse or parent, as appropriate. This will take 2–4 weeks. Nutritional requirements are supplied by the pharmacy in pre-assembled packs. Other stores/supplies are delivered every 4 weeks. An infusion pump, trolley, refrigerator and intravenous stand can be loaned by commercial companies who specialise in home-care delivery systems. The patient's home needs to have suitable facilities for the management of an aseptic infusion system at home, e.g. suitable worktop surface, adequate handwashing and storage facilities, telephone. If necessary, these requirements should be made available through the occupational therapy and social work departments.

The patient reports to hospital on a regular basis in order that checks can be carried out and, where necessary, the nutritional components altered. The patient must be supplied with a 24-hour contact in case of requiring advice or emergency help. The general practitioner must be made aware of these developments and asked to be involved in shared care with the hospital consultant. Funding and finance is an important issue, and should be organised prior to the final decision regarding a patient going home on i.v. nutrition.

Summary

Safe intravenous nutrition has been developed by doctors, pharmacists, biochemists, microbiologists, nurses and nutrition experts. The role of the nurse in this form of therapy (whether undertaken in a specialist centre or in the patient's own home) continues to increase. Ideally, a senior nurse with specific responsibility for nutrition patients is appointed. A high standard of nursing care, including assessment of the patient, meticulous levels of hygiene, close observation, accu-

Table 17.1 Main features of vitamins

Vitamin	Sources	Function	Results of deficiency	Results of excess	Notes/clinical uses
A	Dairy products, e.g. milk, butter and cream. Also in fish liver oils. Can be formed in the body from carotene, a substance found in carrots, green vegetables and liver	Formation of rhodopsin, a pigment in some of the light-sensitive cells (rods) in the retina	Damage to skin and mucous membranes; corneal lesions; night blindness	Poisoning with vomiting and prostration, and over a longer period, painful swelling of bones. High levels may cause birth defects. Women who are, or may become, pregnant should be advised not to take vitamin A supplements except on medical advice. They should not eat liver or liver products	Deficiency in UK is rare
B_1 (thiamine)	Egg, liver, wheatgerm and some vegetables	Essential for certain stages of carbohydrate metabolism			Deficiency may occur in chronic alcoholism and is best treated by parenteral administration of vitamins B and C. Recommended that: use is restricted to essential i.v. injection is administered slowly (over 10 minutes) facilities for treating anaphylaxis should be available Potentially serious allergic adverse reactions may occur during or shortly after administration
B_2 (riboflavine)	Same as vitamin B_1	Necessary for carbohydrate metabolism	Ulceration and infection of mucous membranes and skin		Deficiency only occurs with malnutrition
Nicotinamide	Animal and vegetable protein. Can be manufactured both by the body itself and by bacteria present in the gut		Pellagra		Deficiency rare except in general malnutrition
Pyridoxine		Necessary for metabolism of many amino acids	Peripheral neuropathy, convulsions and anaemia		Naturally-occurring deficiency rare in Britain. An acute deficiency may be induced by treatment with the antituberculous drug, isoniazid, which reacts chemically with pyridoxine thus neutralising any of the vitamin present in the body. Pyridoxine used to treat deficiency and is used in prophylaxis

Table 17.1 Cont'd

Vitamin	Sources	Function	Results of deficiency	Results of excess	Notes/clinical uses
B₁₂ (hydroxo-cobalamin)	See p. 269				
C (ascorbic acid)	Fresh fruit and vegetables	Essential for development of collagen, cartilage and bone, and is concerned in haemoglobin formation and tissue repair	Scurvy – characterised by subcutaneous haemorrhage		Scurvy now rare but mild deficiency states may occur during pregnancy and in patients on restricted diets, particularly the elderly
D (calciferol)	Derived mostly from the diet, especially fish, eggs and liver. Can also be formed in the skin under the influence of sunlight	To promote the absorption of calcium from the intestine	Rickets in children, osteomalacia in adults	Very serious toxic effects – widespread calcification of tissues, particularly in the kidney, severe muscular weakness and abdominal pain	Requirements greatest in childhood and during pregnancy and lactation. Deficiency may arise in some ethnic minority groups who have a poor vitamin intake and cover their skin. In most cases, treatment with the natural dietary vitamin (D₂ calciferol) is adequate. The hypocalcaemia of hypopara-thyroidism requires larger doses
E (tocopherol)	Wheat germ, soya-bean, lettuce and other green vegetables.		In young children with congenital cholestasis, abnormally low concentrations may be associated with neuromuscular abnormalities		Available synthetically as tocopherols. Little evidence to suggest oral supplements are essential in adults even where there is fat malabsorption secondary to cholestasis. Neuromuscular abnormalities caused in children respond only to parenteral vitamin E
K	Green leafy vegetables. Also produced by bacteria in the intestine	Essential to assist manufacture, by the liver, of prothrombin and factor VII, needed for coagulation of blood	Haemorrhage, bruising		True deficiency rare as intestinal bacteria synthesise it in quantity. In newborn, intestinal bacteria are absent and therefore they are commonly given phytomenadione (vitamin K₁) by injection. In adults, deficiency is associated with fat malabsorption from pancreatic disease or obstructive jaundice. Replacement therapy is given in form of menadiol. Oral anticoagulants such as warfarin inhibit the use of vitamin K, thus preventing manufacture of essential clotting factors. Vitamin K may thus be used as an antidote to warfarin if need be

rate recording and prompt reporting, is of fundamental importance. Where care at this level is assured, the maximum benefit to the patient of this technique, which may be life saving, is within reach.

VITAMINS

Vitamins are essential substances which are required in daily amounts ranging from micrograms to milligrams for growth, development and maintenance of the body. Many of them are involved in the control of the body's metabolic processes through participation in enzyme reactions. Others have additional roles as structural components of bone and in electrolyte balance.

A good mixed diet provides adequate amounts of vitamins, and some are also formed by bacteria in the colon so that vitamin supplements are normally unnecessary. Restricted diets or defective absorption or utilisation of food result in vitamin deficiencies which lead to a number of conditions requiring administration of appropriate vitamins. Other factors leading to vitamin deficiencies include anorexia and vomiting, gastrointestinal disease, liver damage and cancerous conditions. They can also arise in alcoholics and in the elderly on poor diets and also when natural demands for vitamins are increased in fevers, pregnancy, breast-feeding and metabolic disorders.

Vitamins present in food can be divided into two classes, the fat-soluble vitamins (including vitamins A, D, E and K) and the water-soluble vitamins (including vitamins B and C). Table 17.1 outlines the main features of these vitamins.

REFERENCES

King's Fund Report 1992 A positive approach to nutrition as treatment. King's Fund Centre.

FURTHER READING

Linderborn K M 1993 Vitamin therapy for independently living seniors. Journal of Gerontological Nursing 19(8): 10–20

18

Drug treatment of musculoskeletal and joint diseases

ANATOMY AND PHYSIOLOGY

Movement of the bony framework results from the contraction of muscles at the joints. Although some joints (e.g. vertebral joints) have only slight movement caused by compression of cartilage, the majority of joints in the body (e.g. the hip joint) are freely movable as the result of the contraction of muscles surrounding them and are known as synovial joints (Fig. 18.1).

The characteristics common to all synovial joints are outlined in Table 18.1.

COMMON CONDITIONS

Rheumatoid arthritis

This is a chronic inflammatory autoimmune disease affecting the synovial membrane. It occurs most commonly between the ages of 40 and 60, but may afflict people of any age. Granulation tissue forms on the articular cartilages of the affected joints. In time this may erode not only the cartilages but also bone and even ligaments and tendons in the area. As the disease progresses there is additional and cumulative damage to the joints, leading to increasing deformity, pain and loss of function.

Another autoimmune inflammatory arthritic disease is *ankylosing spondylitis*, in which the sacro-iliac and vertebral joints become ossified.

Osteoarthritis

This is a degenerative non-inflammatory disease.

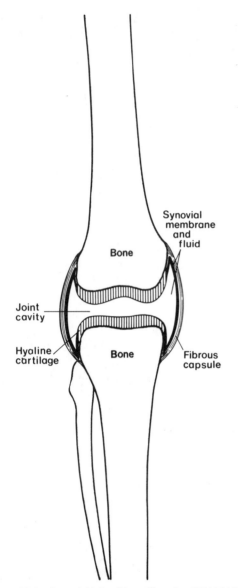

Figure 18.1 Synovial joint. (From Chandler 1991 Tabbner's nursing care: theory and practice, 2nd edn. Churchill Livingstone.)

Articular cartilage gradually becomes thinner because its replacement does not keep pace with its removal. Bone, formed at the margin of the articular cartilage, enlarges and may deform the affected joints and interfere with movement. Involvement of the knee, hip or other joints may become a major disability requiring surgical replacement.

Table 18.1 Characteristics of a synovial joint

Capsular ligament	A surrounding fibrous sleeve which: joins the bones together protects the joint without hindering movement
Articular cartilage	A smooth surface on the parts of the bones in contact, allowing free articulation of the joint
Synovial membrane	A layer of cells secreting a thick fluid, known as synovial fluid, which lubricates the joint, holds the bones in close proximity to one another and provides nourishment for the structures within the joint cavity. As well as lining the capsule, synovial membrane covers the bony surfaces within the joint not covered by articular cartilage
Other structures	Many joints have ligaments continuous with the capsule which provide further stability Muscles or muscle tendons stretch across the joint Movement of bones occurs when the muscle contracts and thus shortens Joint structures and the muscles involved are supplied by both nerves and blood vessels

Gout

This is characterised by higher than normal levels of uric acid in the blood due to either overproduction or defective excretion by the kidneys. Uric acid is a waste product of the breakdown of cell nuclei and is produced in excess when there is large-scale cell destruction, e.g. following trauma, malignancy, treatment with cytotoxic drugs and starvation. The excess uric acid forms sodium urate crystals which are deposited in joints and tendons. Acute inflammation is due to substances released by phagocytes that have ingested the crystals. The joints most commonly affected are in the big toe, ankle, knee, wrist and elbow.

DRUGS USED IN RHEUMATIC DISEASES

There is currently no cure for rheumatic diseases such as rheumatoid arthritis or osteoarthritis. Drug treatments are used to alleviate the symptoms which become more severe as the disease progresses. At an early stage in mild rheumatoid arthritis or osteoarthritis, all that may be required to relieve pain is simple analgesics such as paracetamol, buprenorphine, dihydrocodeine or nefopam. These drugs however have no anti-inflammatory action so that their use is limited. When symptoms become more severe, and are not controlled by simple analgesics, treatment gravitates to the use of non-steroidal anti-inflammatory drugs.

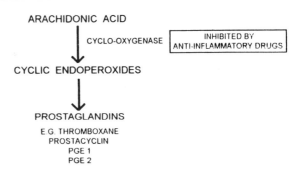

Figure 18.2 Formation of prostaglandins.

NON-STEROIDAL ANTI-INFLAMMATORY DRUGS (NSAIDS)

There are two main actions of the non-steroidal anti-inflammatory drugs – an analgesic effect and an anti-inflammatory effect. The analgesic action occurs quickly and recedes within a few hours whereas the anti-inflammatory effect builds up over a few days and requires regular dosage. NSAIDs are therefore useful for the treatment of continuous pain associated with inflammation, e.g. in rheumatoid arthritis or advanced osteoarthritis.

It is believed that NSAIDSs produce their anti-inflammatory effect by inhibition of prostaglandin synthesis. There are over twenty different naturally occurring prostaglandins which are widely distributed throughout the body since they are synthesised by virtually every tissue. Their release is stimulated by various means, including hormones, mechanical damage and nerve stimulation. Prostaglandins are formed in the body by the enzymatic oxygenation of arachidonic acid and linoleic acid, the enzyme involved being cyclo-oxygenase (Fig. 18.2). Prostaglandins are very potent chemicals with a broad range of activities which include:

- inhibition of gastric acid secretion
- bronchial relaxation
- vasodilator and hypotensive activity including control of blood flow through the renal medulla
- mediation of some aspects of inflammation
- contraction of the iris.

In rheumatoid arthritis it appears that control over the balanced production of prostaglandins is, to some extent, lost, and this results in exces-sive production of prostaglandins involved in inflammation. Administration of NSAIDs blocks the action of the enzyme cyclo-oxygenase which effectively reduces the synthesis of prosta-glandins. The therapeutic outcome is a reduction in pain, tenderness, swelling and temperature in the affected joints, decreased stiffness and increased joint movement.

It is probably the inhibition of prostaglandin synthesis which is responsible for the major side-effects of NSAIDs such as damage to the gastro-intestinal mucosa, peptic erosions and ulcers, and gastrointestinal bleeding. Care should be taken when giving NSAIDs to asthmatic patients.

There is a large number of NSAIDs to select from (Table 18.2). Differences in anti-inflammatory activity are small between the various NSAIDs but differences between individual patient responses are considerable. Approximately 60% of patients will respond to any one NSAID and it may therefore be necessary to try more than one in order to find a suitable NSAID for a patient. First choices may be ibuprofen or diclofenac. Alternatives to these include naproxen, ketoprofen, fenoprofen, flurbiprofen or sulindac. If, in adequate dosage, the first-choice drug does not appear to be working well within 2–3 weeks then a switch to another drug is indicated. Using more than one NSAID simultaneously does not give additional benefit to using one alone and it increases the incidence of adverse effects. The main differences between NSAIDs are in the incidence and type of side-effects (Table 18.3). Orally administered NSAIDs should always be taken after food to reduce the risk of gastrointestinal upset. Certain products

Table 18.2   Non-steroidal anti-inflammatory drugs

Group	Examples
Salicylates	Aspirin Benorylate Diflunisal Salsalate
Arylalkanoic acids	Diclofenac Fenbrufen Fenoprofen Flurbiprofen Ibuprofen Ketoprofen Naproxen
Anthranilic acid	Mefenamic Acid
Pyrazolones	Azapropazone Phenylbutazone
Cyclic acetic acids	Etodolac Indomethacin Sulindac
Oxicams	Piroxicam Tenoxicam

are available in syrup and suppository formulations. Whatever drug is chosen, it is very important to use an adequate dosage. Care should be taken in the elderly who are particularly vulnerable to the adverse effects of these drugs, especially gastrointestinal bleeding.

The duration of treatment depends upon the disease. In osteoarthritis, where there are short-term symptoms in one or two joints, treatment may be tailed off. Prolonged treatment will be necessary where there is chronic pain, stiffness and functional disability in the joints.

DISEASE-MODIFYING THERAPY (OR 'SECOND-LINE') IN THE TREATMENT OF RHEUMATOID ARTHRITIS

Drugs in this group are used when it is clear that the disease is progressing and has not been controlled by NSAIDs. They show the rate of disease progression but have minimal anti-inflammatory activity and are therefore used in addition to NSAIDs. Drugs within this group include penicillamine, gold salts (injection and oral), chloroquine, hydroxychloroquine and sulphasalazine (Table 18.4). They all have a slow onset of action, usually 2–4 months. They have a

Table 18.3   More commonly used NSAIDs

Drug	Formulation	Notes
Ibuprofen	Tablets, capsules, syrup, granules	Fewer side-effects than others but has weaker anti-inflammatory activity
Naproxen	Tablets, suspension, suppositories	Often the NSAID of first choice as many patients find it has the best balance of efficacy and toxicity; administration is only twice daily
Diclofenac sodium	Tablets, controlled-release tablets, injection, suppositories	Action and side-effects similar to those of naproxen
Indomethacin	Capsules, controlled-release capsules, suspension	Action superior to naproxen but incidence of side-effects is higher including headaches, dizziness and gastrointestinal disturbances
Benorylate	Tablets, suspension	Benorylate is a paracetamol-aspirin ester and may be useful in patients experiencing dyspepsia with other NSAIDs. Side-effects include tinnitus, dizziness and mental confusion. Care must be taken not to increase side-effects with purchased drugs containing aspirin
Sulindac	Tablets	Similar in effect to naproxen but does not inhibit renal prostaglandins and may be a safer option in patients with mild renal impairment
Fenbrufen	Tablets, effervescent tablets and capsules	Less gastrointestinal bleeding but high risk of rashes
Ketoprofen	Capsules, controlled-release capsules, suppositories, injection, gel	Modified-release preparation is claimed to cause less gastrointestinal irritation

Table 18.4   Disease modifying drugs

Drug	Formulation	Dose	Notes
Sodium aurothiomalate	Intramuscular injection	Initial 10 mg dose to exclude hypersensitivity; 50 mg weekly until patient responds then interval increased up to 4 weeks. Discontinued if no remission after 1 g	Gold therapy is fairly toxic, and careful supervision is necessary. Rashes occur in 30% of patients and treatment is usually stopped as it can lead to exfoliative dermatitis.Thrombocytopenia and neutropenia can occur and treatment must be stopped. Full blood counts, white cell counts, platelet counts and urine tests are required before each dose of gold
Auranofin	Tablets, 3 mg	3 mg twice daily (if no response after 3 months discontinue). Can be increased to 9 mg daily if no response at 6 months on 6 mg	Less effective but safer than injectable gold. Exhibits side-effects similar to injectable form. The most common side-effect is diarrhoea. The tablet shape is specially designed to improve handling properties for the patient
Penicillamine	Tablets, 125 mg and 250 mg	Initially 125 mg daily, increasing if no response; 500–750 mg daily is the usual maintenance dose	Improvement will take 6–12 weeks to occur. Side-effects occur in up to 50% of patients, the commonest being nausea. Where rashes occur therapy should be stopped and commenced on a lower dosage. Mouth ulcers are an indication for stopping the drug. Renal and haematological side-effects can occur, necessitating regular blood and urine tests. A fall in platelet or white cell count will mean stopping penicillamine treatment
Chloroquine	Tablets, syrup, injection	150 mg daily	Action similar to gold and penicillamine but is better tolerated. Use limited by ocular toxicity. Corneal opacities, reversible on discontinuation of therapy, have been reported in 20–40% of patients. Retinopathy, linked to size of daily dose, may occur. All patients should have a full ophthalmic examination prior to commencement of treatment and subsequently at regular intervals. Other side-effects include gastrointestinal disturbances, depigmentation and loss of hair, and skin reactions
Hydroxychloroquine	Tablets	400 mg daily initially; maintenance 200–400 mg	
Sulphasalazine	Enteric-coated tablets	Initially 500 mg daily. Maximum 2–3 g daily	Effectiveness similar to gold and penicillamine. Side-effects are also similar – full blood counts and liver function tests required throughout therapy. Allergy is common, and sulphasalazine should not be given to patients allergic to sulphonamides or aspirin. Discolours urine and may stain yellow soft contact lenses, particularly extended wear

greater toxicity than the NSAIDs, and close supervision and monitoring are required. Up to 70% of patients will show some improvement but it may be necessary to use more than one second-line agent in sequence.

'THIRD-LINE' AGENTS

This group includes cytotoxic drugs such as azathioprine, cyclophosphamide, methotrexate and chlorambucil. It also includes corticosteroids. These are used when second-line agents fail to produce improvement in severe, progressive disease or toxicity has proved a problem. Second-line agents are not given at the same time as third-line agents, although NSAIDs may still be continued. Cytotoxic drugs carry a greater risk than the second-line agents and are used only after careful consideration. As with second-line agents, the cytotoxics will take 2 to 4 months to provide benefit. Azathioprine is usually the cytotoxic drug of choice and is given in a dose of 2.5 mg per kg per day. Nausea, vomiting, diarrhoea, infection and marrow suppression can be encountered. Full blood counts every month are necessary.

Corticosteroids are potent anti-inflammatory agents but, because of side-effects associated with long-term use and because of disease rebound on withdrawal, they are reserved for:

- patients unresponsive to other treatments
- the elderly with very active disease
- where rapid relief is required in younger patients before slower-acting second-line agents begin to work

Corticosteroids can be given orally or by intravenous or intra-articular injection. Orally, soluble or enteric-coated prednisolone is usually the drug chosen using the smallest dose (e.g. 5–10 mg per day) to produce a beneficial effect.

Large bolus doses of corticosteroids (e.g. methylprednisolone up to 1 g on three consecutive days) can be given intravenously. This form of therapy to suppress highly active inflammatory disease is only given to patients commencing disease-modifying anti-rheumatic drugs and has no place in the routine management of the disease. It appears to shorten the time taken to achieve a response from the disease-modifying drugs. The side-effects of corticosteroids are numerous and include Cushing's syndrome (moon face, hirsutism), diabetes and osteoporosis, particularly of the elderly, peptic ulceration, increased susceptibility to infection and mental disturbances.

Intra-articular injections of corticosteroids can be very effective at relieving inflamed, swollen joints. Methylprednisolone acetate and triamcinolone hexacetonide are of similar efficacy, the drug increasing with increased size of the joint. Repeated intra-articular injections are not recommended as this may lead to side-effects. Care should be taken not to introduce an infection when the injection is administered.

DRUGS USED IN THE TREATMENT OF GOUT

Gout: the disease

Gout is a metabolic disorder in which there is an increase in the amount of uric acid in the body, resulting in a deposition of urate crystals in joints and other tissues. This is caused by an increase in production, or a decrease in renal excretion, or both, of uric acid. The onset of gout is sudden and is characterised by severe pain and inflammation of a single joint, often in the big toe. Although initial symptoms commonly disappear in days or weeks, recurrent attacks are likely with the joints of all limbs becoming chronically affected.

Treatment of acute gout

A non-steroidal anti-inflammatory drug is the treatment of choice for acute gout. Indomethacin is favoured (50–100 mg orally, initially, then 50 mg repeated 4–6-hourly until symptoms are relieved). Alternative NSAIDs include naproxen, azapropazone, diclofenac and ketoprofen (aspirin and salicylates should not be used as they may induce hyperuricaemia). Colchicine is specific and effective in gout but it causes gastrointestinal toxicity which outweighs its therapeutic value.

Long-term management of gout

Long-term management and prophylaxis of gout can be achieved in two ways: (i) blocking the production of uric acid by the administration of a xanthine oxidase inhibitor such as allopurinol, and (ii) increasing the excretion of uric acid by the administration of a uricosuric drug such as probenecid or sulphinpyrazone.

Allopurinol is given orally, the usual dose being 300 mg daily. It is well tolerated but may cause a rash, in which case it should be withdrawn and re-introduced only with caution. It should not be started within 3 weeks of an acute attack of gout as it may precipitate another attack. It is likely that treatment will be life-long. During the commencement of therapy with allopurinol (and also uricosuric drugs), acute attacks of gout may occur. In order to prevent this, indomethacin or colchicine should be given concurrently for the first 1 or 2 months. Allopurinol is well tolerated, but rashes constitute the most common side-effect, in which case it should be withdrawn and re-introduced only with caution or the treatment changed to urico-suric drugs.

Probenecid and sulphinpyrazone increase the excretion of uric acid and should be started at low dosage in order not to overload the excreted urine with acid. This can be aided by increasing fluid intake to at least two litres per day and neutralising the acidic urine with potassium citrate or sodium bicarbonate mixtures. The dosage is increased after the first week and over the next few weeks, with subsequent reduction if the serum uric acid can be maintained in the normal range. Side-effects are infrequent but occasionally include gastrointestinal distur-bances and rashes.

DRUGS CAUSING HYPERURICAEMIA AND GOUT

Certain drugs can precipitate an attack of gout:

- Thiazide and loop diuretics can precipitate on attack of gout by inhibiting the tubular secretion of uric acid.
- Aspirin in low doses inhibits the tubular secretion of uric acid.
- Cytotoxic drugs causing a high rate of cell kill may increase purine production with a consequent increase in the production of uric acid which may result in an acute attack of gout. Allopurinol may be given to prevent this but in the case of mercaptopurine and azathioprine it prevents the clearance of these drugs and increases their toxicity. If allopurinol is given concurrently the dosages of these drugs must be reduced.

DRUGS USED IN NEUROMUSCULAR DISORDERS

Myasthenia gravis

Myasthenia gravis is characterised by muscle weakness arising from defective neuromuscular transmission. It is thought to be caused by an autoimmune mechanism involving the produc-tion of antibodies to the acetylcholine receptors in the neuromuscular junction. Acetylcholine is

therefore blocked at nerve endings and this leads to muscle weakness affecting more commonly the muscles of the eyes, lips, tongue, throat, neck and shoulders. Limb muscles may be affected and movement restricted. These symptoms may be exacerbated by emotional disturbances, stren-uous exercise and pregnancy. Patients may experience temporary or permanent remissions.

Treatment Acetylcholine is broken down by the enzyme cholinesterase. If cholinesterase is inhibited, the concentration of acetylcholine at the motor end plate rises and its action is potentiated. This can be achieved by admin-istering an anticholinesterase such as neo-stigmine. This produces a therapeutic effect for up to 4 hours. It has muscarinic side-effects which include increased salivation, sweating, gastric secretion, motility and diarrhoea. Concurrent administration of an antimuscarinic such as propantheline may be required to counteract these side-effects. Pyridostigmine is preferred to neostigmine because of its longer action and weaker muscarinic action.

Edrophonium has a very brief action and the intramuscular injection is used in the diagnosis of myasthenia gravis. In patients with the disease, a single test-dose usually causes a substantial improvement in muscle power (lasting several minutes). Edrophonium can also be used to determine whether a patient is receiving an optimal dose of cholinergic drug. If treatment is inadequate a transient improvement will be seen on injecting the edrophonium. Conversely, if treatment is excessive, no effect or an intensification of clinical features will be seen.

Skeletal muscle relaxants

Patients with various disorders of the musculo-skeletal system and of the central nervous system suffer from muscle spasm. This spasm may produce pain and deformity. Treatment with drugs is generally only moderately effec-tive. The drugs used in the treatment of muscle spasticity are diazepam, baclofen and dantro-lene. Diazepam has some antispasmodic effect but sedation can be a problem particularly on higher doses. Baclofen acts at the spinal level similar to diazepam. Adverse effects such as sedation and hypotonia can be limiting. Dantrolene acts directly on skeletal muscle. It is used in severe spasticity, multiple sclerosis, spinal cord injury and stroke. Dosage should be increased slowly but if no benefit has been obtained after about 6 weeks the drug should be withdrawn. Drowsiness may be a problem if the patient has to drive or operate machinery.

FURTHER READING

Betts A 1993 Rheumatic disorders. Practice Nursing July/August: 18–19
George E, Dieppe P A 1993 Osteoarthritis. Hospital Update 19(8): 450–456

Scott D 1993 NSAIDs: renewed life for ageing remedies. Care of the Elderly 5(8): 294–296
Star V L, Hochberg M C 1993 Prevention and management of gout. Drugs 45(2): 212–222

19

Drug treatment of eye conditions

ANATOMY AND PHYSIOLOGY

The eye is a spherical organ situated in the orbital cavity whose bony walls and fat help to protect it from damage. The visible part of the eye is only a proportion of the whole so that the eye is best considered in vertical cross section viewed from the side (see Fig. 19.1).

The walls are in three layers. The outermost layer is a fibrous coat consisting of the sclera (the white of the eye) lining all but the anterior part of the eye, which is transparent and known as the cornea.

In the middle is a vascular layer which, like the sclera, lines the posterior five-sixths of the eye and is known as the choroid. The anterior sixth comprises the ciliary body, an essential part of the process of accommodation of the eye, and the iris, the pigmented muscular structure which gives the eye its colour and serves to control the amount of light entering the eye through autonomic nervous stimulation.

In the centre of the eye is the eyeball, which consists of an anterior and a posterior segment separated by the lens. The anterior segment is in turn made up of an anterior chamber and posterior chamber separated by the iris. Both chambers contain a transparent fluid, known as aqueous, secreted by the ciliary glands. Aqueous fluid circulates from the posterior chamber through the pupil into the anterior chamber and back to the general circulation via the canal of Schlemm. In health, the intra-ocular pressure of fluid remains fairly constant. The remaining

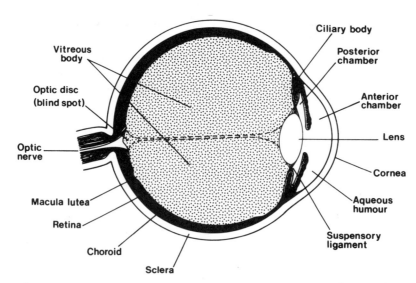

Figure 19.1 The eye. (From Chandler 1991 Tabbner's nursing care: theory and practice, 2nd edn. Churchill Livingstone.)

larger posterior segment of the eyeball is known as the vitreous humour and is filled with a transparent, jelly-like substance which, along with the aqueous fluid, helps keep the shape of the eye.

The eye is protected by accessory organs which include the eyebrows, eyelids and eyelashes, and the lacrimal apparatus.

The lacrimal apparatus (see Fig. 19.2) is essential for the flow of tears. Tears are composed of water, salts and a bactericidal enzyme, lysozyme. Added to this fluid are oily secretions from the Meibomian glands. These combined fluids serve to protect the eye in several ways:

- the constant washing of the fluid over the cornea, through blinking, removes grit
- the lysozyme helps to prevent microbial infection
- the oily nature of the fluid helps to keep the conjunctiva from drying up.

COMMON EYE CONDITIONS

- Red eye
- Eyelid disorders
- Lacrimal disorders

Red eye

Patients often present with a red eye. This rather obvious symptom should be fully investigated to ensure that any very serious condition

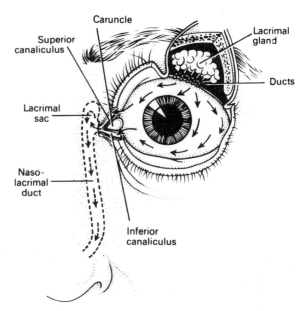

Figure 19.2 The lacrimal apparatus. (From Ross & Wilson 1990 Anatomy and physiology in health and illness, 7th edn. Churchill Livingstone.)

(e.g. glaucoma) does not go undetected. Causes of red eye include:

- conjunctivitis – bacterial or viral
- corneal ulceration due to microbial infection
- episcleritis and scleritis
- acute angle closure glaucoma
- foreign body in the eye.

Eyelid disorders (lumps)

Again, it is important to ensure that any lumps on the eyelid are carefully investigated to exclude serious conditions such as basal-cell carcinoma. Commonly presenting conditions are chalazion (Meibomian cyst), and stye – a local infection of a lash follicle.

Inflammatory eyelid disorders

These include the following:

Blepharitis This is a chronic condition in which the patient complains of sore eyelids. Styes often accompany blepharitis, and the lid margins are inflamed and crusted. The condition may be present in patients suffering from an inflammatory skin disease such as eczema.

Acute inflammatory conditions of the eyelids must be taken as indicating a potentially serious condition which could result in loss of sight or the spread of a life-threatening infection.

Orbital cellulitis This may result from the spread of infection from sinuses. Urgent specialist treatment is required in such cases.

Allergy Allergic reactions can occur as a result of contact with a wide range of allergenic materials from plant or animal sources. Cosmetics may also cause allergic reactions.

Viral infections Infections due to the herpes simplex or herpes zoster virus can result in a vesicular rash on the eyelid.

Drooping of the eyelid (ptosis) This condition may indicate the presence of a serious disease such as myasthenia gravis or a condition that arises due to the ageing process.

Children who present with a drooping eyelid must be very fully investigated by a specialist as the symptoms may indicate a serious condition.

Lacrimal disorders

Excessive tear production Some patients may experience a watering eye due to blockage of the lacrimal sac or nasolacrimal duct. Surgery may be indicated to resolve this problem.

Dry eye syndrome This is a much more common condition, especially in older patients. Patients with this condition suffer considerable discomfort which is due to a deficiency of either aqueous or the mucin component of the tear film. It is often associated with rheumatoid arthritis (Sjogren's syndrome) and autoimmune diseases such as pemphigoid. Certain drugs and infections may be a cause of dry eye syndrome.

EYE INJURIES

Eye injuries can result from a number of causes, notably foreign bodies, blunt injury, or chemical damage. Injuries arising from the use of metal tools on glass, stone or metal can result in penetrating injuries to the eye. Chemical damage to the eye must be treated with copious amounts of a suitable irrigating fluid such as sterile normal saline or sterile water. In emergency situations tap water may have to be used. Eye injuries due to chemicals of alkaline reaction, such as lime, need to be treated very urgently since alkalis have a penetrating action on ocular tissue, causing iritis and cataract formation.

PRE- AND POSTOPERATIVE TREATMENT

Local eye treatment, both pre- and postsurgery, will depend on the condition treated and the surgical procedures used. The main agents used are mydriatics, antibacterials and corticosteroids (see Tables 19.4, 19.5, 19.8, 19.9). Whenever practicable, single-use containers are used to reduce the likelihood of infection.

MEDICAL CONDITIONS AND THE EYE

Many serious medical conditions have ocular symptoms. Examination of the eye may lead to the diagnosis of a serious general condition, e.g.

diabetes mellitus, rheumatoid disease and hypertension. Systemic treatment is indicated in these conditions, the details of which are given in the relevant chapters in this book.

GLAUCOMA

Glaucoma is characterised by a raised intraocular pressure (IOP) which leads to cupping and degeneration of the optic disc. If the condition is untreated, defects in the field of vision enlarge, leading to visual loss. Normal IOP is 16 mmHg ± 3 mmHg. A pressure of 21 mmHg (measured by tonometer), or higher, represents a pathological condition and requires treatment. High IOP causes compression of the vascular supply to the optic disc, resulting in ischaemia, the extent of which will depend on the IOP and vascularity/blood supply of the optic disc. Some eyes can withstand an IOP of 30 mmHg or more without damage due to the presence of a good blood supply to the optic disc. In other eyes a pressure of less than 21 mmHg can cause visual impairment. IOP is maintained as a result of balance between inflow and outflow of aqueous humour which is secreted constantly by the ciliary body. The aqueous humour circulates around the lens before passing through the pupil into the anterior chamber. Aqueous humour leaves the eye through the angle of this chamber by filtering through the trabecular meshwork.

An increased IOP can result from an increased production of aqueous humour or from impaired drainage. In clinical practice most cases of glaucoma diagnosed arise from poor drainage of the aqueous humour from the anterior chamber.

Types of glaucoma

Glaucomas can be divided into two main categories, namely, primary and secondary glaucomas.

Primary glaucomas *Chronic open-angle (simple) glaucoma* is the most common form. Patients may not notice the gradual visual loss taking place, presenting only when serious damage has occurred. A hereditary factor is involved, and diabetics and very short-sighted people are especially at risk of developing this condition.

Acute angle-closure glaucoma. In this condition the affected eye is red and painful, and the presentation is acute. The distinction between open-angle glaucoma and angle-closure glaucoma is made on the basis of the appearance of the anterior chamber angle when examined with a gonioscope. In this form of glaucoma drainage of the aqueous is blocked by the iris. Intraocular pressure builds up very quickly, vision becomes blurred and there is headache and sickness. Older and long-sighted people are especially at risk of developing this condition. Treatment of the glaucomas is summarised in Tables 19.1–19.3. Surgical treatment of glaucoma is beyond the scope of this book. The overall aim of treatment is to reduce intraocular pressure (IOP) thus minimising damage to the optic disc.

Secondary glaucomas These conditions result from developmental abnormalities and acquired defects. A detailed discussion of these conditions is beyond the scope of this book. The developmental abnormalities that can result in glaucoma include inborn errors of metabolism and certain skeletal, cardiovascular and ocular changes that occur in such conditions as Marfan's syndrome. Acquired defects that may result in glaucoma

Table 19.1 Treatment of glaucoma with β-blockers

Drug	Form/dose	Actions/indications	Contraindications/side-effects/nursing points
Betaxolol	Drops 0.5%, twice daily	These drugs release the secretion of aqueous and are used in the treatment of chronic open-angle glaucoma. Long-term treatment is indicated with these drugs so as to achieve prolonged reduction of IOP.	History of cardiovascular disease, asthma. Systemic absorption can occur causing β-blockade. Patient should be encouraged to shut the eyes for several minutes or the punctum should be occluded.
Carteolol	Drops 1% and 2%, twice daily		
Timolol	Drops 0.25%, twice daily		

Table 19.2 Treatment of glaucoma with parasympathomimetics and sympathomimetics

Drug	Form/dose	Actions/indications	Contraindications/side-effects/nursing points
Parasympathomimetics			
Carbachol	Drops 3%, up to 4 times daily	Acts in a manner similar to that of pilocarpine	History of cardiovascular disease. Systemic absorption can occur. Sweating, colic, bronchospasm and hypersalivation can occur (see also p. 50)
Physostigmine	Drops 0.25–0.5%, 2–6 times daily	An anticholinesterase, but the basic action is as for the parasympathomimetics	
Pilocarpine	Drops 0.5 – 4%, 3–6 times daily	Reduces the pupil size and opens up the trabecular network	Pilocarpine should not be used if there is inflammation since vision can be adversely affected
	Ocusert, see p. 19	All these drugs are used in the treatment of chronic open-angle glaucoma; combinations of these drugs are often used	
Sympathomimetics			
Adrenalin	Drops 0.5% or 1%, once/twice daily	Indicated in the treatment of open-angle glaucoma; causes increase in outflow of aqueous and dilates the pupil	Not used for the treatment of narrow-angle glaucoma as closed-angle glaucoma may result. Cardiovascular problems due to systemic absorption. Stinging and redness of the eye
Dipivefrine	Drops 0.1%, twice daily	A pro-drug which is converted into the active drug (adrenalin) in the eye	As for adrenalin, but may be less of a problem due to the pro-drug action
Guanethidine	Drops 5%, once/twice daily	Guanethidine and combination of guanethidine and adrenalin have similar actions/indications to adrenalin	Use with caution in patients with cardiovascular disease; long-term use may cause conjunctival fibrosis
Guanethidine and adrenalin	Drops 1% guanethidine and 0.2% adrenalin OR 3% guanethidine and 0.5% adrenalin, once/twice daily		

Table 19.3 Treatment of glaucoma with carbonic anhydrase inhibitors

Drug	Form/dose	Actions/indications	Contraindications/side-effects/nursing points
Acetazolamide	250 mg tablets or sustained-release capsules 0.25–1 g, daily individual doses	Acetazolamide inhibits carbonic anhydrase. This enzyme regulates bicarbonate production. Bicarbonate anions balance sodium cations involved in aqueous humour secretions	Acetazolamide may induce a mild acidosis. It is contraindicated in idiopathic renal hyperchloraemic acidosis. The drug is also contraindicated in conditions associated with electrolyte level disturbances, e.g. Addison's disease. Careful monitoring of fluid and electrolyte state is required in long-term therapy. Periodic blood cell counts are advisable. Patients should be advised to report any unusual skin rashes. The appearance of significant side-effects should be reported at once. It may be necessary to terminate treatment
Dichlorphenamide	50 mg tablets; 4 tablets initially and 2 tablets every 12 hours until condition is controlled	Action similar to that of acetazolamide. Both of these drugs are used in the treatment of open-angle glaucoma	Patients with hepatic or renal disorders should not be treated with dichlorphenamide. Hypokalaemia can result due to increased potassium excretion. Patients receiving digoxin therapy are especially sensitive to the effects of potassium loss. Carbonic anhydrase inhibitors may potentiate the effects of certain drugs, e.g. antidiabetic drugs. Patients receiving multiple therapy should be carefully monitored

include ocular inflammatory conditions, degenerative conditions, tumours, trauma and postoperative complications. Drug treatment, especially local application of potent corticosteroids (betamethasone and dexamethasone) can cause glaucoma of the chronic open angle type. Any drug which dilates the pupil may result in acute-angle closure glaucoma. Patients with narrow angles only are at risk of developing this dangerous condition. Both local and systemic drugs can cause acute-angle closure glaucoma in susceptible patients. Atropine (parasympathetic blocking drug) and phenylephrine (sympathomimetic) are potential causes of acute-angle closure glaucoma. Systemically administered drugs which have an anti-cholinergic (parasympathetic blocking) action or side-effects can precipitate angle-closure glaucoma. The main groups of drugs that can cause problems are:

Table 19.4   Anti-infective agents – antibacterials

Drug	Form/dose	Actions/indications	Contraindications/side-effects/nursing points
Chloramphenicol	Eye drops 0.5%, 2 drops every 3 hours or more frequently; eye ointment 1%	Used for both treatment and prevention of bacterial infections, e.g. conjunctivitis. Eye ointment useful for application at night (long action). Valuable to prevent secondary bacterial infection in viral conjunctivitis	As with all eye drops there is a possibility of transient stinging on application. Care should be taken to avoid unnecessary long-term use as rare cases of aplastic anaemia have resulted from systemic absorption
Framycetin (also available with hydrocortisone 0.5% where an anti-inflammatory action is required)	Drops 0.5%; eye ointment 0.5%; ophthalmic powder 500 mg for sub-conjunctival infection	Bacterial infections, e.g. conjunctivitis	Most antibacterial agents are applied several times daily, depending on clinical need. All locally applied anti-infective agents have the potential to cause sensitivity reactions. Antibacterial agents combined with corticosteroids should not be applied where viral infections are present – or suspected – since local defence mechanisms will be compromised
Gentamicin	Drops 0.3%; eye ointment 0.3%	Bacterial infections; a broad-spectrum agent	
Norfloxacin	Drops 0.3%	Bacterial infections	May cause local burning/smarting feelings. Patients may notice a bitter taste due to systemic absorption

Table 19.5   Anti-infective agents – antifungal and antiviral agents

Drug	Form/dose	Actions/indications	Contraindications/side-effects/nursing points
Antifungal agents			
Natamycin	Applied locally as a 5% suspension	Fungal corneal ulcers can arise as a result of the inappropriate use of topical corticosteroids.	The treatment of fungal infections of the eye is highly specialised and requires highly skilled treatment
Nystatin	100 000 units/ml	Fungal corneal ulcers and keratomycosis	
Ketoconazole	Oral antifungal agent (see p. 173)		
Antiviral agents			
Acyclovir	Eye ointment 3%, 5 times daily	Herpes simplex infections and herpes simplex keratitis	Treatment must be continued 3 days after healing
Idoxuridine	Eye drops 0.1% applied every hour during the day and every 2 hours at night; eye ointment 0.5% applied every 4 hours	Herpes simplex infections. Acute dendritic ulcers	Contraindicated in pregnancy. Treatment should not be continued for more than 21 days. Antibiotic drops may be used to control secondary infection but the drops should not be mixed

- anti-depressant drugs of the tricyclic group, e.g. amitriptyline
- anti-Parkinson's disease drugs, e.g. benzhexol
- compound antacid preparations containing atropine-like drugs, e.g. Kolanticon gel
- drugs used to treat bronchospasm, e.g. ephedrine

It should be noted that the selective adrenergic drugs, such as salbutamol, do not have any effect on the pupil since salbutamol does not stimulate alpha-adrenoceptors.

Treatment of acute closed-angle glaucoma

This is an acute emergency and must be treated immediately to prevent loss of sight. An intravenous dose of 500 mg acetazolamide is given together with 4% pilocarpine drops to constrict the pupil. Surgical treatment is carried out after the IOP has been reduced.

TREATMENT OF INFECTIONS OF THE EYE

Many infections of the eye are amenable to treatment with topical antimicrobial agents. Wherever possible the drugs used are those which are not used to treat systemic infections so as to reduce the risk of resistance developing. In severe infections it may be necessary to use supporting systemic therapy. Tables 19.4 and 19.5 provide summaries of the main topical anti-infective agents

LOCAL ANAESTHETICS (see also p. 329)

Local anaesthetics (see Table 19.6) are applied to the eye to relieve pain following injury or to reduce discomfort prior to ophthalmological procedures such as tonometry. Hypersensitivity may occur and stinging on application may be a problem. Cocaine eye drops (4%) are still used but their use is declining partly due to high cost, Controlled Drug status and potential side-effects.

Table 19.6 Local anaesthetics

Drug	Form/dose	Actions/indications	Contraindications/side-effects/nursing points
Amethocaine	Drops 0.5% and 1%	Local anaesthetic	Local sensitivity reaction may occur to the drug or preservative used in the eye drops
Lignocaine	Drops 4% with fluorescein 0.25%	Local anaesthetic with staining agent to help in the diagnosis of ocular lesions. The dye (fluorescein) is taken up by the damaged tissue	
Oxybuprocaine	Drops 0.4%	Local anaesthetic	

Table 19.7 Preparations for tear deficiency

Drug	Form/dose	Actions/indications	Contraindications/side-effects/nursing points
Hypromellose	Drops 0.3%, used hourly if necessary	Lubricant in tear deficiency	Frequent applications needed. Inpatients may prefer self-administration of these drops where this can be arranged. The choice of a particular preparation will be determined by acceptability to the patient. Drops such as PVA with a mucomimetic action may provide a longer period of relief from symptoms than drops such as hypromellose
Polyvinyl alcohol (PVA)	Drops 1.4%	Lubricant in tear deficiency	
Acetylcysteine and hypromellose	Drops 5%/0.35%; apply 4 times daily	This product provides lubrication and the acetylcysteine has a mucolytic action which is useful where accumulations of mucus occur	As with other eye conditions, appropriate eye hygiene must be carried out to reduce discomfort from crusting on the eyelid margins

Table 19.8 Anti-inflammatory drugs

Drug	Form/dose	Actions/indications	Contraindications/side-effects/nursing points
Corticosteroid			
Betamethasone	0.1% every 1–2 hours for acute phase. Reduce frequency and use eye ointment 0.1% at night	Indicated for the short-term treatment of inflammatory conditions such as uveitis and scleritis. Also used postoperatively to reduce inflammation	Expert supervision of topical corticosteroid therapy is required since the dangers from topical therapy are significant. Steroid glaucoma may result and undiagnosed herpes simplex infection may be aggravated leading to loss of vision or even of the eye. As in other conditions, therapy with corticosteroids can produce great benefits for patients, but the dangers and side-effects must be guarded against by all concerned with the patient's care.
Other anti-inflammatory drugs			
Antazoline	Drops: antazoline 0.5% with xylometazoline 0.05%; apply 4 times daily	Allergic conjunctivitis	To be avoided in patients with cardiac disease, hypertension, etc. because of possible systemic absorption
Sodium cromoglycate	Drops 2%; apply 4 times daily; eye ointment 4% applied at night	Allergic conjunctivitis; hay fever	Few adverse effects have been reported

Table 19.9 Mydriatics and cycloplegics

Drug	Form/dose	Actions/indications	Contraindications/side-effects/nursing points
Atropine	1% eye drops and eye ointment	Long-acting (7 days) antimuscarinic. Dilates pupil and paralyses ciliary muscle. Used in refraction procedures in young children	As with other eye drops, there are risks of systemic absorption resulting in dry mouth, etc. Patients at extremes of age are more likely to suffer side-effects than other patients. Mydriatics may precipitate acute closed-angle glaucoma
Cyclopentolate	Eye drops 0.5% and 1%	Used for producing cycloplegia for refraction in young children. Effect lasts for up to 24 hours. Also used for relieving pain from pupillary spasm in eye injuries	Similar contraindications to other drugs in this class
Homatropine	Eye drops 1%	Similar to cyclopentolate	
Hyoscine	Eye drops 0.25%	Similar to cyclopentolate	
Tropicamide	Eye drops 0.5% and 1%	Very short-acting mydriatic (3 hours)	

TREATMENT OF TEAR DEFICIENCY

Tear deficiency (see Table 19.7) produces a very troublesome 'dry eye' condition leading to sore, uncomfortable, 'gritty' eyes. Fortunately, the condition can be alleviated by the regular use of water-based lubricant eye drops.

TREATMENT OF INFLAMMATORY EYE CONDITIONS

As in the treatment of skin diseases, the local application of corticosteroids to the eye is poten-tially hazardous (see p. 312). The anti-inflammatory action is however very valuable, as described above. Local application of corticos-teroids in cases of undiagnosed infection (e.g. herpes simplex viral infection) can lead to a rapid worsening of the condition, which may even cause the loss of an eye. Anti-inflammatory drugs are detailed in Table 19.8.

MYDRIATICS AND CYCLOPLEGICS

These drugs (see Table 19.9) dilate the pupil and

paralyse ciliary muscles. The main uses of these drugs are pre- and postoperatively and in diagnostic procedures (e.g. refraction). The pain due to certain eye injuries (e.g. corneal abrasion) can be relieved by the application of homatropine eye drops. Adverse effects are briefly described in Table 19.9. Many eye drops contain highly potent drugs and should be securely stored whenever they are used.

BLEPHAROSPASM

Botulinum toxin, produced by the bacterium *Clostridium botulinum* type A, is one of the most powerful neurotoxins known to man. It can be fatal in severe untreated cases of botulinum food poisoning. The toxin paralyses muscles by blocking the release of acetylcholine from the presynaptic neurones. The effect is irreversible and remains until new nerve end plates form.

A standardised preparation of the toxin is licensed for the treatment of blepharospasm and hemifacial spasm. The potency of the product is expressed in units. The toxin's muscle-weakening action is exploited therapeutically in some dystonias (involuntary muscle spasms), the injection being indicated for blepharospasm and hemifacial spasm. Sufferers typically have uncontrollable blinking spasms in both eyes, symptoms usually starting insidiously in the 50–70 age group. Spasms become more frequent and severe, with both eyes clamping shut, resulting in many patients effectively being blind. Botulinum toxin injection (Dysport) (120 units per affected eye) reduces the intensity of the spasm in 2–5 days and usually lasts for an average of 3–4 months, repeat treatment being required after this. There is no evidence that repeat treatment leads to resistance. However, there are adverse effects, notably blurred vision, local pain and swelling.

20

Drug treatment of ear, nose and oropharynx

This section is concerned mainly with the topical (local) use of medicines.

DRUGS ACTING ON THE EAR

Anatomy and physiology

Sound waves reaching the auricle are channelled through the external auditory canal to the tympanic membrane (ear drum), which vibrates in response. These vibrations are transmitted through the ossicles to the cochlea which converts them into impulses for transmission by the auditory nerve to the brain (Fig. 20.1). The ear is commonly considered as comprising three parts:

outer ear – auricle and external auditory canal
middle ear – tympanic membrane and ossicles
inner ear – cochlea and vestibular labyrinth.

Common conditions

Each part of the ear may be affected by disease. The outer ear may be affected by skin conditions such as eczema, dermatitis and boils, with itching and pain as the presenting symptoms. Inflammation of the external auditory canal is known as *otitis externa*. Wax, secreted by cells in the external auditory canal, may cause some loss of hearing where production is excessive. The ciliated epithelial cells which line the middle ear secrete mucus. Serous otitis media (glue ear) is a condition where the middle ear becomes congested with mucus. Where the mucosa becomes

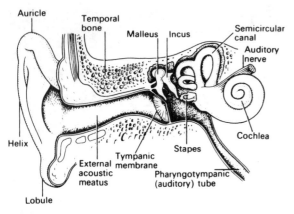

Figure 20.1 The ear. (From Ross & Wilson 1990 Anatomy and physiology in health and illness, 7th edn. Churchill Livingstone.)

infected, resulting in pus formation, the resulting painful condition is known as *acute otitis media*. Occasionally, pressure build-up will cause the tympanic membrane to rupture; this results in pressure release and subsidence of pain. Repeated episodes of infection with recurrent discharge of pus may lead to persistent rupturing of the tympanic membrane and the condition known as *chronic otitis media*. Conditions affecting the inner ear are dealt with in Chapter 10.

Treatment

Otitis externa

As with all ear diseases, aural toilet is a prerequisite. If simple toilet procedures do not produce a benefit, an astringent such as aluminium acetate may be used to treat inflammation. This dries the external ear canal and forms a protective layer on the mucosa. When eczematous non-infected inflammation is present, corticosteroid ear drops such as betamethasone sodium phosphate are recommended. However, these should not be used when inflammation is thought to be secondary to an infection. Topical antibiotics are used to treat infections in courses up to a week – longer may result in resistance or fungal infection. Suitable antibiotics include chloramphenicol and aminoglycosides (framycetin, neomycin, gentamicin). When using aminoglyco-

sides care should be taken that the eardrum is not perforated because of the risk of ototoxicity.

Antibiotic/corticosteroid products are formulated to treat both infection and inflammation. Examples are Sofradex (framycetin/gramicidin/dexamethasone) for uncomplicated infection and Gentisone HC (gentamicin/hydrocortisone) or Betnesol-N (betamethasone/neomycin) for serious infection pending culture results. Clotrimazole is recommended for use in fungal infections of the outer and middle ear. Occasionally, patients may experience mild burning or irritation after applying the solution.

Acute otitis media

Where the condition is caused by viral infection the only treatment needed may be paracetamol to control the pain. Local antibiotic therapy to treat bacterial infections is of value only where the tympanic membrane is perforated. Severe attacks require systemic antibiotics. A decongestant such as xylometazoline is of value in clearing the eustachian tube; this results in reducing pressure in the middle ear and promoting natural drainage.

Chronic otitis media

Regular aural toilet is essential. Antibiotic treatment is of little value, while surgery may be required to reduce the risk of complications.

DRUGS ACTING ON THE NOSE
Anatomy and physiology

The nasal passages are lined by a highly vascular mucous membrane covered with ciliated epithelium which warms and moistens the entering air and traps a certain amount of dust. When the mucous membrane is congested or inflamed there is considerable resistance to inflow and breathing through the nose is correspondingly difficult.

Common conditions

- Nasal allergy, e.g. allergic rhinitis, hay fever

- Nasal congestion, e.g. vasomotor rhinitis, nasal polyps, common cold
- Nasal infection

Treatment

Medicaments are instilled into the nose generally in the form of drops or a spray. The effect however is very transient since the cilia lining the nasal cavities remove them in about twenty minutes.

Nasal allergy

Sodium cromoglycate inhibits the release of chemical mediators such as histamine from mast cells. It is these mediators which, when released in response to exposure to an allergen, cause an allergic reaction. Sodium cromoglycate is therefore used prophylactically, and treatment should be commenced several weeks before the hay fever season commences and continued on a regular basis. Local irritation may occur particularly during initial treatment with insufflations.

In severe rhinitis, administration of a corticosteroid such as beclomethasone directly into the nose decreases inflammation and oedema of the nasal mucosa.

Nasal congestion

All the decongestants are sympathomimetic drugs which cause vasoconstriction of the mucosal blood vessels and provide relief of congestion. The most significant adverse reaction is rebound nasal congestion if treatment is prolonged. Ephedrine nasal drops should be used for no more than 5 to 7 days to avoid rebound congestion. Xylometazoline (nasal drops or spray) is much longer-acting than ephedrine but more likely to cause rebound nasal congestion.

Nasal infection

Local antibiotics have little place in the treatment of nasal infections, but a cream containing chlorhexidine 0.1% and neomycin sulphate 0.5% (Naseptin) is applied locally in the treatment of staphylococcal infections and prophylaxis against nasal carriage of staphylococci.

DRUGS ACTING ON THE OROPHARYNX

Anatomy and physiology

The oropharynx consists of the oral cavity within which there are the gums, teeth, hard palate, soft palate and uvula, tonsils and tongue. The oral cavity is lined throughout with mucous membrane containing small mucus-secreting glands. Three pairs of salivary glands namely parotid, submandibular and sublingual also pour their secretions into the mouth. These combined secretions make up saliva which contains water, mucus, mineral salts and salivary amylase. Approximately 1.5 litres of saliva flow through the mouth in 24 hours; its purpose is to lubricate the oral cavity, initiate the digestion of starches and assist with chewing, swallowing and speaking. The output of saliva is increased by the sight of food, eating and drinking, brushing the teeth, and movement of the jaws.

The lining of a healthy mouth is moist and pink. The teeth are free from caries, the papillae on the tongue are visible and the lips intact. There is no discomfort or odour.

Common conditions

Oral ulceration and inflammation

There are many causes of ulceration in the mouth. Infection, trauma, blood disorders, gastrointestinal disease, nutritional deficiency and drug therapy causing immunodeficiency such as cancer chemotherapy all predispose to a breakdown of the oral mucosa. Treatment of the underlying condition will often resolve the oral problem. Aphthous ulcers are very painful, nonspecific mouth ulcerations which are difficult to treat.

Oropharyngeal infection

Fungal infections of the mouth, principally candidiasis (thrush), are especially likely to arise in patients who are debilitated or immunosuppressed. The commonest groups affected are the very young, the elderly and those receiving a course of broad-spectrum antibiotic or cytotoxic medication.

Viral infections of the mouth include herpes infections.

Reduced salivary flow

Dry mouth may be caused by a reduction in salivary flow such as occurs with:

- certain drugs, e.g. anticholinergics or drugs having anticholinergic side-effects
- radiotherapy near the mouth or throat
- infection of a salivary gland
- inflammation of the mouth or throat
- dental or oral surgery.

Treatment

Oral ulceration and inflammation

Hexetidine solution 0.1% w/v has antibacterial and antiprotozoal activity. It is used in the treatment of gingivitis, pharyngitis and for oral hygiene generally. The solution should normally be used undiluted, although some patients may find the taste rather unpleasant.

Hydrogen peroxide solution 6% w/v is an oxidising agent which, when in contact with organic matter, effervesces, releasing oxygen; this has some mechanical cleansing action. This solution is particularly useful in dealing with anaerobic organisms that cause acute gingivitis, or where the tongue is so heavily furred that other solutions are rendered ineffective. To minimise the likelihood of local irritation the mouth should be well rinsed with water or normal saline when the procedure has been completed.

Aphthous ulcers These are difficult to treat because of the problem of trying to maintain an adequate concentration of drug in contact with the lesions. Box 20.1 gives some drugs which may be prescribed.

Box 20.1 Some drugs used for the treatment of aphthous ulcers

Hydrocortisone lozenges	Held in the mouth as near as possible to the ulcer to reduce inflammation
Triamcinolone dental paste	A specially formulated paste designed to adhere to mucous membranes; contains a potent corticosteroid; care should be taken to treat any concomitant infection that may be present
Benzydamine hydrochloride solution	Used as a mouthwash or spray to relieve pain and inflammation

---

Oropharyngeal infection

Fungal infections Nystatin (suspension or pastilles) is commonly used to treat oral candidiasis. The medication should be retained in the mouth for as long as possible so as to ensure maximum effect. Patients will need to be given guidance on the best way to use the particular product, and the need to avoid eating or drinking for a short time after treatment. With all fungal infections of the mouth, particular attention should be given to cleaning of dentures as these may be a source of re-infection.

Amphotericin, in the form of suspension (or lozenges), is an alternative anti-fungal agent, especially where the infecting organism is resistant to nystatin. Miconazole is an anti-fungal agent with a wide spectrum of activity against pathogenic fungi and some gram-positive bacteria. An oral gel is available containing 125 ml in 5 ml. The gel is retained in the mouth in contact with the lesion for as long as possible.

Viral infections The treatment of choice for herpes simplex virus infections of the skin near the mouth is acyclovir cream. It is not suitable for use on mucous membranes as it may be irritant. Idoxuridine paint (0.1% in dimethylsulphoxide) is a less effective treatment for herpetic lesions of the skin.

Tetracycline mouthwash may be helpful in treating severe herpetic infections of the mouth. The mouthwash is prepared by mixing the contents of a capsule with a small amount of water immediately before use.

Reduced salivary flow

Salivary substitutes are obtainable in the form of a spray or drops and contain small quantities of sodium, potassium, calcium and magnesium salts, sorbitol and carboxymethylcellulose. An alternative approach may be to use a pastille specially formulated to increase salivary flow.

FURTHER READING

Ludman H 1988 ABC of ear nose and throat. British Medical Association, London

21

Drug treatment of skin disorders

THE SKIN

The skin can be described as the body's largest organ in terms of surface area (other than the lungs). The skin provides a waterproof surface and retains essential fluids. It acts as a barrier against infections and is a major controller of body temperature, the heat of the body being regulated by the blood vessels and sweating. It protects underlying organs from physical, chemical and other injuries. The nerve endings in the skin serve as a relay between external influences and internal organs. The skin acts as an organ of expression, betraying the innermost feelings – anxiety by sweating, anger by a red flush and fear by pallor. It is an important store for water, containing 18–20% of the total water content of the body which is distributed mainly in the dermis. This percentage decreases with age.

Anatomy

For practical purposes the skin can be considered in three areas (Fig. 21.1):

- epidermis
- dermis
- other structures, e.g. sweat glands, sebaceous glands and hair follicles.

Epidermis

This consists of four layers. The lowest part is the basal layer where active cells (keratinocytes)

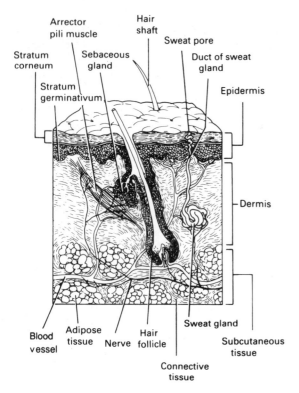

Figure 21.1 Anatomy of the skin. (From Chandler 1991 Tabbner's nursing care: theory and practice, 2nd edn. Churchill Livingstone.)

divide and progress to the surface through the granular layer, changing only in shape and size to reach the stratum corneum or cornified layer. This layer consists of dead skin cells which contain no nuclei and are continuously shed from the surface. Living cells produce keratin which toughens the epidermis and is the basic substance of hair and nails. Melanocytes are a type of cell in the basal layer in which melanin is formed. Melanin is a protective pigment which is released following exposure to sunlight.

Dermis and other structures

The dermis contains different types of nerve endings for sensing pain, pressure and temperature. Sweat glands regulate heat, causing heat loss by evaporation. Sebaceous glands are found all over the body except the palms and the soles of the feet. They are most numerous in the scalp, face, forehead and chin. Their secretion – the

result of decomposition of their cells – is known as sebum, which is discharged through the sebaceous duct into a pilosebaceous (hair) follicle. Sebum contains fatty acids, cholesterol and other substances.

A hair consists of a root containing non-keratinised cells and a shaft composed of keratinised cells. The part below the skin lies in what is called the hair follicle. A pointed projection of the dermis protrudes into the hair bulb and is known as the hair bulb papilla.

SKIN PREPARATIONS

Diseases of the skin are treated by both topical (local) and systemic therapy. A wide range of products is now available ranging from relatively simple emollients to sophisticated formulations containing potent drugs such as corticosteroids.

Emollients and barrier preparations

Emollients are used where a moisturising type of product is likely to be beneficial. They soothe and hydrate the skin and are indicated for dry scaling disorders. Frequent application is required since their effects are short-lived. They are useful in various dermatological conditions such as dry eczematous disorders and, to a lesser extent, psoriasis.

Emulsifying ointment 3% has emollient properties and may be used as a soap substitute to prevent the drying effect of soap on the skin. E45 cream is an effective emollient in conditions such as ichthyosis, traumatic dermatitis, dry eczema, certain types of psoriasis and also where movement of a joint is impaired by dryness or cracking of the overlying skin. E45 cream contains hydrous wool fat (lanolin) which may cause sensitisation in some patients. This should be suspected if an eczematous reaction occurs at the site of application. A wide range of emollient preparations is available. The choice of product will depend on consideration of the patient's condition, the patient's preference and clinical experience.

Barrier creams are used to provide protection against repeated hydration and irritation which can result in napkin rash, sore areas in the elderly, pressure sores and problems in areas surrounding stomata. Zinc and castor oil cream is an effective yet inexpensive emollient and barrier cream with mild astringent properties. However, there is no substitute for diligent nursing care, e.g. with napkin rash, a local dermatitis, the first-line of treatment is to ensure frequent napkin changes and that plastic pants are not too tight or have rough edges which chafe the skin. Rashes may clear when left exposed to the air and an emollient may be helpful. Barrier creams often contain water repellent substances such as dimethicone or other silicones but it is doubtful whether these water-repellent creams are any more effective than traditional compound zinc ointments.

Local anaesthetic and antipruritic preparations

Pruritus or itching may be generalised or localised. Pruritus is considered to be due to the stimulation of the subepidermal nerve plexuses by proteolytic enzymes which are released from the epidermis as a result of either primary irritation or allergic sensitisation reactions. This may be caused by disease, allergy, inflammation or exposure to irritant substances. Itching is a common symptom of many skin disorders including psoriasis, eczema, urticaria and scabies but may also be caused by systemic diseases such as endocrine disease, obstructive jaundice, drug hypersensitivity and certain malignant diseases. Other causes include localised fungal infection or parasitic infection.

Itching in localised parts of the body is often the result of local causes. Itching around the anus may be as a result of threadworm infestations in children or from haemorrhoids. Genital pruritus in women (pruritus vulva) may be caused by vaginal infections such as *Trichomonas vaginalis* or, in older women, by hormone deficiency.

Although scratching may provide temporary relief, it often exacerbates the condition by increasing inflammation. Assessment of the patient with pruritus involves first establishing the underlying cause so that appropriate therapy can be initiated. Where local applications are to

be used for symptomatic relief the patient's history must be checked for previous allergy and the skin inspected for signs of excessive dryness, cracking, weeping or broken areas. The patient must be given instruction on the correct method of application and advice to refrain from scratching or rubbing. This damages the epidermis and creates a vicious circle of lesion, more scratching and further damage.

A number of types of medication are used for the relief of skin irritation. Itching from dry skin is often soothed by a simple emollient. For mild itching arising from sunburn, urticaria or insect bites, a cooling lotion such as calamine, with the possible addition of menthol may be an appropriate treatment. Calamine lotion has astringent, healing, cooling and soothing properties, the addition of menthol increasing the cooling effect. The menthol however may give rise to hypersensitivity reactions in some patients. Oral antihistamines should be used in allergic rashes. Chlorpheniramine is an inexpensive antihistamine which is short-acting and mildly sedating. Where the irritation prevents sleep, a sedating antihistamine taken at night promotes sleep as well as relieves itching. Terfenadine which is longer acting than chlorpheniramine does not cause sedation.

Anal and perianal pruritus commonly occur in patients suffering from haemorrhoids. Control of diet to avoid hard stools as well as careful local hygiene are essential. Bland soothing preparations containing mild astringents such as bismuth subgallate, zinc oxide and hamamelis give symptomatic relief. Postmenopausal pruritus vulvae may be helped by vaginal creams containing oestrogen.

The risk of using preparations for pruritus other than simple emollient and soothing preparations is that prolonged or heavy use may cause skin irritation, resulting in aggravation of the itching. Since itching can be a symptom of many underlying conditions treatment should be reviewed after a week.

Local anaesthetic creams are absorbed through the skin and provide a numbing sensation. EMLA cream, which contains both lignocaine and prilocaine, is recommended for use as a local anaesthetic prior to venepuncture in children. It is applied under an occlusive dressing for a minimum of 1 hour or a maximum of 2 hours before the procedure. Lignocaine is not recommended for recurrent use but is useful in the form of a gel for procedures such as catheterisation.

Topical corticosteroids

Topical corticosteroids are used for the treatment of a wide variety of inflammatory conditions of the skin other than those due to an infection. Corticosteroids suppress various factors causing inflammation but they are not curative since the underlying cause of the inflammation is not affected. When treatment is discontinued the condition is likely to recur unless the underlying condition is successfully treated.

The choice of a topical corticosteroid must be made with care. In most cases a mild corticosteroid is used at the start of treatment. Rule of thumb is to use the minimum amount of the lowest potency corticosteroid. If a patient ceases to respond to a particular corticosteroid another of similar potency may be tried, before resorting to a more potent corticosteroid. Topical corticosteroid preparations are categorised into four groups according to potency (Box 21.1).

Box 21.1 Topical corticosteroids grouped according to potency	
Mild	Hydrocortisone 1%
Moderately potent	Clobetasone butyrate 0.05% (Eumovate)
Potent	Betamethasone 0.1% (Betnovate)
Very potent	Clobetasol propionate 0.05% (Dermovate)

Adequate use of emollients may reduce the need for large quantities of steroids. Where large areas are to be covered by steroids the nurse or patient should wear gloves and the preparation be applied sparingly. Application of excessive quantities of external corticosteroid preparations can result in undesirable local and systemic side-effects. The more potent the preparation, the

more care is required as absorption through the skin can cause severe pituitary adrenal suppression. The body's immune system is suppressed, thus increasing the risk of infection. Absorption is greatest from areas of thin skin and raw surfaces, and the effect is increased by occlusion. Very potent steroids should only be used for short periods. Local side-effects of topical corticosteroids include:

- thinning of the skin, sometimes resulting in stretch marks which may be permanent
- fine blood vessels under the skin surface possibly becoming prominent and resulting in a red rash if the vessels become damaged (telangiectasia); because the skin on the face is especially vulnerable to such damage, topical steroids are not usually prescribed for use on the face
- spread and exacerbation of untreated infection
- increased hair growth
- a possible temporary reduction in pigmentation at the site of application
- acne at the site of application in some patients
- delayed wound healing.

Children, and, in particular, babies, are particularly susceptible to side-effects due to increased absorption owing to their thinner skin and also greater proportion of surface area relative to weight. Potent and very potent steroids should not be used in children or only with great care for short periods. If a mild corticosteroid such as hydrocortisone is prescribed for treating napkin rash or eczema, care should be taken as napkins and plastic pants act as an occlusive dressing and increase absorption.

Some proprietary topical corticosteroid preparations contain antibiotics. These may be prescribed where infection complicates the underlying condition.

Preparations for eczema and psoriasis

Eczema

Eczema (dermatitis) may be caused by a variety of factors. Where possible the underlying cause should be identified and removed but in many cases this may be difficult. Emollients containing zinc oxide and calamine may be effective in treating dry, fissured scaly lesions. Weeping eczemas may be treated by corticosteroids but infection may militate against this. A weak solution (0.01%) of potassium permanganate as wet dressings can be applied, or, where larger areas are involved, potassium permanganate baths should be taken.

Keratolytics such as salicylic acid in yellow soft paraffin are used in chronic eczematous conditions where there is thickening of the skin or scaling. Care must be taken when high concentrations of salicylic acid are applied since salicylic acid is absorbed through the skin and can give rise to salicylate toxicity. Coal tar is more active than salicylic acid and it has keratolytic anti-inflammatory and antipruritic properties. Coal tar in yellow soft paraffin is used in strengths varying from 1% to 5% depending on the severity of the condition, the thicker the eczematous area the stronger the concentration of coal tar required. It has limitations due to unpleasant appearance and smell and its staining action on skin, hair and clothes. It is not suitable for use on the face. More sophisticated preparations containing tars are generally more acceptable to patients than are cruder, traditional preparations.

Psoriasis

Psoriasis occurs in a number of forms but is generally characterised by the accumulation of skin cells resulting in a thickening of the skin covered by silvery scales. It occurs when there is an excessive production of epidermal cells and the shedding of old skin cells remains normal, resulting in the characteristic lesions of psoriasis. For mild conditions an emollient cream may minimise scaling. When this fails to provide adequate relief, additional drug therapy is required.

Salicylic acid preparations are used in scaling conditions to increase the shedding of surface scale. Concentrations of 2% initially may be gradually increased.

The most potent topical preparation available is dithranol, which should be prescribed only by those experienced in its use. Dithranol combines with deoxyribonucleic acid, resulting in the inhibition of nucleoprotein synthesis and so diminishing cellular proliferation. Short-contact applications of 1 hour are effective, the strength of dithranol depending on the patient's condition within a range of 0.1% to 2% in Lassar's paste. Dithranol can cause severe skin irritation and for this reason it must be used strictly in accordance with the prescription. It must be applied only to psoriatic plaques commencing with a low concentration and gradually increasing this to an optimum concentration which produces a therapeutic effect without irritation. Dithranol stains skin purple-brown but this fades in 2 or 3 weeks. Hands should be thoroughly washed after use and it is essential for nurses to wear gloves when applying dithranol preparations. Dithranol should not be used on the face, flexures or scalp. Creams containing dithranol are easier to use than stiff pastes containing dithranol.

For more severe psoriasis not responding to these treatments, more powerful drugs may be prescribed. Acitretin is an oral preparation, available only in hospital and should be prescribed only by or under the supervision of a consultant dermatologist; 25–30 mg is administered daily for 2–4 weeks then adjusted according to response. This will usually be in the range of 25–50 mg daily for a further 6 to 8 weeks; however, a higher dose and longer treatment time may be needed. Side-effects include dryness and cracking of the lips, pruritus and nose bleeds. Acitretin is teratogenic, and contraceptive measures in women who may become pregnant should be commenced at least 1 month before treatment initiation and continued for at least 2 years following cessation of the drug. Another drug used in resistant cases, again under hospital supervision, is methotrexate for its antimitotic activity. It is a folic acid antagonist resulting in the inhibition of cellular proliferation.

Photochemotherapy involves the use of an oral photosensitising agent (psoralens) and exposure to ultraviolet light. This treatment is used for both initial treatment and maintenance therapy. Long-term dangers of this form of therapy are not yet confirmed.

Appropriate treatment of psoriasis improves the appearance of the skin. However, because drugs cannot cure the underlying cause of the disorder, psoriasis tends to recur.

Preparations for acne vulgaris

Acne is a common condition mainly affecting adolescents but it can occur later in life. It is caused by excess production of sebum by the sebaceous glands leading to a blockage of hair follicles by skin debris and hardened sebum. Acne normally affects the skin on the face and neck and less frequently the back and chest. This is characterised by blackheads, papules (inflamed spots) and pustules (raised pus-filled spots with a white centre).

Drugs used to treat acne act in different ways. Most topical preparations are intended to remove follicular plugs and reduce skin flora – these include benzoyl peroxide, salicylic acid, sulphur and tretinoin. Many of these irritate the skin, although this subsides with continued treatment. Benzoyl peroxide and sulphur also have a mild antibacterial effect. Tretinoin reduces sebum production. When applied to the skin it produces an erythematous reaction and skin peeling may occur after application for several days. Topical preparations of erythromycin, tetracycline or clindamycin are useful in patients with mild to moderately severe acne. Topical corticosteroids should not be used for acne. If acne is severe, a course of oral tetracycline or erythromycin may be prescribed – 250 mg 3 times daily before meals for 1–4 weeks then reduced to twice daily until improvement occurs. Several months' treatment or even longer may be required. Female patients must stop tetracycline if they become pregnant since this drug is deposited in teeth and bones. If these measures are unsuccessful, isotretinoin, an oral drug, may be prescribed. This has a similar but more powerful action than tretinoin. It is a hospital-only preparation and should only be prescribed by or under the supervision of a hospital consultant. Side-effects include dry lips, nose bleeds and some loss of hair. Isotretinoin is teratogenic and must not be given to pregnant women.

Contraceptive measures in women who may become pregnant must be effective throughout treatment and for at least 1 month after treatment is complete.

A preparation containing ethinyloestradiol and an anti-androgen, cyproterone acetate, is used to treat women with severe acne refractory to prolonged treatment with tetracyline or other antibiotic. The effect of this combination is probably due to decreased sebum secretion as a result of the anti-androgen effect.

Sunscreens

Sunlight is composed of a spectrum of wavelengths of electromagnetic radiation. Of these, ultraviolet radiation can be particularly harmful to the skin. People vary widely in their sensitivity to ultraviolet radiation. Fair-skinned people have least tolerance and burn easily whereas people with darker skin can withstand exposure for longer periods without noticeable harm. In addition, ultraviolet radiation may be harmful in certain diseases, e.g. lupus erythematosus and rosacea. Certain drugs such as chlorpromazine, demeclocycline and nalidixic acid can increase the skin's sensitivity to sunlight and in all these cases protection may be required from the sun's harmful rays.

Sunscreens contain substances such as aminobenzoic acid and padimate-O (Spectraban) which absorb the damaging portions of the ultraviolet spectrum and in this way provide protection. A range of sunscreens is available, graded according to the degree of protection – the sun protection factor (SPF). This figure indicates the amount of ultraviolet radiation which will be absorbed – the higher the SPF the greater the degree of protection. For skin protection in dermatological conditions an SPF of 15 or more is required. For maximum benefit the sunscreens must be applied frequently. They are applied before sunbathing to prevent erythema while allowing the skin to tan. People with fair skin should start with a sunscreen with a higher SPF. As the skin tans a low SPF may suffice. Because sunscreens filter out only a portion of the harmful rays, patients with sensitive skin should spend as little time as possible exposed to sunlight, even if they are using a sunscreen. Prolonged exposure of unprotected skin to strong sunlight increases the risk of skin cancer, especially among fair-skinned people, and also causes premature ageing of the skin .

Shampoos

Dandruff (pityriasis capitis) is the condition where the accumulation of dead cells on the scalp results in flaky scaling. The regular use of washing with a mild shampoo several times a week may be sufficient to keep the scalp free of dandruff. However, many people find that a medicated shampoo is required. Shampoos containing tar extracts may be useful as they soften the dead scales and make them easier to remove. Shampoos containing zinc pyrithine reduce the formation of dandruff by slowing the growth of skin scales, but are not prescribable. The use of selenium sulphide-containing shampoos is no more beneficial than non-medicated shampoos. Where dandruff is severe and unresponsive to these treatments, weak corticosteroid gels or lotions applied to the scalp may be helpful. Cradle cap in infants is treated with olive oil or arachis oil before shampooing.

Anti-infective preparations

The skin is subject to infection by bacteria, fungi and viruses. In some circumstances topical

Table 21.1   Antibacterial therapy

Drug(s) (presentation)	Indications/notes
Chlorhexidine (solution, medicated dressing)	See wound management, p. 318
Fusidic acid (ointment); mupirocin (ointment)	Useful for superficial infections such as impetigo. Active against *Staphylococcus aureus* and beta-haemolytic streptococci
Povidone-iodine (solution, paint, ointment)	A relatively non-irritant product, the active ingredient being iodine; useful for preventing secondary infection in viral infections. An ointment is used to prevent infection at catheter sites

Table 21.2   Antifungal therapy

Drug(s) (presentation)	Indications/notes
Amphotericin (ointment)	*Candida* infections
Imidazoles, i.e. clotrimazole, ketoconazole. (These drugs are available in a variety of ointments, creams and gels.)	*Candida* infections. Oral candida may require combination therapy using different antifungal drugs. Care must be taken to avoid re-infection from dentures. Athlete's foot is amenable to treatment by imidazoles.
Nystatin (ointment, cream)	*Candida* infections in napkin areas or other areas where there is close contact of skin folds.
Undecenoic acid (ointment, dusting powder)	Athlete's foot

Table 21.3   Antiviral therapy

Drug(s) (presentation)	Indications/notes
Acyclovir (cream) (also available in an oral and parenteral form – see Chapter 11)	Herpes simplex. Recurrent infections may require systemic therapy. As with other infections, in immuno-suppressed patients vigorous systemic treatment is required.
Formaldehyde (formalin) (solution)	Plantar warts. The area surrounding the wart is protected with soft paraffin prior to soaking the wart in formaldehyde solution. Salicylic acid may be used in the treatment of warts since it helps to remove keratinised tissue (keratolytic).
Glutaraldehyde (paint)	Persistent warts. Warts can grow very rapidly in immunosuppressed patients. Any existing warts should be treated prior to commencement of chemotherapy. If warts do develop following chemotherapy highly specialised treatment may be necessary.
Podophyllum resin (paint, ointment)	Genital warts. Due to the irritant nature of podophyllum, care must be taken to protect normal tissue at the time of its application. This drug must not be used in pregnancy.

therapy alone is indicated but where deep penetration of antimicrobial agent is required systemic therapy may be indicated (see also Ch. 11). Anti-infective agents are summarised in Tables 21.1–21.3.

Pediculosis

Contrary to popular belief, head lice are not confined to dirty long hair. In fact they flourish in a clean environment and are passed from person to person when one head touches another. The head louse would appear to have a preference for the blood of children. The reason for this is not understood. As boys get older they are much less susceptible to infestation than are girls. The 'at risk' group includes schoolchildren and some women. Mixing at home, at school or while playing increases the risk to all children. There is never a single case of head lice.

Lice are born, live and die on the host, leaving the head only to transfer to a similar environment. They spend their time feeding off the scalp and reproducing. The eggs laid are glued to the base of a strand of hair and are well camouflaged as they change in colour to match the skin. Once the eggs incubate, each hatches to produce a louse which, left untreated, will eventually sap the person's strength and leave them generally unwell. The empty shells remain firmly glued as the hair continues to grow and they change to a pure white colour distracting attention from any new live eggs which are always laid at the base of a hair. It is the white shell which is left behind that is called a nit.

Nurses in the community, at school and in hospital should exercise diplomacy when dealing with affected patients or explaining the condition to a child's mother. While not wanting to create offence or embarrassment, the nurse in her role as a health educator, must ensure that this particular problem is not allowed to go unchecked.

Treatment of head lice

The only really successful formulations for treating lice are either lotions, which stay on the head long enough to kill eggs as well as lice, or the cream rinse treatments. These wet the hair and the eggs with a conditioner containing the pediculocide which remains when the treatment is washed off. A long contact time is thus achieved with only a short application time.

In order to prevent resistance developing, most health authorities have a rotation policy where only one type of active ingredient will be used in any three-year period, e.g. malathion may be alternated with carbaryl.

When applying a lotion to the head it should be remembered that it is the scalp that has to be treated rather than the hair. The hair should be parted while it is still dry and the lotion sprinkled into the partings until the whole scalp has been moistened, taking care to avoid contact with the eyes. The scalp is massaged gently, paying particular attention to the back of the head and to the areas behind the ears. The hair may then be combed and should be allowed to dry naturally. The application is removed 12 hours later using ordinary shampoo. A fine-tooth comb may be used to remove the nits. If necessary, the treatment is repeated a week later.

If one member of a family is affected, the whole family must be treated to make certain that they are all free of infestation. Classmates should be treated similarly. Mothers should be advised to make a regular check on their children's heads and to encourage combing of the hair especially at bedtime. In summary, regular grooming, prompt detection and effective treatment can help to keep this condition under control.

Disinfectants

Chemical disinfectants play a limited role in helping to achieve the control of infection in both hospital and community practice. The limitations of disinfectants are well known. Poor range of activity and effectiveness, toxicity, inconvenience and high cost all contribute to the declining use of these agents. In addition, the availability of a wide range of sterile disposable equipment, improved physical sterilisation methods and cleaning techniques have further reduced the need for chemical disinfectants. Disinfectants have a limited place in wound management procedures (see p. 320) and in the preparation of skin prior to venepuncture or surgery. Alcoholic solutions containing chlorhexidine 0.5% w/v are often used for such purposes. Chlorhexidine combined with a cleansing agent may be used if the patient's skin is dirty. Hand preparation prior to surgical procedures is generally carried out using a detergent/chlorhexidine combination and a suitable technique. Alcoholic chlorhexidine solution may be useful as a hand rub after washing but this will not achieve decontamination of unwashed skin.

Hard surfaces may be treated with ethyl or isopropyl alcohol in a suitable form (spray or swab). Glutaraldehyde solution has a place in the disinfection of surgical equipment that cannot be heat treated. Careful technique is essential when using glutaraldehyde particularly with regard to the protection of staff and the environment. Whenever possible disinfectants should be used in prepared single-use sachets so as to minimise risks of cross-infection.

Antiperspirants

Hyperhidrosis (overproduction of sweat) may be a localised or a more generalised problem. A generalised problem condition can be treated with anticholinergic drugs, but side-effects (see p. 50) may limit the use of this form of treatment. Localised hyperhidrosis may respond to treatment with a paint containing 20% w/v aluminium chloride in alcohol. The paint is applied overnight to the area affected following careful cleaning and drying. In very resistant cases surgery may be required to remove areas of maximum sweat production.

Table 21.4 indicates some of the potential problems of using certain dermatological prepa-

Table 21.4 Problems associated with some dermatological preparations

Problem	Ingredient causing problem	Methods of risk reduction/precautions
Absorption – systemic	Azelaic acid; corticosteroids (especially potent agents); neomycin; salicylic acid; terbinafine	Avoid contact by using disposable gloves or applicator if available. Wash hands after use (nurse and patient). Occlusive dressings increase absorption – use only when/as prescribed. Discontinue breast-feeding due to risks
Eye irritancy	Aluminium chloride; benzoyl peroxide; carbaryl;dithranol; podophyllum resin; sulphur	Never use on face. Patient should be warned not to rub eyes when (or after) using product. Wash hands after use
Flammable products	Alcohol (especially in high concentrations); collodions; ether	Should never be used near naked flame, electric heaters or other ignition sources
Granuloma	Talc in dusting powders	Avoid contact with broken skin/body cavities
Infection	Many dermatological preparations, especially those containing a high percentage of water and/or prepared by dilution of a proprietary product	All dermatological products should be used with care to avoid contamination/cross-infection. Observe expiry dates/conditions of storage. Single-use packs should be for preservative-free products. Particular care is needed where large areas of broken skin are involved
Irritancy of respiratory tract	Dusting powders; pressurised aerosol	Take care to avoid inhalation, especially in sensitive subjects
Photosensitivity	Antihistamines; coal tar; tretinoin	Patient should be warned to avoid exposure to strong sunlight
Sensitisation reactions	Antihistamines; local anaesthetics; neomycin	Be alert to this possibility. Use of product may have to be discontinued
Skin/fair hair Skin irritancy	Clioquinol; coal tar products; dithranol Dithranol; formaldehyde; malathion; podophyllum resin; sulphur; tioconazole	Patient should be warned in advance Should be applied only to those areas to be treated. Normal skin may be protected by a bland agent, e.g. soft paraffin. Confine application to lesions
Staining of personal linen and the patient's bath	Coal tar products; dithranol; potassium permanganate	Patient should be warned in advance. Particular items of 'old' linen may be advisable when these products are in use

rations. The list should not be regarded as fully comprehensive but does identify the major problem areas.

WOUND MANAGEMENT

A wound can be described as any break in the continuity of the skin resulting from physical, mechanical or thermal damage. Irrespective of the type of wound being treated, the overriding objective is to promote healing and prevent infection. The patients at greatest risk of developing infection are those suffering pre-existing disease or who are in a poor nutritional state. Patients in hospital rather than at home are at increased risk because of exposure to pathogenic microorganisms, many of which have become resistant to antibiotics. While it is not possible to eliminate this risk totally, it can be minimised. Broad principles of wound management are applicable in all settings although the precise management of a wound will depend on the clinical assessment by the individual practitioner. The consensus of opinion today is that the more disturbance, albeit well intentioned, of a wound, the greater the likelihood of infection being introduced and healing being delayed. Consequently, routine changing of dressings is no longer practised.

With the development of the nursing process, hospital nurses are encouraged to assess and treat the patient and his wound(s) on an individual basis, and not as part of a routine dressing round. As a result, the timing of dressings in relation to general ward activities is less easy to define. Nursing and domestic staff have to strive for the best possible compromise in the patients' interests. Rooms set aside for aseptic procedures overcome this difficulty. Wherever possible, whether a single dressing is to be done or several dressings are being done consecutively, a working principle of 'clean to dirty' should be adopted. The main source of infection is the hands of personnel, especially those in close contact with the patient. Correct handwashing technique helps to prevent cross-infections. A non-touch technique for aseptic procedures must also be adopted.

Handwashing procedure

Three forms of handwashing are used in patient care – social, antiseptic and surgical – depending on the procedures to be carried out. The hands should be socially clean before caring for any patient. However, any procedure requiring an aseptic technique, such as the dressing of a wound, involves an antiseptic handwash. Specially formulated preparations containing chlorhexidine or povidone-iodine are suitable as they combine detergency with antiseptic properties. They remove and kill transient organisms on the skin and also have some effect on bacteria in deeper layers of the skin. Organisms on the skin include Gram-positive ones such as *Staphylococcus aureus* and Gram-negative ones such as *Escherichia coli*, both of which are common causes of hospital infection . Regular use of an antiseptic handwash has a cumulative effect and an extremely low level of resident organisms can be achieved. Surgical handwashing is not discussed, although the principles outlined below do apply.

While working with patients, nurses should have short clean nails free of nail varnish and should not wear jewellery or a wrist watch. For each handwash, the hands should be wetted first before the handwashing agent is applied, using an elbow dispenser. All surfaces are lathered, including the wrists. Particular attention should be paid to the backs of the hands and fingers as well as between the fingers. Both hands should be cleaned thoroughly; right-handed people tend to clean the left hand more thoroughly and vice versa. Scrubbing the hands is no longer advocated as this action creates disturbance to the resident flora and can cause trauma. The hands and wrists are rinsed under running water to remove lather and the taps turned off with the elbows or, if necessary, holding a paper towel. Careful drying of the hands with a paper towel is essential to protect the skin from possible breakdown, to make it harder for microorganisms to thrive, and to facilitate putting on gloves. The exact timing of handwashing prior to undertaking an aseptic procedure must be left to the discretion of the nurse.

Preparation of the environment

Potential wound contaminants in the environment take the form of dust and droplets. A few minutes spent in preparing the environment prior to an aseptic procedure reduces these modes of infection. Before setting up the dressing trolley, an explanation should be given to the patient as to what is involved and he should be given the opportunity to make himself as comfortable as possible. Screens should be pulled gently as far in advance of the procedure as possible to allow dust to settle. Sufficient working space is essential so that the procedure can take place safely and efficiently. For example, the floor where the nurse is to be working should be clear; furniture may have to be moved to make way for the dressing trolley, and flowers should be removed from the immediate vicinity. Where the preferred technique involves the wearing of gloves, a flat surface such as the bedtable which later can be cleaned, should first be cleared. Traffic around the patient's bed should be reduced to a minimum.

The spread of droplet infection is another potential hazard. The wearing of masks of suitable specification protects the patient from droplets from the nurse's upper respiratory tract. However, masks – unless of the correct specification and used correctly – can provide a suitable environment for microbial growth. For simple procedures, such as removing sutures or dressing a sealed wound, masks are not required. Only in the case of extensive tissue damage (e.g. burns, skin grafts or deep wounds) or where the patient is immunosuppressed, are masks of high-filter performance used. The same principles apply to the wearing of disposable caps. While the wound is exposed and dressing packs open, conversation should be restricted, the patient having had the reason for this explained at the time of preparation. Nurses with colds and sore throats should never participate in aseptic procedures.

Preparation of the trolley

Trolleys for aseptic procedures should be set aside for the purpose. Before proceeding, the nurse washes her hands and dons a disposable apron. The trolley is cleaned using a small amount of suitable detergent and a damp paper towel. Trolley cleaning includes legs and bars as well as the shelves. It is then dried with a paper towel prior to the application of an alcoholic solution of a disinfectant in the form of a disposable swab, spray or liquid. Alcohol enhances the bactericidal effect of the active agent and is quick-drying. A dry surface is less conducive to the growth of microorganisms than is a damp one. The top shelf is kept clear until the start of the dressing while the necessary requirements for the procedure are placed on the lower shelf. Going through the procedure mentally at this stage ensures that no essential item is omitted.

Packs of sterile equipment and materials should be inspected before use to ensure that they are intact. Further means of determining whether packs are safe for use vary. Satisfactory autoclaving may be confirmed by the indicator on some packs whereas the expiry date or known shelf-life for a specific pack indicates whether it may be safely used. Single-use packs of sterile antiseptic solutions are ideal for wound care. Today the cleansing agent of choice is sodium chloride solution 0.9%.

Preparation of the patient

Having prepared the environment, herself and the trolley for redressing a wound, the nurse assists the patient into a suitable position which, as well as allowing ease of access, is as acceptable to the patient as possible. The patient should be kept warm, comfortable and have privacy. It should be recognised that some patients may prefer not to look at the wound. Conventional analgesia may have been given in advance although sometimes for very painful procedures such as the removal of a large pack, Entonox, a gaseous mixture of 50% oxygen and 50% nitrous oxide, may be given to the patient to inhale during the procedure.

Assessment of the wound

This must be carried out before any specific local

Table 21.5 Wound assessment

Factors	Signs/comments
Presence of infection	Localised heat, swelling, redness, tenderness, pus, foul odour. Swab taken before any antiseptic solution applied
Presence of necrotic tissue	Brown or black appearance
Presence of slough	Yellowish accumulation of dead cells
Presence of granulation tissue	Red appearance due to establishment of new blood vessels. This stage precedes epithelialisation
Epithelialisation	Care is needed to distinguish epithelialisation from slough formation. Epilethelialisation is generally characterised by a pinky-white appearance

Table 21.6 Local wound treatments and their main indications

Product	Main indications
Chlorhexidine solutions	Antiseptic. The very dilute solutions often used have little antibacterial action. May be combined with cetrimide which provides detergency
Hydrogen peroxide 10 volumes	Wound cleansing agent. Not to be used in cavity wounds. Very limited antibacterial effect
Malic acid compound solution (also available as a cream)	Wound cleansing agent
Povidone-iodine spray	Slow release iodine preparation. Wide antibacterial spectrum
Sodium hypochlorite solution (Eusol and Eusol substitutes)	Cleansing and de-sloughing agent. Current opinion suggests this product should only be used for limited periods of time since the healing process can be delayed

treatment is instituted and before the choice of a suitable dressing is made. Specific aspects of the assessment procedure are summarised in Table 21.5.

Having carried out an assessment of the wound it may be necessary to use a local application to assist in achieving the desired result, e.g. de-sloughing local agent (often a solution). Whatever is applied, great care must be exercised in applying the solution to the wound. The technique to be followed will depend on a number of factors but great care must be taken to avoid further trauma.

Having carried out the necessary procedure, e.g. swabbing, the patient is made comfortable and the immediate clinical area is restored to normal. All disposable materials must be placed in the appropriate disposal bag which is sealed ready for disposal. Any re-usable equipment is dealt with in accordance with the local disinfection/sterilisation policy.

Local wound treatments

A range of local treatments is available. These are summarised in Table 21.6. It is emphasised that these products should be used only where clinically indicated.

Prevention of wound infection

Apart from achieving high standards of asepsis during actual wound care procedures, certain preoperative measures are taken to prevent (or reduce the likelihood of) wound infection. Intensive pre-operative skin preparation using a well-defined regimen may be commenced 3 days prior to orthopaedic, cardiac, or other forms of surgery, where the infection risk is great and/or where the consequences of infection are especially dangerous for the patient. Such measures will also reduce the possibility of infection becoming established in underlying tissues.

Apart from the topical approach, irrigation with an antibacterial agent during operative procedures may be carried out. Tetracycline, in the form of a sterile irrigation solution, has been used to reduce infection following abdominal surgery.

Various forms of systemic therapy may also be used to prevent postoperative wound infection. A course of antibiotic or other form of antimicrobial therapy may be given. Gut irrigation procedures with a solution of antibiotics have also been used pre-operatively.

Patients who are poor risks for good wound healing include those with a poor nutritional status; uncontrolled diabetes or obesity; the heavy smoker; and those receiving cytotoxic therapy in combination with surgery. Some of these patients may need additional supportive therapy such as enteral or parenteral nutrition.

Surgical dressings

The purpose of a surgical dressing is generally to stem bleeding, absorb exudate and provide protection so that healing may be allowed to take place. The ideal wound dressing may be considered in terms of the wound, the patient and the dressing itself.

As far as the wound is concerned, the dressing should be:

- of good absorbency
- able to maintain optimal conditions for wound healing, including high humidity at wound/dressing interface, high thermal insulation properties, and gaseous exchange
- impermeable to microorganisms
- able to provide physical protection to the wound
- free from toxic substances and shedding fibres
- removable without causing damage to the newly formed tissues.

As far as the patient is concerned, the dressing should be:

- comfortable, providing a feeling of confidence and sense of security
- non-allergenic.

The dressing itself should be:

- in a sterile presentation, preferably unit pack
- conveniently packaged for ease of removal in aseptic procedures
- compatible with commonly used medicaments
- made so as to allow observation of the wound, and should be radiotranslucent
- economical in use
- easily disposable.

No one dressing has all the above properties, although many dressings developed in the last 25 years combine many of the highly desirable properties listed. The challenge for nurse and doctor is therefore to select a dressing or combination of dressings which will suit a particular wound and the stage reached in the healing process. In order to assist in the selection of a suitable dressing both wounds and dressings can be classified.

Classification of wounds

A wound is first considered according to depth:

- superficial
- cavity.

The state of the wound may then be described:

- clean
- exuding tissue fluid
- sloughing
- clinically infected
- foul smelling.

Having arrived at a clinical description and assessment of the wound, based on the above classification, a suitable dressing can then be selected. Many hospitals have now established written protocols for the treatment of wounds and it is essential that nurses be aware of these and follow the recommendations made.

The work of Winter (1962, 1971) and Bucknell (1984) gave great impetus to the development of surgical dressings which may be described as interactive. Such dressings, the gels and gel-forming products, interact with the wound to create a 'micro-climate' that encourages wound healing. In contrast, the simple woven textiles have no beneficial interactive properties. In the future it is likely that dressings containing biological agents that stimulate the wound healing process will be developed.

Classification of dressings

Dressings can be classified under a number of headings but it is unlikely that one classification system will meet all the needs of the nurse. In Table 21.7 dressings are classified broadly according to the materials used in their manufac-

Table 21.7 Classification of dressings

Material	Example(s)	Main properties/comments
Alginates (derived from certain seaweeds)	Kaltostat; Kaltocarb	Gel-forming on wound surface; haemostatic; simple alginate sheets may require absorbent backing
Collagen	Fibracol in combination with alginate	Gel-forming on wound surface; maintains moist environment to encourage wound healing
Foams	Silastic	Silastic foam is formed by a chemical reaction between two components. This dressing is used to treat cavity wounds.
	Lyofoam	Lyofoam is presented as a foam sheet with a special wound contact surface
Hydrocolloids (gel-forming agents)	Granuflex; Tegasorb	Gel-forming in contact with wound (gel maintains moist environment at wound surface)
Hydrogels	Geliperm; Scherisorb	Provide moist environment which encourages wound healing. Does not provide high absorptive properties. Very costly for routine use
Plastic films (synthetic polymer)	Opsite	Such films protect wound from bacterial contamination and are semi-permeable to allow passage of water vapour, thus preventing maceration of wound
Polysaccharides	Debrisan	Available as beads; draws up tissue exudate. Should be renewed before beads are saturated
Textiles (cotton)	Cotton wool; gauze	Absorptive properties. Do not have any interactive properties

ture. This classification includes an indication of the main properties of the materials.

Alginates

Alginate dressings are manufactured from a variety of seaweeds which, when they come into contact with blood or exudate, turn into a gel. Kaltostat may be used in a wide range of heavily exuding wounds, bleeding or non-bleeding. Kaltoclude comprises a Kaltostat dressing combined with a semipermeable membrane and obviates the need for any additional dressing. It is suitable for moderate to lightly exuding wounds. Kaltocarb also consists of a Kaltostat dressing but has incorporated into it activated charcoal to help absorb odour from wounds which are complicated by bacterial infection, fungating from carcinoma or gangrenous.

Collagen

Dressings containing collagen in combination with alginate have recently been introduced. It is claimed that this combination provides a dressing which maintains a moist wound healing environment through the various phases of wound healing.

Foams

Two types of foam dressings are in use. Silastic foam is produced by a chemical reaction between a base and a catalyst. The foam forms to occupy the wound cavity and is both absorbent and non-adherent. Lyofoam is a polyurethane foam sheet one side of which has been heated to form a hydrophilic surface. It creates a moist environment which encourages wound healing and has significant absorption properties.

Hydrogels

These novel materials contain 96% water. The material is given strength and flexibility by a polymer, polyacrylamide. Geliperm is an example of such material. This interactive dressing provides a moist environment which encourages wound healing. The dressings are very comfortable for the patient and easy to remove. The availability of hydrocolloid dressings and the high cost have limited the use of hydrogel dressings.

Hydrocolloids

Hydrocolloid dressings contain cellulose derivatives which, when they come into contact with the wound, liquefy to produce a pus-like fluid. Examples include Granuflex and Comfeel. As the dressing absorbs moisture from the wound, debridement takes place which may temporarily increase the size of the wound but then allows healing to take place. Although no secondary dressing is necessary, it is important to ensure that the dressing extends at least 2 cm beyond the edge of the wound. In this form of dressing the liquefying process of itself produces a very strong odour about which the patient should be warned.

Plastic films

These plastic film dressings have the advantage of being waterproof, transparent and comfortable. They therefore maintain a moist environment, permit easy observation of the wound and may be used in many sites. Their most appropriate use is for dressing surgical wounds, catheter insertion sites and superficial burns or pressure sores. The heavy exudate associated with leg ulcers and deep pressure sores precludes their use for deep wounds. Examples include Opsite and Bioclusive.

Polysaccharides

Polysaccharides (synthetic sugars) are used in the form of beads, pastes or granules. Debrisan and Iodosorb are examples of bead dressings which when placed in contact with a wound rapidly draw the exudate into the beads which swell to form a gel. Dressings require to be changed before the beads become fully saturated, e.g. once or twice a day. They are suitable only for sloughy, exuding wounds.

Textiles

Simple absorbent pads such as lint, gauze, and gauze and cotton tissue provide protection, keep wounds warm and are of good absorbency. However, they may adhere to the wound surface and shed fibres into the wound. Microbiological protection is limited. Structured dressing pads such as Surgipad and Ete which have an outer sleeve of non-adherent material possess similar properties to the various simple absorbent pads but are generally easier to remove. Some contain a layer of activated charcoal which is useful for deodorising malodorous wounds and ulcers. Tulle dressings are of open weave and are often impregnated with soft paraffin or polyethylene glycol. These are especially suitable in the management of abrasions and superficial burns because of their non-adherent property. They may be impregnated further with, e.g. chlorhexidine or framycetin, thus adding antimicrobial effect.

REFERENCES

Bucknell T E 1984 Factors affecting wound healing. In: Bucknell T E, Ellis H (eds) Wound healing for surgeons. Baillière Tindall, London, pp 42–74
Winter G D 1962 Formation of the scab and rate of epithelialisation of superficial wounds in the skin of the young domestic pig. Nature 193: 293 – 294

Winter G D 1971 Healing of skin wounds and the influence of dressing on the repair process. In: Harkiss K J (ed) Surgical dressings and wound healing. Crosby and Lockwood, London

FURTHER READING

Bale S 1993 Intervention in wound management. Surgical Nurse 6(3): 17–20
Gawkrodger D 1993 Atopic eczema Practitioner 237: 166–171

Johnson A 1993 Wound assessment. Wound Management May/June: 27–30

22

Anaesthetic agents

INTRODUCTION

Detailed knowledge of individual anaesthetic drugs is necessary only for nurses working in the operating theatre or intensive therapy unit. However, all surgical ward nurses should have an appreciation of what comprises a modern anaesthetic. Most important of all is an understanding of the drugs used in the pre- and postanaesthetic management of the surgical patient.

Despite the technological complexity of modern anaesthetic practice, the exact mechanism of general anaesthesia has yet to be elucidated. The fact that compounds as diverse as inorganic gases, ethers and steroids can produce general anaesthesia suggests that their action is non-specific. In contrast, the mode of action of local anaesthetic drugs is well understood: transmission of peripheral nerve impulses is blocked by the reversible 'plugging' of sodium channels, preventing membrane depolarisation.

In adults, general anaesthesia is almost always induced by intravenous injection. The dose is dependent on factors such as age and cardiac output. Babies and young children are often anaesthetised with inhalational agents because small veins are difficult to cannulate. Once the patient is asleep, anaesthesia is usually maintained by a mixture of anaesthetic gases (strictly speaking, *vapours*) in oxygen. However, accurate syringe pumps can be used to deliver intravenous anaesthetic for the duration of the operation. This is known as total intravenous anaesthesia (TIVA). Local anaesthetics can be used alone (as in a spinal or epidural) or in conjunction with general anaesthesia or sedation. Depending on the nature of the operation, a patient will either be allowed to breathe spontaneously, or will be mechanically ventilated while paralysed with a muscle relaxant (or *neuromuscular blocking*) drug.

PRE-OPERATIVE MEDICATION

In the days of ether and chloroform, premedication was essential. Ether caused profuse salivation and tracheobronchial secretions, and therefore atropine was used routinely as a drying agent. In contrast, chloroform predisposed the patient to dangerous cardiac arrhythmias, and heavy sedation was necessary to minimise the risk.

In anaesthetic practice today pre-operative medication is prescribed in response to the specific needs of the patient. Table 22.1 indicates the main drugs used to dry bronchial, pharyngeal and salivary secretions. All these drugs have antimuscarinic actions (see p. 50).

Sedative drugs are no substitute for explanation and reassurance by nursing staff. However, a benzodiazepine such as temazepam or lorazepam given orally helps patients to relax before going to theatre. Children are often prescribed trimeprazine (Vallergan) syrup. The introduction of EMLA cream has allowed pain-free needle insertion. EMLA stands for 'eutectic mixture of local anaesthetic', which is a white cream containing two local anaesthetic ingredients, lignocaine and prilocaine. An hour before venepuncture it is applied to the back of the hand and covered by an occlusive dressing to facilitate penetration into nerve endings in the epidermis.

Many patients undergoing surgery will be taking medicines for conditions unrelated to their operation. Abrupt discontinuation can have adverse effects. The nurse will be guided by the anaesthetist, and should be prepared to administer certain drugs (particularly heart and blood pressure medication) as usual, with a sip of water, even if the patient is 'nil by mouth'. On the other hand, oral hypoglycaemic agents should never be given to a fasting patient. Insulin will be administered with dextrose by intravenous infusion. The anaesthetist may prescribe additional medication such as a nitrate patch (e.g. Transiderm-Nitro) for a patient with angina. Asthmatics should have their salbutamol (or equivalent) inhalers available for use prior to induction of anaesthesia.

Patients who are pregnant or who have a hiatus hernia are at increased risk of inhaling gastric contents, which can cause a fatal pneumonitis. A histamine type 2 receptor antagonist such as ranitidine is given before caesarean section to stop gastric acid secretion. Immediately before induction of anaesthesia, 30 ml 0.3 molar sodium citrate is given by mouth to raise the pH of the stomach contents.

INHALATIONAL AGENTS

Nitrous oxide entered medical practice in the 1840s. The 'ideal' inhalational agent has yet to be developed; the features of such an agent are given in Box 22.1.

Nitrous oxide is supplied in blue cylinders. It is a weak anaesthetic, and has to be administered with at least 30% oxygen. On the anaesthetic machine in the operating theatre, nitrous oxide and oxygen are directed to *vaporisers*, which are filled with potent liquid anaesthetic. Halothane, enflurane and isoflurane are the three agents currently used in the United Kingdom, although desflurane and sevoflurane may be introduced in

Table 22.1 Drugs used to dry secretions

Drug	Adult dose/route	Actions/notes
Atropine	600 μg i.m. or i.v. before induction of anaesthesia	Dries secretions; may cause tachycardia
Hyoscine	400 μg i.m. or i.v. before induction	Dries secretions. Induces amnesia. Less tachycardia than atropine. May cause CNS disturbances
Glycopyrronium bromide	200–400 μg i.m. or i.v. before induction	Dries secretions. Less tachycardia than atropine. Reduces acidity of gastric contents

the near future. The depth of anaesthesia is varied by altering the concentration of vapour carried by the oxygen and nitrous oxide. A 50/50 mixture of oxygen and nitrous oxide is known as Entonox (a trade name registered by the British Oxygen Company). An Entonox cylinder has a blue body with a blue and white shoulder. Entonox is carried by ambulances for use in emergency situations and is used for analgesia during labour and for short potentially painful procedures such as dressing changes. Some patients feel little effect from breathing Entonox, yet others may lose consciousness. Therefore, the mask should always be applied by the patient. Should loss of consciousness occur, the mask will fall away.

Box 22.1 Desirable features of an 'ideal' inhalational agent

It should not form flammable mixtures with oxygen or other agents
The vapour should not be unpleasant to inhale
The drug should be insoluble in the bloodstream, allowing rapid induction and elimination
The drug should be free of organ-specific toxic effects, e.g. renal or hepatic failure, and should not undergo metabolism in the body
Depression of the cardiovascular and respiratory systems should be minimal
The drug should possess analgesic properties

INTRAVENOUS ANAESTHETICS

Intravenous anaesthesia became established in the 1920s. Again, the 'ideal' agent does not exist, but its features are shown in Box 22.2.

Box 22.2 Desirable features of an 'ideal' intravenous agent

The drug should not cause pain on injection
Induction of anaesthesia should be rapid and smooth
Return of consciousness should also be rapid, with no hangover, nausea, vomiting, or unpleasant dreams
Depression of the cardiovascular and respiratory systems should be minimal
Serious adverse reactions should be extremely rare

Thiopentone, a barbiturate, is still widely used after half a century. Methohexitone, another barbiturate, affords a less smooth induction but faster recovery compared with thiopentone. It is used to provide anaesthesia for electroconvulsive therapy. The barbiturates have been superseded for day cases by propofol (Diprivan), which allows a clearer-headed recovery with less nausea or vomiting. In addition, anaesthesia can be maintained by continuous infusion, since recovery is rapid, even after prolonged administration for TIVA. However, the cost of Diprivan is about five times that of thiopentone. Etomidate is the drug of choice for those patients in whom cardiovascular stability is particularly important. Midazolam (Hypnovel) and diazepam (Diazemuls) are benzodiazepines which are available as intravenous preparations. Both can induce anaesthesia, but are mainly used in smaller doses to provide sedation for endoscopies. Flumazenil (Anexate) is a specific benzodiazepine antagonist which reverses the effects of both these drugs. Ketamine increases heart rate and blood pressure, and is favoured for the shocked patient. It is used in military surgery, and for emergency procedures outside hospital such as amputation of a trapped limb. It is rarely used unsupplemented in hospital because recovery is associated with unpleasant dreams and hallucinations, which are minimised if the patient is disturbed as little as possible in the recovery period.

MUSCLE RELAXANTS

Muscle relaxant drugs are used to paralyse a patient's muscles to allow passage of a tracheal tube, to maintain relaxation of the body's muscles for abdominal surgery, and to facilitate artificial ventilation. Suxamethonium (Scoline) is a particularly short-acting drug. It has a common, unique side-effect: pains in muscles not usually associated with strain after exercise, for example, between the scapulae. The complaint is commonest in the muscular young patient who is up and about soon after the operation. A rarer problem is a genetic deficiency of the enzyme needed to break down the drug and terminate its action. A patient scheduled for a short procedure might have to be kept asleep and artificially ventilated for a number of hours until the drug effect wears off. This complication is often called 'Scoline apnoea'. There are a number of other muscle relaxant drugs (Box 22.3) which differ in their onset and duration of action.

Box 22.3 Non-depolarising muscle relaxants

Alcuronium	Atracurium	Gallamine	Mivacurium
Pancuronium	Rocuronium	Tubocurarine	Vecuronium

ANALGESICS

Opioids are naturally occurring and synthetic drugs which produce morphine-like effects. They act on receptors found in the brain and spinal cord. Short-acting synthetic opioids like fentanyl and alfentanil are commonly used as components of the anaesthetic. Longer-acting drugs tend to be used for postoperative analgesia. There is little to choose between equipotent doses of different opioids; morphine is the reference by which all newer drugs may be judged in terms of analgesic efficacy and side-effects. Box 22.4 lists the side-effects common to all opioids. The potential for causing slowing of breathing and respiratory arrest is by far the most important.

Box 22.4 Side-effects of opioids

Respiratory depression
Nausea and vomiting
Dysphoria and hallucinations
Cough suppression
Constipation
Pupillary constriction

Postoperative analgesia has traditionally been prescribed as a fixed-dose intramuscular injection of opioid, to be given no more frequently than 4-hourly. This regime is unsatisfactory, since it does not allow for patients' enormous differences in analgesic requirements after the same operation. Some patients are reticent about asking for analgesia because of fear of the injection, demonstrating apparent failure to cope, or developing addiction. Moreover, drugs given intramuscularly are not well-absorbed when patients are cold after lengthy surgery and skeletal muscle is poorly perfused. If injections are repeated in an attempt to control pain, there is a risk of absorption of dangerously large amounts when the patient warms up.

A recent major advance in the management of postoperative pain has been the development of patient-controlled analgesia (PCA). In response to pressing a button, the patient receives boluses of opioid by the *intravenous* route. The key to understanding PCA is the *'lockout interval'*; this is the period after a bolus during which any further attempts by the patient to receive opioid will be turned down by the machine. A PCA system might initially be set to deliver a 1 mg bolus of morphine with a lockout interval of 5 minutes. Since there are 12×5 minutes in an hour, the patient would be able to receive a maximum of 12×1 mg = 12 mg per hour. Were this to prove inadequate, the anaesthetist would administer a further loading dose and increase the bolus setting. The safety of PCA relies on *only* the patient pressing the button.

Patients' pain, degree of sedation and respiratory rate should be evaluated and recorded as routinely as pulse and blood pressure. Wherever opioids are administered, naloxone (Narcan), which is a specific antagonist, should be immediately available.

Non-steroidal anti-inflammatory drugs (NSAIDs) work by inhibiting enzymes involved in mediating pain from damaged tissue. Diclofenac (Voltarol) and ketorolac (Toradol) are related to aspirin. Their advantage is that there is no risk of respiratory depression. They can be given *in addition to* opioids, improving the quality of postoperative analgesia and reducing the necessary dose of opioid and its side-effects. However, there are important contraindications (Box 22.5).

Box 22.5 Contraindications to NSAIDs

Renal impairment, dehydration or hypovolaemia
Bleeding abnormalities or risk of postoperative bleeding
History of peptic ulcer or gastrointestinal bleeding
Asthma or nasal polyps
Pregnancy, labour, delivery or lactation

If Voltarol is given by intramuscular injection, the site *must* be deep into the gluteal muscle because injection into the thigh can be complicated by nerve damage and abscess formation. The drug is effective given as a suppository.

ANTI-EMETICS

Nausea and vomiting is a frequent minor complication of surgery and anaesthesia. A number of factors contribute to its likelihood (Box 22.6).

Box 22.6 Factors contributing to postoperative nausea and vomiting

Patient age (twice as likely in children) and sex (women have higher incidence, greatest in weeks 3 and 4 of the menstrual cycle)
History of motion sickness or vomiting after previous anaesthetic
Whether anti-emetics are given prior to induction of anaesthesia
Which anaesthetics/analgesics are used (opioids increase the incidence)
Type of operation (e.g. laparoscopy, squint, or middle ear surgery) and duration
Adequacy of postoperative analgesia

Table 22.2 lists examples of anti-emetic agents and their respective modes of action. None is reliably effective, although ondansetron, which is effective in reducing vomiting induced by chemotherapy, shows great promise for postoperative use.

LOCAL ANAESTHETICS

Local anaesthetics work by blocking conduction of nerve impulses conveying pain. The various agents have different durations of action and toxicity. They can be injected anywhere from the site of the incision (local infiltration) to the cerebrospinal fluid (spinal block). Local anaesthetics can be used to provide analgesia following most operations. If catheters are inserted close to nerves running from the area of the operation (*e.g.* brachial plexus for hand surgery) analgesia can be maintained for as long as is necessary by topping up with local anaesthetic when pain returns. Bupivacaine (Marcain) is a longer-acting agent than lignocaine, although more toxic in overdose. Epidurals are increasingly being used for postoperative analgesia following major abdominal, vascular and thoracic surgery. Drugs are injected via a catheter to bathe the nerves outside the spinal cord. Side-effects of epidurals include hypotension (due to block of sympathetic nerves and treatable with ephedrine), block of motor nerves causing inability to move the legs, and urinary retention. The doses necessary for epidural use can be reduced by mixing the local anaesthetic with opioid. Prilocaine (Citanest), the least toxic local anaesthetic, is used for Bier's block. This is a technique which facilitates hand or forearm surgery (a common procedure is reduction of a

Table 22.2 Anti-emetic agents and their actions

Agent	Action
Metoclopramide (Maxolon)	Dopamine antagonist (benzamide)
Prochlorperazine (Stemetil)	Dopamine antagonist (phenothiazine)
Droperidol (Droleptan)	Dopamine antagonist (butyrophenone)
Hyoscine (Scopolamine)	Anticholinergic
Cyclizine (Valoid)	Antihistamine
Ondansetron (Zofran)	5-HT$_3$ antagonist

Table 22.3 Symptoms and signs of local anaesthetic toxicity

Symptoms	Signs
Numbness of tongue or lips	Slurring of speech
Light-headedness	Drowsiness
Tinnitus	Convulsions
Anxiety	Cardio-respiratory arrest

Colles fracture). The arm is held up in order to drain its blood and a tourniquet is inflated. Local anaesthetic is then injected into a vein on the back of the hand. It is crucial that the tourniquet is not released for at least 20 minutes, in order to prevent a large toxic dose of local anaesthetic entering the circulation. The symptoms and signs of local anaesthetic toxicity relate to the drug reaching the brain and heart by either excessive absorption into the bloodstream or inadvertent injection into a blood vessel (Table 22.3).

Treatment of local anaesthetic toxicity

The *immediate* treatment is to call for help, clear the airway and administer 100% oxygen. Ventilation must be started at once if the patient has stopped breathing. With effective oxygenation, cardiac arrest ought not to occur. However, if a patient develops intractable ventricular fibrillation following bupivacaine, bretylium tosylate (5–10 mg/kg) might be effective in restoring normal rhythm.

FURTHER READING

Bruce L 1992 Epidural analgesia-pain relief. Surgical Nurse 5(4): 4–8
Clark E C 1992 Postoperative patient-controlled analgesia. Surgical Nurse 5(4): 20–21

Dale F 1993 Postoperative pain in the elective surgical patient. British Journal of Nursing 2(17): 842–849

23

Palliative care

Although palliative care is made up of several different, but complementary, elements, the effective relief of pain is perhaps the major challenge facing clinical staff. The treatment of acute pain resulting from, say, trauma, presents relatively few problems, but the relief of chronic pain in inoperable cancer requires a high degree of specialist skill. Chronic pain presents in many ways and seldom arises from clearly defined anatomical sites. Multiple pains are often reported by patients with advanced malignant disease. In addition to having pain, the patient may be depressed and emotional. The pain may 'spill over' and affect the patient's family and friends. Just as the presentation of pain can vary, so, too, can the causes of pain and the sites involved. The treatment chosen will be greatly influenced by the nature of the pain. Pain can be classified according to origin, either the anatomical structure(s) involved or the disease process: see, for example, Box 23.1.

Box 23.1 Classification of pain according to anatomical structure(s) involved and disease process

Anatomical	*Disease*
Visceral pain	Deep infection
Bone pain	Gastric distension
Soft-tissue pain	Pain in paralysed limb
Nerve pain	Muscle spasm
Pleural pain	
Headache	
Rectal pain	

Table 23.1 Products used for the relief of pain

Product groups	Examples	Availability
Non-opioids	Aspirin	Tablets
	Paracetamol	Tablets, suppositories
	NSAIDs	Tablets, injections, suppositories, local applications
	Nefopam	Tablets, injection
Weak opioids – limited place in treatment of mild/ moderate pain	Codeine	Tablets, injection
	Dihydrocodeine	Tablets, injection
Strong opioids (long-acting)	Buprenorphine*	Tablets, injection
	Morphine	Tablets, oral solution, injection, suppositories
	Diamorphine	Tablets, injection
	Phenazocine	Tablets, injection, suppositories
	Oxycodone	Suppositories
Strong opioids (short-acting) – not recommended in palliative care	Dextromoramide	Tablets, suppositories
	Dipipanone	Tablets (in combination with cyclizine)
	Pethidine	Tablets, injection
	Pentazocine*	Capsule, injection, suppositories

*Antagonistic effects if used in combination with other opioids and therefore best avoided.
A number of combination products is also available, e.g. paracetamol with a small dose of codeine. Soluble tablets are also available in a number of instances.

Table 23.2 Non-opioids

Drug	Adult dose/route	Notes
Aspirin. Aspirin is a common ingredient of many proprietary preparations that patients may buy. A careful drug history may reveal multiple analgesic use	300–900 mg orally every 4–6 hours. Maximum daily dose 4 g	Gastric irritation may be a problem – should be given after food, and antacids may be prescribed. Soluble forms may be more acceptable to the patient. Risk of drug interactions. Bronchospasm and skin reactions have been reported in hypersensitive patients. Often given in combination with codeine in co-codaprin tablets. Enteric coated tablets available
Paracetamol	500 mg – 1 g orally 6 hourly. Maximum daily dose 4 g	Liver damage is a major concern following overdosage (see p. 39). Available in various forms, including a paediatric elixir and suppository. Doses for children must be carefully assessed.
Nefopam	60 mg orally three times daily. Can increase to 90 mg. 20 mg i.m. every 6 hours	Dose should be reduced to 30 mg in elderly patients
Naproxen	550 mg twice daily *after food*	See p. 37
Ibuprofen	200–600 mg orally, 8-hourly	NSAID of choice for treatment of pain associated with inflammation. Diclofenac is a more potent alternative
Diclofenac	75–150 mg orally, 8-hourly, after food. 75 mg i.m. up to twice daily	As with all NSAIDs, monitor for signs of gastric irritation

TREATMENT

As with any treatment programme, it is vitally important to take a careful history and recognise that the patient will have the expectation of becoming pain-free without reduction in mental alertness. The patient's previous experience may result in fear due to the expectation of pain. Tensions may result which can greatly increase the patient's pain and associated problems. A basic principle is to seek to anticipate crises and avoid having to resort to injections if at all possible. A wide range of products is available for the relief of pain. This reflects the great variation in the presentation and severity of pain. Table 23.1 indicates the range of commonly used products.

Diagnosis/assessment of pain

This is a highly skilled process which calls for consideration of a number of factors including, for example:

- is the pain worsened by movement?
- is the pain periodic in nature?
- does pain follow eating?
- do the symptoms imply a CNS lesion?
- do the symptoms suggest involvement of a peripheral nerve?

Table 23.3 Examples of drugs used in combination therapy

Drug	Adult dose/route	Notes
Chlorpromazine	25 mg orally at night	Useful sedative effect
Prochlorperazine	5 mg orally, 8-hourly	Sedative and anti-emetic
Diazepam	5 mg orally, 8-hourly	May have useful muscle relaxant effect

- are skin symptoms present?
- do sensory changes suggest peripheral neuropathies?

Depending on the diagnosis and severity of pain it may be necessary to add other treatments to the analgesic chosen (see p. 334).

Treatment of mild pain

The non-opioids are the basis of treatment, either singly or in combination. As with other forms of drug therapy, care should be taken to select the dose/route/formulation that best meets the patient's needs. Table 23.2 summarises the main drugs/doses/indications, etc.

There may be advantages in combining small doses of psychotropic drugs with the mild analgesic. Drugs used in combination therapy are detailed in Table 23.3.

Table 23.4 Advantages and disadvantages of morphine

Advantages	Disadvantages
Highly effective in reasonable dose	Controlled drug – record keeping
Active orally	Causes constipation
Wide range of presentations available, e.g. oral solutions, tablets (including slow-release tablets), injection and suppositories	'Morphine myths' There are still concerns in the minds of some clinicians that morphine causes respiratory depression, addiction, tolerance and euphoria. As a result it may be considered as a drug of 'last resort'. In fact, these perceived problems are seldom seen where morphine (and other strong opioids) are used in the treatment of cancer pain
Widely available	
Relatively inexpensive	
Side-effects manageable	
Extensive literature/ research findings	

Treatment of moderate pain

Weak opioids may be useful. Although they achieve an analgesic effect in a manner similar to that of morphine they are less potent. However, side-effects are more likely to be a problem than with morphine because of the high doses needed to achieve pain relief. Weak opioids can be used in combination with other drugs, e.g. aspirin and codeine, paracetamol and codeine.

Treatment of severe pain

Extensive experience has shown that strong opioids are the most valuable drugs in achieving pain relief for many cancer patients with severe pain. Morphine remains the drug of choice for many reasons which are summarised in Table 23.4. The advantages obtained by using morphine

Table 23.5 Determination of morphine dose

Patient's analgesic history	Dose of morphine (oral)
Previously controlled on non-opioid	*2 mg morphine every 4 hours
Previously controlled on weak opioid	*10 mg morphine every 4 hours
Previously on other strong opioids	Calculate equivalent dose of morphine, e.g. the conversion factor for pethidine is 0.125, i.e. 100 mg pethidine ≡ 12.5 mg morphine. If the patient was poorly controlled increase the equivalent morphine dose by 50%
Poor renal function	Doses given (see * above) should be reduced by 50%
Poor hepatic function	Severe hepatic failure has an effect on morphine metabolism but it is rare to need to reduce the dose of morphine on this account

Table 23.6 Dosage increments of morphine

Morphine dosage (4-hourly)	Dosage increment (every 3rd day)
5 mg, 7.5 mg	2.5 mg
10 mg	5 mg
20 mg	10 mg
30 mg	15 mg
60 mg	30 mg

Table 23.7 Non-oral routes for opioids

Route	Notes
Intravenous or intramuscular	Suitable where relief of pain can be achieved by 4-hourly injections. Greater frequency than this is not acceptable. Diamorphine is more soluble than morphine and the dose can be given in a smaller volume of water
Rectal	Morphine can be given rectally in doses similar to oral doses. Oxycodone is a long-acting strong opioid which can be given in suppository form. The rectal route may not be acceptable to some patients
Intrathecal	Combination of low-dose strong opioid and bupivicaine can be given intrathecally. This treatment is suitable for ambulant patients, but spinal catheter care requires special skills
Transdermal	Fentanyl is available as skin patches in the USA. Transdermal systems are expensive and have a slow onset of action

by far outweigh the disadvantages, some of which are more imagined than real.

The decision to use morphine (or other strong opioid) is arrived at when control of pain is lost using a weaker analgesic. Following full consideration of the clinical findings it may be necessary to move to a smaller dose of a more potent drug. The overall aim of treatment is to keep the patient pain-free and alert by keeping the plasma concentration of drug *continuously* within the patient's own effective zone. This is achieved by *regular* administration of the selected dose of the chosen strong opioid. The oral route is preferred whenever possible. The determination of dose will depend on the patient's previous history of analgesic use, and renal function, as outlined in Table 23.5.

Dosage levels

It may be necessary to increase the dose by titration to the patient's pain. Sequential increments will be required depending on current dosage as indicated in Table 23.6.

Care should be taken where there is renal impairment to avoid accumulation of the morphine metabolite M6G (morphine-6-glucuronide).

Dosage intervals

Regular administration (4-hourly) is essential to ensure continuous relief of pain. Controlled-release preparations provide relief when given at 12-hourly intervals. Careful adjustment of dosage can help to ensure that the patient has the benefit of a pain-free, undisturbed night's sleep. Controlled release preparations are useful (12-hourly dosage intervals) or the bedtime dose of morphine solution can be increased by up to

Table 23.8 Drugs used as adjuncts for control of pain

Drug	Adult dose	Indications/notes
Amitriptyline	10–75 mg at night orally	Useful in pain of neuropathic origin. Anticholinergic side-effects may cause problems in higher doses
Carbamezapine	100–200 mg twice daily, orally, increasing if necessary to 1.2 g daily in divided doses	Similar indications to amitriptyline. Side-effects include gastrointestinal disturbances and visual disturbances. If necessary, blood level monitoring can be used as a basis for dosage adjustment
Dexamethasone	8–12 mg twice daily by mouth. Dose should be reduced to lowest level that will control symptoms	Particularly useful for relieving pain by reducing inflammation which may cause nerve compression or raised intracranial pressure. Other benefits of dexamethasone include appetite stimulation. Major side-effects associated with corticosteroids may occur
Hyoscine butylbromide	30–180 mg by subcutaneous infusion over 24 hours	Smooth muscle spasm in bowel or ureter
Baclofen	5 mg every 8 hours, increasing slowly up to 100 mg daily; given after food	Spasm of skeletal muscle. Side-effects may be troublesome. These include sedation, drowsiness, nausea, ataxia, headaches and tremor
Dantrolene Diazepam	25 mg daily 2–15 mg daily	May be worthwhile alternatives to baclofen where this drug is poorly tolerated.

Table 23.9 Other drugs used in palliative care

Drug groups/products	Indications/notes
Laxatives (see p. 63). Co-danthramer is particularly useful. 10 ml at night is given as a routine laxative in patients receiving 10 mg morphine 4-hourly	All opioids cause constipation. Routine laxatives must be prescribed.

Anti-emetics (see p. 140). A wide range of products is available	It may be appropriate to combine the anti-emetic with the analgesic for subcutaneous infusion. The following drugs are compatible with diamorphine:
	    metoclopramide
	    methotrimeprazine
	    hyoscine hydrobromide
	    dexamethasone sodium phosphate
	Other combinations with diamorphine are best avoided

Oral lubricants (see p. 307).	A dry mouth can cause the patient much distress and should be avoided at all costs
Local antifungal agents (see p. 172)	Candidiasis can be effectively treated using appropriate local/systemic antifungal therapy
Products for oral hygiene (see p. 449)	Care of the mouth is particularly important for the cancer patient
Chemotherapeutic agents (see p. 241)	Palliative chemotherapy may be useful in a limited number of patients. The aim is to limit/slow down the spread of the disease without undue side-effects
Nutritional adjuncts	Having corrected any underlying problem, e.g. nausea and vomiting, constipation, etc., there may be a place for the use of appropriate nutritional adjuncts on the advice of the dietitian
Anti-diarrhoeal agents (see p. 64)	Diarrhoea does not affect a high proportion of cancer patients but can be a serious problem for some patients. Careful clinical investigation is called for and it may be necessary to take measures to treat dehydration
Anti-infective agents (see p. 153)	Appropriate anti-infective treatment may be required, e.g. soft-tissue infection, urinary tract infection, etc.

100%. A combination of 4-hourly morphine solution and a controlled dose of tablet at night is not recommended.

Parenteral opioids (and other non-oral routes)

The oral route is preferred wherever possible. However, in the last few days or hours of life, alternatives to the oral route will often have to be considered. Other reasons for using non-oral routes include dysphagia, acute breakthrough pain, and nausea and vomiting. Non-oral routes available are outlined in Table 23.7.

In some patients it may be necessary to use adjuncts where the control of pain cannot be achieved by a first line analgesic agent alone. It should also be borne in mind that radiotherapy, transcutaneous electrical nerve stimulation and surgery may have to be used. Table 23.8 outlines some of the drugs used as adjuncts.

Other drugs used in palliative care

While pain relief is the cornerstone of care it is vitally important not to neglect other symptoms that may trouble the patient. An indication of other drugs used is given in Table 23.9.

FURTHER READING

Doyle D (ed) 1986 International symposium on pain control. Royal Society of Medicine Services Limited, London
Modern Medicine Postgraduate Partwork Series. Palliative care. February 1990 Caring for the dying patient at home. Modern Medicine, London

Regnard C F B, Tempest S 1992 A guide to symptom relief in advanced cancer, 3rd edn. Haigh and Hochland, Manchester
Russell K 1992 Pharmacology of pain. Surgical Nurse 5(6): 18–22

Drug management and the role of the nurse

SECTION CONTENTS

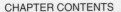

CHAPTER CONTENTS

24

Control of medicines in hospital and the community

INTRODUCTION

The supply, storage and use of all medicinal products are controlled by the Medicines Act 1968. Three classes of products are defined in the Act; these are shown in Box 24.1.

Box 24.1 Classes of products defined by the Medicines Act 1968	
General Sale List (GSL)	Medicines which can be bought in a general store
Pharmacy medicines (P)	Medicines which may be sold only under the supervision of a pharmacist
Prescription-only medicines (PoMs)	Medicines that can be sold or supplied on prescription only

Additional legislation for Controlled Drugs is provided by the Misuse of Drugs Act 1971. The Medicines Act is concerned primarily with regulating the legitimate use of medicines; the Misuse of Drugs Act is concerned with the prevention of the abuse of Controlled Drugs. Certain legal requirements apply to the sale, supply, dispensing and labelling of each class of medicinal product. These requirements are applicable mainly in the community, e.g. sale/supply of medicines by community pharmacists and others. In hospital practice, all medicines are treated in the same way, no distinction being made between the different classes listed above.

However, Controlled Drugs are subject to additional security and recording requirements. The key elements of the legislation that affect nursing practice are described below.

ADMINISTRATION OF PoMs

The Medicines Act provides that 'no one may administer a PoM otherwise than to himself, unless he is a practitioner or is acting in accordance with the directions of a practitioner'. Certain exemptions to this rule are made in the case of life-saving drugs, e.g. adrenalin, certain antihistamines, antidotes, etc.; normally this exemption would not apply in hospitals.

This aspect is normally covered by a health authority policy statement which permits medicine administration *only* in accordance with the written prescription of a medical or dental practitioner. The only exception to this rule is where an agreed local policy has been drawn up (see p. 366).

PRESCRIBING OF PoMs

In hospital practice the in-patient prescription includes directions to the nurse for administration of the medicine. If a prescription is written for an outpatient more details of the patient are required than would be the case for an inpatient, e.g. address of patient and quantity of medicine to be supplied.

EMERGENCY SUPPLY OF PoMs

A community pharmacist can, under specified conditions, supply PoMs in an emergency without a prescription, on the request of a doctor or an individual patient. In hospital practice, situations under which medicines can be supplied without a prescription will be defined in the local code of practice for medicine management.

LABELLING OF MEDICINAL PRODUCTS

Standard labelling requirements are described in the Act. This is largely a matter for the manufac-

turer or pharmacist to comply with. The main particulars included on a label of a medicinal product are listed below:

- the name of the product – this may be an approved name and/or a proprietary name
- the pharmaceutical form, e.g. tablets, capsules, etc.
- the strength of the product, distinguishing between active and non-active ingredients
- the quantity in the container expressed in appropriate terms, e.g. in the case of tablets the number of dosage units and in the case of an ointment the weight contained in the pack
- any special storage instructions
- a date after which the product should not be used (expiry date)
- name and address of supplier and product licence number.

Additional labelling requirements apply to dispensed medicines. It is common in hospital practice for the pharmacist to add further information to labels in response to local need.

STORAGE OF MEDICINAL PRODUCTS IN HOSPTIAL

Although different classes of drugs are recognised under the Medicines Act, in hospital practice *all* medicinal products are treated in the same basic way, i.e. secure storage in locked cupboards. In many instances, the controls applied to the different types of medicines in hospitals exceed the basic legal requirements. This is of course necessary to ensure the protection and safety of both patients and staff. Health authorities have a duty to ensure that regulations are drawn up and applied to all aspects of the use of medicines.

Separate locked cupboards are required for the following:

- internal medicines
- external medicines
- disinfectants/antiseptics
- clinical reagents.

A lockable drug refrigerator is also required. Separate sections will be required within a cupboard or refrigerator, e.g. to segregate oral preparations from injections. Other storage facilities are provided for larger volume sterile solutions.

CONTROLLED DRUGS

The Misuse of Drugs Act 1971 regulates the importation, export, sale and use of narcotics such as morphine, diamorphine and other drugs of addiction. Other aspects covered by the Act include the establishment of an Advisory Council on Misuse of Drugs.

The use of Controlled Drugs in medicine is permitted by the Misuse of Drugs Regulations 1973. Different levels of control are applied within the regulations. The main controls are as follows:

- A licence is needed to import or export.
- Compounding/manufacturing is permitted by a practitioner or pharmacist.
- A pharmacist may supply to a patient on the prescription of an appropriate practitioner.
- These drugs may be administered to a patient by a person acting in accordance with the instructions of a doctor or dentist.
- Safe custody and record keeping are required.
- The following persons are also authorised to be in possession of and to supply Controlled Drugs:
  - medical or dental practitioner
  - matron or acting matron of a hospital or nursing home
  - the sister, or acting sister, for the time being in charge of a ward, theatre or other department.

The authority is limited to obtaining ward stocks from no other source but the pharmacist engaged in dispensing medicines in the particular hospital. In some situations, where there is no on-site pharmacy, the hospital pharmacy normally providing the pharmaceutical service is regarded as being within this provision. Limitations are applied to the authorisations, in that they apply only so far as is necessary for the practice or exercise of their profession. A sister, or acting sister in charge of a ward, theatre or department

may not supply any Controlled Drug other than for administration to a patient in accordance with the prescription of a doctor (or dentist). It should be noted that, apart from health care personnel, other groups of workers are permitted to possess/supply Controlled Drugs, e.g. the Master of a ship, person in charge of a recognised laboratory, manager of an offshore installation.

Barbiturates and appetite suppressants

As from January 1985 certain orders and amendments to the list of drugs controlled under the Misuse of Drugs Act 1971 came into effect. This resulted in certain barbiturates and appetite suppressants (e.g. diethylpropion) becoming Controlled Drugs. All the requirements for prescription writing, ordering, recording and storing Controlled Drugs apply to the following drugs (among others):

amylobarbitone
butobarbitone
cyclobarbitone
methylphenobarbitone
pentobarbitone
quinalbarbitone.

The regulations covering phenobarbitone are not so comprehensive in that the handwriting requirements (see p. 342) do not apply nor do the storage and recording requirements for Controlled Drugs. This is because of the use of phenobarbitone in the treatment of epilepsy.

Supply of Controlled Drugs to addicts

Special regulations are applicable to the supply of Controlled Drugs to persons who are addicted to these drugs. For example, a doctor may prescribe Controlled Drugs for an addicted person only if he holds a licence issued by the Secretary of State. (Any doctor may prescribe Controlled Drugs to an addicted person who is suffering from injury or organic disease). A special prescription is often used to enable addicts to receive daily supplies of Controlled Drugs.

CONTROLLED DRUGS IN HOSPITAL

Certain of the legal requirements concerning drug control do not apply in hospitals. However, health authorities are required to institute safe procedures in accordance with official circulars, reports, etc. Failure to institute or comply with these procedures would leave the health authorities or individual liable to legal action. In practice, a positive attitude to all aspects of safe use of medicines will benefit patients and safeguard health care workers.

Legislation and responsibility of staff

Procedures involved in the handling of Controlled Drugs are drawn up by health authorities against the background of the legal and professional responsibilities defined in the documents listed below and may be supplemented where necessary in accordance with local requirements:

- The Misuse of Drugs Act 1971
- Misuse of Drugs Regulations 1973
- The Aitken Report – Control of Dangerous Drugs and Poisons in Hospitals 1958
- The Roxburgh Report – Control of Medicines in Hospital Wards and Departments 1972
- The Duthie Report – Guidelines for the Safe and Secure Handling of Medicines 1988.

Prescribing

Preparations which are subject to the prescription requirements of the Misuse of Drugs Regulations 1973 are distinguished throughout the British National Formulary by the symbol CD (Controlled Drug).

In-patient prescriptions are normally written on a standard prescription sheet.

For out-patients (or patients on discharge from hospital) detailed information is required. It is not lawful for a practitioner to issue a prescription for a Controlled Drug, or for a pharmacist to dispense it, unless it complies with the following requirements. The prescription must:

- be in writing and signed by the person issuing it with his usual signature and be dated by him
- be in ink or otherwise so as to be indelible
- except in the case of an NHS or local health authority prescription, specify the address of the person issuing it
- have written on it, if issued by a dentist, the words 'for dental treatment only'
- specify (in the handwriting of the person issuing the prescription) the name and address of the person for whose treatment it is issued
- specify (again in the prescriber's own handwriting) the dose to be taken and (a) in the case of preparations, the form and, where appropriate, the strength of the preparation, and either the total quantity (in both words and figures) of the preparation, or the number (in both words and figures) or dosage units to be supplied; (b) in any other case, the total quantity (in both words and figures) of the Controlled Drug to be supplied
- in the case of a prescription for a total quantity intended to be dispensed by instalments, contain a direction specifying the amount of the instalments which may be dispensed and the intervals to be observed when dispensing.

Ordering

Controlled Drug supplies for hospital wards and departments may only be ordered by a sister or acting sister using the order book (Ref No 90–500) provided for the purpose. For each product:

- the name of the preparation (in block letters)
- the formulation
- the strength (in figures and words), and
- the total quantity (in figures and words)

should be entered using a separate page for each product (Fig. 24.1). The nurse places her signature and designation, and dates the order.

The whole order book is sent to the pharmacy department where the pharmacist prepares the order and signs the requisition. The person acting as messenger for the return of drugs to the

Name of Preparation	Strength	Quantity
MORPHINE SULPHATE SLOW RELEASE TABLETS	10mg (TEN)	30 TAB. (THIRTY)

(Each preparation to be ordered on a separate page)

Ordered by _____ *GClark* _____ Date _15/7/94_
(Signature of Sister or Acting Sister)

Supplied by _____ *Rachel Sangster* _____ Date _15/7/94_
(Pharmacist's Signature)

Accepted for delivery _____ Date _15/7/94._
(Signature of messenger)

TO BE RETAINED IN THE PHARMACEUTICAL DEPARTMENT

Figure 24.1   Order form for Controlled Drugs.

ward or department also signs the requisition. The original requisition is then retained in the pharmaceutical department. Replacement order books are obtained from pharmacy departments.

Delivery and receipt

Delivery of Controlled Drugs may be made in a locked box or by a designated messenger. If Controlled Drugs are collected from the pharmacy, the appropriate section should be completed by the messenger. Careful consideration should be given as to persons suitable to act as messengers carrying Controlled Drugs. It is prudent to restrict student nurses, who at times may have to act as messengers, to those who have received theoretical instruction in the handling of Controlled Drugs.

On receipt of supplies of a Controlled Drug and the order book by a ward or department, a registered nurse should check the drugs against the copy requisition. If all is found to be correct, the copy requisition is signed (Fig. 24.2) and the order book retained in the ward or department. If there is any discrepancy, the pharmacy should be notified at once.

An entry is then made in the ward Controlled Drugs record book (Ref No 90–501) with details of the new supply, keeping records of the different forms and strengths of each preparation in separate sections or pages (Fig. 24.3A). The page is headed with the name of the preparation (in block letters), its form and strength. The columns are filled appropriately to include the number of tablets or vials, or the volume of liquid received, the date and the serial number of the requisition. Where there is continuity of use of a page or section, the existing stock balance is added to the new supply. When it is necessary to start a new section or page, the index is amended accordingly.

Name of Preparation	Strength	Quantity
MORPHINE SULPHATE SLOW RELEASE TABLETS	10mg (TEN)	30 TABS. (THIRTY)

(Each preparation to be ordered on a separate page)

Ordered by _____ *G.Clark* _____ Date __15/7/94__
(Signature of Sister or Acting Sister)

Supplied by _____ *Rachel Sangster* _____ Date __15/7/94__
(Pharmacist's Signature)

Accepted for delivery _____ Date __15/7/94.__
(Signature of messenger)

Received by _____ *C. Bowden* _____ Date __15/7/94__
(To be signed in the ward in the presence of the Messenger)

TO BE RETAINED BY THE SISTER

Figure 24.2 Copy order for Controlled Drugs.

Storage

Controlled Drugs are required to be stored in a separate locked cupboard constructed to prevent unauthorised access to the drugs. It is customary for this cupboard to be within another locked cupboard. Preferably, the cupboard should be sited where it is visible to nursing staff on duty. With this recommendation however, there is the disadvantage that 'visible' cupboards are also often in the busiest parts of a ward, for example, at the nurses' station or within the patient area of a Nightingale type ward. These locations are not conducive to a clear, uninterrupted environment in which to concentrate on checking drugs and so extra care is essential. A warning light indicating when the cupboard is open is normally provided. The key(s) to this cupboard must be held in the possession of the trained nurse in charge of the ward.

Spare keys for Controlled Drugs cupboards are generally kept in the hospital pharmacy. If there is no pharmacy on site, local arrangements are usually made for spare keys to be held in the safe keeping of the senior nurse manager concerned. In departments where Controlled Drugs are stored but which do not have 24-hour supervisory cover such as out-patient clinics, arrangements for the safe keeping of the key(s) to the Controlled Drugs cupboard out of working hours must be made.

Loss or suspected loss of keys should be reported in the first instance to the senior nurse manager on duty whose duty it is to inform a senior member of the pharmacy staff and, if necessary, the security officer for the hospital.

As with all other drugs, Controlled Drugs should not be transferred to other containers but must be retained in the orginal container which should not be defaced in any way.

Administration

The basic procedure for giving any medication applies also to the giving of a Controlled Drug. Instructions relating specifically to Controlled Drugs are as follows:

- Two persons must be involved in the administration of a Controlled Drug, one of whom must be a registered nurse or a registered doctor.
- The keys to the Controlled Drugs cupboard are obtained from the nurse-in-charge.
- The stock amount of the drug to be used is checked against the last entry in the Controlled Drugs record book.
- After the dose in selected, the remaining stock is returned to the cupboard, which is then locked.
- The date, the name of the patient, the amount of the drug to be given and the stock balance are entered in the record book (Fig. 24.3A).
- Both persons involved take the prepared drug to the patient, one to administer the drug, the other to act as witness.
- The time of administration and the signatures of the two persons are entered in the record book.
- The keys of the Controlled Drugs cupboard are returned to the nurse-in-charge.

Keeping the ward or department Controlled Drugs record books

Strictly according to the Regulations the sister or acting sister is not required to keep a drug register. However, in practice, the keeping of a drug register at ward or department level is always required by the health authority.

The record book must be kept in accordance with the guidance given on page 346. Replacement record books are available from the pharmacy department.

When Controlled Drugs are dispensed by the pharmacy for a named individual in-patient, each supply should be recorded in a separate section of the ward Controlled Drugs record book.

When arriving at a stock balance of liquid oral medicines it may not always be possible to obtain exactly the theoretical number of doses from each container. Accordingly records may be made as illustrated in Figure 24.3B.

Checking stock balances

By nurses This is undertaken in accordance with locally agreed procedures. Regular checks are part of ward drug management. The intervals vary from on a shift basis or daily to weekly.

By pharmacists These checks are made at least at 3 monthly intervals but may be required more frequently. A written record of the check is made in the ward Controlled Drugs record book by the pharmacist carrying out the check.

Procedure to be adopted if (a) the Controlled Drugs order book and/or ward Controlled Drugs record book and/or (b) Controlled Drugs are missing

In the event of loss or suspected loss of these, the nurse-in-charge of the ward or department should contact the senior nurse manager on duty who will inform the senior pharmacy manager if this becomes necessary.

Disposal of Controlled Drugs

An individual dose of a Controlled Drug which is prepared and is unsuitable for taking back into stock should be disposed of in the ward or department and a record made in the ward Controlled Drugs record book. The destruction must be witnessed by a registered nurse. The same procedure should be adopted where only part of the contents of an ampoule is required for administration. Any accidental breakage should be dealt with in the same way.

Destruction of Controlled Drugs

It is technically illegal to destroy Controlled Drugs (and other medicinal products) by means of the public sewerage system. As stated above it is acceptable to dispose of part of an ampoule or unused dose at ward level. However quantities in excess of this should be returned to the

NAME, FORM OF PREPARATION AND STRENGTH ....DIAMORPHINE INJECTION 1Cmg....

AMOUNT(S) OBTAINED						AMOUNTS ADMINISTERED				STOCK BALANCE
Amount	Date Received	Serial No. of Requisition	Date	Time	Patient's Name	Amount Given	Given by (Signature)	Witnessed by (Signature)		
20 AMP	7/9/94	O7								20 am
			9/9/94	7.10am	A. Patient	1Cmg	J.Milne	J. Sergant		19 am
			9/9/94	11.35am	A. Patient	2Cmg	J.Milne	M Edgar		17 a
			10/9/94	—	STOCK CHECKED and found correct B.Smith, Sister					17 am
1C AMP.	16/9/94	O8								27 a

Figure 24.3A Extract from ward Controlled Drugs record book.

NAME, FORM OF PREPARATION AND STRENGTH MORPHINE in CHLOROFORM WATER 20mg in 5ml

AMOUNT(S) OBTAINED			AMOUNTS ADMINISTERED						STOCK BALANCE
Amount	Date Received	Serial No. of Requisition	Date	Time	Patient's Name	Amount Given	Given by (Signature)	Witnessed by (Signature)	
200ml	16/8/94	06							200ml
			18/8/94	3.20pm	A. Patient	10ml	J. Milne	M. Duncan	190ml
			18/8/94	6.40pm	B. Patient	5ml	June Joovie	M. Duncan	185ml
									✻ 60ml
200ml	23/8/94	11							260ml
			25/8/94	5.20am	C. Patient	10ml	Louise Smith	J. Riddel	250ml

THE ABOVE PROCEDURE TO BE ADOPTED IF THERE IS CONTINUITY OF USE AND AN ACCURATE BALANCE

ALTERNATIVE PROCEDURES WHERE THEORETICAL BALANCE DOES NOT EQUAL ACTUAL BALANCE

									170ml
			19/9/94	9am	F. Brown	10ml	L Armstrong	C. Conway	160ml
									40ml
			23/9/94	stock checked	many strike losses on nursing				30ml
			23/9/94	Balance returned to pharmacy & many					NIL
200ml	23/9/94	14	23/9/94						200ml

(OR)

IF THERE IS CONTINUITY OF USE THE CORRECTED BALANCE SHOULD BE ADDED TO NEW SUPPLY

WHERE LOSSES APPEAR EXCESSIVE PHARMACY SHOULD BE NOTIFIED

Figure 24.3B Extract from ward Controlled Drugs record book.

pharmaceutical department. The pharmacist will arrange for safe destruction within the Duty of Care requirements.

Controlled Drugs brought in by patients on admission

Some problems can arise at ward level with Controlled Drugs brought in by patients on admission. These will have been obtained by the patient on prescription. Technically it is illegal for the ward sister to receive these drugs from the patient. However in such situations the pharmacist may lawfully accept such drugs for destruction. On rare occasions a patient may be in possession of illicit Controlled Drugs. This is obviously a very delicate matter and is dealt with having regard to all clinical and legal considerations. At the present time it is illegal for the pharmacist to receive such drugs and it may be necessary to call in the police to deal with the matter. In such situations medical confidentiality will be observed unless there are compelling reasons to the contrary.

Unwanted or time-expired Controlled Drugs

These should be returned to the pharmacy, having made suitable records in the ward Controlled Drugs record book.

Retention of records

All Controlled Drugs order books and record books must be retained for 2 years after the date of the last entry. After this time, such documents should be destroyed by burning or shredding.

OTHER ASPECTS OF THE CONTROL OF MEDICINES

While legal aspects of the control of medicines remain central to all hospital medicine policies, it is important to recognise the changes that are occurring which make an impact on the way medicines are controlled. Computerised medi-

cine management systems provide the opportunity to follow the movement of medicines from the manufacturer through to the administration of a dose to the patient.

Not only must security be maintained throughout all transactions involving medicines, but it is also vitally important to provide information to the users of medicines as to costs, compliance with formulary, etc. (see p. 364). The Duthie Report (Department of Health 1988) defines the Medicine Trail, which is the path taken by medicines from manufacturers (or other supplier) via the hospital pharmacy to the ward. At each point on the trail appropriate safeguards and procedures are recommended to ensure that there are defined responsibilities, appropriate record keeping and reconciliation (checks on receipts/issues/balances). Many of the responsibilities etc defined in the Duthie Report will be undertaken by the hospital pharmacist.

Some specific points from the Duthie Report which relate to the duties and responsibilities of the nurse (and are not dealt with elsewhere) are summarised below:

Medicines brought into hospital by patients

It will be necessary to establish a local policy to ensure that such medicines are either used safely by the patient or disposed of in accordance with policy requirements. It must never be forgotten that the medicines brought in by patients are the patient's property – and the patient's permission must be sought before any such medicines are destroyed.

Controlled stationery

All medicine order books and stationery must be kept in a safe place on the ward so as to reduce the likelihood of misuse.

Samples and clinical trial materials

It is essential to ensure that all such materials are received from the pharmaceutical department and not direct from a manufacturer.

Medicines liable to diversion

The security of Controlled Drugs is vitally important as is the security of medicines that may be especially attractive to the drug user (e.g. temazepam). Such drugs should be subject to checks as agreed with senior nurse and pharmacy managers.

Operating theatres and accident and emergency departments

Nurses working in operating theatres and accident and emergency departments may face particular problems in ensuring all the necessary records are maintained. This especially relates to the use of Controlled Drugs by anaesthetists. It is essential to establish very clear procedures that all staff will adhere to.

Community clinics, family planning clinics

Just as with wards and departments in hospitals clear guidance is needed for all staff working in clinic settings. Responsibilities must be defined at all stages from ordering to use of the medicine.

Borrowing of medicines

Legislation to remove Crown Immunity (Medicines Control Agency 1992) means that the practice of borrowing medicines between wards is no longer acceptable.

MANAGEMENT OF MEDICINES IN DAY HOSPITALS

The day hospital aims to provide facilities for assessment, diagnosis and rehabilitation of patients who do not require hospital admission as well as to maintain the level of rehabilitation achieved by patients discharged from in-patient care. Such departments have become an accepted component of health care for elderly people and also for psychiatric patients. In the geriatric field, the limited supply of beds in hospital and the need for an immediate service to patients following their discharge from hospital largely account for the development of day hospitals.

Day hospitals operate during daylight hours and cater for the needs of appropriately selected patients allowing them to remain in the community with their spouse, relatives or friends. Facilities are provided for medical examination, nursing treatments, physiotherapy, occupational therapy, speech therapy, diversional therapy, chiropody and hairdressing. Attendance at a day hospital varies with the individual patient, ranging from several times a week to merely once a month.

Practical aspects

The management of medicines in a day hospital is many sided as elderly patients present a wide range of conditions which require to be assessed and treated. On his first visit to the day hospital, the patient should be asked to bring all his medicines with him. It is customary for the patient to be given a full medical examination as part of being assessed. In addition the medicines should be examined by the doctor, and the patient asked in detail what each is being taken for, the number to be taken, the frequency and so on. At this time, the patient should also be asked if he is able to gain access to the medicines or if he is experiencing any other difficulties with them. If there is any doubt about the patient's ability to cope with the medicines at home, appropriate action should be taken by the staff of the day hospital. This may involve contacting a relative of the patient, the general practitioner, the district nurse or the community pharmacist. The use of a suitable compliance aid should be considered. If necessary, the liaison health visitor will be asked to visit the patient at home to try to assist with the problem. Since patients attending a day hospital are out-patients under the care of their GP, the geriatrician does not normally prescribe medicines for them. He may however withdraw medication immediately from a patient for a suspected adverse reaction; suggest to the GP the need for a medicine or a change in prescription; and in response to laboratory results or the severity of symptoms, prescribe a course of antibiotics, for example, when otherwise there might be an unacceptable delay in written advice reaching the patient's own doctor.

On subsequent visits, the patient is normally only required to bring those medicines which have to be taken during the period of the visit. It is tempting for the patient to transfer to smaller containers only those medicines which he will require but this practice is to be discouraged. The contribution made by ambulance personnel and home helps in prompting patients to remember to pick up important items such as their medicines (and door key) before they leave home should not be undervalued.

Some of the patients attending the day hospital may be capable of remembering to take their medicines as well as undertaking the procedure involved. Others, who normally are supervised or assisted in taking their medicines by relatives or a neighbour, will need this support maintained by the day hospital staff. The nurse is in an ideal position to supervise patients taking their medicines giving guidance and encouragement as required. It is especially important that she uses her powers of observation during treatment and that she is alert to the possibility of unwanted side-effects which can have serious consequences in older people.

To provide for those occasions when patients forget to bring their medicines or require to have a symptom dealt with on the spot, a small stock of medicines should be stored securely in the department. Small amounts of medicines for the relief of unexpected discomfort in patients may be held, such as simple analgesics and antacids. Supplies of certain medicines which must never be omitted should also be kept. These may include antibiotics, oral antidiabetic drugs and antihypertensives.

Apart from medicines, other nursing procedures involving pharmaceutical products may have to be carried out. These may include urine testing, catheter irrigation, stoma care and surgical dressings. Resuscitative measures may have to be instigated if a patient collapses and so the nurse must ensure that relevant and updated emergency medicines are available. The importance of keeping accurate records of the medicines which patients attending the day hospital are taking and good lines of communication between all the personnel involved cannot be over-emphasised. The principles and practice of medicine management apply to the day hospital as much as in other situations. The notable feature of the day hospital in this context, however, is that the patients form a mobile and ever-changing group making patient identification and staff stability of the utmost importance.

DISPOSAL OF TIME-EXPIRED AND UNWANTED MEDICINES

Under the Environmental Protection Act 1990 a 'duty of care' requirement was introduced. The effect of this legislation was to place very clear responsibilities on health care staff to ensure that time-expired and unwanted medicines are safely disposed of. Both community and hospital pharmacists must provide the necessary disposal services within the legal framework ensuring environmental hazard and pollution are obviated. Nurses need to be aware of the provisions of the legislation so that in their own practice, and in giving advice to patients and carers, they can be confident of working within the law. The Duty of Care requirements also apply to the disposal of other clinical waste such as used syringes and needles.

CONTROL OF SUBSTANCES HAZARDOUS TO HEALTH

The Control of Substances Hazardous to Health Regulations (1988) (COSHH) are designed to provide a framework of control within which all substances hazardous to health can be used safely. Many substances used in health care are hazardous to health. As an example, glutaraldehyde, a sporicidal disinfectant, is a recognised skin and respiratory sensitiser which can cause occupational asthma. It is important therefore to protect all staff from exposure to glutaraldehyde. At the same time, it is important that controls over the use of this and other disinfectants are not such as to reduce the desired antimicrobial activity of the agent. The administration of cytotoxic drugs presents particular hazards to staff. These are discussed in more detail elsewhere (see p. 232). Key elements of the COSHH regulations are listed below:

- Responsibility for ensuring compliance with the regulations lies with the employer.
- In practice, responsibility is delegated to the manager of a department or safety officer.
- Known health hazards must be given high priority.
- Microbiological hazards are included.
- Having determined that a substance is hazardous the following action must be taken:
  assess the risk in the particular setting
  control the risk
  produce data sheets (on procedures to be followed) for guidance of staff
  introduce and monitor compliance with data sheet requirements
  carry out review of procedures and health surveillance of staff involved.

The assessment of risk should take the form of a written statement and should be carried out in a systematic way. All the controls introduced are designed either to avoid exposure to the hazardous substance or limit the exposure to an accepted safe level. Control methods range from the use of protective clothing to the use of mechanical ventilation systems. An outline of the contents of a COSHH data sheet is given in Box 24.2.

Box 24.2 Contents of COSHH data sheet

Name of substance
Chemical formula
Occupational exposure limit
Form of product
Uses of product
Specific health hazards
Sensitisation
Other harmful effects
Specific hazards
Dealing with spillages
Disposal of surplus material
First aid

As with all procedures it is essential to monitor compliance with the controls and ensure that any equipment used to contain the risk is maintained in good order. All staff share the responsibility of achieving and maintaining safe working practices within the COSHH regulations. In seeking to improve the health of patients every effort must be made to avoid damaging the health of those caring for them. Risks to patients from administered medicines are outside the scope of the COSHH regulations.

HAZARD WARNINGS AND DRUG WITHDRAWALS

Every precaution is taken by manufacturers and distributors of medicines to ensure that all medicines comply with the relevant standards and are safe for their intended use. However mistakes do occasionally occur in either the manufacturing, packaging or distribution process. In order to avoid any risk to patients or staff it is the responsibility of the Health Departments to issue any hazard notification without delay. This is normally done through health service channels. Nurses would be provided with written information on the particular hazard by the pharmacist. It may be necessary to check ward stocks and withdraw the affected product from use. It is very rare for the hazard to be life-threatening; mislabelling is probably the most commonly notified hazard.

Following the receipt and evaluation of clinical data the Medicines Control Agency (MCA) may withdraw a product licence. The effect of this is to remove the product from use. This has been done on a number of occasions, notably the withdrawal of a non-steroidal anti-inflammatory drug following reports of serious side-effects in older patients. If the urgency warrants it, such withdrawals are notified via the public media. This can sometimes cause difficulty to health care professionals when their patients have information to which they do not have access.

REFERENCES

Control of Substances Hazardous to Health Regulations 1988 HMSO, London Statutory Instruments 1988 No 1657
Department of Health 1988 Guidelines for the safe and secure handling of medicines. (Duthie Report)

Medicines Control Agency 1992 Guidance to the NHS on the licensing requirements of the Medicines Act 1968

FURTHER READING

Atwell C 1990 Control of substances hazardous to health. Surgical Nurse 3(6): 10–13
Department of Health/Welsh Office/Scottish Office Home and Health Department 1989 Guide to the *Misuse of Drugs Act 1971* and the *Misuse of Drugs Regulations*

Royal Pharmaceutical Society of Great Britain 1993 Medicines, ethics and practice: a guide to pharmacists.

25

Pharmaceutical services

Safe and effective management of drug therapy depends on many factors, not least of which is the availability of effective pharmaceutical services.

The pharmacist's role as intermediary between prescriber and patient is central, as is the direction of dispensing and supply services. The role is enhanced by the provision of information services to patients, prescribers and nurses. Other specialised technical services designed to contribute to the achievement of optimal drug therapy include the compounding of sterile preparations for total parenteral nutrition, cytotoxic drug therapy and the supply of radiopharmaceuticals for diagnosis and treatment.

DISTRIBUTION OF PRESCRIBED MEDICINES TO WARDS

Several different methods are used to supply medicines to wards. The choice of method used will depend on a number of factors including the extent of medicine use, layout of the hospital, geographical considerations and resources available.

The overall aim of any medicine distribution system is to ensure that the necessary medicines of the required quality are available when required in quantities that reflect both current, and to some extent, future usage. No one method of distribution is likely to be suitable for use in all situations. Each method has advantages and disadvantages.

Stock system

This is the most basic method. The nurse interprets the prescription, checks ward stocks and orders the medicines that reflect the needs of the ward at that particular time. Medicine orders are then made out by the nurse and met by the pharmaceutical department, usually by technical staff, working under the direction of a pharmacist. On receipt of the completed order at the ward, the nurse is responsible for checking the items supplied and ensuring correct storage on the ward prior to administration to the patient.

This stock system (Fig. 25.1) has superficial advantages in that it is simple to operate and can be used on a temporary basis when staff shortages preclude the use of safer methods. It may be the only applicable method where communications are difficult, e.g. in more remote areas. However, the disadvantages of this approach are very significant and outweigh any marginal advantages. The use of this system does not permit the pharmacist to discharge his full professional role as intermediary between prescriber and patient. There is no opportunity to interpret the prescription, check dosage levels or monitor prescriptions for possible drug interactions which may hazard the patient. There is also no opportunity for the pharmacist to advise on aspects of drug therapy prior to decisions being made by the prescriber. In effect, the nurse takes on a role for which she is not fully trained. This is in no way a denigration of the role of the nurse, rather, it is a question of using the specialist skills of health professionals in the most effective way for the benefit of the patient. When using this supply method, the nurse is involved in much clinically unproductive work and at the same time contact on a professional level between nurse and pharmacist is minimal. As a result there is considerable potential for misunderstanding as to the range and quantities of medicines required at a particular time. Although the nurse will be alert to such

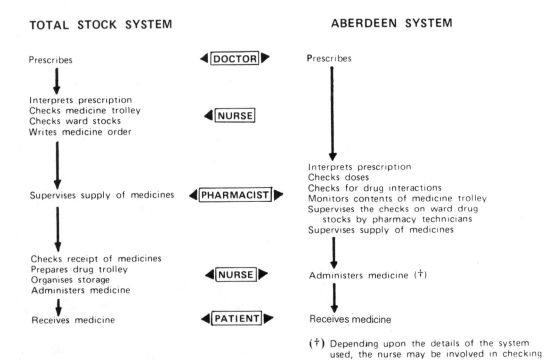

Figure 25.1 Comparison of total stock system and Aberdeen system.

WARD REQUISITION

WARD NAME: CODE: 2968   ORDERED   BY........................

REQUISITION DATE: /   /   NUMBER: A99999/1   AUTHORISED BY....................

Product Description	Stock	Code	Qty	Product Description	Stock	Code	Qty
GROUP 000010 : ORAL (SOLID DOSE) PREPARATIONS							
Amoxycillin 250mg cap 15	8	088536		Aspirin disp 75mg tab 100	2	095958	
Augmentin disp tab 21	2	081728		Augmentin tab 21	6	098345	
Betahistine 8mg tab 20	1	096431		Co-proxamol tab 100	6	072435	
Diazepam 10mg tab 20	1	089796		Diazepam 2mg tab 20	6	088382	
Diazepam 5mg tab 20	6	088501		Diclofenac Sod 100mg SR tab 28	1	066508	
Diclofenac Sod 50mg tab 10	6	080403					
Erythromycin 250mg tab 20	1	092428		Dihydrocodeine 30mg tab 50	2	010715	
Metoclopramide 10mg tab 50	1	098299		Flucloxacillin 250mg cap 20	2	088145	
Paracetamol 500mg tab 50	6	021032		Metronidazole 400mg tab 30	1	088943	
Phenoxymethylpenicillin - 250mg tab 50	1	042331		Paracetamol 500mg sol tab 60	2	089176	
				Prochlorperazine 5mg tab 50			
					1	005479	
Pseudoephedrine 60mg tab 100	1	006246		Ranitidine 150mg tab 20			
				Temazepam 10mg tab 50	3	090840	
Senna tab 100	1	089761			4	072648	
Terfenadine tab 10	1	082031					
GROUP 000020 : INJECTABLE PREPARATIONS							
Adrenaline 1-1000 amp 5ml x 10	1	041912		Amoxycillin 500mg vial 10	1	005010	
Atropine sulph 600mcg amp 1ml x 10	1	027200		Augmentin intravenous 1.2g vial 5	2	073709	
Benzylpenicillin 600mg vial 25	1	092983		Cefotaxime 1g vial 1 (Claforan)	10	057584	
Chlorpheniramine 10mg/ml amp 1ml x 5	1	022500		Diazepam emulsion 5mg/ml amp 2ml x 10	1	072516	
Flucloxacillin 500mg vial 10	1	013366		Frusemide 10mg/ml amp 2ml x 10	1	080845	
				Glycopyrrolate 0.2mg/ml amp 1ml 1 x 10	1	057789	
Glucose 50% vial 50ml	2	042293					
Heparin 1,000u/ml vial 5ml x 1	5	028592		Heparin 5000u/ml vial 5ml x 1 only	5	028606	
Heparinised saline 10u/ml amp 5ml x 10	2	055387		Hydrocortisone sod succ 100mg vial 10	1	073113	
Hyoscine Butylbr 20mg amp 10	1	007552		Metoclopramide 10mg/2ml amp 10	1	094749	
Metronidazole 5mg/ml inf (bag) 100ml	4	025526		Prochlorperazine 12.5mg/ml amp 1ml x 10	2	006882	
Ranitidine 25mg/ml amp 2ml x 5	2	065609		Sodium Chloride 0.9% amp 5ml x 20	2	085790	
Water for Injections amp 10ml x 20	4	085820		Water for Injections amp 5ml x 20	2	085847	
GROUP 000030 : ORAL LIQUID PREPARATIONS							
Dihydrocodeine 10mg/5ml elix 150ml	2	010685		Gaviscon liq 200ml	1	077178	
Lactulose 300ml	2	012149		Mucaine susp 200ml	3	087491	
GROUP 000040 : OPHTHALMIC & AURAL PREPARATIONS							
Chloramphenicol 1% oint 4g	6	008117		Hypromellose 0.3% e/drops 10ml	2	025216	
GROUP 000045 : INHALATION & NASAL PREPARATIONS							
Beclomethasone 50mcg inhaler 80 dose x 1	1	000094		Ipratropium 0.25mg/ml neb sol 2ml x 10	2	079774	
Naseptin cream 15g	4	083046		Salbutamol 100mcg/dose inhaler 80 dose x 1	1	001910	
Salbutamol 5mg/ml respirator soln 20ml	2	001945		Terbutaline Sulph 100 dose inhaler 1	1	071269	
Xylometazoline 0.1% drops 10ml	10	020680					

Figure 25.2 Pre-printed medicine order form.

problems as expiry dates of medicines, the presence of a large relatively uncontrolled ward stock increases the risk of hazard to the patient and may result in wastage of drugs. This method of drug supply is increasingly being replaced by one of the following systems which are designed to overcome the many disadvantages inherent in a system which relegates the role of the pharmacist to that of a specialist storekeeper and that of the nurse to a mail order customer.

CLINICAL PHARMACY

The use of highly structured documentation for recording the prescribing and administration of medicines has made it possible for the pharmacist to discharge his professional responsibilities at ward level. By visiting the ward the pharmacist is able to obtain detailed information on the medicines prescribed for each patient. He is able to contribute his professional skills on all facets

of the use of medicines. As a member of the ward team he is well placed to advise professional colleagues on a wide range of topics related to drug therapy. Interpretation of prescriptions, checking of dosage levels and monitoring prescriptions for possible drug interactions are a vital part of the pharmacist's role but, working at ward level, the pharmacist has access to more information on the patient's clinical condition, special problems, etc, than would be the case if working solely within the pharmaceutical department.

It should be noted that with the Aberdeen system (Fig. 25.1) the prescription remains on the ward at all times thus eliminating errors that might arise due to its absence.

The pharmaceutical service may take complete responsibility for ensuring that the necessary medicines are available both in stock and in the medicine trolley. As with all other distribution methods, computerised management systems

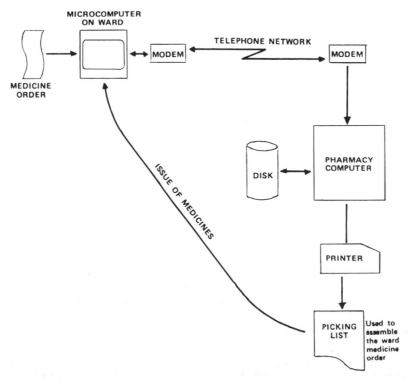

Figure 25.3 Medicine order system using a microcomputer at ward level linked directly to pharmacy computer.

confer many advantages, such as the pre-printed medicine order form (Fig. 25.2).

Portable microcomputers can also be used to assist in supply procedures, either to produce an order for the required medicines at ward level or to input the order directly into the pharmacy computer (Fig. 25.3).

The computer can also produce information on use of drugs, range, quantities, costs, etc, which can be used as a basis on which to establish and monitor ward prescribing policies, ward formularies, or drug stock lists.

Using the Aberdeen system, the nurse is released from clinically unproductive work and is able to concentrate her skills on the nursing care of her patients. The contribution of the pharmacist at ward level is complementary to, and not in conflict with, the role of the nurse and other clinical staff. A clinical pharmacy service is an accepted and vital element of the pharmaceutical service (see Box 25.1).

Clinical pharmacists have developed specialist expertise in response to the needs of oncology patients, older people, children and other patient groups.

Pharmacists working at ward level may encounter some suspicion or even resentment from nurses, who feel that another aspect of their role is being eroded. As clinical pharmacy services have evolved each profession has gained a better insight into the role of the other. This has resulted in the establishment of smooth working relationships which contribute significantly to the safe, effective and economical management of medicines. Pressures on nurses are greater than ever before due to many factors including quicker 'turnover' of patients, a shorter working week and highly-stretched staffing resources. Against this background, nurses have to deal with a wide range of problems arising from the ever increasing complexity of drug therapy. Nurses recognise the clinical pharmacist as a valuable source of practical help, advice and support.

Clinical pharmacy services are compatible with all medicine distribution systems, but the way in which these are provided will vary according to local needs.

Box 25.1   Key elements of a clinical pharmacy service

Review of prescriptions:
  dosage
  route of administration
  adverse drug reactions
  drug interactions
Rapid response to changing needs for medicines
Advice of formulation/presentation of medicines to meet the needs of individual patients
Formulary management systems – development and monitoring
Advice on aids to patient compliance

Pharmaceutical care

The concept of pharmaceutical care developed in the USA is increasingly receiving attention in the United Kingdom. Significant benefits can be achieved for patients in introducing a system whereby the pharmacist exercises control over the drugs used by an individual patient which is governed by a commitment to that patient's best interests. In practical terms the provision of pharmaceutical care follows a problem-solving approach with several key elements which are familiar to nurses:

- evaluation of the patient's drug-related needs
- determination of the patient's actual or potential problems
- development with other health professionals of a pharmaceutical care plan designed to deal with problems identified
- implementation and monitoring of the plan.

The rate and extent to which pharmaceutical care will be developed in the United Kingdom depends on many factors, in particular the availability of adequate resources. Nevertheless, with increasing emphasis on care in the community, plans will be needed for patients receiving complex therapy in their own homes. Co-operative working between pharmacists and community health care staff (especially nurses) will also be essential if effective pharmaceutical care is to be implemented successfully. Table 25.1 outlines the process by which a pharmaceutical care plan can be established.

Table 25.1   Development of a pharmaceutical care plan

Stage	Action by pharmacist	Notes
I	Establish contact with the patient	The need for a good professional working relationship cannot be overstated
II	Collect and interpret information on patient's condition and drug history (including use of non-prescription medicines)	Aspects that will require particular attention include: non-compliance of the patient practical problems with medicine use drug interactions incidence of side-effects poor medicine hygiene/storage
III	List patient's problems in priority order	It will be important to establish the degree of risk involved in order to prioritise the problems
IV	Establish whenever possible the desired *outcome* of each problem identified	In some situations the outcome may be very easy to define – e.g. improve the storage of medicines. Thereafter, outcomes may be less easy to define but every effort must be made to do so
V	Examine alternatives available and choose the best in the particular circumstances	As with all stages, the needs of the *individual patient* will be the paramount consideration
VI	Design and implement a monitoring plan based on patient's needs	The plan should focus on outcomes which can be measured
VII	Implement plan	Effective communication within the health care team is vital, especially between community nursing staff and the pharmacist
VIII	Follow up to determine overall success of the plan	It is emphasised that pharmaceutical care plans have an overall requirement of a long-term commitment to the patient

The introduction of pharmaceutical care plans should not be seen as a threat to the role of the nurse or other health prefessional. As with the development of clinical pharmacy, the overall objective of pharmaceutical care is to utilise the skills of the pharmacist so that the benefits of drug treatment are fully realised for the patient.

Partial stock/individual dispensing system

Under this arrangement prescribed medicines are supplied either as ward stocks, or are dispensed for an individual patient. Confusion can arise at ward level owing to the presence of these two different categories of medicine in the trolley. The decision as to when a medicine becomes an agreed ward stock item may cause friction, especially when an individually dispensed item is retained by the nurse for ward stock. Effective liaison between pharmacists and nurses enables the use of medicines to be closely monitored and agreement reached on the range of stock items required.

Individual patient dispensing

With the increasing emphasis on primary nursing care there is a need for systems of medication distribution which are compatible with an individual approach to patient care. Dispensing for individual patients meets this need. Medicines are supplied, not as communal stock bottles, but for administration only to the patient named on the label of the dispensed medicine. A very limited range of medicines is supplied as ward stock as cover for periods when the pharmaceutical service may be limited.

The dispensed medicines are stored in separate compartments, one for each patient, within a specially designed medicine trolley (Fig. 25.4). A disadvantage of this method of supply is that it is more labour intensive for the pharmacy than a stock system. However, with good organisation, the workload generated can be contained. The trolley can be sent to the pharmacy and the prescribed medicines placed in each compartment as appropriate. Some medicine trolleys are fitted with removable

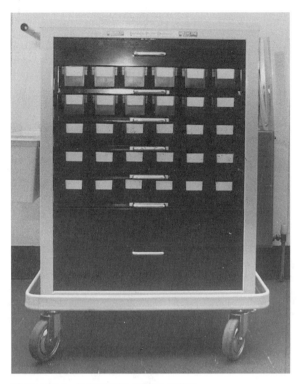

Figure 25.4 Individual medicine trolley.

cassettes (Fig. 25.5) which can be sent to the pharmacy for filling.

Using this system the nurse makes the selection of medicine(s) to be administered from the patient's own medicines. This is in contrast to the stock system where the selection has to be made

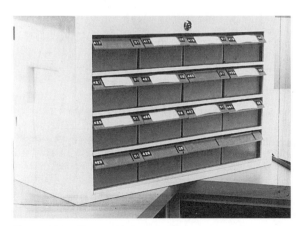

Figure 25.5 Removable cassette.

from the contents of a medicine trolley which may contain 40 or more different preparations (Fig. 25.6). Compared with a stock system, the time taken to administer medicines is reduced by up to 50%. The same care and attention in selecting the medicine against the prescription prior to administration are required as with any other system, but the selection process is greatly facilitated. It also gives the opportunilty to focus on individual patient's medicines as an entity, which is helpful in teaching sessions that may be undertaken at ward level. A further advantage of this system is that it can be used to help the patient develop a better understanding of his medicines and, where appropriate, self-administration of medicines can be facilitated. Other aspects of the self-administration of medicines in hospitals are discussed on page 410.

Individual patient dispensing using unit dose presentation

Although widely used in American hospitals and some continental hospitals, unit dose systems have not been used on a large scale in the United Kingdom. In this system, medicines, both solid and liquid dose forms, are dispensed in unit packs designed to be opened just before administration (Fig. 25.7). As a result, the process of selection of a dose by the nurse prior to administration is greatly simplified. Detailed patient medication records are maintained in the pharmacy and are updated in line with changes in therapy. Using this information the pharmacist is responsible for ensuring that a sufficient number of doses of the correct medicine is available for the individual patient. The pharmacist therefore plays a very central role in the selection of the particular medicine although the nurse still undertakes the final selection prior to administration. Many advantages are claimed to derive from the introduction of this medicine distribution system.

These include reduction of drug errors, reduction in time spent by nurses on non-clinical work, less wastage of medicines and better control generally, since ward stocks are elimi-

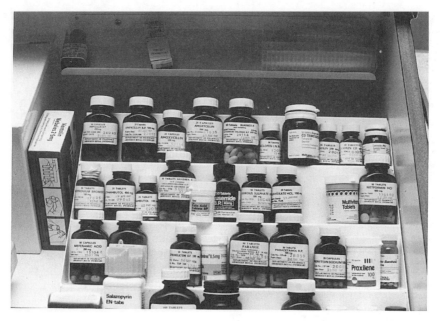

Figure 25.6   Contents of medicine trolley.

nated. Peak demands on pharmacy can be smoothed out as the supply system is very much under the control of the pharmacist. The disadvantages are, however, quite significant. Unit dose packaging must be undertaken in the hospital pharmacy where the technical problems such as product stability in the packaging system chosen must first have been solved. Automated computer-linked unit dose dispensing systems are being evaluated. Such

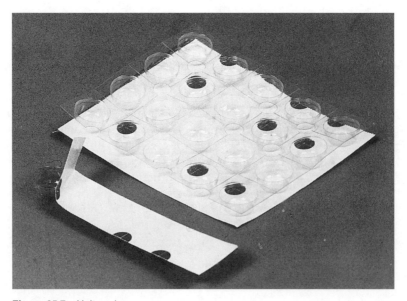

Figure 25.7   Unit packs.

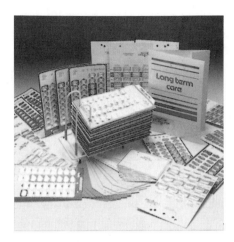

Figure 25.8 Controlled dose systems.

systems have the potential to increase the availability of unit dose systems, since the workload is more manageable than with more conventional packaging methods.

Controlled dose system

This is a more sophisticated form of individual patient dispensing in which medicines (solid dose forms only) are supplied as courses in multi-blister packs. The advantages and disadvantages are similar to those described with the unit dose system (Fig. 25.8).

DISTRIBUTION OF OTHER MEDICINES AND PHARMACEUTICALS TO WARDS

Significant quantities of medicines and related products which are not routinely prescribed are supplied for use in wards. These can be considered broadly as:

- medicines for emergency resuscitation procedures
- products used in nursing care
- substances used in medical diagnosis
- disinfectants/antiseptics.

Resuscitation packs

These are supplied by the pharmacy in accordance with local policy. The packaging and presentation of drugs will be a matter for the pharmaceutical service. It is vital to ensure that the contents are suitably labelled and that adequate checks are made to ensure the contents are not allowed to pass the expiry date.

Nursing care products

In order to avoid multiplicity of products in use for nursing care procedures such as catheter care, skin care and eye bathing, it is desirable to establish a formulary of nursing care products (see p. 437). Such a formulary contains monographs on the products which are available for use by nurses without medical prescription. The items contained in the formulary are supplied on a routine 'top-up' basis.

Diagnostic agents

Clinical reagents are normally supplied on a routine stock basis. Other more specialised agents are supplied on request.

Disinfectants, antiseptics, lotions, etc

It is now standard practice for wards (and departments) to use a range of products as agreed by the control of infection committee. The disinfection policy will contain information on the use of products together with supporting technical information. The products are supplied on a routine indenting or topping-up basis. A discussion of the properties and uses of disinfectants appears in Chapter 21.

DISTRIBUTION OF MEDICINES AND PHARMACEUTICALS TO HOSPITAL DEPARTMENTS

The distribution of medicines and related products to departments (e.g. to operating theatres) often involves considerable bulk, but the product range is less extensive than to wards.

However, it is still important to achieve standardisation since duplication of products is costly and may cause confusion. Pre-printed drug indents facilitate the introduction and maintenance of a standard range of products. Specialised clinical planning services are required in hospital clinical departments, although the scope for individualisation of medication regimes is limited.

Special arrangements are often required in Accident and Emergency departments, such as the provision of 'patient-ready' packs of analgesics and antibiotics which can be issued to patients without nurses having to undertake 'dispensing'.

TECHNICAL SUPPORT SERVICES

The drug distribution arrangements previously described are supplemented by specialist technical support services. These are dispensing services which require pharmaceutical expertise and special environmental conditions such as those provided in an aseptic suite. These central, pharmacy-based services, have been developed in response to the growing complexity of drug therapy and the need to provide the highest possible standards of patient care.

Central intravenous additive services (CIVAS)

The addition of drugs to intravenous fluids is best performed in an aseptic dispensing suite rather than a ward where full aseptic standards are impossible to achieve. By providing these services centrally, nurses are relieved of time-consuming manipulative tasks and are able to concentrate on clinical care. On occasions it will be necessary to make an addition to an intravenous fluid at ward or departmental level but this should only be undertaken where there is no alternative.

Total parenteral nutrition services (see also p. 276)

The administration of nutrients, vitamins and minerals in combination in a single container presented ready for use represents a far safer method of administration than that provided by using a series of separate containers. The 3-litre (or smaller volume) container prepared under strict aseptic conditions within the pharmacy reduces infection risks and helps to ensure accuracy of the therapy.

Cytotoxic reconstitution services (see also p. 232)

The risks inherent in reconstituting cytotoxic drugs without due attention to the safety of the doctor or nurse undertaking this task are well recognised. Full protection of operator and product can be achieved only within a specialised unit having all the necessary facilities such as vertical laminar air flow cabinets, air-conditioning and facilities for staff to change into sterile protective clothing. As with the other specialist services, the donor of the medicine is provided with an accurately compounded, fully labelled, ready-to-use sterile product. Although this greatly reduces hazards, care is required when administering the medicine so as to avoid aerosol formation and spillage which may contaminate the environment.

Radiopharmaceuticals

Major hospital pharmaceutical departments provide a service supplying sterile radioisotope injections for use in specialised diagnostic procedures. The injections are formulated in order to accumulate in a particular organ or part of the body, e.g. phosphate injection becomes concentrated in bone, thiosulphate in the liver, albumin microspheres are temporarily trapped in the lung capillaries. These chemicals are labelled with a short-acting radionuclide such as ^{99m}Tc (half-life 8 hours) which rapidly decays. A camera which is sensitive to the radioactive particles which are emitted by the technetium, scans the organ or part of the body. This illustrates different concentrations within a particular organ and in this way abnormalities can be located.

Drug information services

The provision of information on many aspects of the use of medicines and properties of drugs is an integral part of pharmaceutical services. The organisation of this service and method of provision will vary considerably, depending on circumstances. In larger acute hospitals, a department under the control of a full-time specialist pharmacist, will provide the service on a district, area or regional basis. The pharmacist providing clinical services will also be a source of drug information. All pharmacists have access to the specialist hospital-based services to supplement their own resources. Drug information pharmacists work closely with their clinical colleagues when the nature of the query requires highly specialised information that can only be obtained by a literature search. Pharmaceutical manufacturers are an important source of product information, and professional bodies such as the Royal Pharmaceutical Society of Great Britain provide invaluable support to practising pharmacists.

All specialist drug information services are available to health professionals but are not normally available directly to members of the public. With the rapid development of information technology drug information will become much more widely available to health professionals. Queries received by pharmacists cover a wide range of topics, including dose, route of administration, adverse effects, interactions, contraindications and increasingly information on cost/benefits of particular treatments. Information on medicines is provided in response to specific requests and in regular bulletins.

An important part of the practising pharmacist's work is also to provide patients with the necessary information to enable the patient to use his medicines in the most effective way. This aspect is discussed in more detail in Chapter 26.

PHARMACEUTICAL SERVICES IN THE COMMUNITY

The community pharmacist is responsible for the supply of medicines to patients in the community. In addition, the community pharmacist is responsible for the provision of a wide range of health care products, surgical appliances, dressings, etc.

Medicines are supplied on prescription and, where legislation permits, are also sold over the counter. In many instances, an individual will seek the pharmacist's advice and guidance on a particular health problem. This may result in a medicine being recommended and sold to the client, or the phamacist may suggest self-referral to the general practitioner. Surveys have shown that there is considerable use of proprietary medicines by the public and this should always be borne in mind by health care staff in both community and hospital practice. Members of the public often regard purchased medicines as being little more than ordinary household commodities. As a result, important information on the patient's current full medications may not be readily divulged. The community pharmacist will provide information on the use of medicines to community health care staff and give invaluable support and guidance to his clients.

For many years the community pharmacist has played a vital part in health care provision. There is great potential to extend further the contribution the community pharmacist can make not only in the treatment of illness but in prevention of ill health. With the growing emphasis on self-care and the limitation of prescribing certain products within the NHS, more people will seek the professional advice of the pharmacist for the treatment of minor ailments.

The use of computer technology enables the pharmacist to exercise a monitoring role by maintaining patient medication records, including information on allergies to specific drugs. The provision of information on the use of medicines is of growing importance. The pharmacist is well placed to provide the necessary information in the most suitable form for patients and their carers.

As more patients are cared for in their own homes, and in the community, the community pharmacist's services will be even more important in the years ahead. In addition to providing services to patients suffering from chronic diseases, the community pharmacist provides a range of services to special categories of patients such as drug users.

Participation in health promotion campaigns is an accepted part of the community pharmacist's role. There is great potential for an expansion of this increasingly important role.

FORMULARIES

Drug formularies have been used in medicine for many years. In pre-NHS days, most voluntary hospitals had a drug formulary which was a core list of medicines approved by the medical committee for use in that institution. In most cases the motivation for establishing a formulary appears to have been the need to control prescribing costs. Today, it is widely accepted that a drug formulary is an essential element in the drive to achieve rational prescribing while at the same time controlling costs. Box 25.2 outlines the stages in formulary development which would be followed by a Drug and Therapeutics Committee (D&TC) in hospital with a multidisciplinary membership of doctors, pharmacists, nurses and finance officer.

mation is increasingly by means of a computerised system which also facilitates monitoring of formulary compliance. The choice of drug for inclusion in the formulary is based on safety, efficacy and cost. Increasingly general practitioners are developing formularies – often in consultation with hospital specialists and drug information pharmacists. The classification system used by the British National Formulary (BNF) is generally adopted in local formularies for ease of reference.

Government policy has strongly encouraged the development of drug formularies throughout the NHS. From the evidence available, drug formularies appear to have significant advantages for patient care. However, the introduction of formularies may cause friction and misunderstanding since some prescribers view formulary development as a major threat to their clinical freedom. Some of the advantages and disadvantages postulated are summarised in Table 25.2.

Although opponents of drug formularies may still be heard, there can be little doubt that as the range of drugs available to the prescriber continues to expand and costs continue to escalate, formularies will become even more important. Effective multidisciplinary working methods and consultation will do much to reduce the difficulties outlined above.

Nurses will play an increasingly important

Box 25.2 Stages in formulary development in the hospital setting

Stage I	Request for inclusion of product by consultant(s)
Stage II	Consideration by D&TC
Stage III	Inclusion in formulary (or rejection or suggestion of alternative)
Stage IV	Publication of information on product to prescriber
Stage V	Monitoring of impact/cost/benefits
Stage VI	Depending on outcome, use of drug extended or curtailed

---

The method of presentation of the formulary varies from a simple listing of products to a compendium giving full details of the formulations, actions and uses of each drug, side-effects, dosage levels and costs. Presentation of the infor-

Table 25.2 Advantages and disadvantages of drug formularies

Advantages	Disadvantages
Lowers prescribing costs	Restricts clinical freedom
Encourages generic prescribing	Inhibits introduction of new products :
Improves drug safety	reduces research efforts
Improves patient care	stifles innovation by
Reduces range of products to be stored	pharmaceutical industry
Facilitates drug purchasing in hospitals	Restricts the patient's choice
Educational value	Reduces treatment options
Provides opportunity for multidisciplinary working	
Improves continuity of care especially where a joint hospital/ community formulary is in place	

role, both in formulary development (as a member of the D&TC) and formulary management at ward level. As drug budgets are devolved to ward level, nurses are provided with the incentive to assist in achieving and monitoring formulary compliance. To carry out this important task, the need for accurate, up-to-date information on medicine usage is vital. Pharmaceutical services are provided in such a way that staff who are responsible for the use of medicines receive regular feedback on levels of use of both formulary and non-formulary drugs. The introduction of a formulary system may create problems for nurses when a patient receiving a non-formulary medicine is admitted for inpatient care. The approach to this problem will vary depending on local arrangements. For example, the patient may continue to be given the medicine(s) using supplies he has brought in on admission. This approach needs the support and advice of the clinical pharmacist (and/or prescriber) to ensure that the medicine(s) are suitable for use. When the prescriber considers it to be appropriate another medicine may be substituted. In such situations the nurse can help to explain to the patient the reasons for any change in therapy. On the other hand, the nurse may become the patient's advocate and ask that the patient be maintained on his original therapy where in her professional view it would be disadvantageous to change the patient's therapy. In addition to formularies designed to meet the prescribing needs of doctors, formularies of nursing care products have been developed (see p. 437). Proposals to introduce nurse prescribing in the community using a nationally agreed Nurse Prescribers' Formulary have been postponed.

PATIENT PROTOCOLS

Doctors in general practice and hospitals are developing shared care protocols for the care of patients suffering from chronic illnesses such as asthma, diabetes and hypertension. Patient protocols have strong links with drug formularies, since protocols contain details of drug treatment regimes. Shared-care protocols represent an agreement between consultant, GP and patient on the approach to diagnosis and treatment of a particular illness. The purpose of the protocol is to standardise treatment and to help ensure continuity of care and involvement of the patient. An outline of a shared-care protocol is given in Box 25.3.

Computerisation of the management of patient care greatly assists in the introduction, monitoring and audit of the benefits (or otherwise) achieved by use of the protocol. Shared-care protocols also provide a framework within which the patient can become fully involved in the treatment plan.

Box 25.3   Outline of a shared-care protocol

Brief introduction to the condition dealt with in protocol
Objectives of the protocol
Responsibilities of the consultant, e.g.
    communications consultant ↔ patient ↔ GP
    source of supply of medicines
    treatment regime drug/dose/route/etc
Responsibilities of GP, e.g. prescribing (and
administration) of the drug(s)
Responsibilities of the patient, e.g. attendance at clinic(s)
Contact telephone numbers, etc.

In addition to shared-care protocols, GPs are adopting protocols for use within their own practices on the treatment of such conditions as urinary tract infection (UTI), intractable pain and chronic bronchitis.

Protocols are seen by some doctors as limiting clinical freedom and as a potential threat to innovation. There are also legal implications and concerns that patient protocols may be unduly influenced by cost factors. Advantages claimed for patient protocols include improved patient care, elimination of the wide variation in diagnosis and treatment, and opportunities for the introduction of clinical audit. A protocol for the treatment of UTI in general practice as described by Brooks et al (1992) contained the following elements:

- organisation of care, e.g.
    aims of treatment
    organisation of diagnostic services

- assessment and treatment of the patient
- problem solving and follow-up
- patient checklist
- practice audit.

As protocols are developed there will be many opportunities for nurses to contribute to their development and audit since nurses are well placed to help in the evaluation.

LOCAL POLICIES

In small hospitals with no resident doctor, in specialist units and in some community settings the strict criteria laid down by the UKCC with respect to the administration of medicines either cannot be applied or, if applied, could introduce dangerous delay with consequent risks to patients. In these situations, an agreed local policy may be drawn up for use by nurses. Where a policy of this kind applies it must clearly state:

- the circumstances in which particular 'prescription-only medicines' may be administered in advance of examination by a doctor
- the form, route and dosage range of the medicines so authorised
- which nurse(s) are allowed to be involved in the administration of these medicines.

REFERENCES

Brooks D, Clift T, Dodd A et al 1992 UTI. MIMS Magazine weekly pull-out, October 13

FURTHER READING

Chief Administrative Pharmaceutical Officers' Group 1990 Standards for pharmaceutical services provided from health board premises in Scotland
Department of Health Circular HC(88)54 1988 The way forward for hospital pharmaceutical services
The Scottish Office 1991 The patient's charter. A charter for health
Regional Pharmaceutical Officers' Group 1991 Standards for pharmaceutical services in health authorities in England

Royal Pharmaceutical Society of Great Britain 1992 The future of community pharmacy. Joint working party report on pharmaceutical care
Schumock G T, Leister K A, Edwards D et al 1990 Method for evaluating performance of clinical pharmacists. American Journal of Hospital Pharmacy 47: 127–131
Scottish Office Home and Health Department Circular No. 1988(GEN)32 The way forward for hospital pharmaceutical services

26

Achieving safe and effective drug therapy

INTRODUCTION

This section provides guidance for nurses on the management of medicines. Medicines are subject to a range of controls both in terms of legislation, and local policies and procedures. This is necessary to ensure that:

- medicines are manufactured to the highest standards
- medicines are tested and evaluated before being licensed
- the potential for abuse is minimised
- medicines are stored securely under appropriate conditions
- medicines are used in such a way as to minimise risk to both patient and donor
- medicines are administered appropriately to enable the best possible therapeutic outcome to be achieved.

The manufacture, packaging and distribution of medicines depends on the expertise of the pharmaceutical industry. At local level the pharmaceutical service provides a comprehensive service designed to meet the needs of patients and those providing medical and nursing care. The objectives of achieving successful patient care depend on the integrity and security of all stages of the supply chain from manufacture to patient. All those involved in using medicines for diagnosis, treatment or palliation must be aware of the need to ensure compliance with their legal and professional responsibilities. At the same time the use of medicines has to be considered against a background of ethical and moral issues. When a health professional has to make a judgement on a moral or ethical issue arising from drug treatment the foremost concern must always be the well-being of the patient. Some of the factors that contribute to the concerns nurses and their colleagues have about medicines may also be of concern in other aspects of their professional practice.

Financial factors

While many drugs are relatively inexpensive, there is an increasing number the cost of which is very significant. These include chemotherapeutic agents, antibiotics, parenteral nutrition and certain drugs used in the treatment of patients with immunodeficiency syndrome. Fortunately patients requiring high cost treatments are in the minority. However it may be argued that scarce resources are being used in such a way that very limited benefits are being achieved for the few to the detriment of the rest of the population. More often, it is not a case of whether to prescribe or not but which drug will produce the desired outcome, be acceptable to the patient and also keep costs to the minimum. Choices do have to be made between various forms of treatment. Local drug formularies help the process of choice so that prescribing costs are contained without compromising treatment, safety and efficacy.

Professional factors

Doctors want to be able to help their patients get better. However, there are factors which doctors must consider before deciding which is the best treatment (or indeed whether or not to treat the patient). For example, the decision may be influenced by the likely side-effects, the risk of dependence on the drug, the age of the patient and the patient's prognosis. Difficulties may arise when there are conflicting professional views on prescribing. Medical misadventures can also have a profound effect on a doctor's prescribing behaviour many years after the event. Downward pressure on prescribing costs must not be allowed to compromise patient care.

Well researched prescribing policies and protocols must take into account cost factors, but all health care professionals have a duty to provide the best for their patients in the light of the current state of knowledge. When to withhold treatment can be a much more difficult decision than when to initiate treatment.

Personal factors

The realisation that patients and their families hold, and are entitled to hold, their own beliefs about treatment has been given increased attention with the introduction of the Patient's Charter. The patient (and his family) can only formulate views on a proposed treatment if he is in possession of relevant information about his condition, the nature and effects of the treatment, the alternatives available and the consequences of not accepting treatment. There may be situations where it is in the patient's best interests not to provide information on his drug therapy, e.g. in malignant disease. From time to time it may be necessary to change a patient's drug therapy. The reasons for any changes must be clearly explained to the patient by the prescriber particularly where changes are made for economic reasons. A medicine which has proved to be highly successful in treating a particular condition plays an important part in the patient's life. There may be an understandable reluctance, on the part of the patient, to accept the change. Nurses and pharmacists can play an important part in providing the patient with any necessary reassurance when drug treatment is changed for whatever reason.

Social factors

The ethical issues relating to medicines with which society is confronted raise questions rather than provide answers. For example, should the pharmaceutical industry be making profits out of illness? Some would argue that profits are the result of innovation and great capital investment which must be rewarded. Should animals be used for testing new drugs? Clearly, Animal Rights campaigners think not while others regard such practice acceptable if humanely carried out. What then of clinical drug trials on humans? In the advanced stages of testing there is no practicable alternative. Wider issues about pollution of the environment, with chemical waste arising from the manufacturing processes involved in drug production, may also be a concern. Very strict legislation does provide a high degree of protection, but concerns will always exist. Dependence, addiction and over-reliance on drugs raise doubts in the minds of many health professionals. Nurses are required to enter into the debate on the ethical aspects of the use of medicines as part of their professional role. Guidance is given in the UKCC Code of Professional Conduct. Local ethics committees provide guidance on specific matters particularly on ethical aspects of clinical trials. There may be situations where, on religious grounds, a nurse cannot be involved in a particular form of treatment. This stance has to be respected and accepted by colleagues without any form of sanction being applied. Nurses in such situations will receive the support they need but, as always, the best interests of the patient must be served.

THE ROLE OF THE NURSE

From the earliest day of her career every nurse is involved to some extent in the management of medicines. Although responsibilities increase and change with time, the safe and effective management of medicines remains a high priority for all practising nurses. The importance of establishing a firm basis of learning during pre-registration training is well recognised, as is the need to progress to wider aspects, as part of professional development. Thus the nurse builds upon the knowledge and skills acquired to prepare herself for the particular responsibilities and duties in her chosen speciality. As with all health professionals the nurse has a responsibility to keep up to date and make her contribution to professional issues of the day.

Although it is recognised that the emphasis will vary depending on the speciality in which the nurse works, the role of the nurse in drug therapy can be broadly summarised under the following headings:

- to ensure that the correct dosage is given at the correct time and by the correct route
- to observe/report any side-effects and drug interactions, and to take action to alleviate unavoidable side-effects
- to observe and assess the patient so that medical and nursing decisions can be made
- to participate in education and guidance of patients (and in some cases their relatives) with regard to their drug therapy, in order to promote patient compliance and the achievement of therapeutic objectives
- to take action to help reduce, or remove, the need for drug therapy
- to contribute to the evaluation and development of new treatments, and/or the reassessment of existing treatments
- to follow recognised procedures for the control of medicines and pharmaceutical products at ward or departmental level and to contribute to the development of these procedures and controls in response to changing situations.

The nurse's role is much more than a mechanical achievement of objectives. It is a professional role requiring knowledge, skill, judgement and commitment.

The standards expected of each individual registered nurse (or midwife or health visitor) with respect to medicines are made explicit by the United Kingdom Central Council (1992). To meet such standards, the expectation is that the nurse is personally accountable for her practice and in so doing acts at all times to promote and safeguard the interests and well-being of patients and clients.

Having outlined the current role of the nurse in drug therapy it is important to realise that many changes and developments are taking place within both health care and the health professions. These changes are having, and will continue to have, an increasing impact on the practising nurse whether in hospital or community. Some of the changes are as follows:

- changing patterns in the provision of health care
- increasing complexity of drug therapy in general
- increasing specialisation in the use of drugs, such as cytotoxic therapy and total parenteral nutrition
- the development of new drug delivery systems
- changes in drug presentation, improved packaging, and new drug distribution systems
- increasing concern regarding the side-effects of drug treatment
- a greater interest in alternative medicine
- an increasing emphasis on the need to use resources effectively
- the need to ensure that the person administering the drugs is not harmed by them
- a greater awareness of the need to ensure the safe and effective use of medicines by older people
- the increasing use of computers in clinical practice, both in hopsitals and the community
- an increasing emphasis on self-care
- the development of clinical pharmacy services
- professional aspirations of health care workers generally.

The practising nurse is becoming more aware of the great benefits and potential dangers of drug therapy. As the nurse is accountable for her clinical actions, it is essential that she acquires well-founded confidence in what she does. This confidence is achieved through the mastering of practical skills supported by the necessary theoretical knowledge. No matter how careful and expert the prescribing doctor, or dispensing pharmacist, the consequences for the patient may be disastrous if the nurse is ill-equipped to discharge her vital role to the full.

Knowledge/information

In order to be safe in the administration of medicines and to be able to advise patients appropriately, the nurse requires a knowledge of basic pharmacology as well as physiology. A knowledge of the medicines in use and their management is equally important. In addition, she needs to know and understand the policies and procedures which relate to medicines. Along with this background knowledge the nurse requires to have basic information on each patient including any special points about him which could have a bearing on the successful management of his medicines.

Pharmacology and physiology

Basic pharmacology includes:

- drug absorption mechanisms
- the metabolic action of the liver
- the method by which substances are transported in the bloodstream
- cell transport and activity
- the excretory function of the kidneys.

Without an appreciation of the relevant physiology, the nurse's understanding of how drugs act in the body is incomplete and her safety and effectiveness in practice is therefore open to question. A lack of specialist knowledge of the physiology of extremes of age may hazard the very young or very old patient who is often more at risk from adverse drug reactions than patients in other age groups.

Legal and professional responsibilities

All nurses, including nursing students, have legal responsibilities and are professionally accountable. Every health authority is required to establish policies and procedures which set out in detail instruction and guidance on the administration and storage of medicines. These policies are derived from statutory sources and circulars of guidance issued by the Department of Health (DoH). The nurse must be fully conversant with policies and procedures and adhere to them at all times.

Nurses must also work within the professional standards set by the United Kingdom Central Council for Nurses, Midwives and Health

Visitors (UKCC) and the National Boards for Nursing, Midwifery and Health Visiting, and follow the recommendations made by the Royal College of Nursing (RCN).

The medicines

A working knowledge of the medicines used includes:

- range of presentation of medicines
- ordering/requisitioning procedures
- storage of medicines and disposal of unwanted medicines
- legislation and local hospital policy
- prescribing/recording procedures
- dosage levels
- routes/methods of administration
- rationale for the particular therapy
- safe handling of drugs known to be hazardous
- methods of promoting effectiveness of and/or reducing the need for drug therapy.

The following additional areas of knowledge are also important:

- mode of action of drugs
- recognition of side-effects and methods of minimising/dealing with unavoidable side-effects
- signs and symptoms of drug toxicity
- methods of dealing with effects of drug toxicity
- drug/drug interactions
- drug/food interactions
- effects of disease states on drug therapy
- potential dangers of self-medication
- use of clinical reagents
- aspects of research into drugs
- achieving/improving patient compliance

The patient

It is essential that the nurse is aware of the relevant details about the person who is to receive the medication. The patient's name, age and unit number are necessary for correctly identifying the patient. A knowledge of his medical diagnosis, physical capabilities and mental capacity is essential in achieving safe and effective drug treatment. In addition, the nurse must make herself aware of any special instructions relating to a particular patient's drug therapy. For example, it is important to be aware of hypersensitivity a patient may have to a particular medicine so that it is never given to him. The nurse should be alert to changing circumstances such as the patient who is temporarily to be given nothing by mouth and be able to respond appropriately in terms of medicine administration.

Knowledge and information are vital. Acquiring and using knowledge contributes to safety in medicine administration. By understanding the theory behind medicine administration, the nurse can also act with greater confidence. In the exercise of her professional accountability however, she must be prepared to acknowledge any limitations in her knowledge. It is important too to recognise that information about medicines and their management keeps changing and that practising nurses have a responsibility to keep pace with new developments. Even up-to-date knowledge of course is not of itself sufficient to guarantee safe practice.

Skills

As well as knowledge, a number of skills have to be mastered for the successful management of medicines.

Observation skills

By continual observation a nurse assesses the patient's condition before and after drug treatment, and in so doing helps to establish when treatment is indicated and whether it is being beneficial or otherwise. Nurses routinely measure and record indices such as blood pressure, pulse rate and weight, but it is the ability to note (and report) significant change in these recordings that is important.

Observable changes in a patient receiving specific forms of drug therapy may include:

- allergic reaction, ranging from skin rash to anaphylaxis
- muscular weakness arising from potassium loss in diuretic therapy
- bruising or overt bleeding arising from too high a dose of an anticoagulant
- euphoria associated with corticosteroid therapy
- depression associated with antihypertensive drug therapy
- anorexia in a patient receiving digoxin therapy.

Communication skills

From the moment a person becomes a patient, his continued well-being (and eventual restoration to health) depends on effective communication with him, and between health care personnel. Nowhere is this more important than with all aspects of drug therapy.

At a very early stage, interviewing skills are needed when eliciting a patient's history. This will involve collecting details of current drug therapy, prescribed or non-prescribed, and any difficulties the patient has in taking medicines. The patient may reveal a belief in alternative medicine or some form of lay medicine and this should never be discounted. Information on a patient's medical condition and/or drug therapy may be obtained from the medical pendant or bracelet worn by some patients.

Throughout the patient's stay in hospital other more general communication skills are used. Instructions to the patient should be clear and concise, offered at a suitable pace, and in a voice that can be heard. A conscious effort should be made to avoid the use of medical or nursing jargon. Ensuring that the patient is wearing his spectacles and/or hearing aid may mean the difference between success and failure in communicating with him.

An equally important part of the communication process is a willingness to listen. Patients are often happy to talk about their illnesses and treatments and by appropriate questioning and astute follow-up of cues, the nurse can assess how much comprehension a patient has of his disorder and which problems are most real to

him. By non-verbal means, such as a gesture, facial expression or mood, the patient can convey respectively the nature or location of pain, his like or dislike of taking a medicine, and the likelihood of his actually taking the medicines.

The nurse also needs to be able to give and receive messages about patients and their medicines to and from doctors, pharmacists and other nurses. In addition, the importance of writing out the message in detail serves as an additional check and may also be required in the event of a query arising.

Particular opportunities for communication between nurse and patient arise when medicines are being administered (e.g. when applying a preparation to an area of broken skin the nurse may help to ease pain by engaging the patient in some topic of conversation so as to divert his attention from the procedure). However it is not always appropriate to deal with detailed questions at the time of administration as this may cause too much delay or increase the risk of error in the procedure itself. Nevertheless the patient is entitled to know the name of the medicine, why it is being given, the dose he is to have, how often it is to be taken, and, if possible, the length of the course of treatment. It may also be appropriate to advise the patient of any likely side-effects. If the patient's questions cannot be dealt with fully at the time he should be assured that a more detailed explanation will be given later. Patients may need additional explanation and reassurance when a new treatment is begun or when a medicine is changed or discontinued.

The nurse should also be prepared to learn from the patient. Many patients, especially those suffering from chronic conditions, such as asthma, myasthenia gravis or Parkinson's disease will almost certainly have far more practical experience in managing their condition than the nurse. For example, these patients know by personal experience what the optimum time of administration of their medicine is.

Teaching skills

Linked with observation and communication skills are those associated with teaching. Virginia

Henderson (1966) states that it is part of the nurse's role to improve the patient's level of understanding and thus promote their health. Rodman & Smith (1974) suggest that nurses should aim to teach about drug therapy so that at the time of discharge from hospital, the patient can display a full understanding of his illness and medicines, and can take his medicines in accordance with the prescription. The assumption is that patient teaching promotes independence by facilitating self-administration of the medication, and thus the achievement of therapeutic benefit. By alerting the patient to potentially harmful situations, (e.g. taking aspirin when receiving warfarin therapy) nurses can contribute significantly to the patient's continued well-being. Increased understanding may help the patient in deciding to comply with the prescribed therapy.

The role of 'teacher' is to guide, stimulate and direct. In association with the administration of medicines, it is the nurse who primarily takes this role. She is the person who helps the patient to link what he already knows to that which is unfamiliar to him. The teaching process will include explaining, demonstrating, supervising and drawing diagrams as appropriate. Teaching is an essential part of patient management and time must be found for it in spite of other pressures. Opportunities for teaching need to be recognised and put to use. As so much of what we learn results from copying others, nurses must display a high level of precision and professionalism in all aspects of medicine management and, in so doing, teach by example. Individual factors do, however, influence learning and consequently the approach to teaching. These include the patient's level of intelligence and maturity, knowledge, past experience, physical ability and motivation. Where a patient is unable to master the necessary skill, the nurse may have to teach a relative or friend.

Some practical points to remember when teaching patients and/or relatives are as follows.

Make sure the time is right for teaching

Teaching a patient about his medicines should be carried out at a time mutually convenient to patient and nurse. An explanation of the use of medicines which he is to take when he gets home from hospital should be made well in advance of the time of discharge. In this way, he is less likely to be hurried and there will still be time left to deal with any difficulties which arise (e.g. the occurrence of an unexpected side-effect).

Avoid giving the impression that you are hurried

The flustered nurse whose every second glance is at the ward clock can convey anxiety to her patient which in turn may interfere with concentration. By talking to the patient about his medicines from an early stage and continuing to keep him informed of changes until the time of discharge, the task of administering medicines is made more simple and effective. The patient is more likely to assimilate information when the main points are repeated at appropriate intervals. In this way, teaching becomes an integral part of medicine administration.

Consider whether the patient can hear you

The noise created by equipment used in the ward may prevent instructions from being heard. Patients who wear a hearing aid may require assistance in its use.

Consider whether the patient can see

Many patients need to wear spectacles for reading and at other times. Good lighting is necessary.

Maintain eye contact

This should be achieved as much as possible while talking to the patient.

Avoid creating a mirror image

When demonstrating how to load a syringe, sit or stand alongside the patient rather than face him so that he can observe the procedure from the stance in which he will perform it.

Adopt a positive approach

For example, 'Hold the syringe this way'.

Keep speech and demonstration separate

When learning a skill for the first time, a limited amount of information can be absorbed at one time.

Break the teaching into stages

Do this whenever possible and select important points which require special emphasis.

Do not assume that the patient is literate

Obviously great tact is required to establish the extent of the patient's ability to read and write. People with literacy difficulties often wish to deny them and are skilful at concealing their problems. Conversely do not 'talk down' to patients. Where English is not understood, the help of an interpreter will be required.

It may be of encouragement to nurses to be reminded that one of the best ways of improving one's knowledge of a subject is to teach it to somebody else.

Motor skills

Apart from the situations where hospital inpatients manage their own drug therapy, medicines are administered by nurses using skills acquired through learning and practice. Improvements in drug presentation, (e.g. pre-filled syringes and aseptic dispensing services) have simplified and improved the safety of drug administration. On the other hand, application of modern technology in clinical areas has placed additonal demands on nurses' skills and technical abilities. The use of electronically controlled drug delivery systems, pumps, and other devices requires skills quite different from those traditionally associated with nursing. Against this background however, it is vitally important that the traditional practical skills of the nurse are not neglected.

The degree of skill required in medicine administration varies considerably, depending on the dosage form used, the route/method of administration, and the extent to which the patient cooperates or is able to co-operate.

The giving of a simple tablet to a relatively well, intelligent, and cooperative patient presents few problems. Administering a small volume of a liquid medicine from a dropper to a mentally handicapped, athetoid child presents a greater challenge. To succeed in administering an intramuscular injection to a very agitated and uncooperative patient demands experience, skill and tenacity. The motor skills required include manual dexterity, coordination of hand and eye, coupled with lightness and delicacy of touch. Specialised situations such as those met in dermatology and ophthalmology call for skills which are only acquired through repeated practice.

Numeracy skills

With the increasing potency and specificity of modern drugs it is now more vital than ever to ensure accuracy when administering medicines. It is essential therefore that the nurse has a sound working knowledge of SI units of mass and volume and can calculate in these units. Recognition by pharmacists that it is important to supply medicines to wards and departments in a suitable range of strengths has reduced the need for calculations prior to the administration of medicines. Nevertheless, a nurse may be called upon to calculate how to obtain a dose of say 50 µg from a dosage form that contains 250 µg in 2 ml. Attempts to do this have unfortunately resulted in errors of tenfold or even more. Nurses must also have an understanding of proportions and percentages. It is suggested that these alone represent a minimal level of attainment. Nurses working in intensive care units would be expected to have considerably greater numerical skills and knowledge. Guidance on basic calculations is given in this chapter.

Attitudes

The least tangible part of the nurse's role is her overall attitude to patients and the management of their medicines. Relevant skills and knowledge are vital if the nurse is to discharge her basic responsibilities. However, without an informed respect for drugs generally, the full benefits of drug therapy will not be achieved and drug therapy may fail.

On a professional level, the nurse should have an awareness of the place of all medicines, in the care of the patient. Recognition of the reasons for the need to be systematic in adherence to both national (legal) and local procedural requirements is vital. The recognition should be based on a broad understanding of the principles involved, not merely the mechanical following of a set of rules. An overall sense of the need for security in its widest sense is required, coupled with an appreciation of economic factors. An enquiring attitude of mind associated with a knowledgeable, well-informed approach, will give the nurse confidence to play her full part in ensuring safe and effective drug therapy.

However, it is also important to consider those attitudes which are, to a large extent, linked with personal qualities. These include powers of observation and the ability to keep calm and work under pressure. Being selective in dealing with interruptions during procedures involving medicines calls for judgement, patience and, occasionally, a sense of humour. The nurse must exercise judgement, since a degree of flexibility may be called for on occasions; firmness, linked with tact, is a prerequisite. The balanced assessment of one's own knowledge, or lack of it, is important, as is the willingness to ask and seek advice.

Against this background it should not be forgotten that the nurse has a duty to encourage the patient to regard all medicines with respect, without at the same time causing anxiety. In exercising the necessary skills and demonstrating the correct attitude, the nurse sets an example for the patient to follow when he goes home. Special emphasis on certain aspects, such as the need for safe storage of medicines, can be reinforced by the attitude adopted by the nurse and the care and concern she shows. A patient may be reluctant to take the medicines and/or unable to see the need for them. This demands patience and perseverance by the nurse. Often the problem arises with those in greatest need of the treatment. With a responsibility to act as a role model in health education, the nurse should respect medicines at all times, both in her professional and personal life.

THE ROLE OF THE COMMUNITY NURSE

With the increasing trend towards care in the community, the role of the community nurse in relation to drug therapy has expanded over the last few years. Other factors have contributed to this expanded role not least of which is the ageing population (see also p. 33). With the possibility of nurses prescribing selected items, the community nurse must be even more aware of side-effects, drug interactions, etc. She must also be aware of the legal aspects of drug therapy and accountability. The vital role of the community nurse in relation to drug therapy can be considered under a number of headings.

Storage and safe keeping of medicines in the home

The patient's general practitioner normally prescribes the necessary medicines although in certain situations a consultant may retain this responsibility. It is important to remember that the medicines are the patient's property and should always be regarded as such by the community nurse. Patients should be advised on the safe storage of medicines especially the need to keep all medicines out of the reach of children. Any special storage requirements such as refrigeration should also be borne in mind. On occasions the nurse may need to advise the patient, or patient's relatives, to destroy any accumulations of unwanted medicines. The nurse should not take possession of any unwanted drugs. If controlled drugs are involved the nurse must not take possession of these since she is not authorised to receive Controlled Drugs in this way. In both situations the nurse should give the necessary guidance to the patient or patient's relatives and a record of the destruction should be made. The record should be witnessed and signed by the nurse and a member of the patient's family or carer. On some occasions it may be possible for the patient to sign.

Administration of medicines

Essentially the community nurse has the same responsibilities as the hospital nurse. There is naturally a difference of emphasis but the principles are the same. The detailed guidelines given on pages 381–389 apply equally to the community nurse but of course a second nurse will not be present to carry out the checking procedure. Where appropriate, relatives may be asked to check drugs – helping them to feel part of the caring team instead of being simply bystanders. Full records of medicines administered, normally only parenteral forms, are maintained and signed by the community nurse.

The responsibility for taking oral medicines rests with the patient but in some situations older people may need guidance and help from the community nurse especially when the patient's short-term memory is failing. Despite strenuous and ingenious efforts by the nurse, severely confused patients may be beyond immediate help. Hospital admission may be required in the patient's best interests.

Monitoring drug therapy

The community nurse gets to know her patients especially well and as a result is in a good position to assist in the monitoring of all drug therapy. As part of planning nursing care a note is made in the patient's records of possible side-effects that may arise from the prescribed drug therapy. When planning a visit, this specific information is taken into account by the nurse. This provides a basis on which judgements can be made relating to changes in the patient's condition which may or may not be due to the side-effects of drug therapy. The nurse will be especially concerned about this aspect of her role when a new course of drug therapy is commenced. The occurrence of side-effects should of course be reported to the prescriber so that, if necessary, changes in therapy can be made.

Provision of information to other health care workers

On occasion it may be necessary for the community nurse to provide information on a patient's drug therapy to professional colleagues. For hospital colleagues this is often conveyed via the liaison health visitor. Information can now be transferred, using microcomputer technology, through the public telephone system (Health Net British Telecom) so that a printed message is available without the delay often associated with a letter.

Provision of information to patients

The patient may receive conflicting advice about his medicines from well-meaning neighbours, relatives and friends. This may cause confusion in the patient's mind which may lead to non-compliance. Community nurses are often able to give the patient suitable guidance with the help of the general practitioner and community pharmacist where necessary.

Compliance aspects

Since the general practitioner prescribes the vast majority of all medicines it follows that the scope for improving patient compliance in the community is almost unlimited. Many of the strategies for improving patient compliance discussed in this chapter can be used by the community nurse.

Proprietary and 'lay' medicines

Many patients will purchase proprietary medicines which may in some instances conflict with prescribed medicines. For example aspirin-containing preparations potentiate the effect of oral anticoagulants and should obviously be avoided by patients receiving this therapy. Normally the general practitioner and community pharmacist will give the patient guidance but the patient may be unaware of the presence of aspirin in a proprietary product. The introduction of selected list prescribing under the NHS will no doubt result in more patients buying medicines from a pharmacy. If the community nurse is aware of the proprietary medicines a patient is taking, suitable advice can be given.

Patients may also have faith in a 'lay' remedy or some form of alternative medicine. This aspect is briefly discussed in Chapter 1.

Care of the patient following cytotoxic drug therapy

In order to respond to the special needs of the patient who has received cytotoxic drug therapy in hospital the community nurse will require detailed information on the nature of the therapy.

Administration of Controlled Drugs

The administration of Controlled Drugs varies depending on where the patient stays. In rural areas there is generally no evening or night cover in which case the patient's general practitioner often administers the drugs. In urban areas, 24-hour nursing cover permits more nurse input. In any case, the necessary drugs will be prescribed by the patient's general practitioner and supplied by the community pharmacist. Community nurses, unlike hospital nurses, do not keep stocks of Controlled Drugs. The drugs are kept in the patient's home as is a Controlled Drug form signed by the GP. A copy of the form is kept in the patient's notes in the surgery. The community nurse also keeps a record in the home of doses administered together with the balance of ampoules (or other dosage form) remaining.

Security of medicines and equipment

Normally the community nurse does not carry with her any medicines other than those which may be required in the emergency treatment of anaphylaxis. Community midwives carry pethidine. Checks are made at regular intervals to ensure that these preparations have not passed the expiry date. Syringes and needles are not left in the patient's home and suitable arrangements must be made for safe disposal by the nurse.

Extended role of the nurse in the community

Although it is customary for vaccinations to be administered by health visitors in clinics, the administration of immunological agents by nurses is regarded as part of the Extended Role of the Nurse which requires authorisation from the medical practitioner involved. Other procedures that come into this category include tuberculin skin tests and both intravenous and intra-arterial medication.

Nurse prescribing

The 'Medicinal Products: Prescribing Nurses Act 1992' is an important piece of legislation which will have a significant effect on the professional role of the nurse. The legislation can be seen as a recognition of the fact that many nurses, in particular in community practice, already frequently advise their medical colleagues of the needs of patients especially as regards topical therapy, wound care and symptom relief.

In hospital practice nurses generally have access to a range of medicinal products which they are authorised to use without medical prescription. Written protocols are agreed locally in accordance with the needs of the particular ward or department. Such protocols may take the form of a nursing formulary or symptom relief policy. The use of these protocols is recognised by the UKCC in their publication *Standards for the Administration of Medicines October 1992*. Regulations included in the protocols will be determined jointly by clinical staff having regard to a number of factors, such as patient need, effectiveness and the safety profile of the medicine(s). Clinical pharmacists are well placed to advise on the content, structure and applicability of the protocol.

Nursing formulary

Many current protocols are presented as a formulary of nursing care products. Such formularies include topical applications for the care of the hair, nose and mouth, skin, wounds and bladder. Each product included in the formulary will normally have a data sheet in the following format.

- actions
- indications/limitations as to use
- method of use
- precautions in use with particular emphasis on any hazards
- storage conditions e.g. cool/cold storage
- pack sizes/costs
- date of issue of data sheet (so as to facilitate review).

Symptom relief policy

Symptom relief policy can be considered as a logical development from the nursing formulary. Such a policy gives the nurse the opportunity to further exercise her professional skills in order to meet the needs of the patient. Nurses are well placed both to adjust dosages/frequency of administration and to prescribe certain medicines without the need for medical intervention. It is emphasised that dosage adjustment and prescribing must be in accordance with agreed written policies. Symptom relief will generally include the relief of pain, constipation, sore throat and mild upper respiratory tract problems. Nurses can often prescribe for the relief of gastrointestinal symptoms. They may also prescribe and use local instillations to the bladder especially where indwelling catheters have to be maintained. Whilst the policies on prescribing for symptom relief are applicable widely, a doctor may wish to make certain exceptions in the case of a particular patient. For example, 'symptom relief except laxatives' may be entered on the patient's case notes/prescription sheet.

All medicines administered within the professional remit of the nurse must be recorded on the patient's prescription/recording sheet. There can be no doubt whatsoever that prescribing by nurses, within agreed and well recognised protocols, is greatly to the benefit of patients and enhances the professional role of the nurse.

Prescribing by community nurses

The legislation permitting nurse prescribing within the NHS received the Royal Assent in March 1992, the Act amending the Medicines Act 1968, the National Health Service Act 1968, the NHS Act 1977 and other legislation. This primary legislation has been introduced to permit appropriately qualified nurses working in community practice to prescribe (within the NHS) medicines and appliances (surgical dressings, etc) needed for the nursing care of their patients. Prescribing authority is limited to qualified nurses who have had the necessary additional training. Training programmes envisaged are of two types:

1. a 2-day free-standing module for qualified district nurses and health visitors
2. specific training incorporated into district nurse and health visitor courses.

In both situations nurses will be expected to have a suitable level of background knowledge of clinical pharmacology and therapeutics in order to be able to benefit fully from the training. Training programmes will focus on the need for the nurse to be able to prescribe effectively from the limited list of medicines and appliances, known as the Nurse Prescribers' Formulary which has been approved by the United Kingdom Health Ministers. In addition to knowledge of clinical pharmacology and therapeutics the nurse will be required to demonstrate a knowledge of the relevant legislation and to be fully aware of issues of accountability and professional responsibility. The overall training requirements are summarised below.

Nurse prescribers' training requirements

- basic clinical pharmacology and therapeutics
- legislation
- professional role/accountability
- role of the professions (doctor, nurse, pharmacist)
- principles, practices and procedures of nurse prescribing

- knowledge of actions/uses/hazards of products included in the Formulary
- economic aspects.

Nurse Prescribers' Formulary. At the time of writing the detail of the content of the Formulary is not known. It is expected that prescribing will be restricted to a limited range of medicines and appliances. Community pharmacists will not be able to dispense any prescriptions written by nurses for products outwith the approved range. Products available for prescribing by nurses will probably include laxatives, stoma care products, analgesics associated with minor trauma, bladder instillations, preparations for the treatment of simple skin and ear conditions, surgical dressings and treatments for head lice. It should be pointed out that treatments initiated by nurses should always be fully recorded and communicated to the patient's doctor as soon as possible.

The advent of nurse prescribing within community practice in the NHS will, in time, also have an impact on the role of the nurse in hospital practice. Hospital nurses have always had certain prescribing responsibilities and it seems likely that these will develop in the years ahead. Nurse prescribing can be seen as having special relevance as care in the community gathers momentum. Continuity of care between hospital and the community will be greatly facilitated by nurse prescribing.

Further implications for nurses of the introduction of nurse prescribing. The introduction of nurse prescribing brings into even stronger focus the principles of medicine management and associated responsibilities already familiar to the professional nurse. Nurses authorised to prescribe will be required to utilise to the full their knowledge of the actions and uses of medicines and their skills in observation, communication and recording. Furthermore, nurses will take a greater part in decision-making and thereby have increasing reasons to be accountable for their actions and inactions.

It could be argued that prescribing medicines is simply another medical task that is being devolved to nurses primarily to relieve hard pressed doctors of a time-consuming chore.

However, many nurses and other health professionals would consider that the development of nurse prescribing is part of a logical progression which recognises the needs of patients and how these can best be met. As discussed earlier, nurses have for many years exercised considerable influence on the prescribing process. All the indications are that when nurses assume wider professional responsibilities the outcomes are greatly beneficial to patient care. As always when assuming wider responsibilities nurses will expect to encounter a new set of challenges and opportunities. Prescribing is not a simple mechanistic act. Relationships between patient and prescriber can be subject to tensions and perhaps unreasonable demands on the part of the patient. It will be vitally important to ensure that all parties to the prescribing process have a clear understanding of the remit of the nurse and the constraints of a limited formulary within which the nurse is working. Prescribing, whether by doctors or nurses, should never be seen as a substitute for preventive measures or the use of basic household remedies. Patient education, information and counselling must not be neglected in the new situation that is developing. Community nurses are especially well placed to monitor the patient's total use of medicines both prescribed and non-prescribed. As more potent medicinal products become available without prescription this aspect of the nurse's responsibilities will become increasingly important. Nurse prescribing must not and will not be allowed to become purely a supply service, important though this is. As with all aspects of nursing care, the clinical need of the patient will be uppermost in the nurse's mind when she decides to prescribe for her patient.

The triple duty nurse

The guidelines above apply equally to the triple duty nurse working in remote areas of the country.

Specialised therapy in the home

Apart from haemodialysis and peritoneal dialysis, a discussion of which is beyond the scope of this book, several sophisticated forms of therapy (see below) are now carried out in the patient's own home. The number of patients involved is not large but it would appear that this trend will develop in the years ahead. The extent to which the community nurse is involved in the therapy will depend on several factors. In a number of situations patients will be taught to carry out the technique for themselves but will need support and guidance from the nurse who will also carry out periodic checks on the patient's technique. Technical support services (e.g. equipment maintenance) will also be required by the patient.

Home intravenous antibiotic therapy

Patients suffering from cystic fibrosis or advanced bronchiectasis have been taught to self-administer intravenous antibiotics using an intravenous cannula which was inserted in hospital when treatment was initiated.

Home parenteral nutrition

This form of therapy (see also p. 276) is used for patients with severe intestinal failure. In most instances the therapy is required in the short term where the condition is reversible but in some patients therapy must be continued for life.

Home ambulatory intravenous cytotoxic therapy

Research is currently being undertaken on this aspect of home drug therapy. Community nurses may become involved in the maintenance of Hickman catheters introduced to save frequent venepunctures for out-patients receiving cytotoxic therapy.

Continuous subcutaneous infusion of insulin

The administration of insulin by continuous subcutaneous infusion is made possible by the availability of portable external insulin pumps. There are theoretical advantages in using such a drug delivery system as compared to the traditional daily or twice daily injections. Further evaluation of the use of these pumps will no

doubt be undertaken. Nurses should note and follow local policy as this can vary between one health authority and another.

Continuous intravenous administration of drugs using a syringe driver

This technique is available for use in the patient's home for pain control in terminal care and other specialised forms of therapy such as insulin.

Intermittent intravenous administration of drugs using a syringe pump

A battery-operated syringe pump is also available for the injection of drugs in boluses at regular but infrequent intervals.

Home nebulisers for the treatment of asthma

Nebulisers are occasionally prescribed for asthmatic patients who have been found unresponsive to conventional treatment. Dangers associated with this form of treatment have been identified particularly when the nebuliser in use has not been prescribed.

The forms of home therapy briefly described above have a number of advantages, the greatest of which is the fact that many patients are able to resume a reasonably normal lifestyle with this form of treatment. In addition, home therapy is more economical than hospital-based therapy. Obviously, care in patient selection for any form of sophisticated home therapy is extremely important as is the need for training and continuing support. In certain situations the community nurse will need special instruction on the techniques involved, which can best be provided in the ward where the treatment is initiated. Community nurses, in responding to this technological revolution are working to ensure that their patients receive maximum therapeutic benefit.

THE ROLE OF CARERS

It is important to recognise the role of carers in helping people to manage their medicines in domestic settings. Both home helps and informal carers provide support in a variety of ways. This may range from collection of the prescription and dispensed medicines to helping with administration of both oral and topical medicines. All health professionals should make every effort to support the work of carers by assisting with their training and providing advice on such practical aspects as compliance aids and sources of further help and advice.

THE PRINCIPLES OF ADMINISTRATION OF MEDICINES

A number of basic ground rules apply to the administration of medicines irrespective of the method of administration used.

Following the policy

Policies regarding the storage, checking and administration of medicines are established by health authorities from a number of sources. These include:

- legal requirements
- government health circulars
- UKCC codes of practice
- RCN recommendations.

In addition, local policies which relate to a functional unit, e.g. hospital or ward, may exist within this wider context. Copies of the relevant policies should be readily accessible. It is incumbent on nurses to become fully conversant with these policies and to adhere to them at all times.

Assessing the patient and his medicines

When compiling a profile of any patient, whether newly referred to the district nurse, or on admission to hospital, the nurse is ideally placed to identify actual or potential problems the patient may have in relation to his medicines. It is important to gather personal data including age, address and available family support as these may have a bearing on the likelihood of the patient managing to take his medicines at home.

The patient should be asked if he is taking medicines of any kind – prescribed or non-prescribed – and whether he is experiencing any difficulty with them. The effect that individual drugs are having, or may be suspected of having, on the activities of living should be considered, e.g. the constipating effect of some analgesics may affect elimination; the nauseating effect of an antibiotic may interfere with eating and drinking; a sedative drug may make communication difficult. An examination of medicines brought into hospital by the patient may reveal patient non-compliance. Moreover, through questioning and/or observation, the nurse may be the first to discover that the patient is hypersensitive to a medicine.

The initial assessment of a patient's physical capabilities and mental capacity helps in estimating the degree of dependence he is likely to have on others for assistance including the taking of medicines. The patient's learning needs with respect to his medicines may also be established at this time. Thereafter, assessment of the patient's condition and his needs is carried out on a continual basis. Finally, just prior to the administration of any medicine, the nurse must consider whether, according to the condition of the patient at the time, it is appropriate to proceed.

Some of the difficulties patients have which can interfere with safe and effective medicine management, and the nursing implications, are listed in Table 26.1 using the activities of living categorised by Roper, Logan and Tierney (1985).

Planning drug therapy

Medicines are prescribed by the doctor taking into account the patient's age and other factors including body mass, physical and mental condition, concurrent illness and in some instances, his specific requests or beliefs. The nurse can assist in suggesting times of administration that will fit in with other activities with which the patient is involved. Where the presentation of the medicine (e.g. a large tablet) is likely to pose a problem, the nurse can draw the doctor's attention to the patient's difficulty. It is at this stage of

Table 26.1   Difficulties which can interfere with medicine management

Activity of living	Patient problems and nursing implications
Maintaining a safe environment	Where compliance is likely to pose a problem, it may be necessary to ask a relative or friend to supervise or assist the patient with his medicines on discharge from hospital. Extra emphasis on safety with medicines is essential where there are children. Any drug or medicine sensitivity known to the patient should be clearly entered in nursing and medical records including medicine prescription sheets. Patients should be discouraged from 'hoarding' unused medicines and instructed about safe disposal.
Communicating	Guidance and instruction in the administration of medicines must be matched to the patient's level of understanding. Advice from each member of staff must be consistent. Nurses must help patients to appreciate the importance of taking medicines correctly. Relatives may be asked to provide further support. Many older patients have difficulty seeing their medicines. Small white tablets against a white background or clear liquids in a clear medicine glass can be overlooked. Nurses should ensure that good light is provided and that the patient is wearing his spectacles. The successful taking of medicines depends on receiving accurate instruction, most of which is verbal. When patients are weak and depressed, hearing is less acute.
Breathing	Where severe breathlessness makes swallowing difficult, an alternative route, such as the rectal route, may be used.
Eating and drinking	Inability to swallow will necessitate the use of alternative routes of administration (e.g. via nasogastric tube, per rectum or by injection). Patients with dysphagia may require oral medicines in liquid form. Nausea and vomiting often prevent successful administration of oral medicines. Patients may indicate ways they have devised to overcome this problem. Large volumes of fluid should be discouraged where the daily intake is restricted (e.g. in renal failure). Patients taking certain sulphonamides require to take copious amounts of liquids. The concurrent use of alcohol with prescribed medicines may result in dangerous interactions.
Eliminating	Loss of control of the anal sphincter or faecal impaction may make it impossible for the patient to retain rectal medication. Constipation may interfere with the free flow of urine per urinary catheter and may make bladder irrigation difficult.
Personal cleansing and dressing	Lack of interest in personal hygiene or embarrassment may make a patient reluctant to accept treatment for such problems as body odours or head lice. Some topical applications stain clothing, bedding and the bath, which may be the cause of non-compliance.
Controlling body temperature	Some drugs may affect the heat regulating mechanism, e.g. phenothiazines. Requirements of clothing and room temperature should be adjusted accordingly.
Mobilising	Patients should be in the most upright position possible for taking oral medicines. Great care must be taken to avoid inhalation when giving medicines to patients who have to be nursed in the prone or recumbent position. Restrictions may be imposed on the patient's mobility so that the nurse must adapt her approach to the administration of medicines accordingly. Where there is loss of the use of both hands or where tremor is very severe, considerable assistance will be required with the taking of medicines. Strategies for overcoming the difficulty of mild tremor, stiffness of the hands, or having the use of one hand only, can be taught. The use of an appropriate aid should be considered. Lack of mobility may prevent the patient from obtaining his medicines when at home.

Table 26.1 *Cont'd*	
Activity of living	**Patient problems and nursing implications**
Working and playing	Poorly-motivated patients are less likely to take an interest in their medicines. Encouragement should be given to all patients but especially to those who will have to manage their medicines at home. Importance should be attached to drugs which constitute replacement therapy or control of disease. Those in full-time education or employment may have difficulty maintaining compliance in taking their medicines.
Expressing sexuality	Embarrassment may interfere with the satisfactory insertion or application of certain preparations (e.g. pessaries, vaginal creams). The nurse should be tactful in her approach and ensure maximum privacy. Whenever possible, self-administration should be encouraged.
Sleeping	Very drowsy patients may be unable to cooperate in the taking of medicines, and other routes may have to be used. Special care must be taken to avoid accidental inhalation of medicines.
Dying	In terminal care, injections should be minimised. Where this cannot be avoided, the volume of reconstituting fluid used should be the minimum compatible with the physical and other properties of the drug. A smaller needle may be required for giving an intramuscular injection, e.g. 23G, 1 inch for an adult. Control of pain is achieved through thorough assessment of the pain, careful choice of analgesic, appropriate dosage and administration at regular and suitable intervals. There is no place in terminal illness for 'analgesics as required'.

the process that the clinical pharmacist can be of particular assistance. When an intravenous infusion is to be given, it may be possible to take into account the patient's preference of which arm to use. Here the nurse should act as the patient's advocate as necessary.

Writing the prescription

With few exceptions, responsibility rests with the prescriber to provide the statutory components of a prescription, clearly and indelibly written, authorising the administration of any medicine(s) irrespective of whether he or another person is going to administer the medicine(s). Unless provided for in a specific protocol, or in exceptional circumstances, instruction by telephone to administer a previously unprescribed substance is not acceptable. Any telephone call involving medicines requires the experience of a trained nurse to take the message. She should repeat the order to the doctor to ensure accuracy. An entry should be made by the nurse taking the message on the appropriate prescription sheet.

The prescribing doctor should sign the entry at the earliest possible opportunity. Local policy will demand that in any event the prescription is signed within a set period of time, for example, within 24 hours. New prescriptions for Controlled Drugs must never be ordered by telephone. An alternative to telephoning prescriptions is using facsimile transmission (fax). Computerised prescribing systems are being developed for use in hospitals. In primary care many general practitioners use computers for both acute and repeat prescribing. Whatever the method used, where the new prescription replaces an earlier one, the latter must be cancelled clearly and the cancellation signed and dated by a registered medical practitioner.

Interpreting the prescription

All prescriptions must bear:

- the full name of the patient
- the patient's address if at home or, in the case of an in-patient, the hospital and ward

- the patient's age/date of birth and unit number.

Six items must be present as part of the actual prescription before administration can take place. These are:

- The date (including day, month and year) of prescribing of each individual medicine which should be coincidental with the date of commencement. As far as possible medicines should not be prescribed prospectively although it is recognised that for practical purposes pre-operative medicines and diagnostic agents may have to be prescribed in this way.
- The name of the medicine prescribed written in full in block letters using the approved (generic) name for single ingredient preparations. If the product is a compound formulation (i.e., contains more than one active component), the name of a proprietary (trade) product may be used. In some instances, the name will include the strength of the medicine to be used (for example, glucose 5%).
- The dosage of the medicine to be given each time, prescribed using the metric system. Substitutes for actual dosage (e.g. 1 tab instead of 250 mg; 1 vial instead of 100 mg) must be avoided except in the case of multi-ingredient formulations. Decimal fractions should be avoided (e.g. 250 µg (micrograms) and not 0.25 mg). When writing prescriptions the word 'micrograms' (or nanograms) should be written in full and not abbreviated.
- The route (method) of administration which may be abbreviated as follows:

SL	sublingual
PR	per rectum
TOP	topical
INHAL	inhalation
SC	subcutaneous
IM	intramuscular
IV	intravenous
ID	intradermal

Oral and other forms of administration should be written in full using block letters.

'O' for oral is not a recognised abbreviation and may lead to error if linked to the dose prescribed. Further requirements for giving the medicine may have to be stated specifically. For example:

ORAL after food
TOP to both eyes
INHAL via Lifecare mask 24% at 2 litres per minute

Instructions of any length will obviously require to extend to the next prescription line. When using the documents of the Aberdeen system of prescribing and recording medicines, the code letter opposite the name of the medicine is (as always) the one that is used.

- The time(s) ticked or entered in writing. The prescription must specify the time of administration with the exception of 'as required' prescriptions. In this situation, the prescribing instructions must be written in English stating the symptom(s) to be relieved and the maximum frequency (for example, 'As required for headache every 4 hours'). For once only prescriptions, the actual time should be indicated. A term such as 'monthly' can lead to inaccuracies or omissions and is better to be written as 'four weekly' or 'every 28 days'. Where a specific number of doses or number of days of a medicine is to be given, instructions to this effect must be clearly written. In an out-patient or community setting, the duration of the course of treatment before review should also be stated on the prescription.
- The full signature of a registered (or provisionally registered) practitioner for each individual prescription. Initials do not suffice and an unsigned prescription has no validity.

Additional information may be provided in conjunction with the prescription. For example, if the doctor has agreed to allow the patient to keep a particular medicine within his reach, he should enter this on the prescription. The trained nurse may enter a specific preference of the patient in relation to his medicines. The clinical pharmacist will advise on aspects of the storage of such medicines. The monitoring of prescriptions by the clinical pharmacist working at ward level provides additional safeguards for the patient.

It is emphasised that, although medicines are prescribed by a doctor, the nurse administering them is accountable for her actions (and inactions). If any part of the prescription is unclear, absent or in the nurse's view incorrect, she must seek clarification before administering the medicine. When two nurses are involved in the administration of a medicine, each takes responsibility for reading the prescription, selecting the medicine and witnessing the administration.

Minimising cross-infection

Prior to any procedure involving medicines the hands should at least be socially clean. If the procedure involves an aseptic technique then an antiseptic handwash is required.

As far as possible, the hands should not come into contact with the medicine. Tablets and capsules are tipped out into the cap of the medicine container before being placed in a medicine measure or spoon; medicines from a blister pack are pushed through the foil side of the pack. Gloves should be used when applying creams or ointments. Medicine trays should be washed after use and sticky medicine bottles wiped before being returned to the trolley or cupboard. All storage and preparation areas should be kept clean.

Checking the product

The label and/or packaging nearest to the product must be checked before administration. It is not sufficient to check the outer box or packet in which a bottle or blister pack is contained. If there is any doubt about the legibility of the container information, the medicine must not be used and the container with its contents should be returned to the pharmacy.

Medicines should remain in their original container until required for use. They should not be transferred into another container.

Pharmaceutical products should only be used if they are in date and their colour, appearance/consistency and smell are unaltered. Unsuitable medicines should be returned to the pharmacy and the advice of the clinical pharmacist sought.

Identifying the patient

The patient must be identified correctly. He should be addressed by name or asked to state his name. A check should be made of the name on the bed label or chart kept at the bedside. Factors contributing to ease of identification include knowing the patient in your care, checking medicines with a second nurse and making proper use of identification bracelets/photographs. However, shift work, staff shortages, movement of staff from ward to ward or from team to team and a high turnover of patients can create difficulties in knowing patients well. Not all staff like patients to be 'labelled' (i.e., using identification bracelets) or to ask the patient to state his name. Encouragement of patients to be more mobile and to socialise away from the bedside, in day rooms, can add to the problems, while deafness and confusion can compound them.

Not uncommonly, patients with the same name appear in a ward. It is of paramount importance that the nurse in charge draws the attention of the patients concerned and all staff to this occurrence. The hospital unit number, unique to the patient, is the only safe means of distinguishing patients in this situation.

Positioning the patient

For safety and comfort, patients should be suitably positioned in advance of being given a medicine. For example:

- an upright position will assist the swallowing of a medicine
- for giving an injection, bladder irrigation or rectal medicine, only the area involved should be uncovered
- to facilitate the administration of an injection or a rectal medicine, the nurse should encourage the patient to relax.

Selecting, checking and administering the medicine

Before administering any medicine it is essential to check on the recording sheet that it has not already been given. The prescription is then carefully read and the appropriate form of the medicine identified. These two are compared and any calculation of dose carried out. The medicine is removed from its container and the label re-checked before being returned to the trolley or cupboard. The medicine is finally made ready for administration and the patient identified. There are thus a series of checks to be made on every occasion. Moreover, in the event of another member of staff or the patient himself questioning any aspect of the procedure, the nurse must be willing to make further checks.

Although medicines require to be administered according to the prescription, they are often linked to other aspects of the patient's care. It falls to the nurse to integrate the administration of a patient's medicines with nursing care, investigations and other treatments without departing from the general instructions contained in the prescription. To achieve an optimal outcome, the nurse must base her decision on a sound knowledge of the purpose of medication. However, some medicines do not need to be given at a specific time of day but do need to be given in conjunction with a nursing procedure. For example, topical medicines may need to be applied in association with bathing, a surgical dressing or oral hygiene.

Using discretion

The nurse must be alert to those occasions when it would be unsafe to proceed in giving a medicine exactly as prescribed. For example:

- digoxin is not administered unless the pulse rate is 60 beats per minute or above
- depending on the patient's baseline blood pressure and the severity of pain, it may be inappropriate to administer narcotic analgesics in the early postoperative period
- permission to use an alternative route of administration should be sought following an

upper endoscopy when the throat has been anaesthetised or when a patient is being fasted.

When a dose has to be omitted or reduced (or the medicine is refused by the patient or not immediately obtainable) a record of the fact must be made giving the reason and initialled by the member(s) of staff involved.

Teaching the patient

Through careful explanation prior to the administration of medicines and acting as a good role model in relation to medicines, the nurse gradually builds up the patient's knowledge of, expertise in handling and respect for his medicines. Every opportunity should be taken to teach hospital patients and/or their relatives about the medicines which will require to be continued on discharge home. Self-administration of medicines may be a useful strategy. It may be important, for example, for the patient to increase his fluid intake while taking a particular medicine. Teaching a newly-diagnosed diabetic patient how to administer insulin to himself calls on the nurse's ability to demonstrate the procedure to him, and to provide the necessary encouragement and supervision. It is also the nurse's duty to draw the attention of patients, as appropriate, to patient information leaflets concerning their prescribed medicines.

Promoting the effectiveness of medicines

In addition to administering medicines correctly, the nurse has a responsibility to do her utmost to promote their effectiveness. A knowledge of how medicines act, along with thoughtful prescribing, allow the nurse to play a considerable part in improving efficacy of the drugs the patient is receiving. For example:

- The absorption of some antibiotics (e.g. ampicillin) taken by mouth is decreased by the presence of food in the gut and so it is advisable to give the medicine before a main meal.
- By restricting salt in the diet of those patients receiving diuretic therapy, there is less

sodium to be reabsorbed by the renal tubules. Less water will be absorbed, therefore more urine is produced.

- In the terminal stages of a painful illness where comfort has become the primary concern, careful attention to timing of the giving of analgesics is essential to obtain complete pain relief. By so doing, the medicine can relieve pain just as it is due to break through, the only drawback being that this may mean wakening the patient.

Monitoring the effect of medicines

Indices recorded by nurses which reflect the effect of commonly used groups of medicines are referred to in Table 26.2.

Although the nurse is greatly assisted in monitoring the effect of medicines by these recordings, there is no substitute for using general powers of observation. The nurse is ideally placed to get to know her patients well and, although she may not always fully understand what process is developing, often knows intuitively when even the most minor change in the patient's condition is taking place.

In addition to the indices monitored by nurses, laboratory tests are used as a basis for making adjustments to doses/frequency of administration of certain medicines:

- *Prothrombin times* (PT) indicate the capacity of the blood to clot and are used to monitor the effect of anticoagulant drugs. Daily dosages are calculated according to the prothrombin time. While maximum anticoagulation is the aim in the prevention of thrombus formation, extreme caution is required to prevent over anticoagulation and subsequent bleeding.
- *The white blood cell count* (WBC) reflects the patient's resistance to infection. Frequent checks of the white blood cell count are carried out on patients receiving immunosuppressant or cytotoxic therapy as these drugs can reduce the count to a dangerously low level and hence lower the patient's resistance to infection.

- *Therapeutic drug monitoring* (TDM). Laboratory techniques are also used to determine the level of a particular drug in the plasma. Doses are adjusted to achieve or maintain the desired therapeutic level of drug in the patient's blood. Such monitoring is commonly used in the management of epilepsy and certain psychiatric conditions.

As new technology becomes available analyses can be carried out at ward level obviating the need for samples to be sent to a central laboratory, e.g. blood gas determination.

Not only is time saved by carrying out tests at ward level, a further benefit is the ability to monitor biochemical changes in the patient and adjust drug treatment accordingly.

Maintaining the comfort of the patient

Nursing measures alone are not always sufficient to achieve maximum functioning of body systems and therefore comfort. Nevertheless, it is always better to try simple remedies in non-emergency situations before resorting to the use of medicines. Moreover, the start of a course of drug therapy does not indicate the discontinuation of these measures. In other words, medicines do not *replace* nursing care. Some examples may be cited:

- analgesics
    maintaining good communication
    giving the patient reassurance
    careful positioning
    promoting sleep
    applying local heat or massage
- laxatives
    increasing fluid intake
    providing high fibre foods
    encouraging mobility
    maximising the gastrocolic reflex
    providing privacy for toilet purposes
- hypnotics
    creating peace of mind
    making a comfortable bed
    ensuring a quiet, undisturbed environment
    avoiding caffeine-containing drinks late at night

Table 26.2   The effect of medicines on the patient's vital signs and other indices

Index	Effect

Temperature	Body temperature will be *reduced* when:
	    an appropriate antibiotic is given for bacterial infection
	    an antipyretic is used to control disturbance of the heat-regulating centre
	    an antithyroid drug is used to treat hyperthyroidism

Pulse	The heart rate is *slowed*, steadied and strengthened by:
	    cardiac glycosides
	    (The radial and apical rates may require to be measured by two nurses simultaneously.)
	The pulse is *increased* by:
	    anticholinergic drugs
	    thyroxine

Respiration	The rate and pattern of breathing are likely to be *improved* by:
	    diuretics
	    bronchodilators
	    antibiotics
	    (The forced expiratory volume (FEV) may require to be estimated using a peak flow meter before and after inhaling bronchodilators.)
	
	Analgesics, by relieving pain, may make breathing more comfortable, but in high doses may *depress* respiration to a dangerous level.

Blood pressure	The blood pressure can be *raised* by:
	    corticosteroids
	    (They are often used in the treatment of collapse.)
	High blood pressure is treated with:
	    antihypertensives
	    (They may cause the blood pressure to fall sharply when the patient stands up and therefore close monitoring, including records of lying and standing blood pressure, is essential.)
	
	The blood pressure can be *lowered* when using:
	    strong analgesics
	    (Extreme caution is needed in states of shock and following anaesthetic.)

Weight	Weight *loss* (or lack of it) may reflect the beneficial (or otherwise) effect of a high-dose diuretic. (A careful record of the patient's weight taken at the same time each day in the same clothing should be kept when high doses of a diuretic are being used.)
Urinary output	Urine formation is *increased* with diuretics. Retention of fluid in the tissues with subsequent *oliguria* occurs with corticosteroids. (A record of both intake and output of fluid helps monitor fluid balance.)

Glycosuria	The blood glucose level and consequent presence of glucose in the urine are *lowered* by:
	    insulin
	    sulphonylureas
	and *raised* by:
	    corticosteroids
	    thiazide diuretics
	
	(Monitoring of diabetes is now largely done by testing a sample of capillary blood taken from the thumb or ear lobe several times per day. Patients receiving high doses of corticosteroids or thiazide diuretics may have their urine tested for glucose at regular intervals).

In some patients unavoidable side-effects arise as the result of taking medicines, and precautions therefore have to be taken to minimise these side-effects. Certain groups of drugs are predictable in the nature of the effects they produce. For example:

- Strong analgesics. Drugs such as diamorphine

make patients feel sick and this can be especially distressing postoperatively or, for example, following myocardial infarction, when stress should be kept to a minimum. It is common practice for an anti-emetic to be prescribed for use at the same time.

- Sedatives. Patients may become disorientated as well as drowsy. It may be necessary to erect bed sides and advisable to position the patient's bed within view of the nursing staff, especially at night.
- Diuretics. These are given early in the morning so that urinary frequency has worn off by the middle of the day, allowing freedom of activity for the remainder of the day. Incontinence of urine can be precipitated (as can falling) in an attempt to reach the toilet in time. In geriatric wards with large numbers of dependent patients, arrangements are sometimes made to administer diuretics slightly later to fit in with the number of staff available to provide the necessary assistance with toileting. Where applicable, the patient should be told what to expect, be shown some means of summoning assistance and should have his bed positioned close to the toilet or have a commode placed at the bedside.
- Oral iron preparations. These colour the stools black and the patient should be warned accordingly. This can be especially alarming to him if he has a history of passing blood in the stools and he mistakes the discolouration for a recurrence of bleeding.

Many patients, in spite of having serious conditions and receiving powerful medication, remain relatively well. Their appearance, however, may be deceptive and nurses must be forever vigilant in detecting the onset of adverse reaction.

Disposal of unwanted medicines

In general, doses of medicines removed from their original container for administration to a patient should not be returned to that container. An unopened ampoule may be returned to the box, but great care should be taken to ensure that the ampoule is replaced in the correct box.

The disposal of unwanted medicines must comply with the Duty of Care legislation (see p. 350). The clinical pharmacist and community pharmacist will advise and help to ensure compliance with local policies. The disposal of cytotoxic drugs requires particular care (see p. 234).

Keeping records

A prescription sheet and recording sheet should be raised for all in-patients and, on discharge or transfer, filed with the patient's case records whether or not entries have been made. In hospital, all medicines must be entered on the patient's prescription sheet including any lay medicines the doctor has authorised the patient to continue to receive. On each occasion a medicine is administered, a record to this effect is made and signed or initialled as appropriate by the nurse(s) involved. When a medicine due is not given, for whatever reason, the appropriate recording is made.

Evaluating and reporting back

Maintaining effective drug therapy cannot be assured without some form of feedback by the nurse to the prescriber. A medicine may make the patient feel nauseated every time it is taken or a patient may report that he is gaining little benefit from it. On the positive side, it is equally important to note that a patient is, for example, sleeping better or breathing more easily as the result of his medication. Observing and reporting *any* new clinical features following the start of a course of drug therapy are an essential part of the nurse's role. As the result of the evaluative process, the medicine may be discontinued, exchanged for another, continued as before, or continued with some alteration to the prescription.

CALCULATIONS: BASIC PRINCIPLES

With the development of clinical pharmacy services and the introduction of unit packs, the overall need for nurses to undertake calculations in connection with the administration of medicines and other pharmaceutical products has declined. Situations, however, still arise where the nurse needs to perform basic calculations, and these she must be able to do accurately and with confidence. Apart from the need to calculate how to obtain a particular dose for an individual patient, a sound understanding of SI (Système International) units of mass (weight) and volume as well as percentages is essential if medicines, disinfectants, etc., are to be used safely and effectively. Whenever possible the need to perform calculations should be avoided by appropriate use of the pharmaceutical service, not because the nurse is lacking in the necessary skills, but so as to improve accuracy of dosage. In paediatric practice for example, it is much better to use a paediatric dosage specially dispensed for the purpose, than to attempt to obtain the required dose from a product intended primarily for adult use, although, on occasions, there may be no practical alternative to this approach. It is against this background that the following paragraphs should be studied.

SI units

The international system of units for mass and volume is as follows.

Mass	1 kilogram	(kg)	= 1000 grams
	1 gram	(g)	= 1000 milligrams
	1 milligram	(mg)	= 1000 micrograms
	1 microgram	(μg)*	= 1000 nanograms (ng)*

| Volume | 1 litre | = 1000 millilitre (ml) |
| | 1 millilitre | = 1000 microlitres (μl) |

*It should be noted that these abbreviations should not be used in prescription writing because of the possibility of confusion with other abbreviations.

The mole and the millimole (mmol)

The strength of a pharmaceutical preparation used in electrolyte replacement therapy is normally expressed in millimoles per tablet or millimoles per given volume of solution. (In addition the strength will be expressed as a percentage).

A millimole is one thousandth of a mole, which is the molecular weight of a substance expressed in grams. Nurses will not normally be expected to calculate millimoles from molecular weights, but may have to calculate how much of a given solution to measure to obtain a particular dose. The term millimole is also used to express the strength of substances other than electrolytes.

Percentages

The strength of a pharmaceutical product may be expressed as a percentage, meaning parts per 100 parts. This is expressed in four ways:

- *Percentage weight in volume (% w/v).* The expression 5% w/v indicates that 5 g of active ingredient is present in 100 ml of product.
- *Percentage weight in weight (% w/w).* The expression 5% w/w indicates that 5 g of active ingredient is present in 100 g of product.
- *Percentage volume in volume (v/v).* The expression 5% v/v indicates that 5 ml of active ingredient is present in 100 ml of product.
- *Percentage volume in weight (% v/w).* The expression 5% v/w indicates that 5 ml of active ingredient is contained in 100 g of product.

Expressing the strength of active ingredient(s)

Solid dose forms

In most cases the strength of the active ingredient(s) present in each tablet or capsule will be expressed on the label of the product in grams, milligrams or micrograms, e.g. amoxycillin 250 mg. Quantities of less than 1 gram should always be expressed in milligrams; thus, the expression 500 mg is used and not 0.5 g. Similarly, quantities of less than 1 milligram should always be expressed in micrograms. This approach should always be followed when prescribing, recording the administration, ordering or dispensing medicines. This reduces the need to use the decimal point, which, if incorrectly placed, can lead to massive errors in drug administration. The need for the decimal point to be used remains when doses such as 37.5 mg are required.

Strengths of active ingredients in some solid dosage forms are expressed in units of activity, e.g. halibut oil capsules contain 4000 units of vitamin A.

Products used for electrolyte replacement therapy, in addition to a strength of active ingredient being given in grams or milligrams, will also have the strength quoted in millimoles (mmol). A slow-release potassium chloride tablet, for example, contains 600 mg of potassium chloride or 8 mmol of K^+ and Cl^-.

Liquid oral dosage forms

The amount of active ingredient per given volume is usually given for the strength of preparations such as antibiotic syrups. An ampicillin syrup will bear a label stating that the product contains 250 mg in 5 ml, or a paediatric digoxin elixir contains 50 micrograms in 1 ml. It is in connection with the administration of liquid medicines (oral and parenteral) that calculations are often required.

Liquid parenteral dosage forms

Small volume injections Two main approaches will be encountered depending on the volume of the product:

- Small-volume injections will normally bear a label expressing the strength of the product in a manner similar to that used for oral liquids. For example, an injection will be shown to contain 25 mg per 1 ml but care should be taken to note the volume in each ampoule, since if the ampoule contains 2 ml the amount of active ingredient in the ampoule is 50 mg.
- The strength of some small volume injections of local anaesthetics such as lignocaine are commonly expressed as a percentage w/v.

On the label of parenteral products for electrolyte replacement therapy (large- or small-volume) the strength is frequently expressed as a percentage, mass per given volume, and mmol per given volume.

Examples

A strong sterile solution of potassium chloride contains potassium chloride 15% w/v or approx 2 mmol each of K^+ and Cl^- per 1 ml.

The molecular weight of potassium chloride (KCl) is 74.55. One mole is therefore 74.55 grams. It follows from the definition that *1 millimole* is contained in $\frac{74.55}{1000}$ g of KCl = 0.07455 g or 74.55 mg.

A 15% w/v solution contains 15 g per 100 ml.
OR 15 000 mg per 100 ml
OR 150 mg per 1 ml
OR $\frac{150}{74.55}$ millimoles per 1 ml
OR 2.01 mmol *each* of K^+ and Cl^- per 1 ml
For practical purposes, a figure of 2.0 mmol would be used.

Sodium chloride intravenous infusion contains sodium chloride 0.9% w/v or 0.15 mmol each of Na^+ and Cl^- per 1 ml.

The molecular weight of sodium chloride (NaCl) is 58.45. One mole is therefore 58.45 grams. It follows from the definition that *1 millimole* is contained in $\frac{58.45}{1000}$ of NaCl = 0.05845 g or 58.45 mg.

A 0.9% w/v solution contains 0.9 g per 100 ml.
OR 900 mg per 100 ml
OR 9 mg per 1 ml
OR $\frac{9}{58.45}$ = 0.154 millimoles per 1 ml
OR 0.154 mmol *each* of Na^+ and Cl^- per 1 ml
For practical purposes, a figure of 0.15 mmol would be used.

The strength of adrenalin injections is still frequently expressed as 1 in 1000. This indicates that 1 gram of active ingredient is contained in 1000 ml of product. Of more value to the nurse is the fact that 1 ml of the injection contains 1 mg of adrenalin.

When a product is supplied in an ampoule or rubber-capped vial as a dry powder for reconstitution before use, the label will give the amount of dry powder contained in it. When reconstituting such products prior to injection the total volume produced by adding the diluent to the powder must be known if only a part of the dose in the ampoule or vial is to be administered.

The strength of certain biological materials such as insulin and heparin is expressed in units of activity per given volume e.g. 100 units per 1 ml (insulin) or 5000 units per 1 ml (heparin).

Large-volume parenteral products

Labels on containers of large-volume infusion solutions will generally give information on the strength of the product in percentage terms. For example, solutions of sodium chloride may contain 0.9% w/v, or a glucose (dextrose) infusion may contain 5% w/v. Solutions for electrolyte replacement therapy will also contain information on the number of millimoles per given volume.

Other pharmaceutical products

The strengths of such products as lotions, sterile topical solutions, irrigations, antiseptic solutions, etc., will generally be expressed as a percentage, i.e. liquid preparations as a percentage w/v, solid or semi-solid preparations as a percentage w/w. When very dilute antiseptic solutions are in use the strength may be expressed as the number of parts of active ingredient in a given volume of fluid, e.g. 1 in 5000, 1 in 2000. In the first example, 1 gram of the active ingredient is contained in 5000 ml of product, in the second case 1 gram is contained in 2000 ml of product.

Making a calculation

Two different approaches may be used: either a method based on 'first principles' or a method involving the use of a simple formula. In practice, the nurse may feel more confident using one of these methods rather than the other. For the purposes of checking a calculation it is worthwhile using both methods.

Example

A dose of 50 mg of a drug is required. The product available on the ward contains 200 mg in 5 ml.

Method 1 (first principles)

Firstly calculate the amount of drug in 1 ml of product, that is:

$$\frac{200}{5} = 40 \text{ mg}$$

The product available therefore contains 40 mg in 1 ml. For a dose of 50 mg:

$$\frac{50}{40} \times 1 \text{ ml} = 1.25 \text{ ml}$$

Answer: 1.25 ml must be measured.

Method 2 (formula)

This is based on simple proportion and uses the following formula:

$$\frac{\text{Dose required (mg)}}{\text{Strength available (mg)}} \times \frac{\text{dose volume (ml) of}}{\text{available product}}$$

= volume (ml) containing the required dose

$$\frac{50}{200} \times 5 \quad = \frac{50}{40}$$

$$= \frac{5}{4}$$

$$= 1.25 \text{ ml}$$

Answer: 1.25 ml would be measured.

As a simple memory aid it may be helpful to think of the formula as 'want'/'got'. This of course is no substitute for a clear understanding of this method of calculating.

Solid dose forms

Calculations involving solid dose forms will generally cause few problems, but as with all calculations, the need for accuracy cannot be overstated. Sometimes there will be no alternative but to subdivide a tablet or to give a number of tablets to obtain the prescribed dose.

Example 1

The dose required is 50 micrograms, but the product available contains 100 micrograms.

It is obvious that the tablet must be divided to obtain the required dose since the product available is twice the strength of the dose required. A general formula can be used in situations of this kind.

It is essential that the strengths are expressed in the same units, in this case micrograms.

$$\frac{\text{Dose required}}{\text{Strength available}} \times 1 = \begin{array}{l}\text{proportion of original}\\\text{dosage form to give}\\\text{required dose}\end{array}$$

$$\frac{50}{100} \times 1 = \frac{1}{2} \text{ tablet required.}$$

Example 2

The dose required is 100 micrograms, but the product available contains 25 micrograms.

$$\frac{\text{Dose required}}{\text{Strength available}} \times 1 = \text{number of tablets required}$$

$$\frac{100}{25} \times 1 = 4 \text{ tablets required.}$$

Example 3

A dose of 50 micrograms is required, and the tablets available are labelled 0.1 mg.

On some occasions it is necessary to convert fractions of a milligram into micrograms. This should rarely be required, since for quantities less than 1 milligram the prescriber should use micrograms and the label on the container should bear the strength expressed in micrograms. However, situations do arise where the dose is expressed in micrograms and the product available is labelled in milligrams, or vice versa.

The formula dose required/strength available × 1 can again be used but the dose required and strength available must be expressed in the same terms, in this case micrograms:

1 milligram = 1000 micrograms

0.1 milligram = 100 micrograms (the decimal point is moved one place to the left)

Using the formula:

$$\frac{\text{Dose required}}{\text{Strength available}} = \frac{50}{100} \times 1 = \frac{1}{2} \text{ tablet required.}$$

Example 4

A dose of 0.05 mg is prescribed, and the strength of the product is expressed as 100 micrograms.

Before proceeding it is necessary to convert 0.05 mg into micrograms:

1 milligram = 1000 micrograms
0.1 milligram = 100 micrograms (decimal point moved one place to the left)
0.05 milligram = 50 micrograms (÷2)

The calculation may then be completed as before.

Oral liquids

Calculations involving liquid dosage forms are essentially similar to those for solid dosage forms, being based on either the first principles method or the formula.

Example 1

The dose required is 200 mg but the product available contains 250 mg in 5 ml.

From first principles:
If there are 250 mg in 5 ml, then 1 ml contains 50 mg. So, for a dose of 200 mg:

$$\frac{200}{50} \times 1 \text{ ml} = 4 \text{ ml required.}$$

Using the formula:

$$\frac{\text{Dose required (mg)}}{\text{Strength available (mg)}} \times \begin{array}{l}\text{dose volume (ml) of}\\\text{available product, that}\\\text{is:}\end{array}$$

$$\frac{200}{250} \times 5 = 4 \text{ ml required.}$$

The required dose is contained in 4 ml of the available product. It is important to note that the dose required and the strength available must be expressed in the same units, in this case milligrams.

Example 2

It is required to give a dose of 45 mg but the product available contains 30 mg in 5 ml.

From first principles:
If there are 30 mg in 5 ml, then 1 ml contains 6 mg.

For a dose of 45 mg, $\dfrac{45}{6} \times 1$ ml = 7.5 ml required.

Using the formula:

$\dfrac{\text{Dose required (mg)}}{\text{Strength available (mg)}} \times \text{dose volume (ml)}$

$\qquad$ = volume (ml) to be measured to give required dose, that is:

$\dfrac{45}{30} \times 5 = 7.5$ ml must be measured to give the required dose.

Parenteral products

A similar approach to calculations is applicable here.

Example 1

The dose required is 50 micrograms but the strength available is 500 micrograms in 2 ml.

$\dfrac{\text{Dose required (in micrograms)}}{\text{Strength available (in micrograms)}}$
$\times \text{dose volume (ml) of available product}$

= volume (ml) containing the required dose, that is:

$\dfrac{50}{500} \times 2 = 0.2$ ml of the available product required.

The figures obtained by this means can (and should) always be checked by a second nurse, preferably using first principles.

The strength available is:
500 micrograms in 2 ml,
or ÷ 2, i.e., 250 micrograms in 1 ml,
then ÷ 5, i.e. 50 micrograms in 0.2 ml.

It will be obvious that a sound knowledge of SI units and decimals is essential if these simple calculations are to be performed accurately. As with solid-dose forms, it may be that the dose required is contained in a multiple of the standard dosage form.

Example 2

The dose required is 7.5 mg but the strength available is 5 mg in 5 ml.

$\dfrac{\text{Dose required (mg)}}{\text{Strength available (mg)}} \times \begin{array}{l}\text{dose volume (ml) of} \\ \text{available product}\end{array}$

= volume (ml) containing the required dose, that is:

$\dfrac{7.5}{5} \times 5 = 7.5$ ml contains the required dose.

Checking from first principles, product available contains:
5 mg in 5 ml
or ÷ 5, i.e. 1 mg in 1 ml.
So, for a dose of 7.5 mg, 7.5 ml of the available product is required.

Example 3

The dose required is 17.5 g but the strength available is 5% w/v, i.e. it contains 5 g in 100 ml.

To calculate how to obtain the 17.5 g dose required the general formula can again be used.

$\dfrac{\text{Dose required}}{\text{Strength available}} \times \text{dose volume (ml)}$

= volume (ml) needed to obtain the required dose.

In this situation the formula is expressed as follows:

$\dfrac{\text{Amount of active ingredient required (dose) g}}{\begin{array}{l}\text{Amount of active ingredient in grams} \\ \text{per 100 ml of solution available}\end{array}} \times 100\ \text{ml}$

= volume (ml) to give dose required, that is:

$\dfrac{17.5}{5} \times 100 = 350$ ml required.

Again, the calculation can be checked from first principles:

A 5% w/v solution contains 5 g in 100 ml
or × 3, i.e. 15 g in 300 ml
or ÷ 2, i.e. 2.5 g in 50 ml.
So, 17.5 g is contained in 350 ml.

Example 4

A strong solution of potassium chloride contains 2 mmol each of K^+ and Cl^- in each ml. Calculate the volume required to obtain a dose of 10 mmol of K^+.

$$\frac{\text{Dose required}}{\text{Strength available}} \times \text{dose volume (ml)}$$

= volume (ml) to give required dose, that is:

$\frac{10}{2} \times 1 = 5$ ml required to give a dose of 10 mmol K^+.

Example 5

Heparin injection contains 5000 units per ml. Calculate the volume required to obtain a dose of 3000 units.

$$\frac{\text{Dose required}}{\text{Strength available}} \times \text{dose volume}$$

= volume (ml) to give required dose, that is:

$\frac{3000}{5000} \times 1 = 0.6$ ml required to give 3000 units.

Topical antiseptics

Although antiseptic solutions are commonly produced in a ready-to-use form, calculations may still be required in connection with the dilution of antiseptics.

Example

Chlorhexidine is available as a 5% concentrate, and 1 litre of a 0.05% w/v solution is required for use as an irrigation.

Again, the general formula can be used, on this occasion using the percentages.

$$\frac{\% \text{ required}}{\% \text{ available}} \times \text{volume required (ml)}$$

= volume of concentrate required to be diluted to 1 litre, that is:

$$\frac{0.05}{5} \times 1000 = 10 \text{ ml}.$$

So, 10 ml of a 5% w/v solution must be diluted to 1000 ml to give a 0.05% w/v solution.

Calculations involving reconstitution of injections

When an injection has to be reconstituted from a powder before use, it should be noted that the resulting volume is in excess of the volume of diluent added, due to the displacement effect of the powder. This must be taken into account if a dose less than that contained in the vial is required.

Example

A vial contains 500 mg but the dose required is 200 mg.

The addition of 5 ml diluent yields a volume of 5.25 ml when drawn into the syringe. In this case it is useful to use the general formula.

$$\frac{\text{Dose required (mg)}}{\text{Strength available (mg)}} \times \text{dose volume (ml)}$$

= volume (ml) to be measured, that is:

$\frac{200}{500} \times 5.25 = \frac{2.1 \text{ ml required to obtain a dose of}}{200 \text{ mg.}}$

Dosage calculations involving body surface area

In certain specialised forms of therapy (e.g. cytotoxic drug therapy) drug dosage is based on body surface area. The patient's body surface area is determined from a table (nomogram) using the patient's body weight and height. For example, if a patient's height is 190 cm and body weight is 90 kg, reference to the nomogram indicates the patient's body surface area is 2.3 m². A typical dosage regime for doxorubicin is 60 mg per square metre of body surface area given i.v. every 3 weeks. For a patient with a body surface area of 2.3 m², a dose of 60×2.3 mg (138 mg) would be given every 3 weeks.

ERRORS IN THE MANAGEMENT OF MEDICINES

With the increasing complexity of drug therapy and the need for many patients to receive multiple drug therapy, the potential for errors in the administration of medicines is great. A medical ward with 30 beds may have as many as 60 products in use at any one time and could keep in stock a range of 200 medicinal products excluding lotions, sterile fluids, etc. Factors other than complexity of therapy also contribute to errors in the administration of medicines.

An error in the administration of medicines may be, at best, inconvenient for the patient or, at worst, catastrophic. In order to gain a balanced perspective it is necessary first to form a working definition of an error. This is best done by considering how, in practical terms, the overall objective of drug therapy (i.e. therapeutic benefit for the patient with minimal adverse effects) is most likely to be achieved. The assumption is made that the prescriber has taken all relevant factors into account before prescribing and that the choice of drug, dose, route, etc., is appropriate in every respect. To achieve therapeutic benefit for the patient it is obviously essential to ensure that *the right dose of the right drug is administered at the right time by the right route*. Adherence by all health care staff to recognised drug procedures is clearly a prerequisite at all times.

Adverse drug reactions and interactions should be avoided if at all possible. However, if an adverse drug reaction is unavoidable, the effect on the patient should be minimised. It therefore follows that monitoring of the patient is essential. All adverse reactions to drugs should be reported to the doctor.

A drug error can be identified as *any aspect of commission or omission that militates against the achievement of the therapeutic objective*, i.e. benefit for the patient. Such acts may relate to one or more of the practical aspects discussed above. It is obvious that it is not possible to comply to the letter with *all* aspects of medicine administration throughout *all* courses of drug therapy for *all* patients. Clearly, it is essential that, on every occasion, the correct dose of the correct drug is administered by the correct route. However, it must be recognised that it is often not possible to administer all medicines exactly at the time indicated on the prescription sheet due to the time required to complete a medicine round. This is technically an error but will seldom be of clinical significance. There are occasions however when the timing of the administration of certain medicines is of vital importance to the patient such as, for example, with pre-operative medication. Whatever the pressures, every effort must be made to eliminate errors by maintaining the highest possible standards of practice.

Sources of errors

Errors can arise for many reasons and are often compounded in a cascade-like way. For example, an error in dispensing may not be detected by the checking system in the pharmacy. Medical and/or nursing personnel may either fail to notice or be unaware of the error which may finally result in a patient being given an incorrect dose or even the wrong drug. The failure of professionals to adhere to the rules of good practice has been recognised by Ley (1981) in medical, nursing and pharmaceutical personnel. Such failures are a potential source of major error. Although errors are often compounded, specific sources of errors may be attributed to particular health professionals.

The prescriber

Full responsibility rests with the prescriber to state clearly and without ambiguity the medicines the patient is to be given. Well designed prescribing documents undoubtedly contribute to more accurate drug therapy. However, adherence to the prescribing policy is essential if errors are to be avoided irrespective of the sophistication of the system used. Bad handwriting is probably the commonest potential source of error. Confusion between similar drug names is a well recognised source of error, e.g. Intal, Inderal; quinine, quinidine; chlorpromazine, chlorpropamide. Even when clearly written these words have a similar 'shape'. Unofficial abbreviations for medicines are always open to misinterpretation and should not be used. Those who prescribe, dispense and administer medicines should not accept badly written instructions.

The omission of essential information (e.g. the strength of the drug) may result in assumptions being made about what is required. Where cancellation of a prescription lacks precision, the medicine may continue to be given to the possible detriment of the patient.

Electronic prescribing systems have the potential to improve the overall quality of prescribing.

The pharmacist

Errors in the administration of medicines may be due directly or indirectly to failures in the pharmaceutical service. As with clinical departments and wards, standards and procedures in pharmaceutical departments are designed to ensure that, as far as possible, errors are eliminated. Nevertheless, errors can and do occur which may be due to failures to meet standards and, on some occasions, to lack of effective communication with the prescriber or nurse in charge of a ward or department.

Errors or omissions in the labelling of medicines may cause difficulty, which may lead to an incorrect dose or even a wrong drug being administered. There has been much debate about colour coding of labels/containers, etc, but there can be no substitute for *reading* the label at all times.

On occasion, medicines are required when a full pharmaceutical service is not available. This may result in delay in administering a medicine which may have serious consequences for the patient.

Regrettably, medicines may be supplied to wards with minimal background information as to the actions, uses or dosage of the product. Ward staff may then have to rely on their own limited information sources, especially if the pharmacy-based drug information service is not available. On fairly rare occasions a product or particular batch of a product may have to be withdrawn from use due to a fault or suspected fault. In such circumstances pharmaceutical staff must ensure the rapid flow of accurate information to wards and departments concerned.

When products are issued to wards for use in connection with a clinical trial it is very important that sufficient information is made available (without breaking the code) to the medical and nursing staff to enable the product to be used safely. The interest and cooperation of nurses are gained when the background to, and reasons for, a clinical trial are explained. It is also helpful if the results of the work are discussed with those participating.

The role of the pharmacist in drug therapy has been described as that of 'safety net and overseer'. Any failure to discharge this role has serious implications for the safety and well-being of the patient.

The nurse

Nurses are responsible for the safe and accurate administration of medicines to most inpatients and some patients in the community. (Supervision of medicine taking is also required in certain instances.) In order to discharge these duties the nurse must interpret the prescription, select the correct medicine and make a record of the administration.

The administration of the medicine is the culmination of research, development, manufacture, prescribing and dispensing. All the skill and resources that have gone into making a particular medicine available can, at this stage, contribute nothing. The patient is now dependent on the nurse's skill and attention to detail. The responsibility to ensure safe and accurate administration of a medicine to a patient irrespective of his physical or mental condition should never be underestimated.

Identification of patient

An examination by the authors of drug errors has shown that approximately 50% are due to the nurse's failure to identify the patient correctly. The bracelet is, as yet, the best method developed for identifying patients. However, it is only as safe as those who apply it and refer to it. While every precaution may be taken to insert accurately the information in the bracelet and to attach the bracelet carefully to the right patient, problems can still arise. Sometimes a bracelet has to be removed – for example, when an intravenous infusion is being set up – and it may not be replaced. The patient, unwittingly, may remove the bracelet or he may do so while on weekend leave. The writing on the bracelet may become indistinct with the passage of time. Even when the bracelet remains satisfactorily in position, reference must be made to it. Of course, it was never intended that the bracelet should take the place of effective communication between nurse and patient, or that it would obviate the need for regular updating of staff on the patients under their care.

There can be no doubt about the need for identification bracelets to be used in paediatric units, intensive care units, theatres and in all acute areas where a patient is unable to account for himself. Areas that pose particular difficulty are geriatric units and psychiatric wards. Patients in these wards may understandably have feelings of resentment at being 'labelled'. In addition, staff may feel that this procedure militates against their efforts to reduce any feelings patients may have of being institutionalised and that they know their patients anyway.

The use of regularly updated passport-size photographs (attached to the prescription sheet) are increasingly being used as a more sympathetic aid to patient identification. In any event health authorities must devise workable policies which are in patients' best interests.

Errors in calculations

A study made by MacPherson et al (1983) of 130 nurse learners demonstrated the considerable difficulty some nurses have with basic calculations. This continues to be a cause for concern. Particular problems relate to the use of quantities less than one milligram. Efforts to convert 0.125 mg into micrograms have resulted in gross overdosage of digoxin in paediatric practice. It has been suggested that there might be a place for calculators in assisting those who have such difficulty. If the individual's lack of numeracy is so severe as to call for this level of assistance, there must be grave doubts as to whether a calculator could be used safely. Indeed, the improper use of such equipment may be another source of error. Calculators have a place but should probably only be used to make a final check.

Use of inadequate equipment

Measures for liquid medicines with indistinct markings cannot safely be used. It is especially important in paediatric practice where potent liquid medicines are often used to ensure accuracy.

Using medicines in an unorthodox way may also lead to errors. Some tablets are designed to be broken if a fractional dose is required. Other tablets are not so designed; an attempt to break or divide such a product will almost certainly result in the administration of an incorrect dose. Similarly, the crushing of a slow-release tablet will destroy the essential properties of the formulation, any benefit to the patient being lost. Errors may arise due to the attempted use of an unsuitable presentation such as a very large capsule or tablet which a patient may be unable to swallow.

The patient

The active cooperation of the patient whenever possible is essential in order to achieve the therapeutic benefit of a course of drug treatment. Nurses and their medical colleagues should never take the patient's cooperation for granted or expect this to be given automatically. The patient's right to question or even reject his treatment must be respected. However, nurses must play their part in ensuring that, if a patient does decide to reject a particular treatment, this decision is reached on the basis of a full understanding of the implications for the patient's health and well-being. It would obviously be unfair to attribute the patient's action or lack of action as a source of drug errors, but in some situations the patient will bear some responsibility if the treatment fails. The not uncommon occurrence of finding tablets in the patient's bed or under the cushions of a chair may or may not indicate failure on the part of the patient. This may be the first indication the nurse has that all is not well. Needless to say great tact and perception may be needed to establish the true cause of this rejection.

There are dangers in using medicines brought into hospital by patients on admission. Medicines dispensed for individual patients may have been inappropriately stored in the patient's home. Labels may have been altered or removed causing difficulty in identifying the contents of a container. Nevertheless, in remote areas it may be that on a limited number of occasions it will be necessary to use the patient's own medicines when he is in hospital. The responsibility for using the patient's own medicines when in hospital should not be undertaken lightly. All available means should be used to validate the patient's own medicines before using them in hospital. This will often involve seeking information from the patient himself.

Error avoidance/reduction

Given that drug errors often arise as a result of a series of failures by the health professionals involved, it follows that programmes designed to improve matters must have the active support of prescriber, pharmacist and nurse. The assumption should not be made that actions by nurses alone, important as these are, will be all that is required to eliminate or reduce errors. A non-nursing aspect that is of particular concern to nurses, relates to the minimal amount of curriculum time that appears to be devoted to teaching medical students the procedural aspects of prescribing, administration and recording of medicines. As a result of the low priority given to

this, medical and nursing staff time is often wasted when prescriptions have to be amended to comply with agreed standards. Not surprisingly relationships become strained and drug errors can occur.

The first line manager

The nurse in charge is accountable for the maintenance of standards of medicine administration in her ward.

Insisting on accurate prescribing practice is one of the most demanding aspects of the ward sister's role. It will be to her benefit and the benefit of her patients to make it known that failure to meet the standard is unacceptable.

It is important to ensure that up-to-date relevant information on drugs is readily available at ward level. All wards and departments should have an up-to-date copy of the British National Formulary and local formularies.

Whenever possible, the nurse in charge should avoid delegating the administration of medicines to nurses who are unfamiliar with the identity of patients in the ward. Examples include nurses who have recently been appointed to the ward, have just returned from a period of absence or have been sent to assist on a temporary basis from another ward. It is important also to assign appropriate members of staff to the administration of medicines. It is irresponsible to ask nurses to participate in the administration of medicines unless they have been taught the theoretical aspects of it. The Royal College of Nursing publication *Drug Administration – a Nursing Responsibility* (1983) recommends that the role of the nursing auxiliary or assistant in relation to drug administration is:

'to see that the patient has a drink with which to take the drug, to help the patient into a suitably comfortable position to take the drug, to report to the person conducting the drug round if for any reason the patient fails to take the drug'.

Efforts should be made to discourage discussion with patients' visitors or visiting members of staff during procedures involving the administration of medicines. It may be useful to display a notice on the medicine trolley – DO NOT

DISTURB – with the intention of minimising interruptions during administration of medicines.

In the event of there being duplications in patients' names in a ward, staff and the patients concerned must be alerted. The nurse in charge must also ensure that identification bracelets/photographs are renewed and replaced as necessary.

Great emphasis is rightly placed on the need for the accurate administration of medicines, but it is also essential to ensure that medicines are discontinued when a course of treatment is complete. Where an instruction to discontinue therapy has been given, and where it is clear that the medicine does not constitute replacement or other long-term therapy, the continuing need for the medicine should be questioned. Prime responsibility for discontinuation of treatment must of course rest with the prescriber.

Staff should be encouraged, and if necessary instructed, to keep accurate and legible records of drug administration. Prescribers should be asked to rewrite prescription sheets when they become untidy or when the use of two prescription sheets concurrently could be obviated. 'Kardex' or similar holders for prescribing and recording documents should be kept in good repair and the order of sheets should be rearranged to correspond with the movement of patients within the ward. Nursing staff must adopt a safe and efficient system of storing medicines in the medicine trolley and withdraw medicines which are no longer required. Advice can be sought from pharmacy staff on appropriate levels of ordering, expiry dates, etc, and any other aspects of stock management.

In situations where drug regimes remain unchanged for long periods of time every effort must be made to prevent complacency. Teaching should relate to the procedure only and not to the pharmacological aspects. It is safer when administering medicines to concentrate fully on the procedure and to leave the discussion of uses, actions, side-effects, etc, for a more appropriate time.

The administration of medicines should be kept high on the list of priorities in a ward. The nursing staff's awareness of medicines in use in their ward may be increased by referring to patients' prescription sheets in conjunction with the giving of a verbal report on the patients, for example, at the changeover of staff. If time permits, a separate reporting session specifically about the medicines in use and any related difficulties that the patient or nurse may be having with them can be valuable to the nurse in charge as well as to more junior nursing staff.

Consideration should also be given to the timing and number of medicine rounds required. Standardised systems of prescribing and administration should allow room for flexibility to meet the needs of individual patients. For example, special account may need to be taken of the timing of administration to patients suffering neurological conditions such as Parkinson's disease. Such flexibility of course must reflect the need for effective drug therapy.

Clinical pharmacy services should be fully utilised. Any special needs of the ward will become apparent to the clinical pharmacist but there is no substitute for active cooperation with the pharmacist. A climate of passive acceptance of a service is not conducive to achieving the highest standard of care for patients.

The senior manager

The continuing need to reduce drug errors is the responsibility of those involved in policy making, management and education as well as those in clinical practice.

Nurse managers spend time allocating staff to meet service commitments. Along with the many other demands which they try to meet, greater consideration should be given to staff levels needed at the main medicine round times or when pre- and post-operative medications are to be given.

The extent to which two nurses should be involved in the administration of medicines continues to exercise the minds of nurse managers and nurses in clinical practice. In April 1986 the UKCC was of the view that:

'practitioners whose names are on the first level parts of the register, and midwives, should be seen as competent to administer medicines on their own, and

Box 26.1 The advantages and disadvantages of involving two nurses in the administration of medicines in hospital

Advantages	Disadvantages
Presence of second nurse provides an additional check which should improve patient safety by reducing drug errors.	Blurring of responsibility leading to confusion and perhaps error.
Presence of second nurse helpful if calculations of drug dosage are required.	Nurse learner may be reluctant to 'challenge' a trained nurse, assuming that the trained nurse is always right.
Patient feels reassured that a second person is involved in checking the medicine.	May provide false sense of safety in medicine administration.
Provides important learning situation for procedures of medicine administration.	Medicine round may take longer because of double checking.
Impact of interruptions can be minimised since the medicine round can probably be continued by one nurse.	Dilution of professional responsibility.
	In some situations, e.g. night duty, staffing levels make it impracticable for two nurses to be routinely involved in medicine administration, leading to delay.
Some patients understandably wish to ask questions about their medicines during medicine rounds. This may be difficult for one nurse to cope with although even if two nurses are present some complex questions may have to be noted for answering later.	
Improved security of medicines during medicine rounds. Any emergency arising during the medicine round can be dealt with more promptly.	

responsible for their actions in so doing. The involvement of a second person in the administration of medicines with a first level practitioner need only occur where that practitioner is instructing a learner or the patient's condition makes it necessary or in such other circumstances as are locally determined. Where two persons are involved responsibility still attaches to the senior person.'

Community nurses have, of course, always administered medicines single-handed.

Currently however, it is common for hospital policies to require that two nurses should be involved in the administration of medicines, one of whom is a registered nurse. The possible advantages and disadvantages of this approach are summarised in Box 26.1. It should be noted that there is little evidence in the literature to confirm or otherwise the views expressed – which is not surprising since a valid comparative study would be very difficult to undertake with so many variables to influence the outcome.

Clearly, the advantages and disadvantages outlined in Box 26.1 do not carry equal weight, but will serve as a frame of reference when local policies are being formulated. As with other aspects of nursing care the procedure to be adopted will always be chosen with the best interests of the patient in mind.

The need for two nurses to be involved in the administration of medicines to children is a generally agreed principle.

Equipment and fixtures used in the management of medicines such as medicine trolleys and storage facilities should be chosen with care so that the particular needs of the ward are satisfied. Nurse managers should always be prepared to take time to consult with practising clinical colleagues as to their requirements. Guidance from the pharmacist should also be sought. Policy makers must ensure that the tools of the trade, including prescribing and recording documents, are of similar design and relevant to the drug therapy used in all wards. Mechanisms are needed to ensure that there is an effective means of updating the design of prescription sheets and associated documents in such a way that the needs of particular professional groups are fully met.

Continuing education on the subject is essential for all trained nursing staff along with updating of nurses returning to work after some years' absence. Attendance at regular in-service lectures and seminars on medicine administration should be given a very high priority.

There is also considerable scope for operational research into many aspects of medicine management. Nurse managers have a duty to encourage their staff in this direction.

Nurse managers must ensure that disciplinary procedures applicable in the event of errors in medicine administration are not seen as threatening by nurses.

Apart from actions taken by individuals or within a particular profession, it is essential to ensure that an active multidisciplinary Drug and Therapeutics Committee keeps under review all aspects of medicine management and issues guidance when necessary.

Error reduction/avoidance checklist

Patient

- Pay particular attention to patient identification.
- Take extra care at extremes of age. With individual exceptions, the risks to infants and the very old are greater – partly because of the effects of the drugs but also because they may be unable to speak for themselves.
- Be especially careful when patients are mobile and where large groups of patients are sitting about at random, e.g. in day rooms.
- Whenever possible, increase involvement of patients in their own drug therapy.

Prescription

- Use correct documentation and report any inadequacies in the documentation design/layout.
- Follow the policy and do not accept inadequate, unclear instructions.
- Avoid prospective prescribing whenever possible.
- Avoid use of abbreviations and chemical symbols.
- Take particular care with similar looking drug names.
- Have all calculations checked.

- Be alert to sudden changes in dosage.
- If it appears that a dose has to be made up of several tablets/ampoules, check carefully that all is in order.
- Pay particular attention to doses expressed in micrograms.
- When two nurses are involved in the administration of medicines, read out the details of the prescription and the label so that each is aware of the other's interpretation of them. Also when administering a medicine for which a calculation has to be made, make the calculations independently before making comparison.
- Ask/check/ask again if not satisfied. While wishing to trust colleagues, do not passively take the word of a senior member of staff as necessarily correct.
- Report at once any suspicions you may have that all is not in order regarding the prescription.

Medicine

- Ensure correct storage of medicines, e.g. do not mix different ampoules in the same container.
- Do not alter any labels on containers of pharmaceutical products.
- Do not remove drugs from containers unless for administration.
- Report any apparent abnormalities, e.g. changes in size, shape, colour of a product.
- Use the correct dosage form, e.g. request a supply of 5 mg tablets rather than try to break a 20 mg tablet.
- Where there is no intravenous reconstitution service available and this task has to be undertaken by nursing staff, ensure correct volume of correct diluent is used. (This applies equally to the reconstitution of liquid oral dosage forms.) If in *any* doubt, always ask advice from the pharmacy department.
- Use the correct equipment, e.g. measures, syringes.
- Any drug removed from its container and not used should be disposed of safely.
- Be aware of drug interactions, e.g. drug/drug; drug/food.

- Avoid drug incompatibility, e.g. when adding drugs to intravenous fluids.

Staff

- Be observant. Here is the distinction between seeing and observing. The ability to take in the global view of, say, a chart or the contents of the medicine trolley as well as the details of one prescription or one product has to be acquired.
- When a telephoned order for medicines is unavoidable write the message down and repeat it to the caller.
- Ensure adequate flow of information, e.g. to bacteriology department. Diagnostic tests may be influenced by patients' current or previous drug therapy.
- Report/discuss/seek views of colleagues especially if patient safety is involved, e.g. unexplained side-effects of a drug.
- When two nurses are involved in administering medicines, the more experienced nurse should check the decisions, calculations and actions of the less experienced nurse.
- Whenever possible reduce the ward medicine inventory by encouraging the adoption of a ward formulary or prescribing policy.
- Read the literature and keep up to date; ask for more information if it is not provided.
- Make full use of pharmacy services especially ward/clinical pharmacy service and drug information services.
- Encourage the development of a questioning, enquiring attitude.

Ward management

- Encourage by all practical means adherence to drug policy.
- Integrate verbal report on current ward drug therapy with nursing report.
- Provide suitable drug information source at ward level, e.g. BNF.
- Eliminate borrowing of medicines between wards.
- Reduce interruptions during the administration of medicines.

- Ensure equipment available for medicine administration is suitable in all respects.
- Improve procedures for checking medicines prior to administration.

Hospital management

- Encourage the development of ward prescribing policies, reduction of ward medicine inventory.
- Make careful choice of new equipment, e.g. medicine trolley. Establish regular in-service education for nurses on all aspects of drug therapy.
- Develop clinical pharmacy services.
- Improve nurse staffing levels.
- Establish educational programmes for junior hospital doctors on procedural aspects of ward medicine management including prescribing.
- Promote research/clinical audit into all aspects of medicine use.
- Examine and if necessary improve disciplinary procedure for dealing with errors in the administration of medicines.

Conclusion

However accurate and detailed the prescribing, however efficient the pharmaceutical service, however effective the nursing management, there can be no substitute for the greatest care and attention to detail when a medicine is being administered. Understandably the nurse who undertakes the final act feels in a very vulnerable position. This is because the administration of a medicine is so 'visible' and so final. The medicine has actually been taken by the patient or injected into the patient's tissues. At this stage any second thoughts are not capable of being translated into action (other than reporting the error or suspected error). Unlike written prescriptions, doses actually given cannot be changed. This situation should be recognised by all those who prescribe and dispense medicines and by those who draw up policy and procedure documents. Errors in the administration of medicines are rightly regarded very seriously by nurse managers. However, it may well be that the application of rigid disciplinary procedures may not always be in the best interests of patients, since a tendency to conceal errors may develop.

Every effort must be made to ensure that the nurse who is required to administer medicines has all the skills, knowledge and support necessary to perform this vital duty safely and efficiently. Equally the nurse must adhere to the established procedures at all times. Deviations from this will, sooner or later, result in hazard, or worse, for the patient.

Unfortunately errors in the administration of medicines can never be completely eliminated. However, the development jointly by all the health professionals concerned, of safe, practicable guidelines for medicine management and adherence to these, will help to ensure that patients receive the standard of care to which they are entitled.

COMPLIANCE OF THE PATIENT

An essential component for the successful outcome of any treatment plan, drug or otherwise, is the patient's compliance with the prescriber's advice and directions. The compliance of a patient can be defined as the 'extent to which the patient's behaviour coincides with medical or health advice'. The term 'patient compliance' is often considered to be unsatisfactory, since it has overtones of coercion or compulsion. Alternative, less threatening terms that have been proposed include 'therapeutic alliance' and 'treatment adherence' (Blackwell 1976). For the purposes of this discussion the term 'patient compliance' will be used because it is capable of exact definition, and given appropriate circumstances it can be measured. At no time will the term be used here with any threat, real or implied.

Nurses both in community and hospital practice are well placed to help patients comply with the medical advice and instructions they are given regarding drug treatment. Often, the nurse is the only health professional who has continuing contact with the patient over long periods. As a result, she is able to gain an understanding of the patient's difficulties, offer advice and monitor compliance against this background.

Extent and significance of non-compliance

Some indication of the extent of non-compliance can be obtained when surveys are undertaken on the vast quantities of drugs collected during 'DUMP' (Disposal of unwanted medicines and pills) campaigns. Many studies have been published which demonstrate in detail the extent of non-compliance with directions regarding drug treatment. In long-term therapy, compliance is often very poor, averaging about 50% (Evans & Spelman 1983). With short-term therapy the position may generally be better. Studies by Donabedian & Rosenfeld (1984) and Mushlin (1972) showed that up to 75% of patients complied with their directions. Few studies relate the extent of non-compliance to the failure to achieve the desired therapeutic outcome. Nevertheless non-compliance should always be considered as a possible reason for treatment failure.

Measurement of non-compliance

Many difficulties are presented when measuring, or assessing patient compliance. The methods available vary from the basic tablet count to the use of fairly sophisticated monitoring devices (Norell 1979), and the measurement of the drug (or metabolite) in body fluids. The methods available are listed under two headings, firstly methods that are normally available to the nurse and secondly those methods which require considerable technical back up, and are only applicable in structured investigations into patient compliance.

Methods of compliance assessment available to the nurse

- General impressions of the patient's understanding of the drug regimen.
- Tablet counts at suitable intervals.
- Physiological markers, e.g. pulse rate in digoxin therapy.

- Visible presence of drug or metabolites in urine or faeces, e.g. rifampicin produces a reddish discoloration of the urine.

Methods of compliance determination

- Measurement of drug or metabolite in urine.
- Measurement in body fluids of pharmacologically inert chemical markers added to the medicine.
- Medication monitors that record the withdrawal and time of withdrawal of a dose from the container.
- Some drugs can be detected by chemical analysis of the hair.

Significance of non-compliance

Does it matter that some patients fail to take their medicines as prescribed? There can be no simple answer to this question. Failure to comply may delay a patient's restoration to full health (failure to complete a course of antibiotic therapy), or may be life-threatening (inappropriate use of a corticosteroid by an asthmatic patient). The active extent of non-compliance must also be taken into account since it may well be that for a particular regime an 80% compliance level by the patient may be adequate to achieve the desired therapeutic outcome. No general rules can be established. The whole situation must be assessed, since in many cases the patient's condition will vary and thus his need for medication will change also. Intelligent non-compliance has been described by Weintraub (1976) as occurring when patients either reduce the dose or stop taking a medicine altogether. The reasons for this behaviour may, when examined, be quite rational, such as the adjustment of a drug dose in response to the occurrence of side-effects.

Factors in non-compliance

Many factors have been identified as contributing to patient non-compliance. Haynes (1979) cites more than 200 factors, ranging from doctor/patient relationships to the colour and taste of the prescribed medicine. The factors involved can be classified into three main groups:

- personal factors
- social factors
- factors related directly to the medicines.

Rarely if ever, will non-compliance be due to a single factor. Often it will be attributable to a number of interacting factors. Table 26.3 lists the factors which contribute to non-compliance.

Occupational therapists have an important role to play in advising on the use of the various aids available. Whilst the provision of an aid to compliance will help many patients, equally the mere provision of an aid without more supportive action is unlikely to achieve anything.

The practical problems discussed above, although often contributing to non-compliance according to the strict definitions given, may also jeopardise the safe management of medicines by the patient, e.g. child-resistant closures, once removed, may be left off, with consequent loss of security. Many patients find more unfamiliar presentations, such as suppositories and pressurised aerosols, very difficult to use properly.

The patient's response

Many highly motivated patients, their carers, health personnel and social workers develop their own 'aids to compliance'. A number of approaches have been reported (Williams 1979). The most common is probably the setting out of individual doses, in advance, in household containers such as egg cups, ice trays, egg boxes and the like. Sellotape has been used to stick tablets and capsules to suitable fixtures in the kitchen or living room to act as a reminder that the dose is due. To help the patient select the right medicine, labels on containers are often supplemented by lay terms such as 'water tablets', 'sleeping tablets', 'heart tablets', etc. Instructions on labels may also be modified, additional labels being added often using large print or symbols to reinforce the dosage instructions. The timing of a TV programme may be used by some patients as a signal that a dose is due. A variety of charts, calendars, etc, have also been used to assist the memory.

It would appear that many of these ingenious

Table 26.3 Factors contributing to non-compliance	
FACTOR	**COMMENT**
Personal factors	
Patient's belief as to value of therapy	
Ethnic aspects	May conflict with mainstream Western medicine.
Relationship with health personnel involved	Patient's faith in prescriber, especially, often influences outcome.
Ageing process	Loss of recent memory, physical disability, etc, may contribute to non-compliance.
Some psychiatric illnesses	Schizophrenia, for example, may bring particular problems.
Pressures of a busy life	Especially hard to comply when several daily dosage intervals are involved.
Poor understanding of regimen	
Limited knowledge of condition	
Social factors	
Isolation	May arise from a breakdown in the family structure.
Deprivation	Some patients have to contend with a difficult journey to the surgery or pharmacy. Older people often have to contend with multiple deprivation, and are more vulnerable when things do go wrong with their medicine-taking.
Poverty	Patients who cannot afford prescription charges will probably need help and guidance not only with use of medicines but with the Social Security system also.
Factors directly related to medicines	
Tablets	Large tablets may be difficult to swallow; very small tablets may be difficult for a patient with stiff fingers to pick up.
Liquid medicines	Liquid medicines may have an unpleasant taste, colour or 'feel' in the mouth. Many liquid medicines that are used by older patients are formulated for children. Highly coloured, sweet, sickly flavours are generally not very acceptable to older patients, even if children find them acceptable, which often they do not. Measuring liquid medicines will be difficult for many patients, as will shaking a 500 ml glass bottle of liquid medicine which may weigh almost 1 kg.
Topical preparations	Stiff ointments may be difficult to use or there may be difficulty squeezing creams or ointments out of a tube. Products that stain the patient's linen or bath may prove unacceptable.
Packaging	Child-resistant closures are difficult for many people, although the use of these has reduced accidental poisoning of children significantly.
Labelling	Labelling systems have been improved with the introduction of machine-printed labels for all dispensed medicines, but the small print on some labels may be impossible for some patients to read.
Prophylactic medicines	Medicines prescribed for prophylaxis may not always be taken as prescribed because the patient does not feel the benefit directly.
Unpleasant side-effects	Unpleasant side-effects, such as headache, nausea, etc, may, undoubtedly, be a cause of non-compliance.

aids are of assistance to some patients and such self-help should not normally be discouraged. Equally however there can be no doubt that in some situations the 'home-made' devices will be a further source of problems which may not always be recognised by the patient. By transferring tablets from the original well-closed container, product security and stability will often be lost. For example, if glyceryl trinitrate tablets are not stored in a well-sealed glass jar the volatile active ingredient will be lost. Some products absorb moisture from the atmosphere resulting in loss of activity.

Nurses, pharmacists and doctors can learn from patients' coping strategies since these may highlight inadequacies in the service provided.

Methods for improving patient compliance

Before embarking on a course of action designed to improve patient compliance two main questions must be borne in mind. Firstly, does the patient really need drug therapy or is some other form of therapy more appropriate? Secondly, will improved compliance assist in the achievement of the therapeutic objective(s)? For instance, it may well be that improved compliance will result in an unacceptable level of side-effects. It is also vital to determine the real causes of non-compliance and to ensure that any strategies decided upon are within the patient's capabilities, otherwise further problems will be created for the patient.

The available methods can be considered under four main headings:

- presentation (labelling and packaging) of dispensed medicines
- aids to compliance
- education and counselling
- pre-discharge self-administration of medicines.

In some situations a combination of strategies may be required, the patient being given a suitable aid and counselled as to the importance of therapy. While there is no sure way to identify the potential defaulter, it is essential to make every effort to identify the high-risk patient. Table 26.4 outlines the methods available for improving compliance.

Education and counselling

A study undertaken by the Office of Health Economics in 1980 showed that 50% of patients wanted more information about their prescribed medicines. Of this group, information on side-effects, both short- and long-term, composition of medicines and actions was wanted. Along with their professional colleagues nurses can play a key role in ensuring that patients have sufficient knowledge to enable them to manage their prescribed medicines safely and effectively and thus achieve therapeutic benefit. Herxheimer (1976) has outlined the knowledge needed by patients, or by those responsible for their day-to-day care, in terms of the following questions to the prescriber (see Box 26.2).

Box 26.2	Herxheimer's questions to the prescriber
What for and how?	What kind of tablets are they and in what way do you expect them to help? How should I take them? How many and how often? Will I be able to tell whether they are working? How do I keep them?
How important?	How important is it for me to take these tablets? What is likely to happen if I do not take them?
Any side-effects?	Do the tablets have any other effects that I should look out for? Do they ever cause any trouble? Is it alright to drive when I am taking them? Are they alright with other medicines I may need? Will alcohol interfere with them? What should be done if someone takes too many?
How long for?	How long will I need to continue with these tablets? What should be done with any left over? When will I need to see you again? What will you want to know at the time?

In certain situations, such as when providing palliative care, it may not be appropriate to give

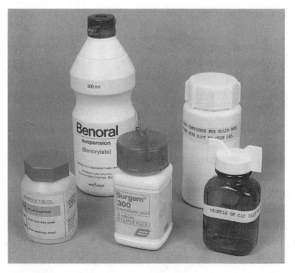

Figure 26.1 Plastic bottles for arthritics.

Table 26.4 Methods for improving patient compliance

PRESENTATION OF DISPENSED MEDICINES	
Appropriate containers and closures	Plastic, lightweight bottles with a cleft for ease of handling by an arthritic patient may be useful (Fig. 26.1). Containers used for tablets should generally be at least the 32 ml size for ease of handling. Plastic containers are generally preferred by patients. Screw caps that can be easily removed have obvious advantages (Le Gallez et al 1984) for some patients although there is great need to ensure that containers fitted with such closures are stored out of the reach of children.
Improved labelling	A wide variety of labelling systems are available, all of which are designed to provide the information required for the patient in a clear unambiguous way. Ideally the label of a dispensed medicine should bear the following information: Full instructions about the drug and its required frequency Approved name of product and strength Name and address of dispensing pharmacist Date of dispensing Quantity dispensed Expiry date of product Lay term (e.g. water tablets) Warning – keep out of reach of children Any special storage instructions Any special precautions in use For external use only and/or other appropriate warnings Examples of the ways in which additonal information, that cannot be included on a label, can be conveyed are illustrated (Fig. 26.2). Blind or partially sighted patients can be helped by using labels with specially large print and/or Braille (Fig. 26.3). The needs of patients whose command of English is minimal will require attention. Labels written in their mother tongue will be required. The needs of the illiterate must be recognised and dealt with in a sympathetic way. Pictorial labels have been developed and these may prove useful in some situations.
AIDS TO COMPLIANCE	
Aids in the management of solid dosage forms	The well known 'Dosett' tray (Fig. 26.4) has certain special features, notably the Braille markings and a detailed labelling facility on the reverse. Other compartmentalised trays of the 'Wiegand' type (Fig. 26.5) are useful since each compartment can be labelled with the contents and any special instructions. The 'Pill Minder' (Fig. 26.6) has some degree of 'child resistance' unlike the other trays described above. Other products available include the 'Medidos' system which has the advantage of being highly portable since each daily tray can be carried separately (Fig. 26.7). Combination products (e.g. diuretic with potassium) may prove useful, since the number of tablets to be taken daily is reduced. Compliance packs (calendar packs) are also made available for some products (e.g. oral contraceptives).
Aids in the management of liquid dosage forms	Measuring liquid medicines with the standard medicine spoon may prove difficult for many patients. Several alternative measuring devices are available (Fig. 26.8). Blind patients may find a special measuring device helpful (Fig. 26.9).
Other aids in the management of medicines	A long-handled ointment applicator has been developed for patients with physical disabilities. A device (Opticare) to aid the instillation of eye drops is available which helps the patient to aim the drop and squeeze the eye drop bottle (Fig. 26.10). Other devices for eye drop instillation include Easidrop for aiming and Autodrop for aiming and squeezing.

the patient all the information listed above, but the list of questions does give much useful guidance to nurses, pharmacists and prescribers.

Patient information leaflets

A wide range of patient information leaflets is available (Sloan 1984) which may be used to

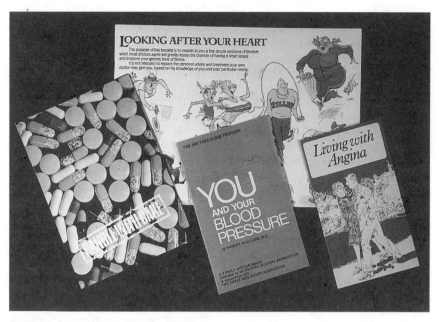

Figure 26.2 Information leaflets.

supplement and reinforce the counselling of patients. These range from general information on a particular condition and associated drug therapy to information packages designed to meet the needs of an individual patient. A study by George et al (1983) found that patients who received a leaflet were more likely to be completely satisfied with the treatment and with the information they had been given. It is vitally important that the information given to patients by different health workers is complementary and does not give rise to confusion.

Education packages

Nurses working in the community play a wider educational role by presenting talks to organised

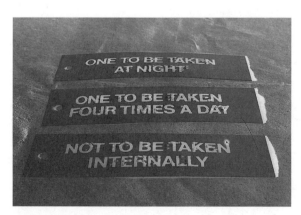

Figure 26.3 Large-print Braille labels.

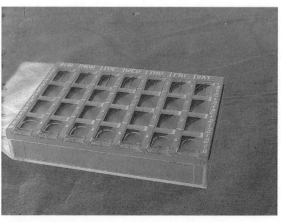

Figure 26.4 Dosett tray.

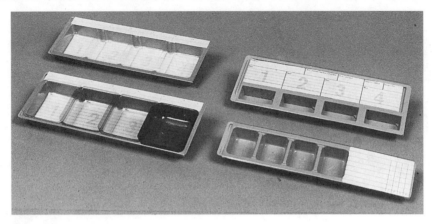

Figure 26.5   Wiegand tray.

groups in the community on aspects of the safe use of medicines. The topics covered by the talks would naturally be selected in line with the interests and needs of the group. In some situations however, a structured presentation in the form of a tape-slide or video package may be appropriate. As an example of this approach, audiovisual packages have been developed for groups interested in the care of older people (Graves Organisation 1984, 1989). An outline of the content is as follows:

- demographic aspects
- extent of use of medicines by older people
- physiology of the ageing process
- factors that cause older people to have difficulty managing their medicines

- practical help in medicine management available to older people.

Self-administration of medicines

A valuable opportunity to improve patient compliance may be presented during a period of inpatient care by instituting a programme of self-administration of medicines. Such methods of medicine administration have been used over the years with particular emphasis on the needs of patients in wards providing rehabilitation, care for older people and care for patients with a mental illness. Increasingly it is being recognised that self-administration systems can be used to advantage in acute wards (Bird 1988). The advantages claimed for systems of self-administration include improved patient compliance on

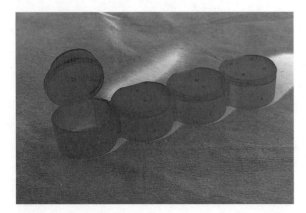

Figure 26.6   Pill Minder.

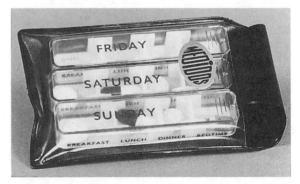

Figure 26.7   Medidos system.

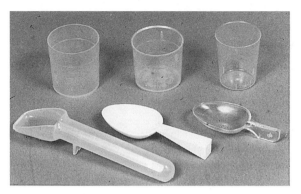

Figure 26.8 Measuring devices.

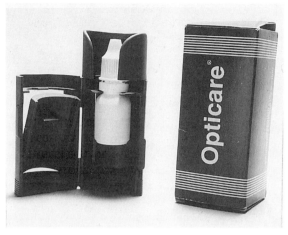

Figure 26.10 Opticare.

discharge from hospital arising from better understanding of the medication(s) and more appropriate timing of medicine administration than can be achieved by the traditional 'medicine round'. Nurses and other professional colleagues may be anxious about the risks that self-administration of medicines may cause, particularly as regards the safety and security of medicines in the ward environment. However, the adoption of a well-structured system will eliminate risk to a very large extent. Well managed self-administration systems are essential to ensure both patient safety and the achievement of the desired therapeutic outcome. The essential components of a system for self-administration of medicines are outlined in Box 26.3.

Box 26.3 Essential components of a system for the self-administration of medicines

- A system which has been fully documented and agreed by all responsible authorities.
- Full patient information made available and the patient's consent obtained.
- A detailed protocol which includes:
  patient assessment
  stages of the process once it has been confirmed that the patient is suitable for self-medication and wishes to undertake this
  detailed documentation including the prescription sheet, a record of self-administration, a record of checks made on the patient's compliance, and any other records of action taken to assist the patient
  clear guidelines on the role of the health care professionals involved especially nurses and clinical pharmacists

---

A number of methods of medicine management have been used to facilitate self-administration of medicines. In limited circumstances patients can be given a small supply of certain medicines to keep in their bedside locker, or patients can be encouraged to ask for their medicines from the medicine trolley. A system that gives the patient full involvement and control is based on using a

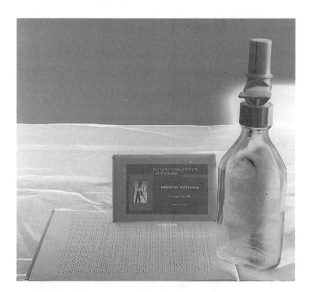

Figure 26.9 Medicine dispenser for the blind.

Box 26.4 Stages in self-administration of medicines

Stage 1	Patient assessed	Patient's knowledge of his medication can be assessed and a general idea of degree of compliance can be established At this stage any special needs patient may have can be identified, e.g. need for compliance aid
Stage 2	Patient given access to bedside medicine cabinet under nurse's supervision	Process of assessment can be continued, frequency and nature of any checks on patient's compliance can be determined on a multidisciplinary basis. Value of any aid to compliance can be evaluated
Stage 3	Patient given key to medicine cabinet and allowed to self-administer with only limited supervision/checks	Further information/education on patient's medicines can be given at this stage as patient's confidence develops
Stage 4	Patient allowed to self-medicate with reduced level of checks (say, weekly) on compliance	During this stage patient can be prepared for discharge and any remaining problems resolved

small lockable medicine cabinet attached to the bedside locker. Access to the medicines is given according to the patient's abilities and needs. Patients who have been shown to be capable of managing their medicines well and whose needs are quite specific may be given the key to the medicine cabinet for the period of their inpatient treatment. In other situations the key may only be made available to the patient at specific times/intervals.

Opportunities to assess and improve patient compliance are presented at all stages of the self-administration process. The stages are summarised in Box 26.4 together with a brief discussion of patient compliance issues.

If at any stage difficulties are identified it may be necessary to review the arrangements which could include discontinuation of the plan or reverting to an earlier stage of the process. This should seldom prove to be necessary if the assessment and checks are made with due care and sensitivity. Patient self-administration of medicines will no doubt play an increasing role in helping patients to achieve good compliance and resulting benefits from their medication.

REFERENCES

Bird C A 1988 Taking their own medicine. Nursing Times 84(45): 28–32

Blackwell B 1976 Treatment adherence. British Journal of Psychiatry 129: 513–531

Donabedian A, Rosenfeld L S 1984 Follow-up study of chronically ill patients discharged from hospital. Journal of Chronic Disorders 14: 847–862

Evans L, Spelman M 1983 The problem of non-compliance with drug therapy. Drugs 25: 63–76

George C F, Nicholas J A, Waters W E 1983 Prescription information leaflets. A pilot study in general practices. British Medical Journal 287: 1193–1196

Graves Organisation 1984 Older people and their medicines. Tape slide presentation

Graves Organisation 1989 Medicines and older people. Videotape presentation

Haynes R B 1979 In: Haynes R B, Taylor D W, Sackett D L (eds) Compliance in health care, John Hopkins University Press, Baltimore, p 1–7

Henderson V 1966 The nature of nursing: a definition and its implications for practice, research and education. Macmillan, New York

Herxheimer A 1976 Sharing the responsibility for treatment. Lancet 2: 1294

Le Gallez P, Bird H A, Wright V et al 1984 Comparison of 12 different containers for dispensing anti-inflammatory drugs. British Medical Journal 288: 699–701

Ley P 1981 Professional non-compliance. A neglected problem. British Journal of Clinical Psychology 20: 151–154

MacPherson W, Andrew M, Brown M et al 1983 Survey of drug administration by learners (unpublished)

Mushlin A I 1972 A study of physicians' ability to predict patient compliance. Master's thesis. John Hopkins University, Baltimore

Norell S E 1979 Improving medication compliance. A randomised clinical trial. British Medical Journal 2: 1031–1033

Rodman M J, Smith D W 1974 Clinical pharmacology in nursing. Lippincott, Philadelphia

Roper N, Logan W W, Tierney A J 1985 The elements of nursing. Churchill Livingstone, Edinburgh

Royal College of Nursing 1983 Drug administration – a nurse's responsibility. RCN, London

Sloan P J M 1984 Survey of patient information booklets. British Medical Journal 288: 915–919

United Kingdom Central Council for Nursing, Midwifery and Health Visiting 1992 Standards for the administration of medicines

Weintraub M 1976 Intelligent and capricious non-compliance. In: Lasagna A (ed) Compliance P39 Futura, Mt Kisco, New York

Williams A 1979 The role of the pharmacist in improving compliance in the elderly patient. Proceedings of the Guild of Hospital Pharmacists 6: 1–22

FURTHER READING

Ashurst S 1993 Nurses must improve their knowledge of pharmacology. British Journal of Nursing 2(12): 608

Bird C A 1990 Patient self-medication. Surgical Nurse 3(1): 22–26

Chief Administrative Pharmaceutical Officers' Group 1992 Medicine self administration guidelines

Davis S 1991 Self-administration of medicines. Nursing Standard 5(15/16): 29–31

Department of Health 1989 Nursing routines and improving efficiency PL/CNO(89) 1

Gatford J D 1990 Nursing calculations, 3rd edn. Churchill Livingstone, Melbourne, ch 1 p 1–15, 20–29, 34–35, 38–39

Ley P 1988 Communicating with patients. Improving communication, satisfaction and compliance. Psychology and medicine series. Croom Helm, London

Presentation to Parliament by the Secretaries of State for Health, Social Security, Wales and Scotland by Command of Her Majesty 1989 Caring for people: community care in the next decade and beyond. Cmnd 849 HMSO, London

27

Administration of medicines

ADMINISTRATION OF MEDICINES BY MOUTH

For the majority of patients, the most convenient and acceptable method of receiving medication is by mouth. Most medicines taken by mouth are intended to be swallowed, and are referred to as oral medicines. Others, known as sublingual, are specifically for dissolving under the tongue; some, known as buccal, are for holding against the mucous membranes of the cheek.

Oral administration

Tablets, capsules and liquid preparations are generally easy to administer and are effective when given orally. If a tablet or capsule sticks in the oesophagus it can cause irritation to the point of ulceration, especially with drugs such as ferrous salts and Slow K. To prevent such an occurrence, patients should ideally take a draught of water (or juice) and then swallow the preparation with a second draught.

Administering oral solids

Patients who have difficulty swallowing tablets may be assisted in a number of ways:

- A drink beforehand moistens the mouth and gets the swallowing process started.
- Where the tablet is large and is scored, it may be split in two or even four. A specially designed tablet splitter (Fig. 27.1) may be helpful.

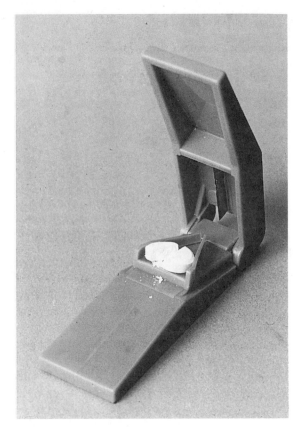

Figure 27.1 Tablet splitter.

- In certain instances the tablet may be crushed using a mortar and pestle or specially designed tablet crusher (Fig. 27.2). Enteric-coated or sustained-release formulations must not be split or crushed.
- Some patients find it helpful to place the tablet at the back of the tongue, take a draught of water and tilt the head back before swallowing. (This stimulates the back of the tongue and produces a swallowing reflex.)
- For those who cannot swallow tablets or capsules, there may be soluble or liquid forms of the medicine available from the pharmacy.
- Dysphagic patients sometimes cope better with semi-solids than with liquids and so may prefer to take their medicines with jam, for example.

Whenever possible, the patient should put the tablet or capsule into his mouth himself. By observing the patient attempting to take a tablet and assessing his capabilities generally, the nurse can decide how best to present further medicines to him. The methods employed are:

- taking directly from a spoon, medicine measure or palm of the hand
- picking up using the thumb and forefinger.

However, some difficulties are incurred by each of these methods. For example:

- A spoon is not advisable for patients with any degree of tremor.
- Medicine measures are not designed with the size of an adult's nose in mind and so access may be difficult!
- Unless the medicine measure is completely dry, tablets can adhere to the measure and go unnoticed.
- Tablets or capsules may be dropped or may stick to the hand if moist.
- Intention tremor and stiff joints may make picking up difficult or impossible.

Generally speaking, patients who are elderly, frail, poorly sighted or confused, are helped if the tablets are placed in a row on the medicine tray accompanied by a glass of water or a suitable beverage. In this way they are more likely to see what they are to take – the colour of the tablets and the number. They can then safely pick each one up themselves and so retain some degree of independence. Hemiplegic patients find this a helpful method especially when more than one tablet have to be taken. Using the unaffected hand, they require to break down the process. For example:

- Pick up glass, take drink, lay down glass.
- Pick up first tablet, place in mouth.
- Pick up glass, take drink, lay down glass.
- Pick up next tablet . . . . . and so on.

White tablets may be overlooked when they are laid out on a white tray and so care must be taken to ensure that none has been missed. If the tray is used in this way, it must be washed before and after use.

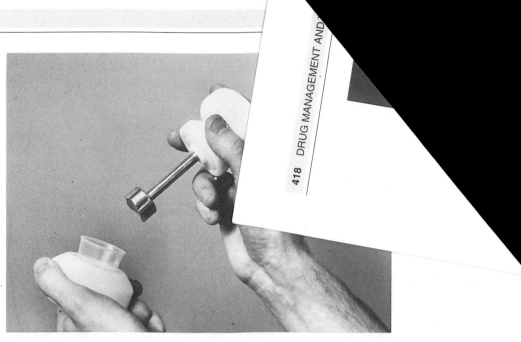

Figure 27.2   Tablet crusher.

Care must be taken, particularly where there is facial paralysis, to ensure that the tablets are swallowed and not retained in the side of the mouth. Patients who do not want to take their tablets are sometimes known to retain the tablet between the gum and the cheek until the staff are out of sight and then reject the tablet, often into the bed.

An adequate volume of fluid, for example, at least 100 ml, ensures transport into the gastro-intestinal tract. Apart from personal tastes and preferences, the choice and volume of liquid to be used will depend on a number of factors. Clearly, for patients on restricted fluids the volume may be critical. Milk may inhibit the absorption of some drugs and acidic fruit cordials tend to cause capsules to swell which may make swallowing more difficult. Improved formulations are a help in disguising the taste of many drugs but children of all ages may welcome the traditional 'spoonful of sugar'.

If a patient rejects part of a dose or vomits after swallowing a dose of medicine, the doctor should be informed along with the time lapse between drug administration and emesis or rejection. Vomitus should be retained for examination of drug content.

Administering oral liquids

- All liquid medicines should be thoroughly shaken before use and measured at eye level in a good light.
- When pouring a liquid medicine the bottle is held with the label in the palm of hand so that if any of the liquid drips down the side of the bottle it will not deface the label.
- Viscous suspensions, syrups, etc, can be more completely administered if taken from a suitable spoon rather than from a medicine measure. A standard 5 ml spoon should normally be used. However medicine spoons of different designs are available, the choice depending mainly on acceptability to the patient. Care should be taken not to overfill a medicine spoon when administering a viscous preparation.
- The formulation of liquid medicines presents many problems not least of which is to achieve an acceptable taste. If particular problems are experienced, the ward pharmacist should be consulted, as dilution or alternative formulation may be of assistance.
- While it is necessary to ensure that soluble tablets are completely dissolved, it is unwise to use an excessive volume of water since an

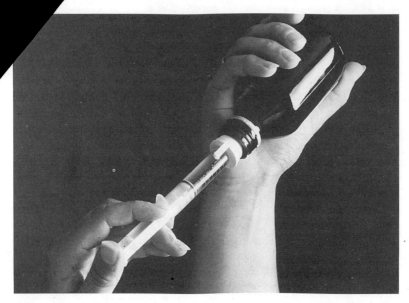

Figure 27.3 Oral syringe.

unpleasant taste may result in rejection by the patient.

- Where the medicine is presented in powder form to be reconstituted, the date of reconstitution or expiry should be marked on the bottle.
- When liquids are being instilled in the mouth from a dropper, a separate bottle and dropper are used for each patient.
- In some instances a specially designed oral syringe may be useful, for example, in paediatrics or where specially potent oral liquid medicines are in use (Fig. 27.3).

The administration of oral medicines is summarised in Box 27.1.

Sublingual administration

First-pass metabolism is avoided when drugs are given by the sublingual route (i.e. under the tongue) since the drug passes directly into the general blood circulation via the blood vessels on the under surface of the tongue. Sublingual tablets are uncoated ready for absorption. Once the tablet has been placed under the tongue, the patient should refrain from swallowing saliva for as long as possible as this contains the drug which will be absorbed. As absorption through the oral mucosa is rapid, the effects of the drug become apparent within a minute or two.

Box 27.1	Administration of oral medicines
Documentation	• prescribing and recording sheet
The medicine	• oral solids (tablet, capsule, lozenge, granules) • oral liquids (mixture, suspension, emulsion, linctus)
The nurse and the patient	• identification of patient • explanation given to patient
Technique	• wherever possible, the patient should be in upright position • whenever possible, the patient should put the medicine into his mouth himself • the nurse should witness the medicine being taken • if required, any fluid taken should be recorded on the patient's fluid balance chart • any medicines rejected should be retained
Hazards	• irritation of gastrointestinal tract • aspiration of the medicine • staining of teeth

Tablets to be given by this route must be prescribed as such. The method of administration is simple requiring no liquid and demanding little effort from the patient. The cooperation of the patient is necessary, however, and a clear explanation of this method of administration should be given to him. Although no harm will ensue if the tablet is swallowed, he will benefit from the drug *only* if it is taken sublingually. The ease with which drugs can be given by this route can be used to advantage in postoperative patients and those who are terminally ill, where swallowing of tablets can be a problem. Buprenorphine, an analgesic, is commonly used in these situations. The sublingual route is also useful when there is risk of symptoms arising unexpectedly and when a rapid effect is wanted, such as in angina pectoris. Patients who are prescribed glyceryl trinitrate tablets for prevention of anginal attacks should be advised to carry with them a small supply of the tablets at all times. The expiry date (8 weeks after *dispensing*) should be carefully noted. Once the individual patient gets to know which activities tend to precipitate an attack, he should get into the habit of placing the tablet under his tongue just before embarking on any of these activities. When the tablet is used to alleviate an anginal attack, it should be taken immediately the pain is experienced and retained under the tongue until the pain is relieved, after which any of the tablet remaining is spat out. This may help prevent headache caused by cerebral vasodilation which often follows administration of this drug.

Buccal administration

When a lozenge or tablet is to be held in the mouth against the mucous membranes of the cheek, the term buccal may be used. It refers to the inside of the cheek where the dosage form dissolves. Tablets for buccal administration are uncoated to facilitate absorption. Hydrocortisone 2.5 mg lozenges are used in this way to treat aphthous ulcers in the mouth. Such medicines are intended to provide a local effect although some of the drug may act systemically when it is swallowed in the saliva.

Medicine rounds

In spite of the gradual disappearance of task allocation in nursing, the majority of medicines issued by nurses in hospital are still administered consecutively to groups of patients in the form of a medicine round (Box 27.2).

Box 27.2 Medicine round	
Documentation	• Kardex system *or* individual prescribing and recording sheet at each patient's bedside
The medicine	• mainly oral medicines (possibly medicines for inhalation also) • stored in alphabetical order according to approved name • trolley padlocked to wall when not in use • unlocked trolley never left unattended • sufficient spoons, medicine measures, oral syringes, etc, available
The environment	• so far as possible, uninterrupted
The nurse and the patient	• each patient greeted and accurately identified
Technique	• nurse works systematically, for example, clockwise round ward or following set order of Kardex • on completion of round, trolley tidied up, non-disposable items washed, sticky bottles wiped and trolley stock replenished as appropriate
Hazards	• medicine(s) given to wrong patient • interruptions leading to error • medicines given too soon or much later than time prescribed • misappropriation of medicines from unsupervised trolley

INJECTIONS

Drugs are given by injection for a number of reasons. For example:

- they may not be absorbed when given by mouth (gentamicin)
- they may be destroyed in the stomach (insulin)
- rapid first-pass metabolism may be extensive (lignocaine)
- a fast onset of action may be required in an emergency

- very precise control over dosage may be needed
- because the patient is unable for whatever reason to take the medicine by mouth.

Since the routes used for administering injections do not involve the gastrointestinal tract, drugs prepared for injection are often described as for *parenteral* use.

Routes of administration

The routes most commonly used for administering injections are:

- subcutaneous (beneath the skin) (Box 27.3)
- intramuscular (into muscle) (Box 27.4)
- intravenous (into a vein)

Unless they have received specific training and are in possession of authorisation to do so, nurses are not permitted to administer medicines via the intravenous route. Intravenous medicines are normally administered only by a doctor. In clinical practice there is increasing use of the intravenous route for the administration of drugs such as antibiotics and diuretics. However, some drugs still require to be given either by the subcutaneous or the intramuscular route and therefore the nurse must maintain the skills involved. Drugs commonly given subcutaneously include:

- insulin
- heparin
- hyoscine
- vaccines

Drugs commonly given intramuscularly include:

- analgesics
- anti-emetics
- corticosteroids

Skin preparation

It is no longer thought necessary to use an alcohol swab to clean the skin prior to the administration of injections. Torrance (1989) cites two studies. One describes a series of 1078 injections given by all routes without any skin preparation and which resulted in no case of systemic or local infections being recorded. The second was a study of 7000 insulin injections given to a group of diabetic patients without skin cleansing with no infection noted. Lipids in the epidermis provide an antibacterial barrier, and so to remove the lipids may be to encourage bacterial colonisation. Clinical evidence suggests that no harm will be caused by pricking the skin *so long as it is socially clean*. Contaminated skin will need preparation to produce a low bacterial count. In this case the site should first be made socially clean followed by a 30 second rub using an 'alcohol swab' and then the skin should be allowed to dry before proceeding. (Alcohol swabs contain 70% alcohol and a disinfectant such as chlorhexidine.) Immunosuppressed patients require to have the skin cleansed in this way as they may become infected by inoculation of a relatively low number of pathogens.

Site

The sites most commonly used for *subcutaneous* injections (Fig. 27.4) are as follows:

- middle outer aspect of the upper arm
- middle anterior aspect of the thigh
- anterior abdominal wall below the umbilicus.

The back and lower loin may also be used.

The sites most commonly used for *intramuscular* injections are as follows:

- upper outer quadrant of the buttock (Fig. 27.5)
- middle outer aspect of the thigh.

It is vital that the injection be confined to one of these areas to avoid damage to the sciatic nerve and to avoid penetrating a major blood vessel. Rotation of the sites used for subcutaneous and intramuscular injections helps to reduce the likelihood of irritation and improves absorption.

Syringes

A syringe consists of a barrel and a plunger (Fig. 27.6). The barrel is graduated. The plunger has a rubber stopper attached. Syringes are available in various sizes, e.g. 2 ml, 5 ml, 10 ml, 20 ml. The choice of syringe is made according to the volume of medication to be injected. The tip of a

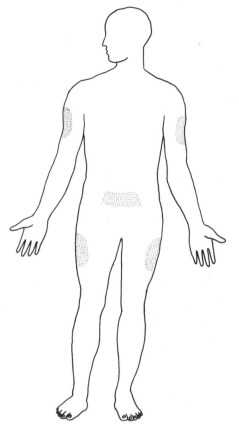

Figure 27.4   Sites for administering subcutaneous injections.

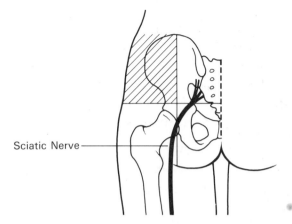

Sciatic Nerve

Figure 27.5   Upper outer quadrant of the buttock.

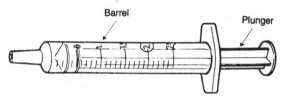

Barrel

Plunger

Figure 27.6   Syringe.

Needles

A needle consists of a hub and a cannula (Fig. 27.7). The cannula is hollow and is made of strong flexible steel that has been siliconised to assist penetration. For the same reason the tip of the cannula is bevelled. Different types of needle have a different bevel (Fig. 27.8). A shorter bevel encourages minimal penetration as is required in an intradermal injection. A longer bevel allows easier deep penetration as needed for an intramuscular injection. The gauge of the cannula is an indication of its diameter. The higher the gauge, the finer the bore. Higher gauges are used for 'watery' solutions and make for less painful injections. Low gauges are essential for injecting viscous (syrupy) solutions. Needle lengths also vary. Selection of length depends on the site of the injection as well as the patient's age and physical build. Each needle is enclosed in a removable guard and individually sealed in a sterile pack. Before use, a check should be made to ensure that the pack has not been damaged.

syringe can vary, with the concentric luer tip being the one used for subcutaneous and intramuscular injections. It is also used for introducing medication via an already sited intravenous cannula. For direct intravenous injections, the eccentric luer tip is used to allow the needle to lie within the vein wall without puncturing the distal wall. The luer tips of syringes interlock to an international standard with needle hubs. Disposable syringes are made of polypropylene which is compatible with most substances to be injected. There are one or two exceptions however. Paraldehyde for example should be administered using a glass syringe since it reacts with plastic and rubber on prolonged contact. Syringes are individually sealed in a sterile pack. Before use, a check should be made that the seal has not been broken.

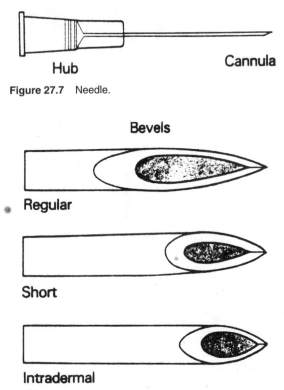

Figure 27.7 Needle.

Figure 27.8 Different bevels on needles.

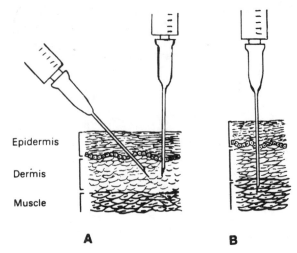

Figure 27.9 Angles for the administration of (A) subcutaneous and (B) intramuscular injections.

For *subcutaneous injections*, a short fine-bore needle is used. For adults, this is normally ⅝ inch (16 mm), 25 gauge, although a ½ inch (12 mm) needle may also be used.

For *intramuscular injections*, the needle used has to be sufficiently long to reach deep into the muscle so as to increase the speed of effect and to reduce the likelihood of the drug seeping back along the needle track. For adults a 1½ inch (40 mm), 21 gauge is normally used. In severely emaciated adults and in small children a 1 inch (25 mm), 23 gauge may be used.

Angle

The angles at which the needle is directed for subcutaneous and intramuscular injections are illustrated (Fig. 27.9). It is now common practice for subcutaneous injections of, for example, heparin or insulin to be given into the abdomen at an angle of 90° using a ½ inch (12 mm), 25 gauge needle.

Volume

When preparing an injection, the nurse should give consideration to the volume which may be effectively accommodated in one site. Apart from the route to be used, the patient's age and physical build are factors which will influence the decision. Normally the following would apply:

for *subcutaneous injections* no more than 2 ml should be injected at one site.

for *intramuscular injections* the volume injected at any one site should normally be of the order of about 2–5 ml.

Where a volume in excess of 5 ml is to be given, two separate sites should be used. The thinner and/or older the patient, the smaller should be the volume. For the fatter and/or younger patient, the volume is less critical.

Pain reduction

Pain caused by injections can be reduced in a number of different ways. First it is important to try to encourage the patient to relax. This may be achieved by explaining to the patient what he should do. The patient should be positioned so that he is at ease. For example, for *subcutaneous injections* the patient should be sitting with the hand resting on the iliac crest; for *intramuscular injections* the patient should be lying *on*, as opposed to leaning over, a couch.

When the buttock is the chosen site for intramuscular injection, administration may be made less painful by asking the patient to adopt the prone position and to point the feet inwards. Internal rotation of the femur helps to relax the gluteus maximus muscle. Alternatively the patient may lie on his side with the lower leg extended and the upper leg flexed.

Fine-bore needles create less pain on puncturing the skin and necessitate slow injection of the fluid. Pain can result from injecting too large a volume of fluid at one site or injecting the drug too quickly, resulting in improper distribution of the drug. The skin may also be cooled using a volatile spray such as ethyl chloride. A further possibility is to use a local anaesthetic agent (see also p. 329)

Subcutaneous administration may be carried out by high-pressure jet injection which pushes the injection through a fine hole into the subcutaneous tissue with the aid of a needle. This technique is particularly useful in mass inoculation programmes.

Rate of absorption

The rates at which drugs are absorbed and take effect after subcutaneous or intramuscular injection depend on two factors. These are the local blood circulation and the nature of the drug solution or suspension. Subcutaneous absorption occurs chiefly through the capillaries and is much faster compared with absorption following oral medication but usually slower than intramuscular absorption because of muscle tissue's excellent blood supply. Absorption following intramuscular injection may be speeded up by massaging the area of injection. However insulin-dependent diabetics are discouraged from massaging the site vigorously in an attempt to preserve the state of the capillaries. An inflamed or oedematous site should be avoided when administering subcutaneous or intramuscular injections so as to prevent a worsening of

the inflammation/oedema and consequently a delay in absorption. In states of shock, blood flow to the skin and superficial muscle may be greatly reduced thus reducing the absorption of drugs from these sites. In this case intravenous injection should be used.

Box 27.3   Administration of subcutaneous injection

Documentation	• as for intramuscular injection
The medicine	• as for intramuscular injection
The environment	• patient seated or in bed • privacy, warmth, comfort
The nurse and the patient	• patient identified • explanation given to patient • patient assisted into supine position if abdomen the chosen site • patient's skin cleanliness assessed
Technique drawing up the injection	• as for intramuscular injection
administering the injection	• nurse ensures hands thoroughly washed • chosen site for injection exposed • skin pinched up between thumb and forefinger • syringe 'cradled' across all four fingers and steadied with the thumb; when 90° angle, use 'pencil grip' – see Box 27.4 • needle with bevel uppermost *pushed gently* through the skin • fluid injected *slowly* and *steadily* • needle *gently* withdrawn • site gently compressed for a few seconds until any oozing stops • patient made comfortable • 'sharps' carefully placed in disposal bin
Hazards	• abscess formation

Box 27.4   Administration of intramuscular injection

Documentation	• prescribing and recording sheet
The medicine	• ampoule or vial containing prescribed drug • ampoule of Water for Injections (or other diluent) if necessary for reconstitution
The environment	• patient in bed or on couch • privacy, warmth, comfort

The nurse and the patient	• patient identified • nurse explains her intentions and indicates how patient may assist • patient assisted into lateral or prone position • patient's skin cleanliness assessed

Technique
drawing up the injection
	• nurse ensures hands are thoroughly washed
	• contents collected into body of ampoule by flicking ampoule with fingers
	• neck of ampoule wiped with alcohol swab
	• ampoule snapped at neck using swab to protect fingers (or by using a plastic sleeve)
	• syringe assembled
	• care taken to prevent needle from touching anything unsterile
	• syringe filled
	• new guarded needle attached
	• air bubbles expelled from syringe by:
	   holding it perpendicular at eye level in a good light
	   pulling plunger back slightly
	   tapping syringe with fingers to collect small bubbles into one
	   pushing plunger until liquid fills needle
	• final volume checked

administering the injection	• nurse ensures hands are washed just prior to administration if involved in positioning patient and on completion of procedure • nurse ensures sufficiently large area of patient's buttock exposed to allow selection of exact site for injection while maintaining maximum privacy • fold of skin and tissue stretched or pinched up • syringe held using 'pencil grip' • needle inserted *quickly* • plunger withdrawn slightly to verify needle has not penetrated blood vessel (if blood appears, needle withdrawn and injection repeated at another site using fresh dose, syringe and needle) • fluid injected *slowly* • needle withdrawn *quickly* • site gently compressed for a few seconds until minor seepage stops • patient made comfortable • 'sharps' carefully placed in disposal bin
Hazards	• abscess formation • nerve damage • injecting medication into large blood vessel

Special aspects of injection procedures

The medicine for injection may on some occasions be presented in a rubber-capped multi-dose vial, especially where the dose is variable. When this occurs, there are some important points to remember. The self-sealing rubber closure must be thoroughly cleaned with an alcohol swab and allowed to dry prior to puncturing it with a needle. Great care is essential in calculating what portion of the total volume is required. To facilitate withdrawal of fluid, the plunger of the syringe is first withdrawn and air injected, the volume of air being the same as the volume of fluid to be withdrawn. It is customary to change the needle after drawing up the injection and before injecting the patient in case a core of rubber is retained inside the needle.

The medicine may be presented in powder form and require reconstitution. Most often this is done using Water for Injections but in certain instances special diluents may be required. It should be recognised that the addition of 1 ml of diluent to 250 mg of a drug will produce a volume in excess of 1 ml. Normally this is of little consequence but may be important if a fraction of the total content of the vial is to be administered. For emaciated patients the volume of reconstituting fluid should be the minimum compatible with the physical and other properties of the drug, e.g. solubility, and any possible local irritancy should be taken into account. On occasion it may be desirable to combine two drugs in the same injection. This may present problems, e.g. physical/chemical incompatibility in the syringe and in the management of any subsequent drug reaction. The prime considerations here should be patient safety and comfort. Clearly, comfort for the patient should not be allowed to detract from safety in drug therapy. Advice of the prescriber and clinical pharmacist will often be helpful in resolving these difficult situations.

When drawing up and injecting antibiotics, disposable gloves should be worn to prevent possible contact with the skin and the development of a sensitivity reaction. The special precautions which require to be taken when handling cytotoxic drugs are given on pages 232 to 236.

The injection may be known to irritate the tissues and stain the skin if its seepage along the needle track to the epidermis is allowed to take place (e.g. iron dextran injection). To prevent this, several precautions should be taken. After the syringe is filled, the needle is changed so that the substance is contained in the syringe only and is less likely to drip from the tip of the needle as it penetrates the skin. To reduce pain as well as the risk of staining, the injection is made deep into the muscle of the upper outer quadrant of the buttock. The arm or thigh do not allow for the depth required and so should not be used. A 21 gauge needle is suitable but it is important that it is long enough to reach the muscle. As a rule of thumb a $1^{1}/_{2}$ inch (40 mm) needle will do for most normal sized adults. Obese patients will require a 2 inch needle. The so-called Z-track technique must be used. This technique involves displacement of the skin and subcutaneous tissue laterally prior to injection (Fig. 27. 10). The injection is made slowly and steadily. Before withdrawing the needle, 10 seconds should be allowed to elapse so that the muscle mass can accommodate the volume of the injection. The site is not massaged otherwise the medication may be forced into the subcutaneous tissue causing irritation.

Patients with haematological conditions such as leukaemia in which the platelet count is likely to be low should never be given intramuscular injections because of the high risk of bleeding into the muscle tissue.

Intravenous injection

Administering a drug directly into a vein avoids all complications of drug absorption and as a result an effective blood level of the drug can be achieved in a matter of seconds. The intravenous route is used:

- in emergency situations such as shock and status asthmaticus
- to administer general anaesthetic agents (e.g. thiopentone sodium)
- for larger volumes (e.g. 5–20 ml)
- where the preparation has irritant properties (e.g. cytotoxic drugs)
- where subcutaneous or intramuscular injections would cause intolerable pain (e.g. aminophylline)

Intravenous injections may however be associated with a number of complications such as:

- a haematoma caused by puncturing through, instead of into, the vein
- necrosis caused by the drug escaping into the surrounding tissues when the needle slips out of the vein and is simply lying in the tissues
- phlebitis at the injection site resulting from a high concentration of an irritant agent, repeated injections or prolonged administration
- because of rapidity of action, intoxication or death if an error is made when calculating or measuring the dose

Except when a nurse has received special training and has been authorised to administer intravenous drugs, this procedure may be carried out only by a doctor. However, it is important that the nurse understands how it is done so that she can, if called upon, play a supporting role.

The standard approach to prescribing , administering and recording medicines is followed. To reduce the risk of introducing microorganisms

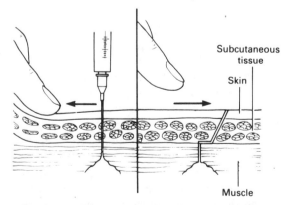

Figure 27.10   Z-track technique. (From Chandler 1991 Tabbner's nursing care: theory and practice, 2nd edn. Churchill Livingstone.)

into the bloodstream, it is essential that the hands are washed, sterile equipment used and an aseptic technique practised. The patient should be given an explanation of what is to be done. He should be in a comfortable position with the site to be used exposed. A vein in the elbow or the back of the hand is normally used. With the help of a tourniquet, the vein is distended to allow access. If indicated, the site of injection is swabbed with a suitable antiseptic and allowed to dry. A syringe with an eccentric nozzle and a 1 inch (25 mm) 20 gauge needle with an intravenous bevel are used for giving an intravenous injection. All air bubbles are expelled from the syringe and the needle filled with drug. Holding the syringe in line with the vein, the needle with the bevel up is pushed through the skin into the vein in the direction of the heart (Fig. 27.11). Before injecting, the position of the needle must be verified by gently pulling the plunger. If no blood is aspirated, the needle must then be withdrawn and another attempt made. After releasing the tourniquet and making an initial injection of 0.1 ml, there should be a pause of at least 30 seconds to observe the response before the remainder is slowly injected (up to 10 minutes). It is dangerous to give a rapid intravenous injection as this exposes tissues and organs such as the heart and brain to high concentrations of a drug which has been poorly diluted with blood. A drug solution injected over 2 minutes will be 60 times more dilute than if injected over 2 seconds. After completing the injection, a sterile swab should be placed over the injection site, the needle slowly removed and gentle pressure maintained to avoid a haematoma.

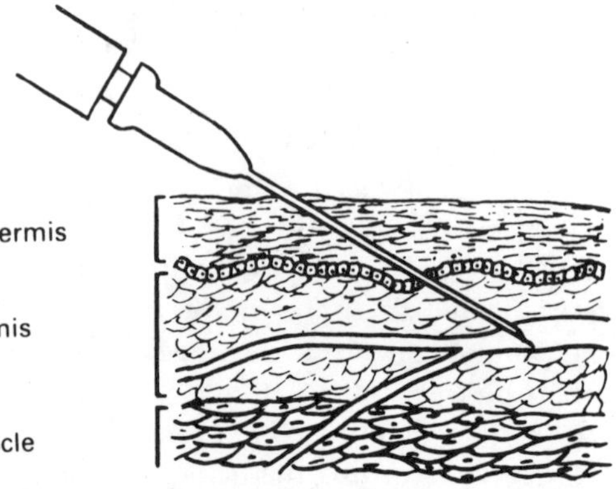

Alternatively, intravenous drugs may be administered intermittently via the side inlet of an indwelling intravenous cannula or into the administration set of an intravenous infusion by means of a three-way stopcock or multiple inlet device. If there is not a continuous fluid infusion to keep the cannula patent, a dilute heparin solution should be injected to prevent blood from clotting in its lumen.

A summary of common routes for injection is given in Table 27.1.

Other routes of injection

Although parenteral administration is normally accomplished by subcutaneous, intramuscular or intravenous routes, occasionally other routes are used to deliver a drug to a particular tissue or organ.

Intra-arterial injection

This route is sometimes used to inject or infuse drugs into an artery supplying the affected organ if the drugs are rapidly metabolised or systemically toxic. Cytotoxic drugs for the treatment of local neoplasms or radio-opaque substances used in arteriography may be injected in this way.

Intra-articular injection

In inflammatory conditions of the joints, particularly rheumatoid arthritis, corticosteroids are given by intra-articular injection to relieve inflammation and increase joint mobility. Insoluble, long-acting compounds such as triamcinolone hexacetonide are used. Corticosteroids should not be injected into infected joints. Tissues or joints injected with corticosteroids have an increased susceptibility to infections. It is therefore essential to observe full aseptic precautions when making these injections.

Epidermis

Dermis

Muscle

Figure 27.11 Intravenous injection.

Table 27.1 Summary of common routes for injections

	Subcutaneous	Intramuscular	Intravenous
Definition	Beneath the skin	Into muscle	Into a vein
Indications	Drug would be destroyed in stomach if taken orally Self-administration desirable	Oral medication cannot be tolerated/used	Emergency situations Irritant medication Anaesthetics
Contraindications	Shock Inflamed or oedematous site	Emaciation Inflamed or oedematous site Shock Low platelet count Irritant substance	Poor venous access Irritant substance
Who may administer	Trained nurse Trainee nurse under supervision of trained nurse	Trained nurse Trainee nurse under supervision of trained nurse	Trained nurse who holds Extended Role certificate
Relative rate of onset of action	Slow	Moderate	Rapid
Maximum volume at one site	2 ml	2–5 ml	5–20 ml
Sites	Outer aspect of upper arm Outer aspect of thigh Abdominal wall, i.e. below umbilicus	Upper outer quadrant of buttock Middle outer aspect of thigh	Forearm Back of hand Antecubital fossa at elbow
Needle: length gauge	5/8 inch (16 mm) 25 g ($\frac{1}{2}$ inch (12 mm), 26g if abdomen used)	$1\frac{1}{2}$ inch (40 mm) 21g	1 inch (25 mm) 20g
Angle	45° to the skin 90° to the skin if using abdominal wall	90° to the skin	As near to parallel to the skin as possible
Hazards	Abscess formation	Nerve damage Abscess formation Injecting into large blood vessel	Cardiac embarrassment caused by very rapid administration Haematoma Extravasation Phlebitis/thrombophlebitis Air or particle embolism Localised infection Septicaemia

Intradermal (intracutaneous) injection

Intradermal injections are small volume injections of the order of 0.02 to 0.1 ml, given with a tuberculin syringe and a $1/2$ inch (12 mm) 26 gauge needle. The most common site used is the anterior aspect of the forearm. The injection is given *just* under the skin holding the syringe about parallel to the skin. The technique is most commonly used for the administration of certain diagnostic agents such as tuberculin PPD and skin testing solutions in the diagnosis of allergy. As the potential allergen is slowly injected a small weal forms.

In testing for allergy a distinct benefit in *not* cleansing the skin beforehand is that there is no risk of causing irritation which could interfere with the interpretation of the result.

Intrathecal injection

It is necessary to administer some drugs intrathecally if they have poor lipid solubility and, as a result, do not pass the blood–brain barrier. In the treatment of meningitis, water-soluble antibiotics are administered by the intrathecal route to achieve adequate concentrations in the cerebrospinal fluid (CSF). Drugs administered by this route include penicillins, the choice of which will depend on the results of bacteriological examination of the CSF. Doses have to be very carefully calculated and are much smaller than would be given by intramuscular or intravenous injection, since in effect, the antibiotic is being introduced into a closed system. Examples of drugs and adult doses administered intrathecally are shown in Box 27.5.

Box 27.5   Examples of adult doses of drugs administered intrathecally

Ampicillin	20 mg	Cloxacillin	20 mg
Benzylpenicillin	6–12 mg	Gentamicin	1 mg
Carbenicillin	20 mg		

Reduced doses are given to infants and children. Methotrexate is administered intrathecally (15 mg at weekly intervals) to treat meningeal leukaemia. In addition, antifungal agents, opioids, corticosteroids and radio-opaque substances, used in the diagnosis of spinal lesions, are sometimes administered by this route. A product specially prepared for the intrathecal route should be used. In many instances intrathecal therapy is supported by a course of the drug given by intramuscular or intravenous injection.

Technique

Drugs for intrathecal injection are normally injected between lumbar vertebrae 3 and 4 into the subarachnoid space of the spinal cord as part of the procedure of lumbar puncture. The role of the nurse is directed towards careful positioning of the patient, assisting the doctor in maintaining an aseptic technique and providing the patient with support and encouragement throughout the procedure.

It is vitally important to maintain full asepsis in this procedure because of the risk of infection being introduced into the CNS. Great care has to be taken with all the manipulations involved. Any diluent (in some instances CSF) used for the drug must of course be sterile and must be free from any bacteriostatic agent or preservative which would damage the delicate tissues of the CNS. The injection as well as being sterile, must not contain particulate matter. A sterile, disposable bacterial filter (0.22 micrometre) must be used between the syringe and needle as a final safeguard for the patient.

INTRAVENOUS INFUSION

When large volumes of fluid (50 ml upwards) require to be administered over a prolonged period, the most effective method is intravenous infusion. The indications for intravenous infusion are:

- to maintain or restore blood volume
- to supply electrolytes or nutrients
- to administer medication, including irritant substances such as certain cytotoxic agents.

Intravenous infusions are packed in either plastic

containers or glass bottles and are delivered to the patient via an intravenous administration set (Fig. 27.12) attached to an intravenous cannula (Fig. 27.13) which has been inserted into the patient's vein. Because of the considerable risk of introducing infection directly into the blood-stream, the infusion fluid, all parts of the administration equipment and any dressings used must be sterile.

Although introducing an intravenous cannula and establishing the free flow of the infusion are the doctor's responsibility, the care of the patient before and after the procedure, and the satisfactory maintenance of the intravenous line rests with the nurse.

Before assembling an intravenous line, it is important to read and check carefully the label of the infusion container against the fluid prescription. The expiry date should be checked. The batch number of each container is always recorded so that in the event of an adverse reaction to the infusion, the offending containers may be identified and withdrawn. The container should also be inspected to ensure it has no flaws and that the fluid is clear and free from particulate matter.

Bottles require an airway to act as a vent as the fluid runs through the administration set whereas plastic containers do not, since they simply collapse as they empty. The rubber cap or entry port is pierced by the spike of the apppropriate administration set, the filter chamber squeezed to fill the set with fluid, air removed from the tubing and the control clamp closed. The free end of the administration set is covered by its sheath until required for use. Once an infusion container is connected to an administration set, it should not hang for more than 24 hours because of risk of contamination through any of the points of entry (Fig 27.14).

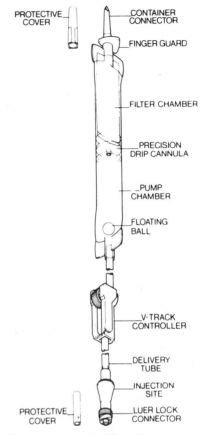

Figure 27.12 Intravenous administration set.

The flow rate is adjusted by means of a roll or screw clamp attached to the tubing. Where accurate control of flow rate is essential, an automatic infusion system (Fig. 27.15) may be used which pumps solutions at a preset rate varying from 50 to 150 ml per hour in adults.

Adjuncts are sometimes used in conjunction with this system, e.g. a calibrated burette may be incorporated in the system into which the infusion drips. One or more drugs can be added to the burette and this is very useful, particularly

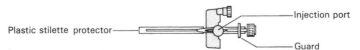

Figure 27.13 Intravenous cannula. (From Jamieson, McCall & Blythe 1992 Guidelines for clinical nursing practices. 2nd edn. Churchill Livingstone.)

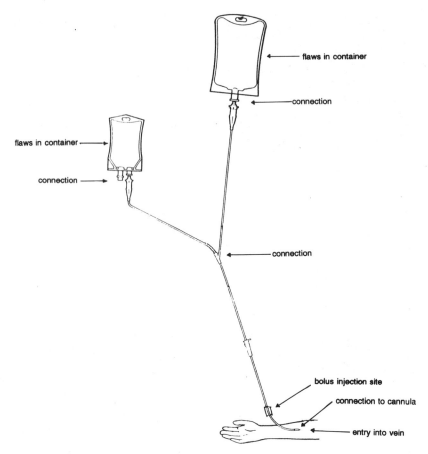

Figure 27.14 Points of entry of contamination.

in intensive care, for intermittent infusion of potent drugs in precise volumes. Drugs may be slowly injected through an additive port in the administration set or can be added to minibottles or minibags usually containing either 5% w/v glucose in water or 0.9% w/v sodium chloride injection. These secondary containers are piggy-backed to the large volume primary container by inserting the needle from the minicontainer administration set into an injection port on the primary administration set (Fig. 27.16). Piggy-back containers may be used to give a higher intermittent blood level of a particular drug than would be achieved if the drug were added to the larger primary container, or to avoid an incompatibility with a drug which may already be present in the primary container.

Drugs commonly given by intravenous infu-

sion include antibiotics, lignocaine, heparin and potassium chloride. The infusion maintains a steady blood level of the drug over a prolonged period of time and the patient is spared the pain of frequent injections. The addition of drugs to intravenous infusion fluids presents a number of hazards (e.g. resulting from interaction between the drug and the infusion fluid). Drugs should not be added to blood, plasma, lipid emulsions, saturated mannitol solutions, sodium bicarbonate solutions, amino acid solutions or dextran solutions because these infusion fluids are particularly likely to be degraded.

In addition to interactions, the fluid infused can be contaminated by microorganisms if admixtures are not carried out under strict aseptic conditions. Ideally, these additions should be made by pharmacy staff using laminar air flow cabinets in

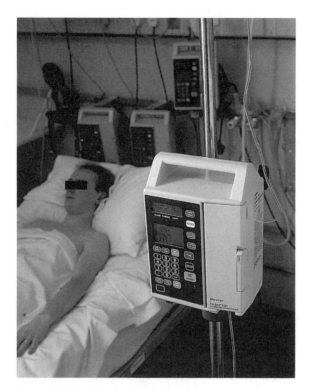

Figure 27.15 Volumetric infusion pump.

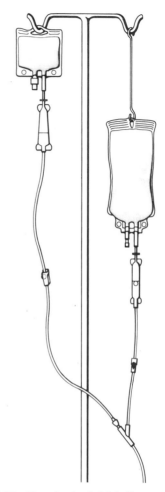

Figure 27.16 Piggy-back administration system.

aseptic rooms and administered within 12–24 hours. Complications such as thrombophlebitis may arise at, and spread beyond the site of cannula insertion. This results from physical or chemical irritation often related to the duration of the infusion or the type of fluid infused. Glucose is mildly acidic and on autoclaving a small quantity is broken down to hydroxy-methylfurfural and these two factors appear to cause a higher incidence of thrombophlebitis when glucose infusions are given. Blood for transfusion should never be mixed with any drug or solution other than 0.9% sodium chloride because of the danger of interaction. If a unit of blood is preceded by a solution such as glucose, agglutination may result. To avoid this, the administration set should be flushed with 0.9% sodium chloride solution or changed.

The standard procedure for prescribing, checking and recording the administration of medicines similarly applies to intravenous infusions. It is important that the patient has an outline of the procedure explained to him in advance and that he is given the chance to have his toilet needs met. A change into a garment with wider sleeves may be required to ensure the infusion flows unobstructed. If possible, whichever arm/hand will make things easier for the patient should be used. The patient should be comfortable, with the site of introduction of the fluid exposed and well lit. Some pain is usually experienced with the insertion of a needle and many patients appreciate having the support and encouragement of the nurse at this time.

The commonest sites of introduction are the forearm, the back of the hand and the antecubital fossa at the elbow. In an emergency, a vein in the foot or the external jugular vein may have to be used. A large straight vein preferably at the junction of two veins and not running over a joint is the one of choice.

The insertion of an intravenous cannula should be regarded as a minor surgical procedure. This together with the fact that a cannula is to be lying in the vein for possibly several days means asepsis is the main objective. The prevention of microbial contamination begins with the appropriate handwashing technique. Careful preparation of the skin is important prior to insertion of the cannula. Atlhough clipping extra long hairs with scissors facilitates the subsequent removal of adhesive tape and is acceptable, shaving the skin is not recommended since it produces tiny abrasions which may become infected. Any visible dirt is washed from the area with soap and water.

Before completing the preparation of the skin, the venous outflow is blocked and the vein distended by applying pressure above the site. This may be achieved in one of three ways:

- the use of a tourniquet
- the use of a sphygmomanometer cuff inflated to 100 mm of mercury
- with the help of an assistant, making sure not to apply too great pressure as this may occlude the arterial supply.

The vein can also be made more prominent in different ways. For example:

- asking the patient to open and close the fist
- gently tapping the vein
- immersing the hand in warm water.

Increased venodilation can also be achieved using glyceryl trinitrate applied in the form of a cream or transdermal patch (see p. 434) distal to the site of cannulation 20–30 minutes before venepuncture is performed.

Finally, the site is rubbed firmly for at least 30 seconds using a 70% alcohol swab and allowed to dry before puncturing the skin. Any further finger contact with the vein should be avoided.

Intravenous cannulae of different gauges are available. A small gauge cannula is sufficient for the delivery of most therapy and limits both the size of the wound and the incidence of intravascular complications. When viscous fluids are to be administered, a large gauge cannula is required.

The cannula is checked to ensure that it is patent and has no obvious defects. With the bevelled edge uppermost, the cannula is firmly entered under the skin a short distance away from the vein, always pointing the cannula proximally towards the heart. It is then gently pushed into the vein making sure to enter the plastic covering on the needle as well as the needle itself into the vein. Some types of cannula show a flash of blood at the hilt of the needle indicating that the needle, but not necessarily the plastic cannula, is in the vein. The tourniquet is then removed and simultaneously the needle withdrawn and the plastic cannula gently advanced into the vein. A well-sited cannula should introduce with little or no resistence. The tubing of the administration set is quickly attached. Gentle pressure on the vein proximal to the cannula tip prevents a leakage of blood through the cannula.

When a small vein is used, the tubing may be attached earlier so that the cannula advances, whilst at the same time infusing fluid through it, thus displacing the walls of the vein. The control clamp is released and the flow rate observed. Subcutaneous swelling around the cannula indicates that it is not in the vein and must be removed.

The cannula is secured using either a sterile gauze dressing or a semi-occlusive transparent dressing. The adjacent tubing is taped so as to prevent any pull on the cannula. A light conforming bandage promotes patient comfort. A splint may be applied and is essential if the cannula has been positioned over a joint.

On completion of the procedure the patient should be made comfortable with the arm supported on a pillow if required. Personal requirements such as a drink, tissues, sickness basin, reading material, etc, should be placed within reach. The call bell should also be to hand and instruction in its use given.

A regimen of fluids to be infused is prescribed by the doctor. The rate of flow required (i.e. the number of drops per minute) can be calculated on the basis that 1 ml equals 15 drops, that is:

$$\text{drops/minute} = \frac{\text{volume of fluid (ml)} \times 15}{\text{duration (min)}}$$

Thus, for 500 ml of fluid to be run through in 4 hours the number of drops per minute is:

$$\frac{500 \times 15}{240} = 31.25$$

For working purposes, this figure may be regarded as 30.

Alternative methods of introducing an intravenous line are either by surgically cutting down on a vein and introducing the cannula under direct vision (e.g. when no veins are visible or patent) or by means of a central venous line (e.g. for prolonged feeding or for central venous pressure measurement). Both of these techniques are specialised procedures which are undertaken by experienced medical staff.

Throughout the ongoing administration of the infusion, the nurse's responsibilities are as follows.

Observing the patient

Each time the patient is attended by the nurse his colour, respirations and general demeanour should be observed. An elevated temperature is noteworthy.

Observing the infusion

A check is made that the infusion is running at the prescribed rate and that the container still has enough fluid in it. The nurse must anticipate the point when the container requires to be changed and estimate how much time will be required to get the next container checked and ready for use.

If the infusion is not running, a systematic list of checks should be made:

- 'drip' stand high enough?
- spike of administration set far enough into bag/bottle?

- in the case of a glass bottle, air inlet in use and patent?
- all connections secure?
- control clamp open!   ·
- tubing kinked or obstructed?
- tape, splint, bandage too tight?
- limb in relaxed position?

Nurses must resist the temptation to try to restart infusions using traditional tricks such as nipping the tubing or winding it round a pair of scissors. These practices create an increase in pressure inside the vein and can damage its wall leading to extravasation. It can also be extremely painful for the patient.

Observing the cannula site

The nurse must be alert to any:

- redness
- swelling
- leakage
- complaints from the patient of pain at or radiating from the cannula site.

Keeping accurate records

The following records must be maintained:

- fluid prescription sheet
- fluid balance sheet
- nursing care plan and progress notes.

Providing nursing care as required

Even the most able patient requires some assistance when one limb is not fully functional. Indeed, patients are to be discouraged from trying to be too independent as this can create movement of the cannula in the vein causing a mechanical phlebitis. Assistance with changing position, toileting, dressing, cutting up food, etc, will often be required.

Reporting abnormalities

Although the infusion is established by a doctor, the doctor depends on the nurse to notify him of any changes in the patient's condition , either of a localised or generalised nature, and any difficulties encountered with the infusion. To reduce the risk of infection it is normally recommended that administration sets are changed after 3 days. However, sets should be changed directly following blood transfusion and in the case of total parenteral nutrition, daily.

The hazards associated with intravenous infusion may be localised or systemic and are potentially very dangerous.

Local hazards are:

- thrombophlebitis
- infection
- extravasation.

Systemic hazards are:

- septicaemia
- cardiac embarrassment caused by too rapid rate
- allergic reaction to fluid or drug
- air or particle embolism.

Consequently, checking procedures, asepsis, careful observation and prompt reporting are vitally important.

TRANSDERMAL ADMINISTRATION

Although most preparations are applied topically to give a local effect, the topical route can also be used to achieve a systemic effect. This is the transdermal route of administration. Drugs administered in this way avoid first-pass metabolism by the liver (see Fig. 2.1, p. 11). The best known is glyceryl trinitrate. Where flexibility of dosage is required this may be achieved with the application of an ointment containing 2% glyceryl trinitrate. Magnitude and duration of effect are directly related to the amount of ointment applied. It is therefore possible by this method to titrate the dosage against the clinical presentation of the patient. To obtain the optimum dosage, 12 mm (0.5 inches) of ointment is applied on the first day, followed by 12 mm increments on each successive day until headache occurs; this length is then reduced by 12 mm. A graduated paper scale facilitates measurement of the dose. When applied to the skin the ointment is covered with a simple dressing. It is not rubbed in.

A more sophisticated transdermal drug delivery system is the transdermal patch. Patches containing a reservoir of glyceryl trinitrate (see Fig. 27.17) are specially designed to achieve a prolonged and constant release of the drug. The main clinical indication for glyceryl trinitrate patches is in the prophylaxis of angina pectoris. The patches have also been used in the prophylactic treatment of phlebitis and extravasation, secondary to long-term venous cannulation.

Patches are available from which the average amount absorbed in 24 hours is either 5 or 10 milligrams. One patch is applied every 24 hours to a hairless area to ensure that it sticks well. The anterior or lateral chest wall is recommended although the upper abdomen and upper arm are other suitable sites. The site should have been washed and thoroughly dried although not powdered before applying the patch.

The sachet in which the patch is packaged should be torn rather than cut open otherwise the patch might get damaged. Without touching the sticky surface (which contains some medicament), the backing is removed and the patch applied pressing firmly for about 5 seconds to ensure complete contact. The patch is then sealed to keep out air or water by running the finger round its edge. A different area should be used each day to avoid skin irritation. Patients who are to be self-administering a transdermal drug for the first time should be counselled in its use. Tolerance to glyceryl trinitrate can develop. There is evidence to suggest that this may be countered by intermittent therapy.

Several other drugs may be administered by this route. For example, a hyoscine patch to prevent motion sickness is placed behind the ear and replaced if necessary after 72 hours behind the other ear; oestradiol used in hormone replacement therapy is applied to unbroken areas below the waistline (not on or near the breasts) and is replaced after 3–4 days. Nicotine transdermal patches are available for weaning addicted smokers off their nicotine dependence.

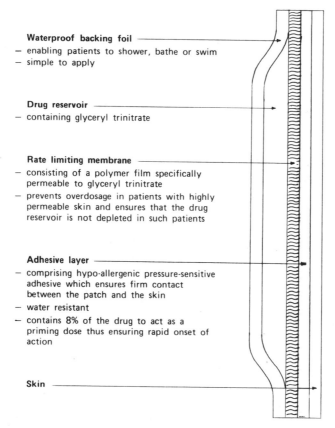

Waterproof backing foil
— enabling patients to shower, bathe or swim
— simple to apply

Drug reservoir
— containing glyceryl trinitrate

Rate limiting membrane
— consisting of a polymer film specifically
permeable to glyceryl trinitrate
— prevents overdosage in patients with highly
permeable skin and ensures that the drug
reservoir is not depleted in such patients

Adhesive layer
— comprising hypo-allergenic pressure-sensitive
adhesive which ensures firm contact
between the patch and the skin
— water resistant
— contains 8% of the drug to act as a
priming dose thus ensuring rapid onset of
action

Skin

Figure 27.17 Transdermal drug delivery system (rate-controlling membrane type).

The transdermal route of administration offers many advantages to the patient and the nurse, since it is non-invasive and convenient. However the high technology involved in developing and producing transdermal systems results in a relatively high cost product. While the number of drugs that can be administered transdermally is gradually expanding there are many problems to be overcome before a clinically effective product can be introduced. Not least of these problems is the efficient barrier to systemic absorption provided by the skin itself.

TOPICAL THERAPY IN SKIN DISORDERS

Although patients with specific skin diseases are often nursed in dermatological wards with specially trained and experienced staff to care for them, many patients in other wards and in the community will, at some time, require nursing care for skin conditions. It is important to recognise that many systemic diseases manifest at least one of their diagnostic features in the skin (Table 27.2). Moreover, the skin acts as a barometer for the general health of the body and this should not be forgotten when treating specific skin diseases.

The comfort of the patient

Treatment of the skin, whether carried out at the bedside or in a treatment room, calls for consideration of a number of factors. First and foremost, privacy must be provided and maintained, and every effort made to ensure that the dignity

Table 27.2 Skin manifestations of systemic diseases

Systemic disease	Skin manifestation(s)
Congestive cardiac failure	Cyanosed; oedematous
Hypertension	May be highly coloured
Chronic obstructive airways disease	Dusky hue or bright pink
Obstructive jaundice	Deep yellow, itching
Hypoglycaemia	Profusely sweating
Diabetic coma	Dry, smelling of acetone
Thyrotoxicosis	Warm; moist
Myxoedema	Dry; coarse
Chronic renal failure	Yellow-brown; uraemic frost
Iron deficiency anaemia	Pale
Pernicious anaemia	Pale lemon-tinted
Viral diseases of childhood	Characteristic rashes; itching

of the patient is preserved. The room should be adequately ventilated but free of draughts.

When caring for patients with a disorder of the skin the nurse should ensure that the environment is conducive to good communication. Here, an individualised approach to the patient is of paramount importance. The management of patients with an apparently similar condition should play no part. Only in a one-to-one situation can there be a satisfactory exchange of views leading to better understanding. The chances of the patient maintaining compliance with the treatment prescribed will be greatly increased if he is helped by the nurse to understand the rationale behind it.

Irrespective of the treatment being followed, all patients with skin conditions need to be cared for with real sensitivity. Feelings of shame, disgust and fear have for long troubled patients with skin diseases often forcing them to hide from the gaze of others. To some extent, this situation has been perpetuated by the attitude of health professionals towards these patients. Sadly, staff may make patients with skin conditions feel 'unclean' by isolating them unnecessarily in single rooms and adopting overprotective measures while treating them. In time, the patient may respond with antisocial behaviour which in turn may affect the attitudes of others until what can only be described as a 'leper complex' develops. Unless it is absolutely necessary to do otherwise, these patients should be shown the same consideration afforded to all other patients. Trust and confidence need to be restored by adopting an open and optimistic outlook. This in itself has a beneficial 'therapeutic' effect.

Assessment

There is no substitute for identifying the cause of the problem and tackling it at source. Since two people suffering from the same condition will rarely present in an identical way it is essential that a thorough assessment is made by examination and questioning. Both visual (often using a hand lens) and tactile examination will be required. Temperature, tension and sensitivity of the skin may be ascertained by careful touching of the affected part(s) using a disposable plastic glove as appropriate. Where it is suspected that a skin condition is due to a reaction to an irritant or allergen, systematic questioning may help to identify the cause, as will carefully managed patch testing.

Treatment selection

Selection of a product by either doctor or nurse requires care, since the choice is very wide indeed. The BNF alone contains several hundred different topical applications. In addition, specially formulated products can be prescribed for patients whose needs cannot be met by an 'off the shelf' formulation. In this case the range of products available is as wide as the prescriber's imagination.

Many skin conditions require the attention of a consultant dermatologist (or other clinician), who will prescribe the treatment. In most primary care, nurses will use their own professional expertise to determine how best to care for a patient's skin problem. The question of where the dividing line lies between the action that it is appropriate for the nurse or doctor to take may create problems. These can be avoided in two ways. Within a particular ward there may be a local agreement that nurses have delegated authority to use certain topical preparations in accordance with written protocols. Another approach, developed in Grampian and other health authorities, is to define, in a formulary of nursing care products, those preparations which are routinely available, without medical prescription, for use by nurses (Table 27.3, Box 27.6).

The formulary illustrated does not include products containing antibiotic, corticosteroid or other potent drugs, since the use of these agents is accompanied by certain risks. Symptoms may be masked by the use of corticosteroids, and the use of certain antibiotics is associated with sensitisation reactions.

Box 27.6   Monograph from nursing care formulary: details for zinc and castor oil ointment

Actions
Zinc oxide 7.5%, Castor oil 50%, Arachis oil 30.5%, White beeswax 10%, Cetostearyl alcohol 2%. Zinc and castor oil ointment is an emollient and a barrier cream with mild astringent properties.

Precautions
1. For external use only.
2. Not for use on eyes.

Availability
Routinely in 15 g tubes.

Storage
Avoid excessive heat and store in a locked cupboard set aside for external preparations.

Table 27.3   Contents of formulary of nursing care products

Type/region of care	Products in formulary
Hair, nose and mouth	Malathion lotion Mouthwash solution tablets Sodium bicarbonate 1–160 aqueous solution Hydrogen peroxide solution
Skin care	Benzalkonium and cetrimide cream (Drapolene) Calamine lotion Chlorhexidine gluconate hand scrub Chlorhexidine gluconate 0.5% in 7% IMS E45 cream Emulsifying wax 3% in water Hexachlorophene dusting powder (Ster-Zac) Alcoholic solution of iodine 2.5% w/v Kaolin poultice BP Lubricating jelly Oilatum emollient Olive oil Paraffin yellow soft Plaster remover Povidone-iodine antiseptic solution Soltan sun cream SPF 25 Talc Thovaline Zinc and castor oil ointment
Wound cleaning and care	Chlorhexidine/cetrimide solution (sachets) Hydrogen peroxide solution Povidone-iodine ointment Sodium chloride sterile solution (sachets)
Local anaesthetic gel	Lignocaine gel (2%)
Medicated dressings	Chlorhexidine acetate gauze dressing
Laxatives	Glycerol suppositories BP Sodium citrate microenema

Prescribing of topical preparations

Unless included in a nursing formulary, topical preparations which contain a specific drug should be regarded in exactly the same way as any other medicine. It follows therefore that prescribing, administration and recording of such products should be in accordance with established policies and procedures for systemic therapy.

Special prescription sheets are required for the prescribing of topical preparations in hospital as it is necessary to incorporate a greater amount of information than the standard in-patient prescription sheet allows. The prescription should include:

- date of the prescription
- name of the preparation; a specially made up formula may consist of several different substances which should be listed
- formulation and its strength; where necessary, details such as aqueous or oily should be given; it is better, where possible, to describe the strength as a percentage; ratios (e.g. 1:9) can be misleading
- quantity to be applied; this may be difficult to quantify; sparingly, liberally, 1 cm or 'a worm' are expressions which may be used; the most commonly used instruction given is 'as sparingly as possible'

- site(s) for application; these should be described specifically (e.g. 'all active areas', 'wherever the skin is dry'); vague expressions such as 'all over' should be avoided
- dressings and bandages to be used; the size of each should be appropriate to the size of the patient's lesion
- number of times of administration; this should span a 24-hour period and should be divided evenly throughout the patient's waking day
- doctor's signature.

Prescribing systemic therapy for dermatological conditions is carried out in the same way as all other systemic prescribing.

Formulation of topical preparations

Several different pharmaceutical preparations (ointments, lotions, etc) are available, each of which has distinctive physical characteristics quite apart from the nature of the active ingredient. In some instances products are used solely for their physical properties, e.g. emollients, barrier preparations and sunscreens. Although a detailed discussion of formulation aspects is outside the scope of this book, certain important principles are emphasised below since they have practical implications for the nurse. Typically, a pharmaceuticul product intended for topical application will have some, or all, of the following components.

Active ingredient(s)

The concentration of the active ingredient(s) will normally be expressed as a percentage weight in weight, e.g. 1% w/w hydrocortisone cream.

Vehicle

The overall characteristics of the product will depend on the vehicle chosen. The vehicle may be aqueous, non-aqueous, liquid or semi-solid depending on the properties required and nature of the active ingredient. Penetration of the active ingredient into the skin is influenced by the properties of the vehicle and nature of the condition being treated. The make up of the vehicle used in proprietary preparations varies greatly. In order to help trace the source of a local reaction to a product it may be necessary to seek information on all the components of the product in order that the source of the problem can be identified.

Antimicrobial preservative agent

The risk of microbial contamination of topical products, especially those containing a high proportion of water, during their use is significant, so it is essential, unless the product is a single-use pack, to include an antimicrobial agent.

Emulsifying/suspending agent

These are required to give a product physical stability, e.g. an emulsifying agent stabilises oil-in-water preparations, and a suspending agent is necessary when insoluble powders of high density are included in a liquid preparation.

Other additives

For example, a buffering agent may be included to give a preparation with a pH approximating to that of normal skin.

Topical preparations and their use

The terms 'cream', 'ointment', 'lotion', etc, are fairly precise but may not always be used in a totally consistent way. Care should always be taken to determine the actual properties of the product which, like other pharmaceuticals, may not always be conveyed by its name.

Creams

Creams are normally oil-in-water emulsions which, since water is the continuous phase, are easily removed, even from hairy areas, by normal cleansing procedures. The evaporation of the water present in the cream produces a useful cooling effect. Drainage from a lesion is facilitated because creams absorb exudates. Drugs normally incorporated into creams include corticosteroids, antibacterial and antifungal agents. Good penetration of the active ingredient into the skin is achieved and may be enhanced due to the presence of a surfactant (emulsifying agent) in the cream. Creams also have a softening effect on thickened tissues.

Although creams normally contain an antimicrobial preservative they should be used with great care to avoid microbial contamination since the antimicrobial agents available for incorporation into creams have a limited spectrum of activity. The antimicrobial agent (and/or active ingredient) may cause skin sensitivity in some patients. Creams are more cosmetically acceptable than ointments especially when applied to the face, as they disappear when rubbed into the skin.

Ointments

It is very important to distinguish between ointments and creams because the two products have different properties. Ointments are normally greasy anhydrous preparations which do not mix with water and therefore should not be applied to exuding lesions. They are occlusive and encourage hydration. Ointments are more difficult to remove from the skin than creams. Soft paraffins are widely used in ointment bases, incorporating liquid paraffin to achieve the required consistency. Ointments soften crusts but are generally not suitable for application to hairy areas. They are particularly useful for application to dry scaly areas.

Being non-aqueous, antimicrobial agents are only occasionally required to be included in ointments and so there is less risk of sensitisation from this source than with creams. However, lanolin wool (wool fat) and derivatives are sometimes included in ointments and may cause contact sensitivity.

Other preparations

Products are also available that combine the properties of both ointments and creams. Such formulations are described as ambiphillic. The formulation is a stable emulsion system with a uniform distribution of fat and water.

Application of creams and ointments

As already stated, ointments and creams generally have different properties and the indications for their use relate to these. However, the guidance given above is not inflexible. A most important aspect is to use a preparation which is acceptable to the patient. These products should be applied as sparingly as possible to affected part(s). If applying a prescribed product the prescriber's instructions must be complied with. Creams and ointments are best applied in the same way as make-up. Small dots of the product are placed at suitable intervals over the area to be treated. Using the tip of the index finger and/or second finger for small areas and the palm of the hand for larger areas, the cream should be spread evenly as far as it will go within the area to be treated. Plain lint or gauze dressings may be required to cover areas to which creams and ointments have been applied.

Pastes

These preparations are essentially similar to ointments but contain a high proportion of powders, have a very stiff consistency, and will adhere to lesions at body temperature. Pastes also have protective properties. Compound zinc paste for example contains 25% by weight of zinc oxide and 20% by weight of starch with 50% white soft paraffin.

Application of pastes

Pastes should only be applied to specific lesions, e.g. in psoriasis, and not to the surrounding skin. Where a paste contains a highly active ingredient (e.g. dithranol), it will be necessary to protect the skin adjacent to the lesion with a bland product such as yellow soft paraffin. If the paste is soft enough (temperature will obviously influence the consistency of the product), it may be applied with the finger(s) of a gloved hand. Pastes which cannot be applied in this way may be applied with a wooden spatula. Pastes will seldom be required to be covered with a dressing, except where it is necessary to protect the patient's linen from staining by the active ingredient. They are not popular with patients as they are messy and difficult to apply.

Dusting powders

Dusting powders are of two main types, medicated and non-medicated. All dusting powders have a basis of starch (absorbent) and talc (lubricant). Non-medicated powders are used in general nursing care to reduce friction and absorb moisture between skin folds. The skin should be clean and well dried before each application. Excessive use should be avoided since 'caking' in skin folds may result causing local irritation or trauma.

Medicated powders have a limited place in the active ingredient of skin diseases since it is generally not possible to achieve a satisfactory concentration of active ingredient at the site of the lesion for any length of time. Dusting powders containing suitable active ingredients are mainly used in prophylaxis (e.g. the prevention of athlete's foot, or the prevention of neonatal staphylococcal cross-infection). Dusting powders containing antibiotics are occasionally used in the treatment of superficial bacterial infections such as impetigo when the powder will tend to stick to the lesions.

Lotions

Lotions are normally simple formulations containing active ingredients in an aqueous solution or suspension. Occasionally oily lotions are used, but such preparations have very different properties to a lotion with an aqueous base since they are water-in-oil emulsions. Lotions with an aqueous base are used in weeping eruptions where they cool and dry the skin by evaporation. In very acute conditions lotions are used to relieve superficial inflammation and assist in the removal of crusts. When the presence of fine solid particles cannot even be tolerated by the patient, lotions which are simple solutions are used until the most acute phase of the condition has passed. Then lotions containing powders in suspension can be used. The cooling properties of a lotion may be enhanced by the addition of alcohol to the vehicle, but this may cause stinging. (Excessive cooling due to the use of lotions must be avoided especially in the elderly.)

Lotions may be useful for the application of a drug to a hairy area of the body where the use of a greasy ointment or stiff paste would be inappropriate or impracticable. In very acute conditions lotions may be applied as wet dressings using lint or other closely-woven fabric. As with all dressings, care should be taken on removal so as to avoid damaging the epithelium. Any dressings that have dried out should be thoroughly wetted with the lotion before being carefully removed. Lotions may also be applied to small lesions using cotton wool or to larger areas using a suitable flat brush.

Paints

Paints are solutions of the active drug in a suitable solvent, such as water, alcohol or a mixture of solvents, depending on the nature of the active ingredient. Application to the skin is normally by means of a brush.

Pressurised aerosols

Pressurised aerosols are widely available for the application of drugs to the skin in such conditions as superficial bacterial infections. Protective applications can also be applied in this way. It is important to use the product in accordance with the manufacturer's recommendations, and to ensure safe disposal of the empty canister. Pressurised aerosols are convenient to use, and confer the advantages of 'no touch' technique, but are relatively expensive.

Nail varnishes

A varnish formulation containing an antifungal

agent is available for the treatment of fungal infections of the nails. The varnish ensures prolonged contact of the antifungal agent with the infected tissue.

Paste bandages

A range of bandages is available which are impregnated with a zinc oxide paste combined with either coal tar, calamine, ichthammol or hydrocortisone. Paste bandages are used for the treatment of such conditions as eczema, leg ulcers and chronic dermatitis.

Special procedures

Skin cleansing

Before applying a topical preparation the skin should be clean. To prevent accumulation, previous applications to the skin should be removed. This is especially important where drugs such as corticosteroids are involved. In order to remove creams, paints, powders or lotions, the patient, or the site, should be bathed using simple soaps and warm water. (Perfumed toilet soap should be avoided.) Pastes, ointments and certain paints are best removed with cotton wool soaked in liquid paraffin or olive oil.

Bathing

Often nurses are not completely satisfied with their work unless all their patients have been bathed. With increasing changes in the skin towards dryness after about the age of 35, the tendency should be towards a reduction in the frequency in bathing. Soaking in a hot bath makes the skin dry due to loss of natural oils and causes epidermal cells to shrink on drying. Any itching of the skin is increased. A conscious effort should be made to adjust routine and not to overwash patients, particularly elderly people and those patients whose skin is noticeably dry. With the shift of emphasis towards individualised nursing care, nurses are well placed to make an assessment of the patient's skin and decide on the care required.

Patients with skin conditions should be advised to resist the temptation to use any cosmetic bath additives. Detergents or antiseptics may cause the patient further problems and should be avoided. To occlude the skin and thus prevent drying by evaporation, liquid paraffin or olive oil may be used. An emollient such as emulsifying ointment may be added to the bath water. This also acts as a mild occlusive and helps to retain moisture in the skin. An oily bath is obviously exceedingly dangerous and therefore it is vitally important that the patient is forewarned of the risk of slipping. The nurse should make a careful judgement as to whether the patient can be safely left to get out of the bath unaided. In any case, the bath should be emptied before the patient climbs out. A secure bath mat should be made available. After using an emollient, the bath needs careful cleaning. It should be filled full with hot water and have a suitable detergent added having first ensured that there are no patients in the vicinity who may mistakenly think that the bath has been filled for their use. The bath is then allowed to empty and as it does so, the water should be agitated and the sides cleaned to remove all traces of the emollient.

Scalp treatment

Shampoos may be used for cleaning or for treatment purposes. Triethanolamine lauryl sulphate 40% forms the basis of some shampoos. It has no additives and is the least irritant. It is therefore useful as a simple cleansing agent for the scalp. Psoriasis of the scalp may be treated with either a tar-based or a desquamative shampoo. Antiseptic shampoos are available for the infected scalp.

Precautions have to be taken to protect the eyes and face from contact with shampoos used as treatment. The patient should be warned to keep his eyes closed throughout the procedure. With gloved hands, two applications are made – the first, a thorough wash to cleanse the scalp; the second, active treatment. Between applications and at the finish, the shampoo should be rinsed out of the hair. The hair is dried with a hair-dryer as soon as possible. Some scalp applications are flammable and when using such products patients should be warned not to dry the hair near a naked flame.

Applying topical preparations (Box 27.7)

Topical preparations should not be applied to normal skin as this wastes time, wastes the product and may do harm. Generally speaking, if the condition is acute then the frequency of the treatment and the strength of the active ingredient(s) may be increased rather than the amount applied. It is only the active ingredient(s) in contact with the affected skin which is going to aid healing – not the layers on top. A 'little can do a lot of good, a lot can do a lot of harm' is a maxim worth remembering.

Box 27.7   Application of topical preparations

Documentation
Special prescription sheet for topical medicines

The medicine
Creams, ointment, pastes, dusting powders, lotions, paints as prescribed

The environment
Such as to ensure privacy
Adequately ventilated but free of draughts

The nurse and the patient
Patient identified
Explanation given to patient
Willingness of nurse to listen to what patient wants to say
Patient given realistic encouragement

Technique
Hand hygiene before and after administration
Polythene gloves worn by nurse
Preparations applied gently and sparingly
Dressing kept to minimum size necessary

Hazards
Irritation of the skin
Infection from contaminated containers

Patients' response to treatment

In-patients undergoing treatment for a skin condition should be given the opportunity at least every 48 hours to express how they feel their condition is responding, and the comments should be recorded in the patient's progress report. In order to gain an account which truly reflects the patient's view of his progress the nurse must be prepared as far as possible to listen to him when he chooses to raise the subject. The opportunity will often arise during a treatment session. It is not sufficient for the nurse to express her view of progress being made. Whatever the nurse observes about the patient himself or his skin, it is important to record what the patient says even if it is simply that he is feeling better or worse.

Patient compliance

Skin conditions are frequently of a chronic or recurring nature which often necessitates teaching patients and/or relatives how to continue treatment. Advice given may include appropriate skin cleansing and the method of application as well as any special precautions such as skin protection and protection of personal linen. Teaching should be realistic and helpful if a reasonable degree of compliance is to be assured. There would be little point in asking a patient to apply a tar preparation before going out in an evening because of its antisocial effect. To most patients, a large unsightly dressing would be equally unacceptable. For the application of an ointment, some disabled patients may find a long-handled ointment applicator of assistance in reaching inaccessible parts of the body. Where there is a degree of difficulty in applying skin preparations, in the absence of a capable family member, it is essential to arrange for the treatment to be carried out by the district nurse.

Safety and storage

In hospitals topical applications must be kept in a locked cupboard set aside for external preparations, careful attention being paid to expiry dates. To prevent cross-infection patients should be supplied with individually dispensed skin applications. Where this is not possible, a quantity of the preparation should be removed from its container with a spatula. If more of the preparation is required, a new spatula should be used. Since rolling up a collapsible tube to expel the contents may obliterate the label it is preferable to squeeze the tube progressively along its entire length.

Hazards

The nurse should be aware of the potential hazards inherent in treating skin conditions. Moreover, she should take the opportunity given to her to set a good example to the patient when carrying out treatments. The precautions to be taken are as follows:

- Skin preparations should be applied in accordance with the prescription.
- Polythene gloves should be worn when applying any preparation to the skin (unless a spatula or brush is being used) so that the nurse does not risk absorbing the active ingredients.
- Creams, especially those prepared by dilution of a primary product, may support bacterial growth and should therefore be used with care to avoid contamination. All creams will bear an expiry date after which the preparation should not be used.
- Topical corticosteroid preparations should be used with extreme caution to avoid the possibility of skin damage and systemic absorption, that is:
  applied gently wearing polythene gloves in exact accordance with the prescription never to treat a minor skin problem supported by counselling of patients, relatives and carers as appropriate.

ADMINISTRATION OF INHALED DRUGS

The fact that drugs can be introduced directly into the pulmonary system is highly advantageous. Not only is their absorption through the lungs rapid but high concentrations of drugs can be obtained in the bronchial mucosa and smooth muscle with minimal systemic side-effects. Inhalation of drugs can be accomplished with the help of inhalation devices such as the:

aerosol inhaler
   spacer devices
   Nebuhaler
   breath-actuated autohaler
dry powder inhaler
wet nebuliser
   Porta-Neb.

Aerosol inhalers

How they work

Most commonly, drugs are delivered to the lungs as sprays from pressurised aerosol dispensers (aerosol inhalers). The drug and its inert propellant, such as freon, are maintained under pressure in a small canister. When the valve is activated, a measured quantity of propellant carrying the drug is released through the mouthpiece.

Administration

Maximum benefit is obtained by the patient only when the proper technique of inhalation is used. Surveys have shown that up to 75% of patients are unable to use aerosol inhalers properly and that 80% of cases of inadequate asthma control are partly due to inhaler technique. This arises because: (i) patients may not be adequately taught to use the devices prescribed; (ii) the technique is difficult for some patients to master; (iii) patients who are competent often develop poor technique and need reassessment and education.

Inhaler technique

Counselling the patient on proper technique is vitally important, with periodic checks to ensure efficiency is being maintained.

Instruction in inhaler technique takes time. Oral instruction should be backed up by demonstration, using a placebo inhaler, and written guidelines.

First, the cover should be removed from the mouthpiece and the inhaler shaken vigorously. With the inhaler held upright, the patient breathes out gently and then places the mouthpiece in the

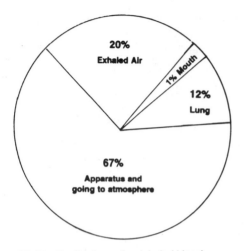

Figure 27.18 Destinations of an inhaled 'dose'.

mouth and closes his lips around it. He should breathe in through the mouth, press the canister to release the medication and continue to breathe in steadily and deeply. The breath is held while the inhaler is removed from the mouth and should continue to be held for as long as is comfortable. The patient should breathe out slowly. If a second puff is to be taken, the inhaler should be kept upright and, after a pause of 0.5–1 minute, the procedure repeated. On completion, the cover is replaced. People lacking the necessary power to depress the canister may find it easier to use both hands.

The dose delivered from the inhaler can be seen as a fine mist. If any can be seen escaping from the mouth or nose the inhaler is not being used correctly. For patients with an ideal technique only about 12% of the dose enters the lungs (Fig. 27.18). Even although this is only a tiny fraction of the oral dose it is enough to be effective. The remainder of the dose lands on the tongue or the back of the throat and is swallowed, but in such a small quantity that it has no systemic effect.

Spacer devices

Spacer devices are particularly useful for:

patients with poor inhalation technique
patients requiring higher doses
children

patients susceptible to candidiasis with inhaled corticosteroids.

A spacer device attached to the inhaler improves the dose delivery to 15%. Spacer devices provide a space between the inhaler and the mouth so allowing for a reduction in the velocity of the aerosol. There is thus less impaction of particles on the oropharynx and this, together with the greater time for evaporation of the propellant, results in a larger proportion of particles reaching the lungs. In utilising a spacer device, coordination of inspiration and actuation of the aerosol is less important. Spacing devices range in size from the Bricanyl Spacer, a foldaway extended mouthpiece, to larger devices with a one-way valve. The latter devices include the Nebuhaler.

Nebuhaler

The Nebuhaler, a plastic cone of 750 ml capacity, increases efficiency to about 20% (Fig. 27.19). A pressurised aerosol is fitted at one end, and the patient breathes in through a one-way valve at the other. On expiration the valve returns to the closed position and a hole in the mouthpiece allows the escape of gas which prevents rebreathing and build-up of carbon dioxide. The Nebuhaler is designed in a cone shape to minimise deposition of bronchodilator on the walls, and the patient can inhale when ready. There is no need to coordinate firing of the canister with inhalation.

Breath-actuated autohaler

When used correctly the inhaler is automatically activated by breathing in, and a click is heard so

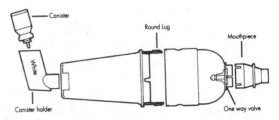

Figure 27.19 The Nebuhaler.

that the patient knows that medication is being received.

Nursing points

With the exception of the Nebuhaler, aerosol inhalers are easily carried in the pocket or handbag, helping the patient to be independent. Nurses supervising patients using this type of device should observe discreetly the patient's inhaling technique but avoid giving any impression of hurrying him in the process. The patient needs to concentrate on what he is doing at this time and so cannot engage in conversation.

Patient education

Compliance is more likely to be achieved if the patient is well informed.

The patient should know:

how to use the inhaler
the dose to be taken
the time interval
the maximum number of inhalations which should be taken in 24 hours.

More cooperation can be achieved if the patient is informed about the disease, the purpose of the therapy, how to recognise deterioration in his condition and what to do if deterioration is suspected.

It is the responsibility of doctors, nurses and pharmacists to promote understanding of the technique involved by teaching, demonstrating and checking the patient's performance at intervals. On this basis, alterations in the choice of device may be made so that the patient derives maximum benefit.

Dry powder inhalers

For those who cannot coordinate aerosol inhalation, alternative methods of administration include a dry powder inhaler (e.g. Rotahaler – salbutamol or beclomethasone dipropionate, Spinhaler – sodium cromoglycate).

How they work

Gelatine capsules containing the active drug, diluted with a suitable inert powder such as lactose, are placed in this small hand-held device which is twisted to break the capsule. With the mouth placed on the mouthpiece, the patient inhales through the device, causing drug particles to be entrained and drawn into the respiratory system. No coordination of hand movement and breathing is required.

Administration

It should be remembered that twice as much drug from a dry powder inhaler is needed for the same effect compared with an aerosol. Some dry powder inhalers occasionally cause coughing due to irritation of the throat and trachea caused by inhalation of the dry powder.

Patient types

Young children can be trained to use dry powder systems but they should be encouraged to use aerosols as soon as they are old enough to do so.

For the chronic asthmatic or bronchitic who is very breathless, a dry powder inhaler may be easier to use than a pressurised aerosol but it is particularly in these patients that wet nebulisers should be considered.

Wet nebulisers

For the treatment of acute breathlessness and wheeze in patients with airflow obstruction, e.g. chronic obstructive airways disease (COAD) and asthma, the method of choice for administering bronchodilator drugs is by inhalation via a mini-nebuliser (Fig. 27.20). Nebuliser solutions contain the same type of active ingredients that are used in an aerosol inhaler. However, the doses used are up to 25 times greater than those in inhalers, which is why the nebuliser is used in states of acute bronchoconstriction.

How they work

A nebuliser is an apparatus for converting

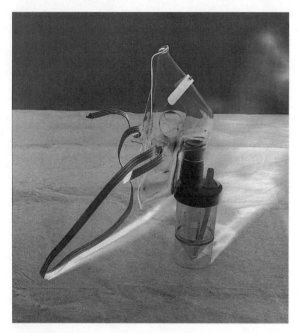

Figure 27.20 The mini-nebuliser ready for use.

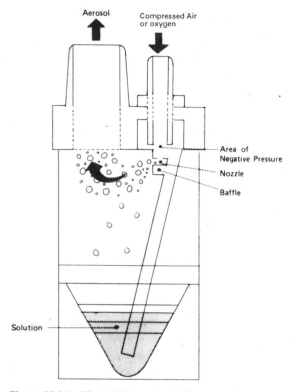

Figure 27.21 Wet nebuliser – in detail.

a liquid into a fine spray. A high-pressure gas source is used to suck up the broncho-dilator solution from a reservoir. The particles of drug produced impinge on a baffle. Particles of the correct size pass on and are breathed in by the patient via a face mask, while larger particles fall back to be nebulised again (Fig. 27.21).

Because a nebuliser has a 'dead space', a quantity of respirator solution has to be nebulised to fill this space before the particles start to leave the nebuliser and achieve a therapeutic effect. Depending on the design of the nebuliser this volume of solution may be 1–2 ml, and for the nebuliser to function efficiently it must have a starting volume of fluid of not less than 4 ml. In order to achieve this volume, sufficient diluent must be added to the bronchodilator solution(s). Sterile 0.9% w/v sodium chloride is chosen since it is isotonic, non-irritant and compatible with commercially available bronchodilator solutions; 25 ml sachets of 0.9% w/v sodium chloride solution are available for this purpose. Water would result in hypotonic solutions which may cause bronchoconstriction.

The carrier gas

The carrier gas used may be either **compressed air or oxygen**. The choice of air or oxygen, however, depends on each individual patient's clinical status.

Oxygen

Studies have shown that oxygen, when used in patients with chronic carbon dioxide retention, may cause acute CO_2 narcosis. Oxygen is acceptable, however, for young asthmatics. Patients with a severe attack of asthma benefit from oxygen during nebulisation since beta$_2$-adrenoceptor stimulants can cause an increase in arterial hypoxaemia.

Patients receiving controlled oxygen should have this discontinued only for the duration of the nebulisation.

Air

The use of air in patients with respiratory failure

without carbon dioxide retention will aggravate their hypoxia. Air should be used for patients with chronic bronchitis and evidence of carbon dioxide retention.

Administration

Patients who are to receive nebulised drugs should preferably be in the sitting position, either in bed or in a chair. By her gentle approach, the nurse can encourage the patient to relax. The patient should be advised to breathe through the mouth.

As with the administration of any medicine, the patient is identified, the prescription carefully read and the expiry date checked. Where a multidose bottle is being used, it must be discarded one month after opening. The nurse should therefore record the date opened on any container used.

Sodium chloride sachets used to give the necessary volume to the bronchodilator solution may be used for more than one patient during a medicine round but must be discarded immediately thereafter.

The required amount of each solution used is drawn up using a sterile syringe and needle to avoid bacterial contamination. As there is no patient contact, there is however no need to change the syringe and needle when drawing up the same drug for use in a number of patients.

To produce particles of the correct size, a minimum **flow rate** of 6 litres per minute is required. This flow rate will deliver at least 65% of the droplets in a size which enables drug penetration into the distal airways. During nebulisation, it is helpful to tap the nebuliser periodically so that large droplets may be shaken down and to ensure maximum delivery of the drug. Optimal nebulisation of 4 ml takes approximately 10 minutes. A proportion of respirator solution will remain in the nebuliser chamber.

Nebuliser care

On completion of the procedure, the nebuliser should be washed in warm, soapy water and dried using a paper towel to reduce the risk of bacterial contamination and prevent a build-up of crystallised drug in the nebuliser. It should be stored in a bag bearing the patient's name.

The Porta-Neb

The Porta-Neb is a portable nebuliser unit designed to allow greater mobility and independence, and therefore suitable for use by patients at home.

How it works

The unit consists of an electrically driven compressor which provides clean breathable air; nebuliser; mask; mouthpiece; and supply tube. In addition a 12 volt connection cable and adaptor are available for operating the unit from a car, boat or caravan.

Typical drug regimens

For administration via a wet nebuliser: (i) beta$_2$-adrenoceptor stimulant respirator solution made up to 4 ml with 0.9% sodium chloride solution, *or* (ii) anticholinergic bronchodilator solution made up to 4 ml with 0.9% sodium chloride solution, *or* (iii) a combination of beta$_2$-adrenoceptor stimulant and anticholinergic bronchodilator solutions.

It is common practice in patients receiving a combination of beta$_2$-adrenoceptor stimulant and anticholinergic bronchodilator solutions for the drugs to be mixed in the same nebuliser and administered concurrently. Other combinations of drugs should not be mixed without consulting the pharmacy.

Nebulised drugs are normally administered 4-hourly. In severe cases of airways obstruction, however, provided pulmonary function tests show reversibility of the obstruction to be possible, the frequency may be increased to 2-hourly or even hourly. Where the obstruction is irreversible artificial ventilation must be begun.

ORAL HYGIENE

The need to carry out oral hygiene in one form or

another to rid the mouth of debris is part of everyday living. When illness presents, the need for oral hygiene is much greater. For example, in anorexia, vomiting, constipation, fever and dehydration, the tongue and the teeth become dry and coated, and if left uncared for result in a foul taste, bad smell and the development of oral sepsis.

Where fluid intake has to be restricted the mouth quickly becomes dry, as it does when a patient is mouth-breathing or receiving continuous oxygen therapy. Patients who are immunosuppressed, as the result of a disease such as leukaemia or treatment such as radiation or cytotoxic drugs, are prone to mouth infections. The cells of the oral mucosa and salivary glands divide at a moderately rapid rate. Anti-cancer treatments aimed at rapidly replicating malignant cells are unfortunately not sufficiently selective and so the mouth is often adversely affected. Diuretics, psychotropics and insulin as well as sympathomimetic and parasympathomimetic agents all alter salivary function. Antibiotics may encourage opportunistic bacteria to flourish in the mouth by reducing the resident flora. The many situations regarded as 'high risk' for developing some form of discomfort of the mouth is evidence of how important this procedure is for nurses.

Some patients can be left to attend to this aspect of their care, some simply need to be prompted or given encouragement. Other patients are capable of carrying out the procedure for themselves but may need assistance in gathering together the necessary equipment. Many patients are wholly dependent on the nurse to meet every need. The purpose is to remove, and prevent the build up of, plaque, to stimulate the flow of saliva and reduce the risk of complications such as candidal infection and parotitis. The three direct methods employed are:

- brushing the teeth with toothpaste and water
- rinsing the mouth with mouthwash solution
- swabbing the mouth (Box 27.8).

Wherever possible patients should be encouraged to brush their teeth in the usual way or have their teeth brushed for them. Some authorities

---

Box 27.8 Swabbing the mouth

The medicine
  sodium bicarbonate solution 1:160
  mouthwash solution tablets
  Vaseline

The environment
  privacy, warmth, comfort

The nurse and the patient
  patient given explanation, if appropriate, of what is
    involved
  patient assisted, if necessary, into position which
    allows ease of access

The technique
  nurse ensures hands are socially clean before and
    after procedure
  patient's dentures removed if appropriate
  mouth examined using spatula and torch to identify
    area requiring greatest attention, e.g. tongue
  solutions prepared
  excess solution squeezed from each swab before use
  oral cavity gently and systematically wiped from inside
    using sodium bicarbonate solution
  each swab used for one wipe only and then discarded
  process repeated using mouthwash solution
  mouth re-inspected
  Vaseline applied sparingly to lips if indicated
  dentures thoroughly brushed before being replaced
  discarded material carefully disposed of
  patient made comfortable
  observations noted on nursing records

Hazards
  infected mouth
  spread of infection to other patients
  inhalation of swab or solution by unconscious patient

---

claim that a soft toothbrush could and should be used more often not only for cleaning teeth but to deal with the problem of a heavily coated tongue and in edentulous patients for cleaning the gums and cheeks also. The act of cleaning one's teeth is an important and beneficial part of any programme of rehabilitation for disabled patients. Stroke patients, for example, can be helped to regain independence and to overcome a lack of awareness which many of them have of one side of the face. Patients with a reduced platelet count whose gums are very liable to bleed are nevertheless also encouraged to use a toothbrush although it must be a soft one.

Mouthwashes are easier for the patient to manage when he feels weak and unwell.

Swabbing with the finger, though not a pleasant procedure for the patient, is essential for those who are acutely ill, unconscious, or in the terminal stages of their illness. This approach needs to be gentle yet effective. The airway of the unconscious or semiconscious patient must be protected at all times. Because of the danger of inhalation, any excess of the solution used for cleaning the mouth should be wrung out of the swab before use. Man-made woven swabs are less inclined to fray and are therefore safer. Care must be taken to ensure that the sponge of an applicator is not retained in the mouth by accident. With conscious patients, the tongue and roof of the mouth should be touched carefully not to make the patient 'gag'. Although oral hygiene is not a sterile procedure, sterile disposable equipment is used for each patient to prevent cross-infection. Gloves are worn by the nurse for her own protection and care should be taken to dispose of soiled materials safely. Ideally, food debris should be removed from the teeth after each meal. Patients appreciate being given the opportunity to rinse dentures after meals. It should be remembered that many patients do not like to be seen without their dentures and so privacy should be provided. Very ill patients will require to have the mouth cleaned at least every 2 hours. Whichever method is applied the aims of oral care are the same, i.e. to cleanse and moisten the mucosa.

There are additional ways of helping to keep the mouth of conscious patients clean and moist. Apart from encouraging and facilitating nasal breathing, imaginative ideas of suitable food and drinks, if permitted, may be put into practice. Flavoured ice lollies or cubes, boiled sweets and chewing gum may help. Fruit juices, especially those containing lemon, stimulate the flow of saliva and are cleansing and refreshing but may cause the mouth or lips to sting if the mucosa is irritated or broken.

In summary, the role of the nurse in oral hygiene is:

- to assess the state of the patient's mouth
- to select the appropriate method of oral hygiene for the patient
- to estimate the amount of assistance the patient requires with the procedure
- to assist the patient with oral hygiene as required
- to observe, report and record details of the condition of the patient's mouth
- to teach aspects of oral hygiene to patients and relatives.

As with other fundamental nursing procedures, most patients are highly appreciative of the care given to make the mouth feel more comfortable. The contribution mouth care can make to improving the appetite and boosting morale cannot be overemphasised. It is a nursing responsibility to ensure that oral hygiene is accorded the high priority it so often warrants.

Special measures taken to keep a patient's mouth clean and comfortable are generally only required for as long as the patient is acutely ill. As the patient's general state of health improves there is usually a concurrent improvement in the condition of the mouth.

Preparations used in general care of the mouth

The preparation selected for use will depend on local guidelines as contained in a nursing formulary (see p. 437) or laid down in some other way, although it cannot be overemphasised that the frequency and standard of mouth care are every bit as important as the individual mouthwash solutions used. The properties of two commonly used preparations are described below.

Thymol

Mouthwash solution tablets One tablet dissolved in 60 ml of water yields an aromatic, pleasant-tasting alkaline solution containing thymol which has mild antimicrobial and deodorant properties.

Compound thymol glycerin This product, when diluted with three times its volume of water, yields a solution with similar properties to that produced by dissolving a mouthwash solution tablet. Both solutions are used to freshen the mouth and for mechanical cleansing. Most patients with a sore mouth appreciate the soothing properties of warm mouthwashes. However, some patients, especially if they are pyrexial, welcome the refreshing effect of a cold mouthwash.

Care must be taken to avoid microbial contamination of thymol mouthwashes by rejecting any unused solution on completion of the procedure. Thymol, in the concentrations normally present in mouthwash solutions, is only a very weak antimicrobial agent. If solutions become contaminated, bacterial growth can occur with consequent risk of infection especially in immunosuppressed patients.

Sodium bicarbonate aqueous solution 1 in 160 (0.625% w/v)

The action of sodium bicarbonate would seem to be to render mucus less viscous, thus facilitating mechanical cleansing. Unfortunately this solution does not have a particularly pleasant taste but is very economical in use.

Preparations used in the care of the mouth in special situations

Tonsillectomy

Mouthwashes are administered after tonsillectomy to remove blood clots from the throat. Using the mouthwash as a gargle may help to clear the throat by mechanical action. The solutions used in this situation are intended to:

- detach blood clots and debris (hydrogen peroxide solution)
- ease pain using local analgesic (benzydamine hydrochloride solution) (see p. 306)
- treat or prevent infection (povidone-iodine solution)
- cleanse and refresh (thymol mouthwash solution).

Epistaxis

Patients who have had an epistaxis appreciate rinsing the mouth with a thymol preparation to rid the mouth of the foul taste caused by blood which has run down the back of the nose.

Post-radiation inflammation of the throat

This may be soothed without aggravating the existing reaction by using sodium bicarbonate solution or povidone-iodine solution as a mouthwash or gargle.

ADMINISTRATION OF EYE PREPARATIONS

The eye is a delicate and vital structure which protects itself in several ways. The immediacy of the blink reflex is evidence of the protective response made to the slightest threat to the eye. An ophthalmic procedure, be it the application of eye drops or of ointment, is approached against this background. Despite the fact that many patients may tolerate more painful procedures with equanimity, procedures involving the eye can cause particular anxiety. Ophthalmic treatment calls for a manner which conveys confidence to the patient, helping to ensure he is relaxed before, during and after the procedure. As with all procedures a clear explanation is given to the patient to gain his cooperation.

Infection risks must be guarded against by washing the hands with a suitable antiseptic cleansing solution before and after each procedure. A damaged eye is particularly susceptible to infection, so that whenever possible a single-use presentation of the eye drop is used. This is especially important when a suspected corneal abrasion is being examined using fluorescein. Where single-dose units are not available, or when larger volumes are required, a separate multi-dose container should be used for each patient. Care must be taken not to contaminate the dropper or nozzle of eye preparations.

When applying eye medication the standard procedures for administering and recording medicines are followed. All containers should be labelled with the patient's name and the date of opening. The label on the eye preparation should be compared with the prescription. The special points to note are:

- the name of the medication, the strength (usually expressed as a percentage)
- the amount
- which eye is to be treated if not both
- the time
- the frequency of administration
- that the preparation is in date.

As with other forms of medication, eye drops may be administered once only (including pre-operatively), or on a regular basis. Intensive treatment may also be indicated such as in the case of an infection. In order to convey all the necessary information it may be necessary to use a prescription sheet specially designed for the purpose (Fig. 27.22).

In order that the medication be administered safely and effectively, it is important to position the patient suitably. The head requires to be tilted back and maintained in a steady position so that the risk of the patient damaging the eye by contact with the equipment in use is minimised. To achieve this, the patient should be lying or else sitting, in which case the head should be supported by a pillow or the back of the chair. Where possible the nurse should work from the affected side so that she is close to the working area and in greater control of the procedure.

As always, safety aspects should be considered. Good lighting is essential for carrying out procedures on delicate structures such as the eye. Light should be from above and behind the nurse. With photophobic patients, consideration must be given to light reaching the patient, otherwise he may be unable to open his eyes. Movements of the hand should be gentle and controlled. Gloves are not worn, as the disposable type are seldom close fitting and therefore in danger of causing damage if they are allowed to touch the sensitive corneal surface of the eye. In all cases, the nurse must be alert to any sign of adverse reaction to a drug used locally in the eye. This may take the form of a worsening of inflammation or spread of inflammation to surrounding skin.

In the event of the wrong preparation having been administered or the wrong eye treated, the doctor must be notified *at once* so that any corrective action may be ordered without delay.

Teaching patients to administer eye medications

Nurses play an important role in teaching patients to master the technique of self-administration of eye medications. Compliance and independence will be more readily achieved where the patient is provided with motivation and encouragement.

When teaching a patient to administer an eye medication the special points to emphasise are:

- the need to wash the hands thoroughly first
- the need to avoid contamination
- the importance of using only the prescribed medications.

Because of the systemic toxicity of many ophthalmic drugs it is especially important that all eye preparations are kept out of the reach of children. Similarly, safe disposal of any remainder when treatment is discontinued, or the container changed, is essential.

Patients may be helped to select for themselves a suitable position in which to administer the medication. To instil eye drops, some patients find lying flat and feeling for the lower lid is a successful method with gravity assisting. This may be inconvenient or impossible for others and they may prefer to work in front of an upstanding mirror although coordination of the hand and eye may take time to master by this method. Self-application of an eye ointment and removal or insertion of a contact lens or artificial eye are best performed in front of a mirror.

Compliance aids

A number of patients experience problems using eye drops due to difficulty in aiming the drops and squeezing the plastic bottle (Winfield et al 1991). Aids to the instillation of eye drops are available which assist patients to use their eye

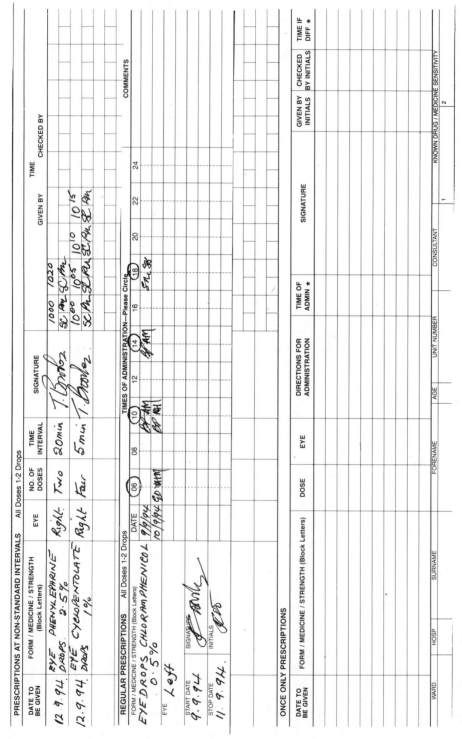

Figure 27.22 Ophthalmic prescription sheet.

drops in accordance with the prescriber's directions. The type of aid needed by the patient will depend on his particular needs. If the patient has difficulty in aiming the bottle, an 'Easidrop' or 'Autodrop' should be considered. These devices are designed to help the patient to position the dropper to expel a drop. Squeezing the bottle can be a particular problem for older patients whose grip strength may be reduced. For patients who have difficulty in both aiming and squeezing the bottle, the Opticare device (Fig 26.10, p. 411) or Autosqueeze may be useful. Whichever device is selected the patient should be given guidance and instruction in its use. In some circumstances it may be appropriate for the patient to use the selected device in the ward for a period prior to discharge so as to help ensure continuity of treatment. The use of a compliance aid often helps the patient gain benefit from the treatment and at the same time achieve greater independence. There is also potential to achieve better use of resources if the number of visits by a district nurse to instil eye drops can be reduced.

Eye drops

Eye drops are sterile aqueous solutions or suspensions, presented in multiple application dropper bottles which may be of glass fitted with a removable glass dropper and teat. An alternative presentation is a flexible plastic container with orifice through which drops are expelled with pressure of the fingers. Both types of container are used by individual patients in the community. Although eye drops in multiple application containers contain preservatives there is always risk of contamination in use. A multiple application container should be used for not more than one month, after which the original container should be rejected and a new container started.

Single-application containers should always be used in surgical procedures. However, solutions presented in this way do not contain preservatives and so a new single-use unit should be used for each application.

The question of the number of drops which can be instilled into the eye requires clarification. One drop from an eye dropper is 50 microlitres (μl) and will overload the average conjunctival sac, which has a capacity of 25 μl (Lessar & Fiscella 1985). To overcome this, where more than one drop of the same preparation is to be instilled (or another preparation used) an interval of 5–10 minutes should elapse before instilling the second drop. This may present difficulties in ophthalmology units where a considerable number of patients may be receiving several different forms of drops in succession. If there is a high rate of tear secretion, aqueous solutions will be quickly diluted or eliminated from the eye into the nasolacrimal duct, thus becoming unavailable for ophthalmic absorption but available for systemic absorption. This may result in systemic side-effects (e.g. dry mouth with atropine). Some practitioners recommend pressure over the punctum after administration as a means of restricting tear flow into the duct. The frequency of instillation of drops varies and will depend on, for example, the degree of infection or inflammation. In the treatment of acute glaucoma, a very intensive regime of instillation is followed initially which is then gradually reduced in frequency to hourly, continuing until the intraocular pressure is controlled and the pupil pinpoint.

Every effort is made to avoid causing irritation to the eye. Drops used straight from the refrigerator cause discomfort for the patient. If eye drops have been refrigerated, sufficient time should be allowed for the drops to gradually attain room temperature before use. A drop instilled from a height greater that 2.5 cm directly onto the cornea will cause stinging. Any irritation caused by faulty technique will result in increased tear secretion with consequent loss of therapeutic benefit due to a dilution effect. In addition, the patient will often react by squeezing the lids in an accentuated blink reflex, expelling the solution between the lids or down the nasolacrimal duct.

If, after the instillation of drops, the patient complains of irritation of the skin or a feeling of heat and tightness, an allergic reaction should be suspected and the doctor informed.

Instillation of eye drops (see Fig 27.23)

Where the eyes are sticky, this procedure is preceded by bathing the eyes using sterile sodium chloride 0.9% solution. There is some debate about the aspect of the eye into which drops should be instilled. Since the tears pass from lacrimal glands situated on the lateral aspect of each eye across the eyeball before draining into the nasolacrimal duct, it would seem logical to instil drops into the outer aspect of the lower fornix so that they are washed across with the tears, allowing time to take effect before draining away. However, some authorities advocate using the middle or the inner aspect. The method which can be achieved by nurse and/or patient may be the deciding factor (Box 27.9).

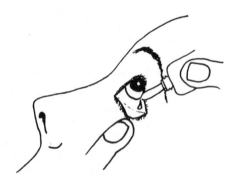

Figure 27.23   Instillation of eye drops.

Box 27.9	Administration of eye drops	
Documentation	•	prescription and recording sheet
The medicine	•	eye drops in accordance with prescription and at room temperature
The environment	•	well-lit location with no 'through traffic'
The nurse and the patient		
general	•	identification of patient and comparison with prescription
	•	cooperation and relaxation of patient achieved by careful explanation and gentle approach
	•	patient discouraged from rubbing eye/reassurance given that blurring of vision is normal and will soon pass
	•	general comfort of patient on completion of procedure
specific	•	encouragement to open eye and look upwards

Box 27.9	Cont'd	
Technique		
general	•	patient's head supported/nurse working from patient's affected side
	•	hand hygiene before and after each treatment and before treating the eye
specific	•	eversion of lower eyelid
	•	adequate warning to patient prior to actual instillation
	•	instillation from correct height
	•	extreme care to avoid touching any part of the eye
	•	immediate replacement of cap if multiple application bottle in use
	•	excess medication mopped from face
Hazards	•	physical trauma
	•	infection
	•	systemic absorption
Special features	•	self-medication with or without compliance aid

Eye ointments

In addition to the more commonly used eye drops many ophthalmic drugs are available as eye ointments. Eye ointments are essentially dispersions of the active ingredient in a sterile bland base, such as soft paraffin or polyethylene glycol. Useful properties of eye ointments include:

- duration of action longer than that of eye drops
- an emollient soothing action
- ease of application
- long shelf-life.

Eye ointments soften crusts, thus preventing adherence of eyelids and eyelashes when the patient is asleep. However, there may be some interference with vision due to the smearing of the cornea with the ointment base (Box 27.10).

Rodding

This procedure is done to prevent formation of adhesions between the eyelid and the eyeball which can arise as the result of chemical burns of the conjuctiva. In the first few days after injury the procedure is likely to be uncomfortable and a local anaesthetic such as amethocaine 0.5% eye drops is instilled in advance. Sterile petroleum jelly is used to lubricate the rod in most cases, although sometimes an antibiotic ointment may be prescribed. By passing the rod under the upper eyelid then moving it from side to side exerting slight pressure outwards, any adhesions are broken down and a film of grease is left between the two surfaces.

Box 27.10   Administration of eye ointment (see Fig. 27.24)

Documentation	• as for instillation of eye drops
The medicine	• eye ointment in accordance with prescription
The environment	• as for eye drops
The nurse and the patient	
general	• as for eye drops
specific	• patient encouraged to close eyes for approximately one minute after application of ointment
Technique	
general	• as for eye drops
specific	• ointment squeezed along lower lid from inner canthus outwards
Hazards	• physical trauma
	• infection

Cleansing the eye

The eye may be cleansed by bathing and irrigating.

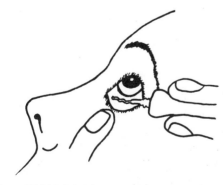

Figure 27.24   Administration of eye ointment.

Eye bathing

This procedure (Box 27.11) may be used to soothe the eye(s) and to remove crusts from the eyelid(s).

Box 27.11   Eye bathing

Documentation	• nursing care plan
The medicine	• sterile 0.9% sodium chloride solution
The environment	• as for instillation of eye drops
	• tray or trolley cleaned, pack and solution prepared as for surgical dressing
The nurse and the patient	• as for eye drops
Technique	
general	• as for eye drops
specific	• uninflamed, uninfected or operated eye bathed first
	• upper lid bathed with patient looking down; lower lid with patient looking up
	• sterile technique
	• each eye swabbed from inner canthus out to prevent infection of the punctum, the lacrimal apparatus or the other eye
	• each swab used once and discarded
	• dry wool never used as it may leave wisps attached to the eyelashes; swabs always well rung out
Hazards	• physical trauma
	• infection

Irrigation of the eye

This procedure (Box 27.12) is carried out mostly in accident and emergency departments and occupational health centres for the emergency removal of irritant chemicals. The volume and nature of the irrigation solution and the equipment used is dependent on the agent which has caused the injury.

Box 27.12   Irrigation of the eye

Documentation	• dependent on condition being treated – nursing care plan or standard prescribing and recording sheet

The medicine	• sterile sodium chloride 0.9% solution (sachet, plastic bag or prefilled disposable undine) *or* special irrigation solution
	• as prescribed at body temperature
The environment	• as for eye bathing
The nurse and the patient	• as for eye drops
Technique general specific	• as for eye drops
	• sterile technique
	• patient holding receiver firmly against appropriate cheek with head tilted slightly towards receiver
	• patient allowed to become accustomed to temperature of solution by pouring a little over cheek first
	• eyelids held apart using thumb and forefinger
	• solution directed in steady stream over eyeball from inner canthus outwards
	• patient asked to move eyeball up, down and from side to side so that entire eye is cleansed
	• eyelids and cheek left dry
	• eyepad applied if instructed
Hazards	• physical trauma
	• infection

Care of an artificial eye

Patients who have had enucleation of an eye performed and have been fitted with a temporary shell or prosthesis, should have the prosthesis removed twice a day, or according to the surgeon's preference, to allow it and the socket to be cleaned with sterile normal saline. The prospect of this activity calls for some degree of fortitude on the part of the nurse but quickly her mind will be concentrated on the technique involved and on the great need to provide the patient with encouragement.

At first the patient is likely to be understandably tense and frightened that the procedure will be painful. He should be warned that he will feel the presence of something in the socket but that there will be no pain.

After a few days, when it is felt that the patient is ready to look at himself in a mirror, and, when he feels he wants to become involved in the care

of his eye, the nurse must be prepared to spend time with the patient. About 3–4 days following the operation, the prosthesis is replaced with an artificial eye. He should be allowed to handle the artificial eye and become familiar with its shape. The notch on the nasal side of the eye which accommodates the trochlea serves as a guide for positioning.

To remove the artificial eye, the patient should be seated. He is asked to look up and using the little finger, the lower edge of the artificial eye is eased up while the lower margin is drawn down. Gentle pressure exerted on the upper lid will allow it to slip out.

To insert an artificial eye, the upper lid is raised and the upper edge of the artificial eye is slipped under. It is then held in place whilst the lower lid is drawn down and the lower edge of the eye is slipped into the lower fornix.

The patient may be taught to carry out eye toilet in front of a bathroom mirror. Until he becomes fully confident, a towel may be placed in the washhand basin to protect the artificial eye from damage should it slip through his fingers. By the time the patient is discharged, he should be quite confident with the procedure. When the socket is completely healed, the patient will be able to rinse his artificial eye under running water and come to no harm.

When a patient with an artificial eye requires to have the eye stored for any length of time, for example, during surgery, it should be placed in a container of sodium chloride 0.9% solution so that it does not dry out and become rough.

Contact lenses

Because of the increased use of contact lenses and the very discreet nature of many of them, nurses must make a conscious effort to ask patients whether they wear contact lenses or to observe whether they are in use. This should be done on the patient's admission to hospital. Lenses should be removed for safekeeping before any general anaesthetic. They should also be removed prior to any eye procedure to prevent irritation and so as not to be spoiled, unless medical advice has been given to the contrary. Great care must be taken in storing them since they are easily damaged, and are both costly and inconvenient to replace. They are normally kept in a specially supplied contact lens case although in an emergency a suitable alternative may have to be found. The container should be labelled with the patient's name, ward and unit number and stored in a safe place. Handling of lenses should be kept to a minimum and they should not be allowed to dry out because of the danger of cracking. Lens solution is normally brought into hospital by the patient but if this is not available sterile normal saline serves just as well, provided that the case with lens and solution are regularly subjected to heat treatment (e.g. 80°C for 40 minutes) to reduce microbial contamination.

To remove a lens, the hands should be washed, rinsed and dried leaving no trace of soap which could be conveyed to the lens and irritate the eye. The patient is asked to tilt his head back as recommended for any eye procedure and to look up. Using the index finger, the lens is gently slid downwards on to the bulbar conjunctiva and then lifted off the conjunctiva with the thumb and index finger. The utmost care is required not to drop a lens as it may then be very difficult to find.

Drugs and contact lenses

Consideration needs to be given to contact lenses and the concurrent administration of medicines. Some patients find that inserting contact lenses is painful and so they may be prescribed local anaesthetic eye drops to instil in advance. It is now well recognised that plastic materials, notably PVC, can absorb certain preparations instilled into the eye. Coloured eye drops such as rose bengal will stain soft contact lenses permanently. Adverse effects from drugs taken systemically have been reported. For example, anticholinergic drugs may cause a reduction in tear secretion and blurred vision while oral contraceptives may also cause ocular complications. Rifampicin, used in the treatment of tuberculosis, colours body secretions, including the tears, an orange-red leading to pigmentation of the contact lens. In certain conditions, however, the water absorption property of the lens can be used to advantage; a soft hydrophilic lens may be inserted to avoid repeated instillation of drugs such as pilocarpine in the treatment of glaucoma.

ADMINISTRATION OF EAR AND NOSE PREPARATIONS

Procedures relating to disorders of the ear and nose involving the use of drugs follow somewhat similar lines. As always, the standard procedure for prescribing and recording medications must be followed. To prevent cross-infection, the hands should be washed before and after each procedure and each patient should have a separate medicine container. When checking ear and nose preparations against the prescription, special note should be made of the strength of the medication and, for example, the number of drops to be instilled and whether both ears/ nostrils are to be treated. Explanation of the procedure is important in order to gain the patient's cooperation so that the medication is allowed to take maximum effect with minimal discomfort. Correct positioning of the patient helps to minimise discomfort and ensure penetration of the medication to the part where it is intended to take effect. Ear and nose procedures are usually carried out with the nurse working at the side being treated. Before instilling ear or nose drops, instructions may be given by the doctor to mop the ear canal or nasal passage using a cotton-tipped applicator for better penetration of the medication. Care should be taken when patients have a history of epistaxis. Because of the delicate membranous structures involved it is important to administer such preparations at a suitable temperature. Ear drops should be used in the temperature range between room and body temperature. If ear drops are instilled from a bottle recently stored in a refrigerator they may cause a mild vertigo. Patients at home may prefer to warm the drops by holding the bottle in the hand or standing it in a bowl of hot water for a few minutes. Nasal drops do not have to be warmed as this will happen as the drops pass over the nasal mucosa although they should be allowed to reach room temperature prior to instillation if previously stored in the refrigerator.

The patient may be helped to feel more secure throughout the procedure if he is given an absorbent tissue to hold. If, for any reason, he has to rise quickly, the tissue may be used to mop excess medication which would otherwise run out of the ear or nose. For patients receiving ear drops who are unable to maintain the required position, a wisp of cotton wool may be *gently* placed in the ear canal to ensure that the drops remain in contact with the epithelium. The prescribed volume of ear drops may range from 2–5 ml. On every occasion it is important to check that the top of the glass dropper used is not chipped or cracked. Patients using any of these preparations at home should be reminded to use only a preparation intended for themselves, to keep it away from children, and to safely discard the container and any remaining medication at the end of the course of treatment (Boxes 27.13 and 27.15).

Ear drops

Ear drops are solutions or suspensions of active ingredient(s) in water, propylene glycol or other suitable vehicle.

Box 27.13	Instillation of ear drops
Documentation	• standard prescribing and recording sheet
The medicine	• prescribed ear drops • separate bottle for each patient • at room temperature, at least
The nurse and the patient	• patient identified • patient given explanation • patient assisted as necessary into position either sitting with head tilted to one side or lying on side with ear to be treated uppermost • patient's clothing protected • patient made comfortable

Box 27.13	*Cont'd*
Technique	• if instructed, external auditory meatus gently mopped with cotton-tipped applicator • hand hygiene before and after actual instillation of drops • bottle shaken if it contains a suspension and required amount drawn into dropper • cartilaginous part of pinna gently pulled up and back (for a child, down and back) • drops instilled in external canal without allowing dropper to come into contact with ear • gentle massage applied over tragus to help work in drops • patient encouraged to maintain position for several minutes to allow drops to reach eardrum • cotton wool ball lightly placed in external meatus if necessary • excess medication wiped away

Ear ointments

Ear ointments have similar properties to ointments in general. Some *eye* ointments may also be prescribed for ear conditions. The customary way of introducing an ointment into the ear is to insert ribbon gauze which has been impregnated with the ointment. The wick is left in for 24 hours. Oral analgesics may be required prior to removal of the wick each day.

Syringing the ear

This procedure (Box 27.14) is carried out to remove plugs of wax which block the ear causing discomfort and deafness, or when closer inspection of the eardrum is required (Fig. 27.25). Syringing with warm water may be sufficient to dislodge and remove the wax. However, where the wax is impacted or difficult to remove, the syringing is often preceded for several days by a course of wax-softening drops such as olive or almond oil or sodium bicarbonate ear drops. Cerumol ear drops contain an organic solvent which may cause sensitisation and should be used only where sodium bicarbonate ear drops

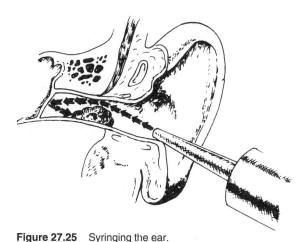

Figure 27.25   Syringing the ear.

have failed. Because of the potential danger of perforating the tympanic membrane, either the ear is examined by a doctor using an auriscope before syringing takes place or enquiries from the patient are made to ensure that there is no history of perforation.

Box 27.14 *Cont'd*		
	•	meatus inspected periodically using auriscope to check that wax has been removed and ear has not been damaged
	•	external auditory meatus gently but thoroughly mopped dry
Hazards	•	infection of the middle ear resulting from rupture of the tympanic membrane
	•	otitis externa

Nasal preparations

Nasal preparations usually take the form of nasal drops. Instead of instilling nasal drops, they may be sprayed into the patient's nose in powder form using a nasal insufflator. A nasal spray is also available which is inserted into the anterior nares. The container is squeezed two or three times to instil the medication.

Box 27.14 Syringing the ear		
The medicine	•	tap water at body temperature (38°C)
The environment	•	usually GP's clinic/surgery by practice or district nurse
The nurse and the patient	•	hand hygiene before and after procedure
	•	patient given clear explanation of what is involved
	•	patient's understanding checked as he may not have heard
	•	patient informed that there may be some discomfort
	•	privacy, warmth, comfort
	•	patient seated in upright chair with towel over appropriate shoulder
	•	patient asked to hold receiver against neck just below ear to be treated
Technique	•	syringe filled with water and air expelled
	•	pinna pulled up and back
	•	fluid directed along roof of auditory canal without undue force but at a steady rate
	•	content of returned fluid observed
	•	procedure repeated until all wax removed

Box 27.15 Instillation of nasal drops		
Documentation	•	standard prescribing and recording sheet
The medicine	•	nasal drops as prescribed
The nurse and the patient	•	patient identified
	•	explanation given to patient
	•	patient assisted into supine position with head hyperextended, e.g. with head over edge of bed or with pillow under shoulders
	•	patient left comfortable on completion of procedure
Technique	•	hand hygiene before and after instillation of drop
	•	patient assisted if necessary to close off one nostril at a time and drop(s) inserted in the other without touching any part of the nose with the dropper
	•	patient encouraged to sniff liquid into back of nose or, if unable, to maintain position for about one minute. Patient instructed not to blow nose. Patient offered bowl into which excess drops collected can be spat out

Packing the nose

Nasal packs may be used to control severe epistaxis and as a rule are inserted by the doctor. The patient is understandably often very alarmed by the blood loss and requires a nurse to stay with, and reassure, him. Diazepam may be given orally and may be continued until the acute episode is over and the pack is removed. The insertion of a nasal pack is done with the patient sitting up with clothing suitably protected. Using a suitable size of nasal speculum, the doctor inserts sterile half-inch (1 cm) ribbon gauze which has been soaked in Vaseline with the aid of forceps.

Alternatively, a Brighton catheter or a Foley catheter may be inserted into the nose and inflated to stop the bleeding. Patients appreciate a mouthwash after a nose bleed and may get rid of clots from the back of the throat by gargling. It is often advisable to administer an oral analgesic prior to removal of a nasal pack, which with drying becomes painful to remove. To begin with, only half of the packing should be gently pulled out to see what happens. If there is no bleeding the remainder can be removed, but if the first stage has caused bleeding, the remainder of the pack should be left in place and a further attempt made later.

BLADDER IRRIGATION

Indwelling catheters, even when introduced into the bladder under the most rigorous aseptic conditions, are an important source of urinary tract infection. In the course of time, crystallisation around and within the lumen of the catheter increases the risk of infection further, by obstructing the flow and causing stasis of urine. By-passing of urine then follows, leading to discomfort, embarrassment and skin breakdown. Patients who produce haematuric urine can also develop severe drainage problems and discomfort, especially when the catheter is blocked by blood clots. Special responsibility therefore rests with nurses involved in the care of patients with a urinary catheter.

The indications for washing out the bladder are:

- to reduce and treat urinary tract infections
- to prevent and clear obstruction of the eye(s) and lumen of the catheter by debris, crystals or blood clot.

The methods most commonly used for introducing fluid into the bladder are:

- intermittent bladder irrigation, either by instillation from an irrigation device such as the Uro-Tainer, or by mechanical irrigation using a form of suction
- continuous bladder irrigation.

The method used will depend on the reason for carrying out the irrigation.

Intermittent irrigation (Box 27.16)

The Uro-Tainer system (Fig. 27.26).

This system has greatly improved the management of indwelling urinary catheters in hospital

Box 27.16	Intermittent bladder irrigation
Documentation	• standard prescribing and recording sheet • fluid balance chart
The medicine	• sterile irrigating solution in either Uro-Tainer or 500 ml bottle • solution as prescribed, visibly clear and at room temperature
The environment	• as for any aseptic procedure • privacy
The nurse and the patient	• patient identified as corresponding to prescription • explanation as to what is involved • patient assisted into relaxed position with only catheter exposed; patient kept warm • clothes and bedding protected • patient made comfortable on completion of procedure
Technique	• aseptic (gloves not required with Uro-Tainer) • observation of returned fluid • new drainage system attached to catheter after irrigation completed • all urine measured and recorded • administration recorded
Hazards	• infection

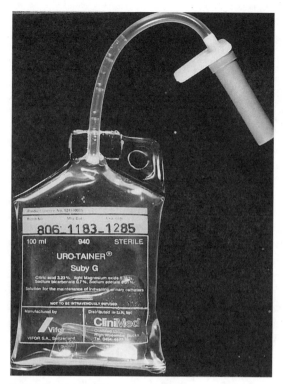

Figure 27.26 The Uro-Tainer system.

and at home. The simple technique involved saves nursing time and can be mastered by patients or their relatives for use at home. Solution G and chlorhexidine solution are available in the form of a ready-to-use irrigation device. Solution G is weakly acidic and is used for flushing out and for preventing crystal formation, or for dissolving crystals already formed in the catheter. Aqueous chlorhexidine solution (0.02% w/v) has a bacteriostatic action against many of the common urinary tract pathogens. Some clinicians recommend routine use of chlorhexidine solution immediately prior to the removal of all urinary catheters. The solution is left in the bladder until such time as the patient wishes to void.

Clot retention is usually treated by irrigation with sterile sodium chloride solution (0.9% w/v) although, where clots prove to be obstinate, alternative methods of irrigation may have to be employed. Sterile sodium citrate solution 3% may also be used to break up clots. The volume

of solution in each Uro-Tainer is 100 ml, although the amount instilled into the bladder is not critical, rather the time the solution is left in the bladder, which may be up to half an hour. Gloves are not necessary when this method of irrigation is used. However, thorough hand-washing is esssential, and care must be taken to join the catheter and irrigation tubing without contaminating them. A regime in current use for patients with long term catheters involves alternate use of a urinary antiseptic, such as chlorhexidine (0.02% w/v), with a decrystallising solution, say, every Tuesday, the other solution every Friday.

Mechanical irrigation using suction

In the event of a catheter becoming completely blocked by blood clots, the catheter may be washed out in an effort to break down the clots by a form of suction using a catheter-tipped syringe and irrigating solution from a bottle or plastic bag. Where blood clots are especially troublesome a large volume of sterile sodium chloride solution (0.9% w/v) will be required. This method is based on first introducing approximately 50 ml of solution which is left in the bladder. This acts as a physical buffer to allow further volumes of fluid to be instilled under pressure then withdrawn by suction through the catheter, depending on the severity of the blockage. The nurse wears gloves for this procedure because of the many manipulative processes involved. It may take a considerable time until the catheter drains freely. The patient, who may already be in pain and be losing blood into the bladder, can find this a tedious and uncomfortable experience. He should therefore be kept warm and as comfortable as possible. As with all such procedures the encouragement and support of the nurse are vital throughout.

Continuous irrigation

Continuous irrigation of the bladder is commonly employed following prostatic surgery to rid the bladder of blood clots and prostatic debris. A three-way catheter, or alternative combination of catheters, is inserted in theatre. This allows one inlet for inflating the catheter balloon and another for the entry of irrigating solution, and an outlet for drainage of the bladder contents. Sodium chloride solution (0.9% w/v) is introduced into the bladder from a 3-litre bag suspended from an infusion stand, via an administration set connected to the catheter. In the immediate postoperative period the control clamp is left open fully to allow for continuous flushing of the bladder and of the eyes of the catheter. After several hours, depending on the degree of haematuria, the rate may be decreased. Volumes of irrigating solution ranging from 15–45 litres may be required to treat the patient during the first 24 hours. The flow of such large volumes of fluid demands frequent attention by the nurse in maintaining input, discarding output and keeping records of both. In urological wards, anticipating needs and finding adequate storage space for large volumes of irrigation solutions can present problems. These may, to some extent, be alleviated by active involvement of the ward pharmacist who can, among other things, help to ensure that supply keeps pace with demand.

It should be remembered that hypertension (resulting from absorption of sodium) and perforation of the bladder may each result from this form of irrigation. Trained nurses in urology wards have particular responsibility therefore to ensure that close monitoring of the blood pressure and pulse (every half-hour at first), fluid balance, and pain is carried out. If the patient complains of pain, no matter how mild, irrigation should not proceed without seeking further advice. While it is important not to alarm junior nursing staff, and hence patients, at this time, the possibility of perforation, especially following transurethral resection of the prostate gland, must never be forgotten.

General principles of bladder irrigation

When using any form of bladder washout the broad principles of medicine administration

apply. The details of the solution are checked against the prescription, and the fluid visually examined before use, to make sure it is free from any particulate matter. Any container whose contents are not clear should be rejected. In view of the high risk to the patient of microbial contamination, all procedures are carried out using a strictly aseptic technique. Ideally, solutions should be warmed to body temperature before use in a solution-warming cabinet. Improvised methods of warming solutions are not recommended since control of the solution temperature is impossible to achieve. In the absence of a solution-warming cabinet it is probably best to use the solution at room temperature.

Patients with an indwelling catheter which has been on continuous drainage for weeks or months, may have difficulty in tolerating the instillation of volumes of solutions in excess of 50 ml because of reduced bladder capacity or bladder irritability. When the bladder is irritated by infection or is reduced in capacity by tumour, it may only be possible to tolerate very small volumes of fluid. On occasion, a volume as small as 10 ml is as much as the patient can hold. Infected fluid is never re-injected. When the patient indicates that the bladder feels uncomfortable, and as though it cannot take in more fluid, then this must be taken as the maximal amount that can be instilled. As soon as possible following any manipulations of a catheter, the catheter should be attached to a sterile closed drainage system. The drainage tubing should be stiff enough to reduce the likelihood of kinking, and the drainage bag should be adequately supported on a floor stand positioned for ease of observation of the colour, consistency and volume of urine drained. Bag holders can become distorted, for example, when lowering the height of the patient's bed. This increases the risk of the tubing becoming kinked. Also, the drainage tap may come into contact with the floor, with obvious risk of contamination.

Details of sterile solutions used in bladder irrigation and some of the drugs used in bladder instillations are given in Chapter 13).

ADMINISTRATION OF VULVAL AND VAGINAL MEDICATIONS

Gynaecological conditions are judged by many women to be a source of extreme embarrassment and fear. Patients express these feelings in different ways. Some are hesitant to ask for further explanation of their condition or treatment, showing a natural reservation about intimate matters. Others fear being thought of as unclean, embarrassed by odour, itching and perhaps staining of underclothes from vaginal discharge. Patients may fear discovery of a malignant condition or that they have developed an infection which has been sexually transmitted. Knowledge of anatomy and physiology of the female genital tract in some instances may be scant and attitudes to bodily functions may have been influenced by folklore.

Nurses working in gynaecological wards and clinics become accustomed to carrying out intimate procedures and discussing very personal issues with their patients. They may need to remind themselves of the importance of maintaining sensitivity to the feelings of each new patient. General ward nurses and district nurses are required to care for patients with gynaecological disorders from time to time, and so they should be ready to turn their attention to the special needs of these patients.

In all cases, embarrassment or attitude on the part of the nurse should never be allowed to interfere with establishing and dealing with the full nature of the problem. Tact, patience and gentleness are essential at all times.

Vulval and vaginal preparations which contain a drug should be prescribed, administered and recorded according to local policy. The genital area should be clean and traces of previously applied cream should be removed. Whenever possible, the patient should apply the preparation herself. The nurse must guarantee privacy for the patient whether she is explaining self-administration or actually carrying out the treatment. It is important to explain to which particular area the treatment is to be directed, the recommended times of administration and the need to complete the course. Disposable gloves should be worn by the nurse when administering vulval and vaginal preparations both to protect the patient and nurse from acquiring infection or the nurse from absorbing any of the medication. Whether nurse or patient carries out the procedure, the hands should be washed before and after. Applicators should be washed in warm soapy water, rinsed and dried. A separate treatment kit should be assigned to the individual patient (Box 27.17).

Box 27.17	Insertion of vaginal pessaries
Documentation	• prescribing and recording sheet
The medicine	• pessary as ordered, with applicator
The environment	• privacy, warmth, comfort
The nurse and the patient	• patient identified • patient given explanation of what is involved and advised to empty bladder • patient assisted if necessary into supine position, with knees flexed and thighs abducted, or left lateral position
Technique	• nurse attends to own hand hygiene and applies disposable gloves • pessary inserted, using applicator, as high as possible along posterior vaginal wall in an upwards and backwards direction for the full length of the vagina • patient's vulval area wiped dry and sanitary pad applied to prevent staining of clothes (tampons should not be used in the presence of infection) • applicator washed in warm, soapy water, rinsed and dried.
Hazards	• pessary can easily be dislodged and so is best inserted on retiring to bed

ADMINISTRATION OF RECTAL MEDICINES (Box 27.18)

Drugs can be administered via the rectum:

- in solid form, as a suppository which melts at body temperature
- as a solution, suspension or foam in the form of an enema.

Box 27.18   Administration of medications by the rectal route

Documentation
- prescribing and recording sheet

The medicine
- suppository or enema as prescribed

The environment
- patient in bed
- privacy, warmth, comfort
- incontinence pad(s) to protect clothes and bedding
- call bell to hand
- commode positioned at bedside if appropriate

The nurse and the patient
- patient identified
- explanation given of what is involved and patient instructed as to how he can relax and assist procedure
- patient assisted into left lateral position with head on one or two pillows, buttocks in line with edge of bed and knees drawn up towards chin

Technique
- nurse ensures hands are socially clean before and after procedure
- disposable gloves worn for insertion of suppositories

Suppositories	Enemas
suppository lubricated using, e.g. 'KY Jelly' or tip melted in hot water as directed on packet	enema nozzle lubricated after air expelled
anus carefully located avoiding external haemorrhoids if present	anus carefully located avoiding external haemorrhoids if present
suppository slowly and gently inserted	enema nozzle inserted for 4–6 cm and then pack slowly rolled up to introduce contents
finger withdrawn smoothly	nozzle withdrawn gently
anal region wiped and patient left comfortable	anal region wiped and patient left comfortable
for evacuant medications, patient encouraged to postpone first urges to defaecate and to make medication work; for retention medications, elevating foot of bed may help patient to retain medication	for evacuant medications, patient encouraged to postpone first urges to defaecate and to make medication work; for retention medications, elevating foot of bed may help patient to retain medication

Hazards
- local irritation
- trauma

The rectal route may be utilised for local or systemic action when:

- drugs cannot be swallowed (e.g. because of vomiting, coma, stricture)
- drugs cause severe irritation of the upper gastrointestinal tract (e.g. indomethacin)
- a prolonged action is desired (e.g. oxycodone)
- the drug must be delivered close to the site of the lesion(s) (e.g. corticosteroid).

The absorptive surface area of the rectum is small, although the blood supply is extremely efficient and therefore absorption can be rapid. However, the presence of faeces may slow absorption, and irritation may cause early evacuation. Laxatives are administered in order to evacuate the rectum and are retained there for approximately 20 minutes. All other drugs given rectally are for retention and are normally administered on retiring to bed so that they may be retained overnight. Given the option, perhaps more patients on long-term drug therapy would choose this route of administration. It is debatable whether doctors in the United Kingdom will follow continental practice in the years ahead by more frequently prescribing drugs for rectal administration. Where this is the chosen method, patients should be encouraged to insert suppositories themselves and may be taught self-administration of a small disposable enema containing a soluble form of prednisolone (Predsol) in the treatment of colitis.

STOMA MANAGEMENT

Stoma care involves the active participation of a number of health carers, with the nurse taking a central part not only in giving nursing care but also in the coordination of care which others provide. The overall aim, is to rehabilitate the patient so that he may care for himself within the framework of a near-normal way of life. There will, however, be situations where self-care alone is inadequate, not because of any failing on the part of the patient, but because the patient's needs make it so. Obviously special care is required for new stoma patients and the terminally ill. Some older patients may become wholly dependent on the nurse for the care of their stoma due to the ravages of the ageing process. On the other hand, many patients will manage very well from day to day provided they have continual general support and access to specialist help and advice when they require it.

The medical knowledge and practical expertise of stoma care are included in every basic nursing course, and the advent of the stoma care sister or nurse provides the nurse with the opportunity to enhance her skills and knowledge. This will help to build confidence in the nurse which must be evident to the patient if the care is to succeed.

Types of stoma

A stoma is usually created when it has been necessary to form a surgical diversion of faeces or urinary flow. There are three main types:

- An operation which necessitates removal of the rectum and sigmoid colon results in the formation of a colostomy. At this point in the intestinal tract, the faeces are generally well formed and evacuation fairly predictable.
- When the large intestine has been entirely removed, or diverted, the stoma is made at the lower end of the small intestine and is known as an ileostomy. With this type of stoma, waste is looser because more of the intestine has been removed, or diverted, resulting in loss of reabsorptive capacity.
- In the treatment of certain bladder disorders, the ureters may be transplanted into a short segment taken from the ileum to form an ileal conduit or they may have been brought to the skin surface in the formation of a ureterostomy. Waste in these cases is urine. In all forms of stoma, since no voluntary muscles are involved, the excretory flow cannot be controlled at will. Management therefore is directed towards modifying waste where this is possible and applying some form of device for its collection.

The newly formed stoma

Postoperative recovery as well as successful management and acceptance of the stoma are influenced by what happens pre-operatively. Time must be found by both medical and nursing staff to explain to the patient (the ostomist) the operation and its implications. More than one discussion is needed as patients understandably do not always retain all the information given on one occasion. Opportunities should also be given to an immediate relative of the patient to ask questions. Privacy is essential when selecting the site of the stoma and when allowing the patient to try various appliances. The patient may be glad to meet with an ostomist and is usually appreciative of being given some literature to peruse at his own pace.

During the immediate postoperative period, in addition to the standard care and support given, the nurse should make regular and frequent checks of the stoma itself. It is important to observe its colour so that early signs of strangulation of its blood supply may be noted and reported. Excessive bleeding or sinking of the stoma must be reported also, as a return to theatre may be indicated. From the start the nurse's attitude to the patient should be positive, being gentle yet firm. Nurses will have to come to terms with any feelings of revulsion which they may have when dealing with the stoma. The thought of having to face such operations is, at first, repugnant to many patients, although given the right psychological support, most patients will find a stoma preferable to the discomfort of the illness they previously suffered. Acceptance of the stoma is the first and greatest hurdle to be overcome. One of the hardest moments for the patient is looking at the stoma for the first time and nurses can be of great support during this difficult period. 'Ready to leave hospital' for the ostomist should mean that he is ready to care for the stoma, no longer being regarded as a patient but as an individual who happens to eliminate in a different way. Each person, naturally, will have his own particular problems and individual methods of overcoming them.

Diet

For those who have a colostomy or ileostomy, correct diet comes before anything else. The aim is to produce faeces which are as well formed as possible without causing constipation. Sensible eating can help to achieve this aim and can minimise other problems for the ostomist (e.g. odour, flatus and excoriation of the skin). Dietetic advice is always available and aims to help the person find a diet which is as near normal as he can possibly manage. At first, a certain amount of experimentation may be required with food combinations. In time, the person usually finds that most foodstuffs can be taken in moderation with a few exceptions. Wind-producing foods are soon identified. Highly spiced foods and onions are to be avoided as they can produce loose and odorous faeces, and much flatus. Pulse foods and Brussels sprouts can cause flatus and noise although not so much odour. The timing of liquid in relation to food is important. It is safer not to drink immediately before, during or until about half an hour after a meal, so as to avoid loosening the faeces. Fizzy drinks are to be avoided and advice on which alcoholic drinks may be safely taken should be sought.

Odour

Odour is caused by either faeces or flatus and therefore good dietary management helps to keep it to a minimum. Very careful hygiene is essential of course, although deodorants also may be used. Deodorant drops or powders are available for placing in the stoma appliance although care should be taken not to allow liquid deodorants to touch the stoma or surrounding skin otherwise they may cause severe irritation. Some ostomy bags have a small vent at the top for inserting deodorant liquid or have a charcoal filter incorporated. A deodorising spray may be used at the time of emptying the appliance and a deodorising air device may be placed as appropriate.

Appliances

No single appliance is suitable for all those who have a stoma and this is reflected in the wide range of products currently available. The aim is to find a device which not only serves the purpose of satisfactorily collecting the waste but is discreet, rustle-free and acceptable. A detailed description of all the different appliances is beyond the scope of this book but there are several aspects which should be understood when considering appliances generally. Stoma bags may or may not be disposable and/or drainable. They are available either as one- or two-piece systems. One-piece appliances consist of a disposable collection bag complete with its own seal. Two-piece appliances comprise an adhesive flange to which a disposable collection bag may be fitted. The flange may be left attached for 3–4 days while the bag is replaced as often as necessary.

The type and site of the stoma, manual dexterity and skin sensitising, all influence the choice of appliance. Many modern appliances involve the use of protective adhesives such as Hallihesive, Stomahesive, Comfeel etc, which, because of their malleability and skin protection properties, provide a good skin seal. Microporous adhesives may also be used and are mostly well tolerated. A belt may be attached to some appliances for added support. Filter pastes are useful for filling dips and creases peristomally thus making the surface level prior to putting on an appliance. These pastes must not be used on sensitive skin as they are spirit-based.

Many permutations of apparatus have been produced, and ostomists themselves make adaptations to suit their own needs.

Skin protection

In the same way as a person who is paraplegic lives with the threat of pressure sores, the ostomist must constantly take care to prevent irritation and breakdown of the skin which surrounds the stoma. A routine of changing the appliance right to the skin will be followed by each individual. Care must be taken to remove plasters without tearing the skin. The area around the stoma is washed using cotton wool, for example, and warm, soapy water, taking care to remove all traces of faeces, mucus, and skin applications. It is important to rinse off all soap to reduce irritation and to pat the skin dry. Any traces of adhesive should be removed using an adhesive solvent. Additional applications of barrier cream and skin gel may be used for protection of the skin. Creams should be applied sparingly to a radius of about 10 cm from the stoma but not on the stoma itself.

Skin breakdown

In the event of the skin becoming red and weepy, adhesives may have to be temporarily replaced with some form of dressing. This may be left in position for several days with the appliance being placed on top of the dressing. Efforts should then be made to identify the cause of the excoriation. It may be that the motions are too loose, calling for a change in diet or a bulking agent. Changing the bag more promptly helps to reduce faecal contact with exposed skin. The size of the aperture may be too big causing a similar problem and may have to be reduced. Ideally there should only be about 0.5 cm of a gap between the stoma and the appliance. Antiseptic solutions tend to be painful when applied to sore skin, causing further irritation, and are best avoided in preference to soap and water, thorough rinsing with cool water, and careful drying.

Disposal of appliances

Ostomists should be encouraged not to allow the care of the stoma to 'take over'. Bearing in mind that he is likely to be one of a family with others in the home to consider, stoma equipment should be kept together, preferably out of sight. A travelling kit may be kept at the ready. The question of disposal of appliances and their contents is an important one for all concerned. Today, many patients dispose of the contents of the bag down the lavatory and as it is flushed they 'sluice' the bag. The empty bag is then wrapped in newspaper and sealed with tape to make a small package. If this is disposed of among ordinary domestic waste in the usual way there will be no

problem. All ostomists are entitled to free prescriptions for all their stoma needs.

Medicines and ostomists

Certain precautions have to be taken by doctors prescribing medicines for patients with an ileostomy or colostomy. Nurses should also be aware of these and other problems relating to medicines that may arise for the ostomist.

Patients with an ileostomy

Diarrhoea with subsequent loss of water and potassium is a very real threat to the ileostomist at any time, and may be exacerbated by taking medicines.

Digoxin The improvement in renal perfusion which results from digoxin therapy may cause additional potassium depletion. Potassium supplements may be needed when digoxin therapy is indicated.

Diuretics These should be avoided whenever possible owing to the risk of dehydration and potassium loss. If diuretic therapy is essential a potassium-sparing diuretic should be used.

Bowel washouts Any form of washout is contraindicated because of the severe risk of dehydration rapidly occurring.

Tablets Those with slow-release properties are unsuitable. Such preparations are designed to release the drug from the tablet during its passage through the digestive tract over a period of 3–6 hours. In ileostomy patients this period is shortened, with the result that drug release may be incomplete leading to under dosage. For this reason, if potassium replacement therapy is required, a liquid form is used to ensure full absorption of potassium.

Patients with a colostomy

Constipation may be a problem for many colostomy patients and should always be borne in mind in their management. For the treatment of constipation, colostomy patients should increase their fluid intake or make some dietary adjustments in preference to taking medication.

If this approach does not help then bulk-forming laxatives such as ispaghula husk or methylcellulose may be used. These act by increasing faecal mass which stimulates peristalsis and effects expulsion of faeces provided sufficient fluid intake is maintained. These medicines are supplied in tablet and granule form. Tablets may be broken up and should be chewed with a little water half an hour before a meal. Liquids are then withheld until about half an hour after the meal. Because these preparations have a hygroscopic action, the timing of fluid is important otherwise the medication absorbs fluid recently taken instead of the fluid content of the faeces. Not all patients find the granular form of these agents manageable as there is a tendency for the granules to swell in the mouth and thus be difficult to swallow. Lactulose, which is an osmotic laxative, is another useful preparation in this situation.

Antacids Those containing aluminium salts may cause the colostomy patient to become constipated.

Antidepressants The anticholinergic effects of some antidepressants can lead to a number of troublesome side-effects including constipation.

Narcotic analgesics Analgesics such as dihydrocodeine are especially constipating. Other narcotic analgesics such as codeine and morphine may also be troublesome.

Patients with ileostomy or colostomy

For any patient with an ileostomy or colostomy, oral antibiotics. oral iron preparations, and antacids containing magnesium salts, should be avoided whenever possible because of the likelihood of diarrhoea. If necessary, concurrent intestinal sedatives such as codeine phosphate may be given.

Conclusion

There can be no doubt that the formation of a stoma brings change to the individual's way of life. The prospect of such an operation for the individual and his family is a daunting one.

With the practical and psychological support of a team of staff through the peri-operative, rehabilitative and independent phases of stoma management, the individual has a very real chance of being able to pursue a career, raise a family, and resume many previously enjoyed activities. The ostomist has to acquire and maintain confidence in his ability to cope in order to lead a full life. Membership of associations and clubs for ostomists can generally help by providing an opportunity to offer and accept support against the background of a common, shared experience. In time, the need for such participation may diminish, but for many, the benefits of membership will continue to be enjoyed over the years.

REFERENCES

Lessar T S, Fiscella R G 1985 Antimicrobial drug delivery to the eye. Drug Intelligence and Clinical Pharmacy 19: 642–654
Torrance C 1989 Intramuscular injection. Part 2. Surgical Nurse 2(6): 24–27

Winfield A J, Williams A, Jessiman D et al 1991 Assisting patients with their eyedrops: 1. Identifying the problems. British Journal of Pharmaceutical Practice 13: 10–14

FURTHER READING

Conaghan P 1993 Subcutaneous heparin injections – bruising. Surgical Nurse 6(2): 25–27
Dougherty L 1992 Intravenous therapy. Surgical Nurse 5(2): 10–13
Dunne A, Winfield A J, Williams A et al 1991 Eye irrigation – practice, procedures and problems. Hospital Pharmacy Practice October: 1–4

Heals D 1993 A key to wellbeing. Oral hygiene in patients with advanced cancer. Professional Nurse 8(6): 391–398
Peate I 1993 Nurse-administered oral hygiene in the hospitalised patient. British Journal of Nursing 2(9): 459–462
Torrance C 1990 Oral hygiene. Surgical Nurse 3(4): 16–20
Williams A, Winfield A J 1990 Topical medication for eye patients. Nursing Times 86(27): 42–43

Index

U

V

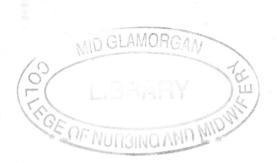